INTERVENTIONAL CARDIOLOGY

CONTEMPORARY CARDIOLOGY

CHRISTOPHER P. CANNON, MD
SERIES EDITOR

INTERVENTIONAL CARDIOLOGY

Percutaneous Noncoronary Intervention

Edited by

HOWARD C. HERRMANN, MD

Professor of Medicine
Cardiovascular Division, Department of Medicine
University of Pennsylvania School of Medicine

Director
Interventional Cardiology and Cardiac Catheterization Laboratories
Hospital of the University of Pennsylvania

Philadelphia, PA

Foreword by

EUGENE BRAUNWALD, MD

Brigham and Women's Hospital, Boston, MA

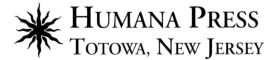

HUMANA PRESS
TOTOWA, NEW JERSEY

© 2005 Humana Press Inc.
999 Riverview Drive, Suite 208
Totowa, New Jersey 07512
www.humanapress.com
For additional copies, pricing for bulk purchases, and/or information about other Humana titles,
contact Humana at the above address or at any of the following numbers: Tel.: 973-256-1699;
Fax: 973-256-8341, E-mail: humana@humanapr.com; or visit our Website: http://humanapress.com

Cover illustrations: Figure 7, Chapter 2, by T. E. Feldman et al.; Fig. 6A, Chapter 5, by F. G. St. Goar et al.;
Fig. 3F, Chapter 10, H. Patel et al.; Cribier-Edwards equine pericardial valve photo courtesy of Edwards Lifesciences.
.
Cover design by Patricia F. Cleary.

This publication is printed on acid-free paper. ∞
ANSI Z39.48-1984 (American National Standards Institute) Permanence of Paper for Printed Library Materials.

Printed in the United States of America. 10 9 8 7 6 5 4 3 2 1

Library of Congress Cataloging-in-Publication Data
Interventional cardiology : percutaneous noncoronary intervention / edited by Howard C. Herrmann.
       p. ; cm. — (Contemporary cardiology)
   Includes bibliographical references and index.
   ISBN 1-58829-367-X (alk. paper) eISBN 1-59259-898-6
   1. Cardiac catheterization. 2. Percutaneous balloon valvuloplasty. 3.
   Heart—Surgery.
   [DNLM: 1. Heart Valve Diseases—therapy. 2. Balloon Dilatation. 3.
   Blood Vessel Prosthesis Implantation. WG 260 I61 2005] I. Herrmann, Howard
   C. II. Series: Contemporary cardiology (Totowa, N.J. : Unnumbered)
   RD598.35.C35I585 2005
   616.1'20754—dc22   2004016767

FOREWORD

The development of catheterization of the right side of the heart was a milestone in the twentieth century. Following the bravado of Werner Forssman's self-catheterization and the subsequent systematic application of the technique by Cournand and Richards and then many others, by the early 1960s, catheterization had emerged as the premier cardiac diagnostic technique for congenital and valvular heart disease.

A number of seminal technical developments followed. These included percutaneous access to the venous and arterial vascular beds, a variety of approaches to catheterization of the left side of the heart, and of course the perfection of coronary arteriography. During the 1970s, therapeutic applications of cardiac catheterization were first introduced, including percutaneous transluminal coronary angioplasty by Gruntzig. Less well known was atrial septostomy for transposition of the great arteries by Rashkind. These were the "opening shots" of a revolution in cardiac therapy using catheter-based techniques which is still ongoing and gathering momentum. Simultaneously, echocardiography was developed and its role as an important diagnostic technique became established.

By the end of the twentieth century, the role of cardiac catheterization had changed drastically. Just as echocardiography and other non-invasive imaging techniques displaced catheterization as the premier cardiac diagnostic method, so were catheter-based approaches displacing surgery as the principal method for repairing anatomic cardiac and vascular abnormalities. Of course, percutaneous coronary interventions have been the mainstay of interventional cardiology. However, beginning with atrial septostomy and then percutaneous mitral balloon valvuloplasty, progress in noncoronary intervention has been accelerating rapidly and on many fronts. Most visible have been the procedures to improve valve function, including percutaneous valve replacement. However, advances in closure of patent foramina ovale as well as atrial and ventricular septal defects are quite impressive. A variety of adjunctive coronary interventions including alcohol septal ablation are gaining a foothold. Disorders of the aorta, carotid, and peripheral arteries, long the domain of the vascular surgeon, are now increasingly managed through catheterization techniques.

Dr. Herrmann, a pioneer in interventional cardiology, has made a major contribution by editing this fine book, *Interventional Cardiology: Percutaneous Noncoronary Intervention*. He has brought together world leaders who have contributed their enormous expertise to this field which is growing rapidly in importance. Although this volume is as current as last month's meetings, it is nonetheless carefully edited, finely illustrated, and well referenced.

Dr. Herrmann and his talented coauthors deserve the thanks of the growing number of interventional cardiologists who are looking beyond the coronary vascular bed and to the growing number of patients who can benefit from percutaneous noncoronary interventions.

Eugene Braunwald, MD
Boston, Massachusetts

PREFACE

From its beginnings, the field of interventional cardiology has been defined by coronary interventions. Today, percutaneous coronary intervention with balloon angioplasty, bare metal, and drug-eluting stents has become the predominant form of coronary revascularization and the most frequent therapeutic intervention in the modern cardiac catheterization laboratory. However, as this field has matured, cardiologists have found novel ways to apply their expertise with wires, guide catheters, balloons, and stents to a number of other vascular beds and structural cardiac diseases.

Specifically, in the area of valvular heart disease, percutaneous noncoronary intervention began with the pioneering work of Jean Kan and Kanji Inoue, who demonstrated the usefulness of balloon valvuloplasty for stenotic valvular heart disease. Part I of *Interventional Cardiology: Percutaneous Noncoronary Intervention* focuses on valvular heart disease and is introduced by reviews of balloon valvuloplasty for mitral stenosis (Chapter 1) and for aortic and pulmonary valve stenosis (Chapter 2). In this regard, one of the most exciting current areas of clinical investigation in valvular heart disease involves a new treatment for aortic stenosis with a stented percutaneously inserted aortic valve as described in Chapter 6. Advancements are also being made in the treatment of regurgitant valvular disease, particularly mitral regurgitation. Chapters 3–5 describe the pathophysiology of mitral regurgitation, and percutaneous approaches either through the coronary sinus or by direct leaflet modification.

Part II describes new interventions for structural heart disease focusing on septal defects at both the atrial and ventricular level. These chapters include descriptions by experts in the field on the use of closure devices for atrial and ventricular septal defects. Although no one would dispute the value of closing a large, hemodynamically significant atrial or ventricular septal defect, the use of devices for closure of patent foramen ovale and to exclude the left atrial appendage in order to reduce the risk of stroke is more controversial. In this regard, Chapter 7 describes the neurologic considerations in PFO closure prior to a discussion of closure devices in Chapters 8, 9, and 12.

Although one goal of this book was to avoid discussion of conventional coronary revascularization, many new and novel devices are being developed as adjunctive therapies during coronary interventions. Nowhere is this more apparent than in the area of myocardial infarction (Chapter 13) and for cardiogenic shock where new percutaneous mechanical assist devices are being utilized (Chapter 14). The use of alcohol septal ablation to modify hypertrophic obstructive cardiomyopathy is another example of a coronary intervention that falls outside of the usual revascularization procedure (Chapter 15). Finally, the last chapter in this section describes myocardial regeneration and therapeutic angiogenesis via both coronary and myocardial approaches.

Probably the most frequent and successful of the noncoronary interventions to date involves the use of angioplasty techniques to treat extracardiac vascular disease. Chapters 17 and 18 describe peripheral intervention in the renal, iliac, and carotid territories. Aortic stent grafting is currently a mostly surgical field as described in Chapter 19, but it is likely that technologic advancements in the future will allow diseases of the aorta to be treated percutaneously in the cardiac catheterization laboratory.

The last section of the book deals with the important adjunctive imaging modalities utilized in these new percutaneous noncoronary interventions. Echocardiography, whether transthoracic, transesophageal, or intracardiac, is more and more frequently being utilized during interventional procedures and is well described in Chapter 20. Improvements in angiography such as 3-dimensional reconstruction, as well as the use of magnetic resonance, round out this section on associated imaging modalities.

Percutaneous coronary intervention will remain the mainstay of most cardiac catheterization laboratories for the foreseeable future. However, percutaneous noncoronary intervention is occupying an ever-increasing niche in many laboratories and for many interventionalists. I am hopeful that *Interventional Cardiology: Percutaneous Noncoronary Intervention* will help to expand this field and provide a forum for future advances and discussion of these modalities. I am grateful to all of the contributors for their expertise and effort in making their knowledge available on a widespread basis. I would also like to thank my wife Deborah and our children Stephanie, Jessica, and Jason for their support and understanding as I completed the editorial process.

Howard C. Herrmann, MD

CONTENTS

Part I.   Valvular Disease

Part II.   Septal Defects

Part III. Adjunctive Coronary Interventions

Part IV. Peripheral Interventions

Part V.   Associated Imaging Modalities

COLOR PLATE

These illustrations are printed in color in the insert that follows page 236:

Chapter 3
Figure 2, p. 51: Image of a human mitral valve annulus and leaflets created with real-time three dimensional echocardiology.
Figure 10, p. 60: Echocardiographic images.

Chapter 8
Figure 5, p. 136: Internal autoadjusting spring mechanism of the CardioSEAL-STAR-Flex system.

Chapter 10
Figure 2C, E, and L, pp. 168–169: Intracardiac echocardiographic images.

Chapter 14
Figure 7, p. 246: Transesophageal imaging of flow across the transseptal cannula in the TandemHeart.

Chapter 19
Figure 4, p. 352: Significant migration of a Talent endograft at 4 yr follow-up.

CONTRIBUTORS

BRIAN H. ANNEX, MD • *Division of Cardiology, Department of Medicine, Durham Veterans Administration and Duke University Medical Center, Durham, NC*

FABRICE BAUER, MD • *Department of Cardiology, Charles Nicolle Hospital, University of Rouen, Rouen, France*

PETER C. BLOCK, MD • *Division of Cardiology, Emory University School of Medicine, Atlanta, GA*

HEIDI N. BONNEAU, RN, MS • *Division of Cardiovascular Medicine, Stanford University School of Medicine, Stanford, CA*

HARAN BURRI, MD • *Cardiology Service, University Hospital of Geneva, Geneva, Switzerland*

QI-LING CAO, MD • *Departments of Pediatrics and Medicine, The University of Chicago Children's Hospital, The University of Chicago Pritzker School of Medicine, Chicago, IL*

JOHN D. CARROLL, MD • *Division of Cardiology, University of Colorado Health Sciences Center, Denver, CO*

MICHAEL T. CAULFIELD, MD • *Cardiology Division, Massachusetts General Hospital, Boston, MA*

S-Y JAMES CHEN, MD • *Division of Cardiology, University of Colorado Health Sciences Center, Denver, CO*

HOWARD A. COHEN, MD • *Cardiovascular Institute, University of Pittsburgh Medical Center, Pittsburgh, PA*

ALAIN CRIBIER, MD • *Department of Cardiology, Charles Nicolle Hospital, University of Rouen, Rouen, France*

MILIND Y. DESAI, MD • *Division of Cardiology, Department of Medicine, Johns Hopkins University School of Medicine, Baltimore, MD*

SIMON R. DIXON, BHB, MBChB • *Division of Cardiology, William Beaumont Hospital, Royal Oak, MI*

RONALD M. FAIRMAN, MD • *Department of Surgery, University of Pennsylvania School of Medicine, Philadelphia, PA*

JAMES I. FANN, MD • *Division of Cardiothoracic Surgery, Stanford University Medical Center, Stanford, CA*

TED E. FELDMAN, MD • *Cardiology Division, Evanston Northwestern Healthcare, Evanston, IL*

PETER J. FITZGERALD, MD, PhD • *Division of Cardiovascular Medicine, Stanford University School of Medicine, Stanford, CA*

DHARSH FERNANDO, MBBS • *Cardiology Division, Massachusetts General Hospital, Boston, MA*

ANTHONY FURLAN, MD • *Division of Stroke and Neurologic Intensive Care, Department of Neurology, Cleveland Clinic Foundation, Cleveland, OH*

JOSEPH H. GORMAN III, MD • *Department of Surgery, University of Pennsylvania School of Medicine, Philadelphia, PA*

ROBERT C. GORMAN, MD • *Department of Surgery, University of Pennsylvania School of Medicine, Philadelphia, PA*

NATHAN E. GREEN, MD • *Division of Cardiology, University of Colorado Health Sciences Center, Denver, CO*

CAMERON HAERY, MD • *Department of Cardiovascular Medicine, Cleveland Clinic Foundation, Cleveland, OH*

ALI H. M. HASSAN, MD • *Division of Cardiovascular Medicine, Stanford University School of Medicine, Stanford, CA*

HOWARD C. HERRMANN, MD • *Cardiovascular Division, Department of Medicine, University of Pennsylvania School of Medicine*

ZIYAD M. HIJAZI, MD • *Departments of Pediatrics and Medicine, The University of Chicago Children's Hospital, The University of Chicago Pritzker School of Medicine, Chicago, IL*

RALF HOLZER, MD • *Departments of Pediatrics and Medicine, The University of Chicago Children's Hospital, The University of Chicago Pritzker School of Medicine, Chicago, IL*

YASUHIRO HONDA, MD • *Division of Cardiovascular Medicine, Stanford University School of Medicine, Stanford, CA*

G. CHAD HUGHES, MD • *Division of Cardiovascular and Thoracic Surgery, Department of Surgery, Duke University Medical Center, Durham, NC*

FUMIAKI IKENO, MD • *Division of Cardiovascular Medicine, Stanford University School of Medicine, Stanford, CA*

SCOTT E. KASNER, MD • *Division of Stroke and Critical Care, Department of Neurology, University of Pennsylvania School of Medicine, Philadelphia, PA*

MICHAEL J. LANDZBERG, MD • *Boston Adult Congenital Heart Disease Service, Department of Cardiology, The Children's Hospital and Brigham and Women's Hospital, Boston, MA*

ALBERT C. LARDO, PhD • *Division of Cardiology, Department of Medicine, Johns Hopkins University School of Medicine, Baltimore, MD*

MARTIN B. LEON, MD • *Cardiovascular Research Foundation, Columbia University, New York, NY*

JOAO A. C. LIMA, MD • *Division of Cardiology, Departments of Medicine and Radiology, Johns Hopkins University School of Medicine, Baltimore, MD*

BERNHARD MEIER, MD • *Department of Cardiology, Swiss Cardiovascular Center Bern, University Hospital, Bern, Switzerland*

STEVEN R. MESSÉ, MD • *Division of Stroke and Critical Care, Department of Neurology, University of Pennsylvania School of Medicine, Philadelphia, PA*

JOHN C. MESSENGER, MD • *Division of Cardiology, University of Colorado Health Sciences Center, Denver, CO*

SURESH R. MULUKUTLA, MD • *Cardiovascular Institute, University of Pittsburgh Medical Center, Pittsburgh, PA*

WILLIAM W. O'NEILL, MD, FACC • *Division of Cardiology, William Beaumont Hospital, Royal Oak, MI*

IGOR F. PALACIOS, MD • *Cardiac Unit, Department of Medicine, Massachusetts General Hospital, Harvard Medical School, Boston, MA*

HITENDRA PATEL, MD • *Division of Pediatric Cardiology, Children's Hospital, Oakland, CA*

MARK REISMAN, MD • *Cardiovascular Research and Cardiac Catheterization Laboratory, Swedish Medical Center, Seattle, WA*

KENNETH ROSENFIELD, MD • *Cardiology Division, Massachusetts General Hospital, Boston, MA*

TIMOTHY A. SANBORN, MD • *Cardiology Division, Feinberg School of Medicine, Northwestern University, Evanston Northwestern Healthcare, Evanston, IL*

ULRICH SIGWART, MD • *Cardiology Service, University Hospital of Geneva, Geneva, Switzerland*

FRANK E. SILVESTRY, MD • *Cardiovascular Division, Department of Medicine, Hospital of the University of Pennsylvania, Philadelphia, PA*

FREDERICK G. ST. GOAR, MD • *Cardiovascular Institute, Mt. View, CA*

CHRISTOPHE TRON, MD • *Department of Cardiology, Charles Nicolle Hospital, University of Rouen, Rouen, France*

NICHOLAS VALETTAS, MD • *Department of Medicine, Henderson General Hospital, Hamilton, Ontario, Canada*

OMAIDA C. VELAZQUEZ, MD • *Department of Surgery, University of Pennsylvania School of Medicine, Philadelphia, PA*

ANDREAS WAHL, MD • *Department of Cardiology, Swiss Cardiovascular Center Bern, University Hospital, Bern, Switzerland*

STEPHAN WINDECKER, MD • *Department of Cardiology, Swiss Cardiovascular Center Bern, University Hospital, Bern, Switzerland*

EDWARD WOO, MD • *Department of Surgery, University of Pennsylvania School of Medicine, Philadelphia, PA*

JAY S. YADAV, MD • *Department of Cardiovascular Medicine, Cleveland Clinic Foundation, Cleveland, OH*

COMPANION CD-ROM

This book is accompanied by a CD-ROM that contains movies of selected procedures described in the text.

I VALVULAR DISEASE

1

Percutaneous Mitral Balloon Valvuloplasty for Patients with Rheumatic Mitral Stenosis
Immediate and Long-Term Follow-up Results

Igor F. Palacios, MD

CONTENTS

INTRODUCTION

Since its introduction in 1984 by Inoue et al. *(1)*, percutaneous mitral balloon commissurotomy or valvotomy (PMV) has been used successfully as an alternative to open or closed surgical mitral commissurotomy in the treatment of patients with symptomatic rheumatic mitral stenosis *(2–20)*. PMV produces good immediate hemodynamic outcome, low complication rates, and clinical improvement in the majority of patients with mitral stenosis *(2–20)*. PMV is safe and effective, and it provides sustained clinical and hemodynamic improvement in patients with rheumatic mitral stenosis. The immediate and long-term results appear to be similar to those of surgical mitral commisssurotomy *(2–20)*. Today, PMV is the preferred form of therapy for relief of mitral stenosis for a selected group of patients with symptomatic mitral stenosis.

From: *Contemporary Cardiology: Interventional Cardiology:*
Percutaneous Noncoronary Intervention
Edited by: H. C. Herrmann © Humana Press Inc., Totowa, NJ

PATIENT SELECTION

Selection of patients for PMV should be based on symptoms, physical examination, and two-dimensional (2D) and Doppler echocardiographic findings. PMV is usually performed electively. However, emergency PMV can be performed as a life-saving procedure in patients with mitral stenosis and severe pulmonary edema refractory to medical therapy and/or cardiogenic shock. Patients considered for PMV should be symptomatic (NYHA ≥ II), should have no recent thromboembolic events, have less than 2 grades of mitral regurgitation by contrast ventriculography (using the Seller's classification), and have no evidence of left atrial thrombus on 2D and transesophageal echocardiography. Transthoracic and transesophageal echocardiography should be performed routinely before PMV. Patients in atrial fibrillation and patients with previous embolic episodes should be anticoagulated with warfarin with a therapeutic prothrombin time for at least 3 mo before PMV. Patients with left atrium thrombus on 2D echocardiography should be excluded. However, PMV could be performed in these patients if left atrium thrombus resolves after warfarin therapy.

TECHNIQUE OF PMV

Percutaneous mitral balloon valvuloplasty is performed in the fasting state under mild sedation. Antibiotics (500 mg dicloxacillin po q/6 h for four doses started before the procedure, or 1 g Cefazolin intravenously at the time of the procedure) are used. Patients allergic to penicillin should receive 1 g Vancomycin intravenously at the time of the procedure.

All patients carefully chosen as candidates for mitral balloon valvuloplasty should undergo diagnostic right and left and transseptal left heart catheterization. Following transseptal left heart catheterization, systemic anticoagulation is achieved by the intravenous administration of 100 units/kg of heparin. In patients older than 40 yr, coronary arteriogaphy should also be performed.

Hemodynamic measurements, cardiac output, and cine left ventriculography are performed before and after PMV. Cardiac output is measured by thermodilution and Fick method techniques. Mitral valve calcification and angiographic severity of mitral regurgitation (Seller's classification) are grade qualitatively from 0 grade to 4 grades as previously described (3). An oxygen saturation diagnostic run can be performed before and after PMV to determine the presence of left to right shunt after PMV.

There is not a unique technique of PMV. Most of the techniques of PMV require transseptal left heart catheterization and use of the antegrade approach. Antegrade PMV can be accomplished using a single-balloon (2,3,6) or a double-balloon technique (3–5,7). In the latter approach, the two balloons could be placed through a single femoral vein and single transseptal puncture (3,5,7) or through two femoral veins and two separate atrial septal punctures (4). In the retrograde technique of PMV, the balloon dilating catheters are advanced percutaneously through the right and left femoral arteries over guide wires that have been snared from the descending aorta (21). These guide wires have been advanced transseptally from the right femoral vein into the left atrium, the left ventricle, and the ascending aorta. A retrograde nontransseptal technique of PMV has also been described (22,23).

The Antegrade Double-Balloon Technique

In performing PMV using the antegrade double-balloon technique (Fig. 1), two 0.0038-in., 260-cm-long Teflon-coated exchange wires are placed across the mitral valve

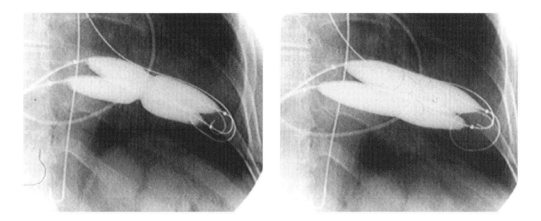

Fig. 1. Double-balloon PMV. Two guide wires are advanced into the ascending and descending aortas with the tip at the level of diaphragm. Two balloon catheters are placed straddling the stenotic mitral valve; markers identifying the proximal end of the balloons are inflated by hand until the waist produced by the stenotic valve disappears.

into the left ventricle, through the aortic valve into the ascending, aorta, and then the descending aorta *(24)*. Care should be taken to maintain large and smooth loops of the guide wires in the left ventricular cavity to allow appropriate placement of the dilating balloons. If a second guide wire cannot be placed into the ascending and descending aorta, a 0.038-in. Amplatz-type transfer guide wire with a performed curlew at its tip can be placed at the left ventricular apex. In patients with a mechanical aortic valve prosthesis, both guide wires with performed curlew tips should be placed at the left ventricular apex. When one or both guide wires are placed in the left ventricular apex, the balloons should be inflated sequentially. Care should be taken to avoid forward movement of the balloons and guide wires to prevent left ventricular perforation. Two balloon dilating catheters, chosen according to the patients' body surface area, are then advanced over each one of the guide wires and positioned across the mitral valve parallel to the longitudinal axis of the left ventricle. The balloon valvotomy catheters are then inflated by hand until the indentation produced by the stenotic mitral valve is no longer seen. Generally one, but occasionally two or three inflations are performed. After complete deflation, the balloons are removed sequentially. (A video of the double-balloon technique is shown as video 1 on the accompanying CD-ROM.)

The Inoue Technique of PMV

Percutaneous mitral balloon valvuloplasty can also been performed using the Inoue technique (Fig. 2) *(1,15–17)*. The Inoue balloon is a 12 French shaft, coaxial, double-lumen catheter. The balloon is made of a double layer of rubber tubing with a layer of synthetic micromesh in between. Following transseptal catheterization, a stainless-steel guide wire is advanced through the transseptal catheter and placed with its tip coiled into the left atrium and the transseptal catheter removed. A 14 French dilator is advanced over the guide wire and is used to dilate the femoral vein and the atrial septum. A balloon catheter chosen according to the patient's height is advanced over the guide wire into the left atrium. The distal part of the balloon is inflated and advanced into the left ventricle with the help of the spring wire stylet, which has been inserted through the inner lumen of the catheter. Once the catheter is in the left ventricle, the partially inflated balloon is moved back and

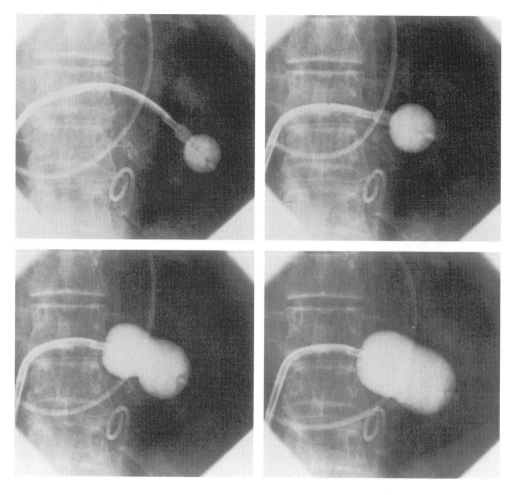

Fig. 2. Inoue technique of PMV. A partially inflated Inoue balloon catheter is placed into the left ventricle (upper left); it is then gently pulled against the mitral plane until resistance is felt (upper right). The balloon is therewith rapidly inflated by hand, an indentation is seen in the balloon's midportion (lower left) straddling the stenotic mitral valve, and the balloon inflated until the waist produced by the stenotic valve disappears (lower right).

forth inside the left ventricle to ensure that it is free of the chordae tendinae. The catheter is then gently pulled against the mitral plane until resistance is felt. The balloon is then rapidly inflated to its full capacity and then deflated quickly. During inflation of the balloon, an indentation should be seen in its midportion. The catheter is withdrawn into the left atrium, and the mitral gradient and cardiac output measured. If further dilatations are required, the stylet is introduced again and the sequence of steps described above repeated at a larger balloon volume. After each dilatation, its effect should be assessed by pressure measurement, auscultation, and 2D echocardiography. If mitral regurgitation occurs, further dilation of the valve should not be performed. (Video 2 demonstrates the Inoue technique of balloon mitral valvuloplasty on the accompanying CD-ROM.)

The Metallic Valvotomy Device Technique of PMV

A reusable metallic valvotomy device was developed by Cribier et al. with the goals of both improving the mitral valvotomy results and decreasing the cost of the procedure.

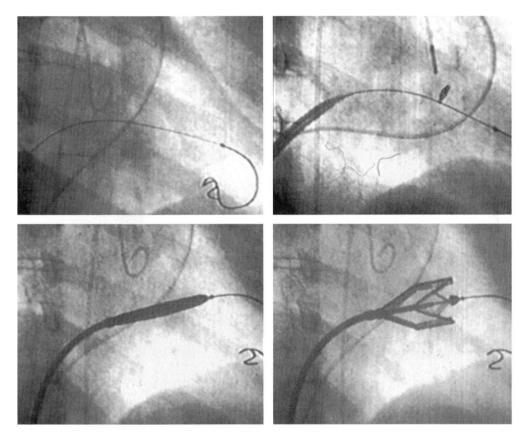

Fig. 3. Metallic dilator technique of PMV. Following transseptal catheterization, a guide wire is placed into the left ventricle apex (upper left), a 14 French dilator is advanced over the guide wire, and the interatrial septum dilated (upper right). The metallic dilator is then carefully advanced over the guide wire and placed straddling the stenotic mitral valve (lower left) and opened to a predetermined measure (lower right) to open the stenotic mitral valve.

The device consists of a detachable metallic cylinder with two articulated bars screwed onto the distal end of a disposable catheter whose proximal end is connected to an activating pliers. By the transseptal route, the device is advanced across the valve over a traction guide wire (Fig. 3). Squeezing the pliers opens the bars up to a maximum extent of 40 mm. The initial clinical experience consisted of 153 patients with a broad spectrum of mitral valve deformities. The procedure was successful in 92% of cases and resulted in a significant increase in mitral valve area, from 0.95 ± 0.2 to 2.16 ± 0.4 cm^2. No increase in mitral regurgitation was noted in 80% of cases. Bilateral splitting of the commissures was observed in 87%. Complications were two cases of severe mitral regurgitation (one requiring surgery), one pericardial tamponade, and one transient cerebrovascular embolic event. In this series, the maximum number of consecutive patients treated with the same device was 35. The results obtained with this new device are encouraging and at least comparable to those of current balloon techniques. Multiple uses after sterilization should markedly decrease the procedural cost, a major advantage in countries with limited resources and high incidence of mitral stenosis *(25)*. [A video (3) demonstrating commissurotomy with the metallic valvulotome is shown on the accompanying CD-ROM.]

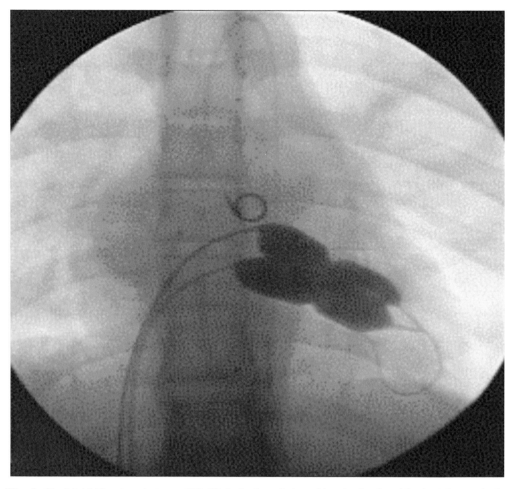

Fig. 4. The Multi-Ttrack technique of PMV. A single soft-tip guide wire is placed in the left ventricular apex. Subsequently, two balloon catheters (one over the wire and the other rapid exchange) are placed straddling the stenotic mitral valve; markers identifying the proximal end of the balloons are inflated by hand until the waist produced by the stenotic valve disappears.

The Multi-Track Technique of PMV

The Multi-Track System is a simplified double-balloon technique for percutaneous mitral valvuloplasty (Fig. 4). The Multi-Track catheter has a short distal tip for connection to the guide wire. This leaves the rest of guide wire free to receive other catheters. Various catheters can be introduced over the same guide wire. The balloons are introduced one after the other, allowing a smaller size of vascular access and transseptal passage. Furthermore, simultaneous pressure measurements in the left atrium and left ventricle are possible through a simple venous access, allowing avoidance of arterial puncture. Worldwide experience between June 1994 and February 2000 included 153 patients with mitral stenosis. In 12 cases, the procedure was done using the exclusive venous approach. The mean mitral valve area increased from 0.75 ± 0.22 to 2 ± 0.33 cm^2 and the mean left atrial pressure dropped from 27 ± 8 to 11 ± 4 mm Hg. Four patients had a significant increase in mitral regurgitation, requiring surgical treatment in two patients. There was no mortality. The

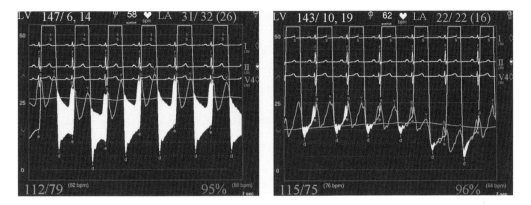

Fig. 5. Hemodynamic changes produced by a successful PMV in one patient with severe mitral steno0sis. Simultaneous left atrium (LA) and left ventricular (LV) pressures before **(right panel)** and after **(left panel)** PMV.

Table 1
Changes in Mitral Valve Area

Author	Institution	No. of pts.	Age (yr)	Pre-PMV	Post-PMV
Palacios	MGH	860	57 ± 12	0.9 ± 0.3	2.0 ± 0.2
Vahanian	Tenon	1514	45 ± 15	1.0 ± 0.2	1.9 ± 0.3
Stefanadis	Athens University	438	44 ± 11	1.0 ± 0.3	2.1 ± 0.5
Chen	Guangzhou	4832	37 ± 12	1.1 ± 0.3	2.1 ± 0.5
NHLBI	Multicenter	738	54 ± 12	1.0 ± 0.4	2.0 ± 0.2
Inoue	Takeda	527	50 ± 10	1.1 ± 0.1	2.0 ± 0.1
Inoue Registry	Multicenter	1251	53 ± 15	1.0 ± 0.3	1.8 ± 0.6
Farhat	Fattouma	463	33 ± 12	1.0 ± 0.2	2.2 ± 0.4
Arora	G.B. Pan	600	27 ± 8	0.8 ± 0.2	2.2 ± 0.4
Cribier	Ruen	153	36 ± 15	1.0 ± 0.2	2.2 ± 0.4

Multi-Track System is a valid user-friendly and cost-effective alternative for the treatment of mitral stenosis. It is a rapid and effective procedure associated with low risks *(26)*.

MECHANISM OF PMV

The mechanism of successful PMV is splitting of the fused commissures toward the mitral annulus, resulting in commissural widening. This mechanism has been demonstrated by pathological *(6,27)*, surgical *(27)*, and echocardiographic studies *(28)*. In addition, in patients with calcific mitral stenosis, the balloons could increase mitral valve flexibility by the fracture of the calcified deposits in the mitral valve leaflets *(6)*. Although rare, undesirable complications such as leaflets tears, left ventricular perforation, tear of the atrial septum, and rupture of chordae, mitral annulus, and papillary muscle could also occur.

IMMEDIATE OUTCOME

Figure 5 shows the hemodynamic changes produced by PMV in one patient. PMV resulted in a significant decrease in mitral gradient, mean left atrium pressure, and mean pulmonary artery pressure and an increase in cardiac output and mitral valve area. Table 1 shows the changes in mitral valve area reported by several investigators using

Table 2
Baseline Characteristics

Number of patients	879 (939 PMV)
Age (yr)	55 ± 15
Female	719 (82%)
Atrial fibrillation	430 (49%)
Previous commissurotomy	143 (16%)
Mitral regurgitatio ≥2+	57 (6.5%)
Fluoroscopic calcium ≥2+	230 (26%)
NYHA Class	
Class I	12 (2%)
Class II	212 (24%)
Class III	539 (61%)
Class IV	116 (13%)

Table 3
Hemodynamic Changes Produced by PMV

	Pre-PMV	Post-PMV	p-Value
Mitral valve area	0.9 ± 0.3	1.9 ± 0.7	<0.0001
Mitral gradient	14 ± 6	6 ± 3	<0.0001
Cardiac output	3.9 ± 1.1	4.5 ± 1.3	<0.0001
Mean PA	36 ± 13	29 ± 11	<0.0001
Mean LA	25 ± 7	17 ± 7	<0.0001

Note:

EBDA/BSA	3.62 ± 0.49 CM^2/m^2
PMV success	72%
Post-PMV MR 3+	56 (6.0%)
Post-PMV MR 4+	32 (3.4%)
QP/QS > 1.5 : 1	50 (5.3%)

the double-balloon and the Inoue techniques of PMV. In most series, PMV is reported to increase mitral valve area from less than 1.0 cm^2 to ≥2.0 cm^2 (2–22,28–30).

Eight hundred seventy-nine consecutive patients with mitral stenosis underwent PMV at Massachusetts General Hospital between July of 1986 and July of 2000 (19). The baseline patient characteristics of this patient population are given in Table 2. As shown in Table 3, in this group of patients, PMV resulted in a significant increase in mitral valve area from 0.9 ± 0.3 to 1.9 ± 0.7 cm^2.

A successful hemodynamic outcome (defined as a post-PMV mitral valve area ≥1.5 cm^2, ≤2 grade increase in mitral regurgitation by angiography, and a QP/QS < 1.5/1) was obtained in 72 % of the patients. Although a suboptimal result occurred in 28 % of the patients, a post-PMV mitral valve area ≤1.0 cm^2 (critical mitral valve area) was present in only 7% of these patients.

PREDICTORS OF INCREASE IN MITRAL VALVE AREA AND PROCEDURAL SUCCESS WITH PMV

Univariate analysis demonstrated that the increase in mitral valve area with PMV is directly related to the balloon size employed, as it reflects in the effective balloon dilating area (EBDA) and is inversely related to the echocardiographic score, the presence of atrial fibrillation, the presence of fluoroscopic calcium, the presence of previous surgical commissurotomy, older age, NYHA pre-PMV, and presence of mitral regurgitation before PMV. Multiple stepwise regression analysis demonstrated that the increase in mitral valve area with PMV is directly related to balloon size ($p < 0.02$) and inversely related to the echocardiographic score ($p < 0.0001$), presence of atrial fibrillation ($p < 0.009$), and mitral regurgitation before PMV ($p < 0.03$).

Univariate predictors of procedural success included younger age ($p = 0.0001$), male gender ($p = 0.0003$), absence of previous commissurotomy ($p = 0.0078$), lower NYHA functional status at presentation ($p = 0.0001$), lower fluoroscopic mitral valve calcification ($p = 0.0001$), lower echocardiographic score ($p = 0.0001$), normal sinus rhythm ($p = 0.0001$), larger pre-PMV mitral valve area ($p = 0.0001$), lower pre-PMV mitral regurgitation ($p = 0.0001$) and lower pre-PMV mean pulmonary artery pressure ($p = 0.001$), and the technique of PMV (double-balloon technique; $p = 0.05$). Multiple stepwise logistic regression analysis identified pre-PMV mitral valve area (odds ratio [OR] = 138; confidence intervals (CIs) = 43.8–466, $p < 0.0001$), echocardiographic score ≤8 [OR = 1.92; CI = 1.26–2.94, $p = 0.002$], male gender [OR = 2.32; CI = 1.37–4.16, $p = 0.002$] absence of previous surgical commissurotomy [OR = 1.79; CI = 1.09–2.94, $p = 0.01$], and younger age [OR = 6.25; CI = 2.5–16.6, $P = 0.0002$] as independent predictors of procedural success.

The Echocardiographic Score

This score is the most important predictor of the immediate outcome of PMV. In this morphologic score, leaflet rigidity, leaflet thickening, valvular calcification, and sub-valvular disease are each scored from 1 to 4 *(12,28)*. A higher score would represent a heavily calcified, thickened, and immobile valve with extensive thickening and calcification of the subvalvular apparatus. Among the four components of the echocardiographic score, valve leaflet thickening and subvalvular disease correlate the best with the increase in mitral valve area produced by PMV. The increase in mitral valve area with PMV is inversely related to the echocardiographic score. The best outcome with PMV occurs in those patients with echocardiographic scores ≤8. The increase in mitral valve area is significantly greater in patients with echocardiographic scores ≤8 than in those with echocardiographic score >8. Suboptimal results with PMV are more likely to occur in patients with valves that are more rigid, more thickened, and with more subvalvular fibrosis and calcification (Fig. 6).

Balloon Size and EBDA

The increase in mitral valve area with PMV is directly related to balloon size. This effect was first demonstrated in a subgroup of patients who underwent a repeat PMV *(9)*. They initially underwent PMV with a single balloon, resulting in a mean mitral valve area of 1.2 ± 0.2 cm^2. They underwent a repeat PMV using the double-balloon technique, which increased the EBDA normalized by body surface area (EBDA/BSA) from 3.41 ± 0.2 to 4.51 ± 0.2 cm^2/m^2. The mean mitral valve area in this group after the repeat PMV was 1.8 ± 0.2 cm^2. The increase in mitral valve area in patients who underwent PMV at the Massachusetts General Hospital using the double-balloon technique (EBDA of 6.4 ± 0.03 cm^2) was significantly greater than the increase in mitral valve area achieved in patients who underwent PMV using the single-balloon technique (EBDA of 4.3 ± 0.02 cm^2). The mean mitral valve areas were 2.0 ± 0.1 and 1.4 ± 0.1 cm^2 for patients who underwent PMV with the double-balloon and the single-balloon techniques, respectively. However, care should be taken in the selection of dilating balloon

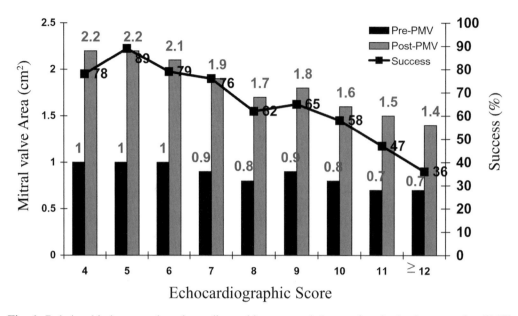

Fig. 6. Relationship between the echocardiographic score and changes in mitral valve area after PMV (bar graphs) and relationship between the echocardiographic score and PMV success (line with filled rectangles). Numbers at the top of bar graphs represent mean mitral valve areas before (black bars) and after PMV (shaded bars) for each echocardiographic score. Percentages on right axis represent PMV success rate at each echocardiographic score.

catheters so as to obtain an adequate final mitral valve area and no change or a minimal increase in mitral regurgitation.

Mitral Valve Calcification

The immediate outcome of patients undergoing PMV is inversely related to the severity of valvular calcification seen by fluoroscopy. Patients without fluoroscopic calcium have a greater increase in mitral valve area after PMV than patients with calcified valves. Patients with either no or 1+ fluoroscopic calcium have a greater increase in mitral valve area after PMV (2.1 ± 0.1 and 1.9 ± 0.1 cm^2, respectively) than those patients with 2, 3, or 4+ of calcium (1.7 ± 0.1, 1.5 ± 0.1, and 1.4 ± 0.1 cm^2, respectively).

Previous Surgical Commissurotomy

Although the increase in mitral valve area with PMV is inversely related to the presence of previous surgical mitral commissurotomy, PMV can produce a good outcome in this group of patients. The mean mitral valve area in 102 patients with previous surgical commissurotomy was 1.7 ± 0.1 cm^2 compared with a valve area of 2.0 ± 0.1 cm^2 in patients without previous surgical commissurotomy. In this group of patients, an echocardiographic score ≤ 8 was again the most important predictor of a successful hemodynamic immediate outcome.

Age

The immediate outcome of PMV is directly related to the age of the patient. The percentage of patients obtaining a good result with this technique decreases as age increases. A successful hemodynamic outcome from PMV was obtained in only less than 50% of patient ≥65 yr old *(14)*. This inverse relationship between age and the immediate outcome from PMV is likely the result of the higher frequency of atrial fibrillation, calcified valves, and higher echocardiographic scores in elderly patients.

Atrial Fibrillation

The increase in mitral valve area with PMV is inversely related to the presence of atrial fibrillation; the post-PMV mitral valve area of patients in normal sinus rhythm was 2.1 ± 0.1 cm^2 compared with a valve area of 1.7 ± 0.1 cm^2 of those patients in atrial fibrillation. The inferior immediate outcome of PMV in patients with mitral stenosis who are in atrial fibrillation is more likely related to the presence of other clinical and morphological characteristics associated with inferior results after PMV. Patients in atrial fibrillation are older and present more frequently with echocardiographic scores >8, NYHA functional class IV, calcified mitral valves under fluoroscopy, and those with a previous history of surgical mitral commissurotomy.

Mitral Regurgitation Before PMV

The presence and severity of mitral regurgitation before PMV is an independent predictor of unfavorable outcome of PMV. The increase in mitral valve area after PMV is inversely related to the severity of mitral regurgitation determined by angiography before the procedure. This inverse relationship between the presence of mitral regurgitation and immediate outcome of PMV is in part the result of the higher frequency of atrial fibrillation, higher echocardiographic scores, calcified mitral valves under fluoroscopy, and older age in patients with mitral regurgitation before PMV.

COMPLICATIONS

Table 4 shows the complications reported by several investigators using the double-balloon and the Inoue techniques of PMV *(1–20,29–32)*. Mortality and morbidity with PMV are low and similar to surgical commissurotomy. There is less than 1% mortality. Severe mitral regurgitation (4 grades by angiography) has been reported in 1–5.2% of the patients. Some of these patients required in-hospital mitral valve replacement. Thromboembolic episodes and stroke has been reported in 0–3.1% and pericardial tamponade in 0.2–4.1% of cases in these series. Pericardial tamponade can occur from transseptal catheterization and, more rarely, from ventricular perforation. PMV is associated with a 3–16% incidence of left to right shunt immediately after the procedure. However, the pulmonary-to-systemic flow ratio is ≥2 : 1 in only a small number of patients.

We have demonstrated that severe mitral regurgitation (4 grades by angiography) occurs in about 2% of patients undergoing PMV *(30,31)*. An undesirable increase in mitral regurgitation (≥2 grades by angiography) occurred in 12.5% of patients *(30,31)*. This undesirable increase in mitral regurgitation is well tolerated in most patients. Furthermore, more than half of them have less mitral regurgitation at follow-up cardiac catheterization. We have demonstrated that EBDA/BSA ratio is the only predictor of increased mitral regurgitation after PMV. The EBDA is calculated using standard geometric formulas. The incidence of mitral regurgitation is lower if balloon sizes are chosen so that the EBDA/BSA ratio is ≤4.0 cm^2/m^2. The single-balloon technique results in a lower incidence of mitral regurgitation but provides less relief of mitral stenosis than the double-balloon technique. Thus, there is an optimal balloon size between 3.1 and 4.0 cm^2/m^2, which achieves a maximal mitral valve area with a minimal increase in mitral regurgitation *(33)*. An echocardiographic score for the mitral valve that can predict the

Table 4
Complications of PMV

Author	No. of pts.	Mortality	Tamponade	Severe MR	Embolism
Palacios	860	0.3%	0.6%	3.3%	1.0%
Vahanian	1514	0.4%	0.3%	3.4%	0.3%
Stefanadis	438	0.2%	0.0%	3.4%	0.0%
Chen	4832	0.1%	0.8%	1.4%	0.5%
NHLBI	738	3.0%	4.0%	3.0%	3.0%
Inoue	527	0.0%	1.6%	1.9%	0.6%
Inoue Registry	1251	0.6%	1.4%	3.8%	0.9%
Farhat	463	0.4%	0.7%	4.6%	2.0%
Arora	600	1.0%	1.3%	1.0%	0.5%
Cribier	153	0.0%	0.7%	1.4%	0.7%

development of severe mitral regurgitation following PMV has recently been reported by Padial et al. *(34)*. This score takes into account the distribution (even or uneven) of leaflet thickening and calcification, the degree and symmetry of commissural disease, and the severity of subvalvular disease. The mechanisms for mitral regurgitation with the Inoue technique may differ and appear to be related to disruption of the valve integrity, including chordal rupture and leaflet tearing *(35)*. Careful balloon positioning may help avoid chordal rupture, and heavily calcified posterior leaflets may be at greater risk of tearing *(35)*.

Left to right shunt through the created atrial communication occurred in 3–16% of the patients undergoing PMV. The size of the defect is small, as reflected in the pulmonary-to-systemic flow ratio of <2 : 1 in the majority of patients. Older age, fluoroscopic evidence of mitral valve calcification, higher echocardiographic score, pre-PMV lower cardiac output, and higher pre-PMV NYHA functional class are the factors that predispose patients to develop left to right shunt post-PMV *(36)*. Clinical, echocardiographic, surgical, and hemodynamic follow-up of patients with post-PMV left to right shunt demonstrated that the defect closed in 59%. Persistent left to right shunt at follow-up is small and clinically well tolerated. In the series from the Massachusetts General Hospital, there is only one patient in whom the atrial shunt remained hemodynamically significant at follow-up. This patient underwent percutaneous transcatheter closure of her atrial defect with a clamshell device. Desideri et al. *(37)* reported atrial shunting determined by color flow transthoracic echocardiography in 61% of 57 patients immediately after PMV. The shunt persisted in 30% of patients at 19 ± 6 mo (range: 9–33) follow-up *(37)*. They identified the magnitude of the post-PMV atrial shunt (QP/QS > 1.5 : 1), use of Bifoil balloon (two balloons on one shaft), and smaller post-PMV mitral valve area as independent predictors of the persistence of atrial shunt at long-term follow-up *(37)*.

CLINICAL FOLLOW-UP

Follow-up studies after PMV are encouraging *(11,14–20,30,35–42)*. Following PMV, the majority of patients have marked clinical improvement and become NYHA Class I or II. However, long-term changes in skeletal muscle and the lungs precludes immediate

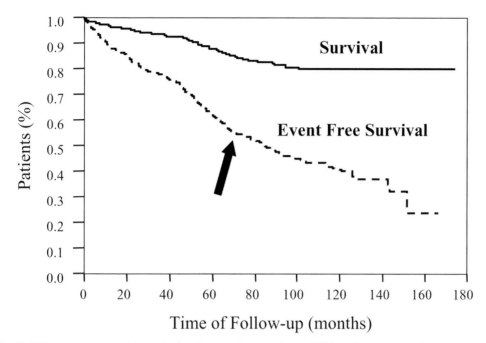

Fig. 7. Fifteen-year actuarial survival and event-free survival of 732 patients undergoing PMV at the Massachusetts General Hospital.

enhancement of exercise performance in some patients who may benefit from exercise training after PMV *(43)*.

The symptomatic, echocardiographic, and hemodynamic improvement produced by PMV persists in intermediate and long-term follow-up. The best long-term results are seen in patients with echocardiographic scores ≤8. When PMV produces a good immediate outcome in this group of patients, restenosis is unlikely to occur at follow-up *(11,14–20,30,35–42)*. Although PMV can result in a good outcome in patients with echocardiographic scores >8, hemodynamic and echocardiographic restenosis is frequently demonstrated at follow-up despite ongoing clinical improvement *(11,14–20,30,35–42)*. Figures 7–11 show the long-term follow-up results of patients undergoing PMV at Massachusetts General Hospital. We reported 110 deaths (25 noncardiac), 234 MVR and 54 redo PMVs accounting for a total of 398 patients with combined events (death, MVR, or redo PMV). Of the remaining 446 patients who were free of combined events, 418 (94%) were in NYHA class I or II (Fig. 7). End-point events occurred less frequently in patients with Echo Score ≤8 and included 51 deaths, 155 MVRs, and 39 redo PMVs, accounting for a total of 245 patients with combined events at follow-up. Of the remaining 330 patients who were free of combined events, 312 (95%) were in NYHA Class I or II (Figs. 8–10). End-point events in patients with Echo Score >8 included 59 deaths, 79 MVRs, and 15 redo PMVs, accounting for a total of 153 patients with combined events at follow-up. Of the remaining 116 patients who were free of any event, 105 (91%) were in NYHA Class I or II (Figs. 8–10).

Figure 8 shows estimated actuarial total survival curves for the overall population and for patients with Echo Score ≤8 and >8. Actuarial survival rates throughout the follow-up period were significantly better in patients with Echo Score ≤8. Survival rates were 82% for patients with Echo Score ≤8 and 57% for patients with Echo Score >8

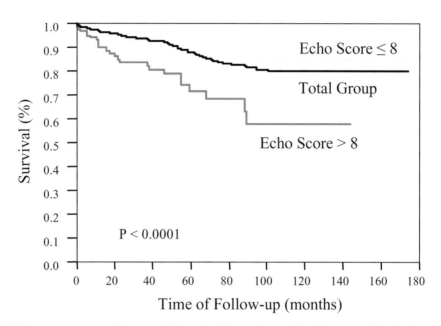

Fig. 8. Fifteen-year comparative actuarial survival for patients with echo score ≤8 and >8 undergoing PMV at the Massachusetts General Hospital. (From ref. *19.*)

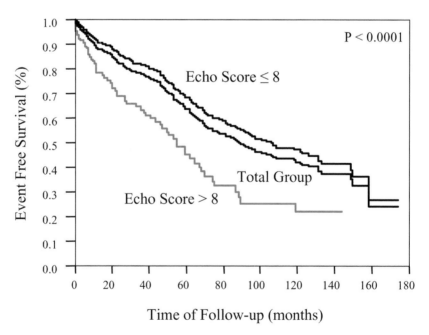

Fig. 9. Fifteen-year comparative actuarial event-free survival for patients with echo score ≤8 and >8 undergoing PMV at the Massachusetts General Hospital. (From ref. *19.*)

at a follow-up time of 12 yr ($p < 0.001$). Survival rates were 82% and 56%, respectively, when only patients with successful PMV were included in the analysis. Figure 9 shows estimated actuarial total event-free survival curves for the overall population

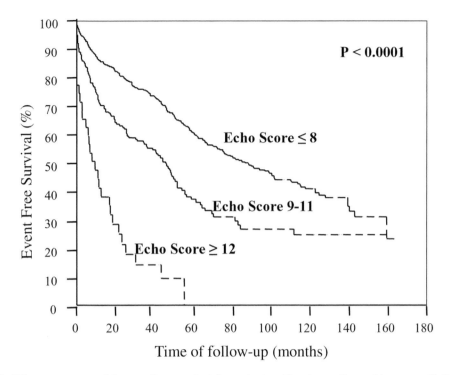

Fig. 10. Fifteen-year actuarial event-free survival for patients with echocardiographic scores ≤8, 9–11, and ≥12 undergoing PMV at the Massachusetts General Hospital.

and for patients with Echo Score ≤8 and >8. Event-free survival (38% vs 22%; $p < 0.0001$) at 12 yr follow-up were also significantly higher for patients with Echo Score ≤8. Event-free survival rates were 41% and 23%, respectively, when only patients with successful PMV were included in the analysis.

Cox regression analysis identified post-PMV MR ≥ 3+, Echo Score >8, age, prior commissurotomy, NYHA functional Class IV, pre-PMV MR ≥ 2+, and post-PMV pulmonary artery pressure as independent predictors of combined events at long-term follow-up *(19)*.

Echocardiographic Score

Patient selection is fundamental in predicting immediate outcome and follow-up results of PMV and surgical commissurotmy procedures. In addition to clinical examination, echocardiographic evaluation of the mitral valve and fluoroscopic screening for valvular calcification are the most important steps in patient selection for successful outcome. The evaluation of candidates for PMV requires a precise evaluation of both valve morphology and function for preprocedure decision-making and follow-up of the patients. Two-dimensional echocardiography is currently the most widely used noninvasive technique for the evaluation of the morphologic characteristics of the mitral valve, subvalvular apparatus, and the valve annular size. An important predictor of the immediate and long-term results of PMV is a morphologic echocardiographic score developed at Massachusetts General Hospital *(28–31)*. In this score, leaflet mobility, leaflet thickening, valvular calcification, and subvalvular disease are each scored from 1+ to 4+, yielding a maximum total echocardiographic score of 16. A higher score would represent a heavily calcified, thickened,

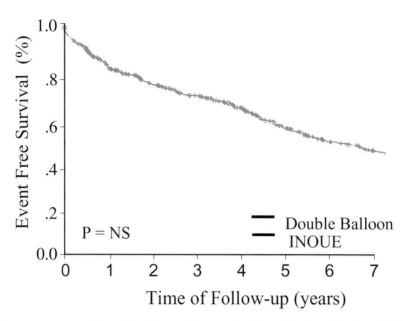

Fig. 11. Seven-year comparative actuarial event-free survival for patients undergoing PMV using the double-balloon technique versus those undergoing PMV using the Inoue technique at the Massachusetts General Hospital.

and immobile valve, with extensive thickening and calcification of the subvalvular apparatus. Among the four components of the echocardiographic score valve, leaflets thickening and subvalvular disease correlate the best with the increase in mitral valve area produced by PMV. An inverse relationship between the immediate and long-term results produced by PMV and the echocardiographic score has been demonstrated *(11,12,15,19)*. Patients with lower echocardiographic scores have a higher likelihood of having a good outcome from PMV with minimal complications and a hemodynamic and clinical improvement that persist at long-term follow-up (Figs. 6 and 9).

Other Predictors of PMV Outcome

The reliability of the echocardiographic score for predicting results of PMV is not optimal because the results of PMV are also related to other factors, such as the presence of fluoroscopic mitral valve calcification, the age and gender of the patient, the presence of atrial fibrillation, pre-PMV mitral regurgitation and pulmonary hypertension, a history of previous surgical commissurotomy, the technique of PMV (double balloon vs Inoue), the severity of mitral stenosis before PMV, and the effective balloon dilating area *(8–11)*.

Follow-up in the Elderly

Tuzcu et al. *(14)* reported the outcome of PMV in 99 elderly patients (≥65 yr). A successful outcome (valve area ≥1.5 cm² without ≥2+ increase in mitral regurgitation and without left to right shunt of ≥1.5 : 1) was achieved in 46 patients. The best multivariate predictor of success was the combination of echocardiographic score, NYHA functional class, and inverse of mitral valve area. Patients who had unsuccessful outcomes from PMV were in a higher NYHA functional class, had higher echocardiographic scores, and had smaller mitral valve areas pre-PMV compared to those patients who had a successful outcome. Actuarial survival and combined event-free survival at 3 yr were significantly better in the successful group. Mean follow-up was 16 ± 1 mo. Actuarial survival (79 ± 7% vs 62 ± 10%; $p = 0.04$), survival without mitral valve replacement (71 ± 8% vs 41 ± 8%; $p = 0.002$), and event-free survival (54 ± 12% vs 38 ± 8%; $p = 0.01$) at 3 yr were significantly better in the successful group of 46 patients than the unsuccessful group of 53 patients. Low echocardiographic score was the independent predictor of survival, and lack of mitral valve calcification was the strongest predictor of event-free survival.

Follow-up of Patients with Calcified Mitral Valves

The presence of fluoroscopically visible calcification on the mitral valve influences the success of PMV. Patients with heavily (≥3 grades) calcified valves under fluoroscopy have a poorer immediate outcome, as reflected in a smaller post-PMV mitral valve area and greater post-PMV mitral valve gradient. Immediate outcome is progressively worse as the calcification becomes more severe. The long-term results of PMV are significantly different in calcified and uncalcified groups and in subgroups of the calcified group *(38)*. The estimated 2-yr survival is significantly lower for patients with calcified mitral valves than for those with uncalcified valves (80% vs 99%). The survival curve becomes worse as the severity of valvular calcification becomes more severe. Freedom from mitral valve replacement at 2 yr was significantly lower for patients with calcified valves than for those with uncalcified valves (67% vs 93%). Similarly, the estimated event-free survival at 2 yr in the calcified group became significantly poorer as the severity of calcification increased. The estimated event-free survival at 2 yr was significantly lower for the calcified than for the uncalcified group (63% vs 88%). The actuarial survival curves with freedom from combined events at 2 yr in the calcified group became significantly poorer as the severity of calcification increased *(38,44)*. Similar results have been reported from the Inoue Multicenter Registry *(45)*. These findings are in agreement with several follow-up studies of surgical commissurotomy that demonstrate that patients with calcified mitral valves had a poorer survival compared to those patients with uncalcified valves *(45–48)*.

Follow-up of Patients with Previous Surgical Commissurotomy

Percutaneous mitral balloon valvuloplasty also has been shown to be a safe procedure in patients with previous surgical mitral commissurotomy *(10,49–51)*. Although a good immediate outcome is frequently achieved in these patients, follow-up results are not as favorable as those obtained in patients without previous surgical commissurotomy *(49–51)*. Although there is no difference in mortality between patients with or without a history of previous surgical commissurotomy at 4 yr follow-up, the number of patients who required mitral valve replacement (26% vs 8%) and/or were in NYHA Class III or IV (35% vs 13%) were significantly higher among those patients with previous commissurotomy. However, when the patients were carefully selected according to the echocardiographic score (≤8), the immediate outcome and the 4-yr follow-up results were excellent and similar to those seen in patients without previous surgical commissurotomy *(10,49–51)*.

Follow-up of Patients with Atrial Fibrillation

We and others recently reported that the presence of atrial fibrillation is associated with inferior immediate and long-term outcome after PMV as reflected in a smaller post-PMV mitral valve area and a lower event-free survival *(52,53)*. The freedom from death, redo

PMV, and mitral valve surgery at a median follow-up time of 61 mo was 32% with versus 61% without in patients atrial fibrillation ($p < 0.0001$) *(52)*. Analysis of preprocedural and procedural characteristics revealed that this association is most likely explained by the presence of multiple factors in the atrial fibrillation group that adversely affect the immediate and long-term outcome of PMV. Patients in atrial fibrillation are older and presented more frequently with NYHA Class IV, echocardiographic score >8, calcified valves under fluoroscopy, and history of previous surgical commissurotomy. In the group of patients in atrial fibrillation, Leon et al. identified severe post-PMV mitral regurgitation (>3+) ($p = 0.0001$), echocardiographic score ≥8 ($p = 0.004$), and pre-PMV NYHA Class IV ($p = 0.046$) as independent predictors of combined events at follow-up *(52)*. The presence of atrial fibrillation *per se* should not be the only determinant in the decision process regarding treatment options in a patient with rheumatic mitral stenosis. The presence of an echocardiographic score ≤8 primarily identify a subgroup of patients in atrial fibrillation in whom percutaneous balloon valvotomy is very likely to be successful and provide good long-term results. Atrial fibrillation is associated with a lower cardiac output, but the long-term outcome of balloon valvuloplasty is independent of the initial cardiac rhythm *(53)*.

Follow-up of Patients with Pulmonary Artery Hypertension

The degree of pulmonary artery hypertension before PMV is inversely related to the immediate and long-term outcome of PMV. Chen et al. *(54)* divided 564 patients undergoing PMV at Massachusetts General Hospital into 3 groups on the basis of the pulmonary vascular resistance (PVR) obtained at cardiac catheterization immediately prior to PMV: group I with PVR ≤ 250 dynes s/cm^{-5} (normal/mildly elevated resistance) comprised 332 patients (59%); group II with PVR between 251 and 400 dynes s/cm^{-5} (moderately elevated resistance) comprised 110 patients (19.5%); group III with PVR ≥ 400 dynes s/cm^{-5} comprised 122 patients (21.5%). Patients in groups I and II were younger, had less severe heart failure symptoms measured by NYHA class and a lower incidence of echocardiographic scores ≥8, atrial fibrillation, and calcium noted on fluoroscopy than patients in group III. Before and after PMV, patients with higher PVR had a smaller mitral valve area, lower cardiac output, and higher mean pulmonary artery pressure. For group I, II, and III patients, the immediate success rates for PMV were 68%, 56%, and 45%, respectively. Therefore, patients in the group with severely elevated pulmonary artery resistance before the procedure had lower immediate success rates of PMV. At long-term follow-up, patients with severely elevated pulmonary vascular resistances had a significant lower survival and event-free survival (survival with freedom from mitral valve surgery or NYHA Class III or IV heart failure).

In 18 women with mitral stenosis and pulmonary hypertension, Mahoney and colleagues administered inhaled nitric oxide (NO) to examine the reversibility of pulmonary vascular resistence before PMV *(55)*. Inhaled NO, but not PMV, acutely reduced PVR, suggesting that a reversible, endothelium-dependent regulatory abnormality of vascular tone is an important mechanism of elevated PVR in mitral stenosis *(55)*.

Follow-up of Patients with Tricuspid Regurgitation

The degree of tricuspid regurgitation before PMV is inversely related to the immediate and long-term outcome of PMV. Sagie et al. *(56)* divided patients undergoing PMV at the Massachusetts General Hospital into three groups on the basis of the degree of tricuspid regurgitation determined by 2D and color flow Doppler echocardiography before PMV. Patients with severe tricuspid regurgitation before PMV were older, had more severe heart failure symptoms measured by NYHA class, and had a higher incidence of echocardiographic scores >8, atrial fibrillation, and calcified mitral valves on fluoroscopy than patients with mild or moderate tricuspid regurgitation. Patients with severe tricuspid regurgitation had a smaller mitral valve area before and after PMV than the patients with mild or moderate tricuspid regurgitation. At long-term follow-up, patients with severe tricuspid regurgitation had a significant lower survival and event-free survival (survival with freedom from mitral valve surgery or NYHA Class III or IV heart failure).

Follow-up of the Best Patients for PMV

In patients identified as optimal candidates for PMV, this technique results in excellent immediate and long-term outcomes. Optimal candidates for PMV are those patients meeting the following characteristics: (1) age <65 yr, (2) normal sinus rhythm, (3) echocardiographic score ≤8, (4) no fluoroscopic mitral valve calcification, and (5) pre-PMV mitral regurgitation ≤1+ Seller's grade. From 780 consecutive patients undergoing percutaneous mitral balloon valvuloplasty (PMV) we identified 202 patients with optimal preprocedure characteristics. In these patients, PMV results in an 81% success rate and a 3.4% incidence of major in hospital combined events (death and/or MVR). In these patients, PMV results in a 97% survival and 76% event-free survival at a median follow-up of 61 mo *(57)*.

Double-Balloon Versus Inoue Technique of PMV

Today, the Inoue and double-balloon techniques of PMV are most widely used. However, there is controversy as to which technique provides superior immediate and long-term results. We compared the immediate procedural and the long-term clinical outcomes after PMV using the double-balloon technique ($n = 621$) and Inoue technique ($n = 113$). There were no statistically significant differences in baseline clinical and morphological characteristics between the double-balloon and Inoue patients. The double-balloon technique resulted in superior immediate outcome, as reflected in a larger post-PMV mitral valve area (1.9 ± 0.7 vs 1.7 ± 0.6 cm^2; $p = 0.005$) and a lower incidence of 3+ mitral regurgitation post-PMV (5.4% vs 10.6%; $p = 0.05$). This superior immediate outcome of the double-balloon technique was observed only in the group of patients with echocardiographic score ≤8 (post-PMV mitral valve areas 2.1 ± 0.7 vs 1.8 ± 0.6; $p = 0.004$). Despite the difference in immediate outcome, there were no significant differences in event-free survival at long-term follow-up between the two techniques (Fig. 11) *(30)*.

Echocardiographic and Hemodynamic Follow-up

Follow-up studies have shown that the incidence of hemodynamic and echocardiographic restenosis is low 2 yr after PMV *(11,13,15–17,37)*. A study of a group of patients undergoing simultaneous clinical evaluation, 2D Doppler echocardiography, and transseptal catheterization 2 yr after PMV reported that 90% of patients were in NYHA Classes I and II and 10% of patients in NYHA Class ≥ III *(13)*. In this study, hemodynamic determination of mitral valve area using the Gorlin equation showed a significant decrease in mitral valve area from 2.0 cm^2 immediately after PMV to 1.6 cm^2 at follow-up. However, there was no significant difference between the echocardiographic mitral valve areas immediately after PMV and at follow-up (1.8 cm^2 and 1.6 cm^2, respectively; $p = $ NS). Although there was a significant difference in the mitral valve area after PMV determined by the Gorlin equation and by 2D echocardiography (2.0 cm^2 vs 1.8 cm^2), there was no significant difference between the mitral valve area determined by the Gorlin equation and the echocardiographic calculated mitral valve area (1.6 cm^2 for both) at follow-up. The discrepancy between the 2D echocardiographic- and Gorlin-equation-determined post-PMV mitral valve areas is the result of the contribution of left to right shunting (undetected by oximetry) across the created interatrial communication, which results in both an erroneously high cardiac output and an overestimation of the mitral valve area by the Gorlin equation *(58)*. Desideri et al. showed no significant differences in mitral valve area (measured by Doppler echocardiography) at 19 ± 6 mo (range: 9–33) follow-up between the post-PMV and follow-up mitral valve areas. Mitral valve areas were 2.2 ± 0.5 cm^2 and 1.9 ± 0.5 cm^2, respectively *(37)*. Echocardiographic restenosis (mitral valve area ≤1.5 cm^2 with >50% reduction of the gain) was seen in 21% of the patients *(38)*. Predictors of restenosis included age, smaller post-PMV mitral valve area, and higher echocardiographic score *(37)*. With the Inoue technique, Chen et al. *(16)* showed no significant differences in mitral valve area determined by 2D Doppler echocardiography in 85 patients at a mean follow-up of 5 ± 1 yr (range: 43–79 mo). Post-PMV and follow-up mitral valve areas were 2.0 ± 0.4 and 1.8 ± 0.5 cm^2, respectively (NS).

PMV Versus Surgical Mitral Commissurotomy

Results of surgical closed mitral commissurotomy have demonstrated favorable long-term hemodynamic and symptomatic improvement from this technique. A restenosis rate of 4.2 to 11.4 per 1000 patients per year was reported by John et al. in 3724 patients who underwent surgical closed mitral commissurotomy *(59)*. Survival after PMV is similar to that reported after surgical mitral commissurotomy. Although freedom from mitral valve replacement (87% vs 92%) and freedom from all events (67% vs 80%) after PMV are lower than reported after surgical commissurotomy *(30,37,59–67)*, freedom from both mitral valve replacement and all events in patients with echocardiographic scores ≤8 are similar to that reported after surgical mitral commissurotomy *(30,37,59–67)*.

Restenosis after both closed and open surgical mitral commissurotomy has been well documented *(59–67)*. Although surgical closed mitral commissurotomy is uncommonly performed in the United States, it is still used frequently in other countries. Long-term follow-up of 267 patients who underwent surgical transventricular mitral commissurotomy at the Mayo Clinic showed a 79%, 67%, and 55% survival at 10, 15, and 20 yr, respectively. Survival with freedom from mitral valve replacement were 57%, 36%, and 24%, respectively *(68)*. In this study, age, atrial fibrillation, and male gender were independent predictors of death, whereas mitral valve calcification, cardiomegaly, and mitral regurgitation were independent predictors of repeat mitral valve surgery *(68)*. Because of similar patient selection and mechanism of mitral valve dilatation, similar long-term results should be expected after PMV. Indeed, prospective, randomized trials comparing PMV and surgical closed mitral commissurotomy have shown no differences in immediate and 3 yr follow-up results between both groups of patients *(69,70)*. Furthermore, restenosis at 3 yr follow-up occurred in 10% and 13% of the patients treated with mitral balloon valvuloplasty and surgical commissurotomy, respectively *(70)*.

Interpretation of long-term clinical follow-up of patients undergoing PMV as well as their comparison with surgical commissurotomy series are confounded by heterogeneity in the patient population. Only a few randomized studies have compared the results of PMV with those of surgical open commissurotomy. Farhat et al. *(71)* reported the results of a randomized trial designed to compare the immediate and long-term results of double-balloon PMV versus those of open and closed surgical mitral commissurotomy in a cohort of patients with severe rheumatic mitral stenosis. This group of patients were, from the clinical and morphological points, of view, optimal candidates for both PMV and surgical commissurotomy (closed or open) procedures as demonstrated by a mean age of less than 30 yr, absence of mitral valve calcification on fluoroscopy and 2D echocardiography, and an echocardiographic score ≤8 in all patients. Their results demonstrate that the immediate and long-term results of PMV are comparable to those of open mitral commissurotomy and superior to those of closed commissurotomy. The hemodynamic improvement, in-hospital complications, and long-term restenosis rate and need for reintervention were superior for the patients treated with either PMV or open commissurotomy than for those treated with closed commissurotomy.

A comparison between PMV and surgical commissurotomy techniques is difficult in view of differences in patient clinical and mitral valve morphology characteristics among different series.

In patients with optimal mitral valve morphology, surgical mitral commissurotomy has favorable long-term hemodynamic and symptomatic improvement. Similar to PMV, patients with advanced age, calcified mitral valves, and with atrial fibrillation had a poorer survival and event-free survival. Several studies have compared the immediate and early follow-up results of PMV versus closed surgical commissurotomy in optimal patients for these techniques. The results of these studies have been controversial, showing either superior outcome from PMV or no significant differences between both techniques *(72–74)*. Patel et al. randomized 45 patients with mitral stenosis and optimal mitral valve morphology to closed surgical commissurotomy and to PMV *(72)*. They demonstrated a larger increase in mitral valve area with PMV (2.1 ± 0.7 vs 1.3 ± 0.3 cm^2). Shrivastava et al. compared the results of single-balloon PMV, double-balloon PMV, and closed surgical commissurotomy in 3 groups of 20 patients each *(73)*. The mitral valve area postintervention was larger for the double-balloon technique of PMV. Postintervention valve areas were 1.9 ± 0.8, 1.5 ± 0.4, and 1.5 ± 0.5 cm^2 for the double-balloon, the single-balloon, and the closed surgical commissurotomy techniques, respectively. On the other hand, Arora et al. randomized 200 patients with a mean age of 19 ± 7 yr and mitral stenosis with optimal mitral valve morphology to PMV and to closed mitral commissurotomy *(74)*. Both procedures resulted in similar postintervention mitral valve areas (2.39 ± 0.9 vs 2.2 ± 0.9 cm^2 for the PMV and the mitral commissurotomy groups, respectively) and no significant differences in event-free survival at a mean follow-up period of 22 ± 6 mo. Restenosis documented by echocardiography was low in both groups: 5% in the PMV group and 4% in the closed commissurotomy group. Turi et al. *(69)* randomized 40 patients with severe mitral stenosis to PMV and to closed surgical commissurotomy. The postintervention mitral valve area at 1 wk (1.6 ± 0.6 vs 1.6 ± 0.7 cm^2) and 8 mo (1.6 ± 0.6 vs 1.8 ± 0.6 cm^2) after the procedures were similar in both groups *(69)*. Reyes et al. randomized 60 patients with severe mitral stenosis and favorable valvular anatomy to PMV and to surgical commissurotomy *(70)*. They reported no significant differences in immediate outcome, complications, and 3.5-yr follow-up between both groups of patients. Improvement was maintained in both groups, but mitral valve areas at follow-up were larger in the PMV group (2.4 ± 0.6 vs 1.8 ± 0.4 cm^2).

Although these initial randomized trials results of PMV versus surgical commissurotomy are encouraging and favors PMV for the treatment of patients with rheumatic mitral stenosis with suitable mitral valve anatomy, there was a need for long-term follow-up studies to define more precisely the role of PMV in these patients. The article by Farhat et al. *(71)* provides this long-term follow-up in a cohort of optimal candidates for PMV and clearly establishes the role of PMV in the treatment of these patients. The immediate and long-term results of PMV in these patients are similar to those obtained with open surgical commissurotomy and significantly superior to those obtained with closed surgical commissurotomy. Because open commissurotomy is associated with a thoracotomy, need for cardiopulmonary bypass, higher cost, longer length of hospital stay, and a longer period of convalescence, PMV should be the procedure of choice for the treatment of these patients *(75)*.

PMV in Pregnant Women

Surgical mitral commissurotomy has been performed in pregnant women with severe mitral stenosis. Because, the risks from anesthesia and surgery for the mother and the fetus are increased, this operation is reserved for those patients with incapacitating symptoms refractory to medical therapy *(76,77)*. Under these conditions PMV can be performed safely after the 20th week of pregnancy, with minimal radiation to the fetus *(78,79)*.

CONCLUSIONS

Percutaneous mitral balloon valvuloplasty produces a good immediate outcome and good clinical long-term follow-up results in a high percentage of patients with mitral stenosis. The immediate and long-term outcomes of patients undergoing PMV is multifactorial. The use of the echocardiographic score in conjunction with other clinical and morphological predictors of PMV outcome allows identification of patients who will obtain the best outcome from PMV. These factors include pre-PMV variables (MVA, history of previous surgical commissurotomy, age and MR) and post-PMV variables (MR ≥ 3+ and PA pressure). Patients with echocardiographic scores ≤8 have the best results, particularly if they are young, are in sinus rhythm, and have no evidence of calcification of the mitral valve under fluoroscopy. The immediate and long-term results of PMV in this group of patients are similar to those reported after surgical mitral commissurotomy. Patients with echocardiographic scores >8 have only a 50% chance to obtain a successful hemodynamic result with PMV, and long-term follow-up results are not as good as those from patients with echocardiographic scores ≤8. In patients with echocardiographic scores ≥12, it is unlikely that PMV could produce good immediate or long-term results. They preferably should undergo open heart surgery. However, PMV could be performed in these patients if they are non-risk/high-risk surgical candidates Surgical therapy for mitral stenosis should be reserved for patients who have ≥2 grades of Seller's mitral regurgitation by angiography and for those patients with severe mitral valve thickening and calcification or with significant subvalvular scarring.

REFERENCES

1. Inoue K, Owaki T, Nakamura T, et al. Clinical application of transvenous mitral commissurotomy by a new balloon catheter. J Thorac Cardiovasc Surg 1984;87:394–402.
2. Lock JE, Kalilullah M, Shrivastava S, et al. Percutaneous catheter commissurotomy in rheumatic mitral stenosis. N Engl J Med 1985;313:1515–1518.
3. Palacios I, Block PC, Brandi S, et al. Percutaneous balloon valvotomy for patients with severe mitral stenosis. Circulation 1987;75:778–784.
4. Al Zaibag M, Ribeiro PA, Al Kassab SA, Al Fagig MR. Percutaneous double balloon mitral valvotomy for rheumatic mitral stenosis. Lancet 1986;1:757–761.

5. Vahanian A, Michel PL, Cormier B, et al. Results of percutaneous mitral commissurotomy in 200 patients. Am J Cardiol 1989;63:847–852.
6. Mc Kay RG, Lock JE, Safian RD, et al. Balloon dilatation of mitral stenosis in adults patients: post-mortem and percutaneous mitral valvuloplasty studies. J Am Coll Cardiol 1987;9:723–731.
7. Mc Kay CR, Kawanishi DT, Rahimtoola SH. Catheter balloon valvuloplasty of the mitral valve in adults using a double balloon technique. Early hemodynamic results. JAMA 1987;257:1753–1761.
8. Abascal VM, O'Shea JP, Wilkins GT, et al. Prediction of successful outcome in 130 patients undergoing percutaneous balloon mitral valvotomy. Circulation 1990;82:448–456.
9. Herrman HC, Wilkins GT, Abascal VM, et al. Percutaneous balloon mitral valvotomy for patients with mitral stenosis: analysis of factors influencing early results. J Thorac Cardiovasc Surg 1988;96:33–38.
10. Rediker DE, Block PC, Abascal VM, Palacios IF. Mitral balloon valvuloplasty for mitral restenosis after surgical commissurotomy. J Am Coll Cardiol 1988;2:252–256.
11. Palacios IF, Block PC, Wilkins GT, Weyman AE. Follow-up of patients undergoing percutaneous mitral balloon valvotomy: Analysis of factors determining restenosis. Circulation 1989;79:573–579.
12. Abascal VM, Wilkins GT, Choong CY, et al. Echocardiographic evaluation of mitral valve structure and function in patients followed for at least 6 months after percutaneous balloon mitral valvuloplasty. J Am Coll Cardiol 1988;12:606–615.
13. Block PC, Palacios IF, Block EH, et al. Late (two year) follow-up after percutaneous mitral balloon valvotomy. Am J Cardiol 1992;69:537–541.
14. Tuzcu EM, Block PC, Griffin BP, et al. Immediate and long term outcome of percutaneous mitral valvotomy in patients 65 years and older. Circulation 1992;85:963–971.
15. Nobuyoshi M, Hamasaki N, Kimura T, et al. Indications, complications, and short term clinical outcome of percutaneous transvenous mitral commissurotomy. Circulation 1989;80:782–792.
16. Chen CR, Cheng TO, Chen JY, et al. Percutaneous mitral valvuloplasty with the Inoue balloon catheter. Am J Cardiol 1992;70:1455–1458.
17. Hung JS, Chern MS, Wu JJ, et al. Short and long term results of catheter balloon percutaneous transvenous mitral commissurotomy. Am J Cardiol 1991;67:854–862.
18. Cohen DJ, Kuntz RE, Gordon SPF, et al. Predictors of long-term outcome after percutaneous mitral valvuloplasty. N Engl J Med 1991;327:1329–1335.
19. Palacios IF, Sanchez PL, Harrell LC, et al. Which patients benefit from percutaneous mitral balloon valvuloplasty? Prevalvuloplasty and postvalvuloplasty variables that predict long-term outcome. Circulation 2002;105:1465–1471.
20. Iung BL, Garbarz E, Michaud P, et al. Late results of percutaneous mitral commissurotomy in a series of 1024 patients. analysis of late clinical deterioration: frequency, anatomic findings and predictive factors. Circulation 1999;99:3272–3278.
21. Babic UU, Pejcic P, Djurisic Z, et al. Percutaneous transarterial balloon valvuloplasty for mitral valve stenosis. Am J Cardiol 1986;57:1101.
22. Stefanides C, Kouroklis C, Stratos C, et al. Percutaneous balloon mitral valvuloplasty by retrograde left atrial catheterization. Am J Cardiol 1990;65:650–654.
23. Stefanides C, Stratos C, Pitsavos C, et al. Retrograde nontransseptal balloon mitral valvuloplasty. Immediate results and long term follow-up. Circulation 1992;85:1760–1767.
24. Palacios IF, Lock JE, Keane JF, Block PC. Percutaneous transvenous balloon valvotomy in a patient with severe calcific mitral stenosis. J Am Coll Cardiol 1986;7:1416.
25. Cribier A, Eltchaninoff H, Koning R, et al. Percutaneous mechanical mitral commissurotomy with a newly designed metallic valvulotome immediate results of the initial experience in 153 patients. Circulation 1999;99:793–799.
26. Bonhoeffer P, Hausse A, Yonga G, et al. Technique and results of percutaneous mitral valvuloplasty with the multi-track system. J Interv Cardiol 2000;13(4):263–268.
27. Block PC, Palacios IF, Jacobs M, et al. The mechanism of successful percutaneous mitral valvotomy in humans. Am J Cardiol 1987;59:178.
28. Wilkins GT, Weyman AE, Abascal VM, et al. Percutaneous mitral valvotomy: An analysis of echocardiographic variables related to outcome and the mechanism of dilatation. Br Heart J 1988;60:299–308.
29. Ruiz CE, Zhang HP, Macaya C, et al. Comparison of Inoue-single balloon versus double balloon techniques for percutaneous mitral valvotomy. Am Heart J 1992;123:942–947.
30. Leon MN, Pathan A, Lopez JC, et al. Immediate outcome of Inoue vs. double balloon percutaneous mitral valvotomy: The Massachusetts General Hospital experience. Circulation 1997;96(Suppl I):2224.
31. Abascal VM, Wilkins GT, Choong CY, et al. Mitral regurgitation after percutaneous mitral valvuloplasty in adults: evaluation by pulsed Doppler echocardiography. J Am Coll Cardiol 1988;2:257–263.

32. The National Heart, Lung and Blood Institute Balloon Valvuloplasty Registry. Complications and mortality of percutaneous balloon mitral commissurotomy. Circulation 1992;85:2014–2024.

33. Roth RB, Block PC, Palacios IF. Predictors of increased mitral regurgitation after percutaneous mitral balloon valvotomy. Cathet Cardiovasc Diagn 1990;20:17–21.

34. Padial LR, Freitas N, Sagie A, et al. Echocardiography can predict which patients will develop severe mitral regurgitation following percutaneous mitral valvulotomy. J Am Coll Cardiol 1996;27:1225–1331.

35. Herrmann HC, Lima JAC, Feldman T, et al. Mechanisms and outcome of severe mitral regurgitation after Inoue balloon valvuloplasty. J Am Coll Cardiol 1993;22:783–789.

36. Casale P, Block PC, O'Shea JP, Palacios IF. Atrial septal defect after percutaneous mitral balloon valvuloplasty: immediate results and follow-up. J Am Coll Cardiol 1990;15:1300–1304.

37. Desideri A, Vanderperren O, Serra A, et al. Long term (9 to 33 months) echocardiographic follow-up after successful percutaneous mitral commissurotomy. Am J Cardiol 1992;69:1602–1606.

38. Palacios IF, Tuzcu EM, Newell JB, Block PC. Four year clinical follow-up of patients undergoing percutaneous mitral balloon valvotomy. Circulation 1990;(Suppl III):545.

39. Babic UU, Grujicic S, Popovic Z, et al. Percutaneous transarterial balloon dilatation of the mitral valve. Five year experience. Br Heart J 1992;67:185–189.

40. The National Heart, Lung and Blood Institute Balloon Valvuloplasty Registry Participants. Multicenter experience with balloon mitral commissurotomy. NHLBI balloon valvuloplasty resgistry report on immediate and 30 day follow-up results. Circulation 1992;85:448–461.

41. Pan M, Medina A, de Lezo JS, Hernandez E, et al. Factors determinig late success after mitral balloon valvotomy. Am J Cardiol 1993;71:1181–1185.

42. Herrmann HC, Kleaveland P, Hill JA, et al. The M-heart percutaneous balloon mitral valvuloplasty registry: initial results and early follow-up. J Am Coll Cardiol 1990;15:1221.

43. Marzo KP, Herrmann HC, Mancini DM. Effect of balloon mitral valvuloplasty on exercise capacity, ventilation, and skeletal muscle oxygenation. J Am Coll Cardiol 1993;21:856.

44. Tuzcu EM, Block PC, Griffin B, et al. Percutaneous mitral balloon valvotomy in patients with calcific mitral stenosis: immediate and long term outcome. J Am Coll Cardiol 1994;23:1604–1609.

45. Post JR, Feldman T, Isner J, Herrmann HC. Inoue balloon mitral valvotomy in patients with severe valvular and subvalvular deformity. J Am Coll Cardiol 1995;25:1129–1136.

46. Harken DE, Ellis LB, Ware PF. The surgical treatment of mitral stenosis. I. Valvuloplasty. N Engl J Med 1948;239:801.

47. Williams JA, Littmann D, Warren R. Experience with the surgical treatment of mitral stenosis. N Engl J Med 1958;258:623–630.

48. Scannell JG, Burke JF, Saidi F, Turner JD. Five-year follow-up study of closed mitral valvotomy. J Thorac Cardiovasc Surg 1960;40:723–730.

49. Medina A, Delezo JS, Hernandez E, et al. Balloon valvuloplasty for mitral restenosis after previous surgery. A comparative study. Am Heart J 1990;120:568–571.

50. Davidson CJ, Bashore TM, Mickel M, et al. Balloon mitral commissurotomy after previous surgical commissurotomy. Circulation 1992;86:91–99.

51. Jang IK, Block PC, Newell JB, et al. Percutaneous mitral balloon valvotomy for recurrent mitral stenosis after surgical commissurotomy. Am J. Cardiol 1995;75:601–605.

52. Leon M, Harrell L, Mahdi N, et al. Immediate and long term outcome of percutaneous mitral balloon valvotomy in patients with mitral stenosis and atrial fibrillation. J Am Coll Cardiol. 1998;(Supplement).

53. Tarka EA, Blitz LR, Herrmann HC. Hemodynamic effects and long-term outcome of percutaneous balloon valvuloplasty in patients with mitral stenosis and atrial fibrillation. Clin Cardiol 2000;23:673–677.

54. Chen MH, Semigran M, Schwammenthal E, et al. Impact of pulmonary resistance on short and long term outcome after percutaneous mitral valvuloplasty. Circulation (submitted for publication).

55. Mahoney PD, Loh E, Blitz LR, Herrmann HC. Hemodynamic effects of inhaled nitric oxide in women with mitral stenosis and pulmonary hypertension. Am J Cardiol 2001:87:188–192.

56. Sagie A, Schwammenthal E, Newell JB, et al. Significant tricuspid regurgitation is a marker for adverse outcome in patients undergoing mitral balloon valvotomy. J Am Coll Cardiol. 1994;24:696–702.

57. Lopez-Cuellar JC, Leon MN, Pathan A, et al. Ten-year follow-up of optimal candidates for percutaneous mitral balloon valvuloplasty. Circulation. 1997;96(Supplement I):2225.

58. Petrossian GA, Tuzcu EM, Ziskind AA, et al. Atrial septal occlusion improves the accuracy of mitral valve area determination following percutaneous mitral balloon valvotomy. Cathet Cardiovasc Diagn 1991;22:21–24.

59. John S, Bashi VV, Jairaj PS, et al. Closed mitral valvotomy: early results and long term follow up of 3724 patients. Circulation 1983;68:891–896.

60. Ellis LR, Harken DE, Black H. A clinical study of 1,000 consecutive cases of mitral stenosis two to nine years after mitral valvuloplasty. Circulation 1959;19:803.
61. Elis FH, Kirklin JW, Parker RL, et al. Mitral commissurotomy: an overall appraisal of clinical and hemodynamic results. Arch Intern Med 1954;94:774.
62. Hoeksema TD, Wallace RB, Kirklin JW. Closed mitral commissurotomy. Am J Cardiol 1966; 17:825–828.
63. Kirklin JW. Percutaneous balloon versus surgical closed commissurotomy for mitral stenosis. Circulation 1991;83:1450–1451.
64. Higgs LM, Glancy DL, O'Brien KP, et al. Mitral restenosis: an uncommon cause of recurrent symptoms following mitral commissurotomy Am J Cardiol 1970;26:34–37.
65. Glover RP, Davila JC, O'Neil TJE, Janton OH. Does mitral stenosis recur after commissurotomy? Circulation 1955;11:14–28.
66. Hickey MSJ, Blackstone EH, Kirklin JW, Dean LS. Outcome probabilities and life history after surgical mitral commissurotomy: Implications for balloon commissurotomy. J Am Coll Cardiol 1991;17:29–42.
67. Scalia D, Rizzoli G, Campanile F, et al. Long-term results of mitral commissurotomy. J Thorac Cardiovasc Surg 1993;105:633–642.
68. Rihal CS, Schaff HV, Frye RL, et al. Long-term follow-up of patients undergoing closed transventricular mitral commissurotomy: a useful surrogate for percutaneous balloon mitral valvuloplasty. J Am Coll Cardiol 1992;20:781–786.
69. Turi ZG, Reyes VP, Raju BS, et al. Percutaneous balloon versus surgical closed commissurotomy for mitral stenosis: a prospective, randomized trial. Circulation 1991;83:1179–1185.
70. Reyes VP, Raju BS, Wynne J, et al. Percutaneous balloon valvuloplasty compared with open surgical commissurotomy for mitral stenosis. N Eng J Med 1994;331:961–967.
71. Farhat MB, Ayari M, Maatouk F, et al. Percutaneous balloon verus surgical closed and open mitral commissurotomy: seven year follow-up results of a randomized trial. Circulation 1998;97:245–250.
72. Patel JJ, Sharma D, Mitha AS, et al. Balloon valvuloplasty versus closed commissurotomy for pliable mitral stenosis: a prospective hemodynamic study. J Am Coll Cardiol 1991;18:1318–1322.
73. Shrivastava S, Mathur A, Dev V, et al. Comparison of immediate hemodynamic response of closed mitral commissurotomy, single-balloon, and double-balloon mitral valvuloplasty in rheumatic mitral stenosis. J Thorac Cardiovasc Surg 1992;104:1264–1267.
74. Arora R, Nair M, Kalra GS, Nigam M, Kkhalillulah M. Immediate and long-term results of balloon and surgical closed mitral valvotomy: a randomized comparatve study. Am Heart J 1993;125:1091–1094.
75. Palacios IF. Farewell to surgical mitral commissurotomy for many patients. Circulation 1998;97:223–226.
76. Bernal Y, Miralles PJ. Cardiac surgery with cardiopulmonary bypass during pregnancy. Obstet Gynecol Surg 1986;41:1.
77. Vosloo S, Reichart B. The feasibility of closed mitral valvotomy in pregnancy. J Thorac Cardiovasc Surg 1987;93:675.
78. Palacios IF, Block PC, Wilkins GT, et al. Percutaneous mitral balloon valvotomy during pregnancy in patients with severe mitral stenosis. Cathet Cardiovasc Diagn 1988;15:109.
79. Mangione JA, Zuliani MF, Del Castillo JM, et al. Percutaneous double balloon mitral valvuloplasty in pregnant women. Am J Cardiol 1989;64:99.

2

Balloon Aortic and Pulmonic Valvuloplasty

Ted E. Feldman, MD
Timothy A. Sanborn, MD
and William W. O'Neill, MD

CONTENTS

INTRODUCTION

Valve replacement for aortic valve stenosis has been the gold standard of therapy for decades. The prognosis of symptomatic severe aortic stenosis is well known, with very high annual mortality and a clearly limited life-span. Surgical aortic valve replacement with a mechanical prosthesis, bioprosthetic, or homograft valve prolongs life in this patient cohort.

The development of balloon catheter aortic valvuloplasty in the mid-1980s initially promised to provide an alternative to valve replacement in patients suitable for this procedure. Early experience with the procedure showed balloon catheter therapy to have limited durability, with restenosis a near certain finding in most adult patients undergoing the procedure *(1–4)*. Accordingly, balloon aortic valvuloplasty (BAV) has found a place in the therapeutic armamentarium for aortic stenosis only among those patients for whom surgical aortic valve replacement is either contraindicated or carries extremely high surgical risk *(5)*. These older patients with symptomatic aortic stenosis have a 1-yr survival of 55–75% and a 1-yr event-free survival of only 40–50% *(2–4)*.

From: *Contemporary Cardiology: Interventional Cardiology:*
Percutaneous Noncoronary Intervention
Edited by: H. C. Herrmann © Humana Press Inc., Totowa, NJ

Table 1
Balloon Valvuloplasty in the Young Adult Age ≤21 Years

Class I
  Symptoms with peak gradient >50 mm Hg
  Gradient >60 mm Hg
  New ECG changes at rest or with exercise >50 mm Hg
Class IIa
  Gradient >50 mm Hg in patient who desires competitive sports or pregnancy
Class III
  Gradient <50 mm Hg with no symptoms or ECG changes

PATIENT SELECTION FOR BALLOON AORTIC VALVULOPLASTY

Patient selection for BAV is challenging. The American Heart Association–American College of Cardiology task force guideline recommendations for therapy with BAV defines a narrow patient population (6). Balloon valvuloplasty is the treatment of choice for aortic stenosis in children and young adults age 21 yr or less with aortic stenosis. Table 1 provides a list of specific indications. In the younger population, valve stenosis severity is defined by gradient, because many of these patients will be growing and have a variable valve area. BAV in this group of patients is durable, and an expectation for good long-term results is extremely different than that seen in older adult patients with aortic valve stenosis. When patients present under 30 or 40 yr of age, it is likely that they have congenital aortic stenosis. When these patients present beyond age 21 or 22 yr, the results of valvuloplasty are less satisfactory. The valve leaflets at this point are usually fibrotic but not calcified and do not respond as well to balloon dilatation as in patients age 21 yr and younger. Patients who present at age 55–70 are likely to have bicuspid aortic stenosis. When the bicuspid valve is heavily calcified BAV might have an outcome similar to patients with calcified degenerative aortic stenosis.

A second group in whom long-term results of BAV can be expected to be durable are those with rheumatic aortic valve stenosis. When patients present with symptoms and aortic stenosis between ages 40 and 60 yr, the disease might be rheumatic in origin. This is an uncommon group of patients, especially in the United States. Because commissural fusion is the mechanism of stenosis in these patients, BAV yields anatomic results that are similar to balloon mitral commissurotomy. Long-term results of BAV are probably better than in senile calcific aortic stenosis. Few data are available on this particular subset, but adult patients in the United States who present under age 60 without a bicuspid valve might often be inferred to have rheumatic stenosis.

The typical patients treated with BAV in the United States are older adults with calcific aortic stenosis. Because results with aortic valve replacement are well established, valvuloplasty is applied generally only when aortic valve replacement is either relatively contraindicated or strategically better to defer. Table 2 presents the Joint Task Force recommendations on the use of balloon valvuloplasty in adult patients (6). There are no Class I indications in this group.

The guidelines recommend balloon valvuloplasty as a bridge to aortic valve surgery in hemodynamically unstable high-risk patients, so that they can be stabilized. Patients who present in cardiogenic shock or who are "stuck" on pressor agents in an intensive care unit are typical of patients in this group. Palliation for patients with serious comorbid

Table 2
Balloon Valvuloplasty in Adults with Aortic Stenosis

Class I
  There are no Class I indications
Class IIa
  Bridge to surgery in unstable, high-risk patients for valve replacement
Class IIb
  Palliation in patients with serious comorbid conditions
  Prior to urgent noncardiac surgery
Class III
  Alternative to aortic valve replacement surgery

conditions is, in practice, probably the most common use of BAV in older adults. Patients who are felt to be at high risk for general anesthesia, those who are elderly and have already had prior sternotomy and bypass, and patients who are simply very elderly represent the typical patients in this setting. Patients with prior bypass surgery, prior mitral valve replacement or repair, a heavily calcified or "porcelain" aorta, severe chronic lung disease, or multiple comorbidities are typical. The ambulatory but very elderly are the best candidates. BAV is also used prior to noncardiac surgery in patients found to have tight aortic valve stenosis on preoperative screening. Those who require extensive cancer surgery are typical of this group. BAV is specifically contraindicated as an alternative to aortic valve replacement. Patients who simply say they wish not to have valve replacement, who are otherwise a good candidate for valve replacement, are prototypic of this situation.

A group in whom BAV should be used with extreme caution comprise those who appear to be in the terminal stages of aortic valve stenosis. Patients who have deteriorated over a long period of time, are very elderly, and are intensive care unit bound with the early stages of multiple-organ failure or sepsis cannot realistically be expected to respond to BAV in many cases. Patient selection in this last group is exceedingly important, and it is critical to try to offer this therapy to patients with multiple comorbid conditions early in their course, before they are no longer salvageable. Procedure timing is similarly crucial in the hemodynamically unstable patient where the early benefit of BAV must be weighed against the risk of further multiorgan failure that could result from delaying surgery.

One situation not clearly addressed by the guidelines are those patients who present with low gradient and low cardiac output, in whom it is uncertain whether aortic valve replacement will result in improved left ventricular function. Among those patients who have a poor response to valve replacement, mortality is extremely high. BAV offers a potential opportunity to see if relief of the aortic stenosis will result in improved left ventricular function, although no studies have assessed or validated this approach. These patients are similar to those described in Table 2 as having BAV as a bridge to surgery. In those who improve, valve replacement surgery might be contemplated. BAV is thus used as a therapeutic trial or as a diagnostic test. Among those in whom ventricular function has deteriorated beyond the point where recovery is possible or who have left ventricular dysfunction because of an etiology other than aortic stenosis, lack of improvement is a signal that valve replacement surgery will not offer functional improvement and should not be pursued further.

ASSESSMENT OF AORTIC STENOSIS SEVERITY

Of critical importance is proper assessment of aortic stenosis severity in potential candidates for BAV. Many times, these patients present with multiple comorbid illnesses, including chronic lung disease. Many also have severe left ventricular failure and depressed left ventricular systolic function and associated hemodynamic lesions, including mitral regurgitation, pulmonary hypertension, and depressed cardiac output. Accordingly, the assessment of the severity of aortic stenosis is a key element in the evaluation of patients for this procedure.

A variety of technical and practical limitations make measurement of valve area difficult. The technical challenges include the inaccuracies of the commonly used disposable pressure transducers, measurement artifacts because of temporal delay of pressure transmission in fluid-filled catheter systems, nonsimultaneous pressure recordings, pressure damping, and the effect of a catheter across the stenotic aortic valve.

The ideal methods for measurement of transvalvular gradient utilized simultaneous acquisition of left ventricular and central aortic pressure with high-fidelity transducers *(7,8)*. This approach is not practical, and a variety of compromises are made in the assessment of aortic valve stenosis.

In practice, the most common method for assessment of aortic stenosis severity is the simultaneous use of a left ventricular pigtail passed retrograde across the valve, compared to a femoral arterial sheath. Use of a pigtail one French size smaller than the sheath and use of a longer-length sheath helps minimize pressure damping in the sheath and pressure amplification in the iliofemoral system. Nonetheless, in cases where the gradient and cardiac output are low, this may yield results significantly different from those obtained when two central aortic catheters are used. Bilateral femoral arterial access may be used to place a left ventricular and central aortic catheter simultaneously. Alternatively, transseptal access to the left ventricle via the venous system with a central aortic catheter placed via the femoral artery will yield excellent results without the additional risks of a second arterial puncture *(9)*. A recent report described a silent cerebral embolism after retrograde catheterization of the aortic valve among patients with valvular stenosis *(10)*. In this randomized study, typical methods to cross the valve retrograde were used in 152 patients. Twenty-two percent who underwent retrograde catheterization had focal diffusion imaging abnormalities on magnetic resonance scans. The transseptal approach eliminates this issue.

The use of a 0.014-in. pressure wire has been described to simplify high-quality central pressure measurements *(7)*. After the aortic valve is crossed retrograde with a conventional 4F or 5F diagnostic catheter, a pressure wire can be passed into the left ventricular apex and the diagnostic catheter withdrawn into the aortic root. This yields remarkably high-quality pressure tracings, visually comparable to those achieved with a high-fidelity micromanometer catheter system.

Patients with low gradient and low cardiac output are the most difficult to evaluate. In addition to scrupulous attention to the quality of pressure recordings and using central aortic pressure compared to left ventricular pressure, a dobutamine infusion to increase the cardiac output by 20–30% will often help in establishing a more accurate measure of the severity of aortic valve stenosis. In some cases, the valve area will appear to increase with increased cardiac output *(11–13)*. This illustrates the so-called flow dependence of the Gorlin equation. In cases of a truly tight aortic valve strength, the valve area will remain constant or sometimes even appear to diminish with an increase in cardiac output.

RETROGRADE TECHNIQUE FOR BALLOON AORTIC VALVULOPLASTY

The retrograde technique basically involves passing a balloon catheter via the femoral arteries retrograde through the aortic arch and across the valve *(14,15)*. The major limitations of the technique are the requirement for a large caliber arterial sheath and the difficulty in maintaining balloon position in the aortic valve during balloon inflations.

After arterial access is gained, using a relatively small caliber (6–8 French) sheath, femoral arteriography is performed to verify the position of the sheath in the common femoral artery. Unless a superficial femoral artery is of exceptionally large caliber, placement of the sheath below the femoral bifurcation precludes use of that puncture for passage of a larger valvuloplasty sheath. Preclosure using a suture closure system can be performed at this point *(16,17)*. Using the existing small caliber sheath, a 6 French or 10 French Perclose device can be preplaced in the arteriotomy and the sutures left dangling. A wire is replaced in the Perclose device, and the device is exchanged for a 12.5 up to 14 French arterial sheath.

A diagnostic catheter is used to pass a wire retrograde across the aortic valve. The technique for crossing the valve retrograde merits some discussion. The use of a specially shaped curved diagnostic catheter (Aortic Stenosis Catheter; Cook Inc., Bloomington, IN) has the advantage of being able to orient the tip of the catheter and thus the direction of wire passage toward the center of the aortic root. The catheter has a gentle curve similar to that of an Amplatz shape and, in addition, has a very soft distal end and side holes *(14)*. The soft distal end allows the catheter to track more easily over a wire, once the wire has been passed into the left ventricle. The side holes permit ventriculography if needed. The catheter is positioned above the aortic valve and gently rotated until the tip of the catheter is as close to the center of the root as possible. The pattern of calcification in the aortic leaflets helps with catheter positioning. Figure 1 shows the diagnostic catheter with the tip pointing just to the right of the orifice of the aortic valve in a left arterior oblique (LAO) projection. The best working projection varies depending on the distortion of the aortic root in a given patient, but is usually a shallow angulation such as an LAO 10°–20° angulation. A movable-core straight guide wire can be used with a softened tip to probe the aortic valve. Gentle clockwise rotation of the catheter usually moves it more superior along the aortic valve, and it is often possible to align the tip of the catheter with the orifice defined by the calcified leaflets. Using this method, the valve can typically be crossed in less than a minute or two *(14)*.

An extrastiff wire must be used to provide adequate support for passage of the balloon. Placing a large curve on the end of the wire facilitates stability of the wire in the left ventricular apex and diminishes the risks for a wire perforation of the left ventricular apex. It is necessary to curve the wire over the edge of a hemostat or pair of scissors, much in the way that one would put a curl on a piece of wrapping paper ribbon (Fig. 2). After the stiff wire has been passed retrograde across the valve, the diagnostic catheter is removed and an aortic valvuloplasty balloon is passed retrograde across the valve. Considerable forward pressure must be used to keep the balloon in position across the valve while it is being inflated. Because these balloons tend to inflate relatively slowly, maximally dilute saline contrast mixture should be used. A dilution of seven parts saline to one part contrast will minimize the inflation fluid viscosity while still allowing enough radio-opacity to visualize the balloon. The balloon should be inflated and then deflated as rapidly as possible. Using a large syringe, it is not possible to fully distend balloons of this size, and a sidearm stopcock with a "booster" smaller syringe on the side should

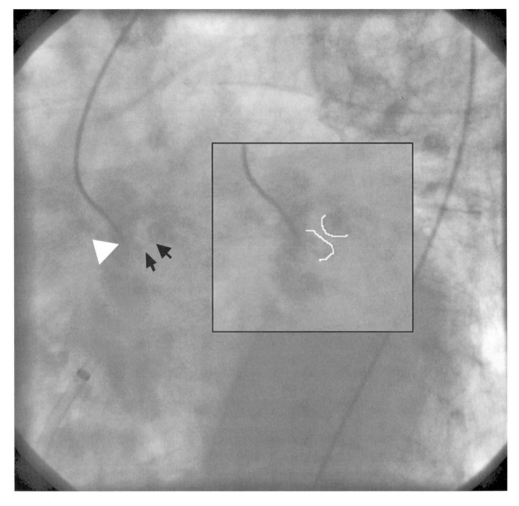

Fig. 1. Technique for crossing the aortic valve. Left anterior oblique projection of the aortic root with an aortic stenosis catheter positioned close to the central orifice of the calcified aortic valve leaflets. The white arrow denotes the position of the tip of the aortic stenosis catheter. The small black arrows show the left ventricular side of the aortic leaflet calcifications on either side of the aortic valve orifice. The inset shows the calcified edges of the thickened aortic valve leaflets outlined in white, with the stenotic orifice in between the two white lines.

be used to complete the inflation *(18)*. Typically, a first inflation can be performed without boosting to full inflation volume to test the patient's tolerance of aortic outflow tract occlusion. Second and third inflations can be attempted if the patient appears to tolerate the first inflation. The balloon could rupture in as many as one-third of patients when it is fully inflated.

One major challenge during retrograde BAV is maintaining the position of the inflated balloon within the valve. The force of left ventricular contraction, even in some poorly functioning ventricles, tends to eject the balloon as it is being inflated. Maintaining a stable position requires an extra-stiff guide wire and coordination between the primary operator and the assistant. It sometimes takes repeated attempts to successfully inflate the balloon. When the balloon fully engages the valve, it "locks" into position. This also

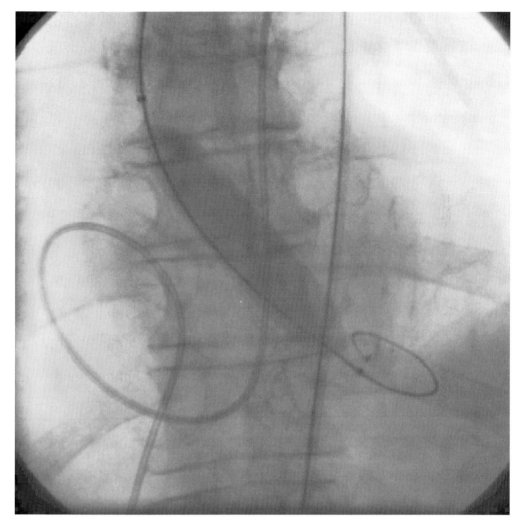

Fig. 2. Retrograde aortic valvuloplasty is accomplished by passing a balloon catheter via the aorta across the aortic valve. The wire is looped in the left ventricular apex. The inflated balloon catheter traverses the stenotic aortic valve. A pulmonary artery pressure monitoring catheter is looped in the right atrium. The curl in the guide wire is placed by running the guide wire over the end of the hemostat in a manner analogous to curling a ribbon for gift-wrapping.

clearly demonstrates that the balloon is of adequate size to apply pressure to the leaflets. If the balloon will not maintain a stable position in the valve even when fully inflated, it may be undersized. Cribier has recently described a technique that will facilitate balloon stability. The right ventricle apex can be paced at 200 beats a minute with a temporary pacing wire while the balloon is inflated. This does not prolong hypotension beyond the time that the inflated balloon would ordinarily cause this to occur, and it allows positioning of the balloon in the aortic annulus.

In some cases, arterial pressure recovery after a first balloon inflation is slow, and in the face of poor left ventricular function, it must be determined whether it is safe to continue with additional balloon inflations. Using this approach, there is no good way to monitor the reduction in transvalvular pressure gradient in between balloon inflations.

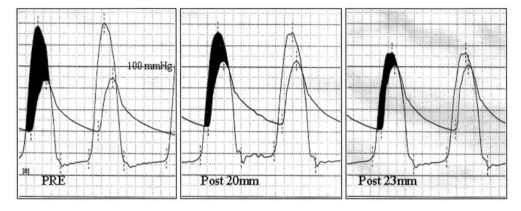

Fig. 3. Hemodynamic changes after aortic valvuloplasty. Before balloon dilatation, a large transaortic valve pressure gradient is noted. The mean gradient is 34 mm Hg. The cardiac output is about 3 L/min, and the aortic valve area is 0.6 cm^2. After inflations of a 20-mm-diameter balloon catheter, the mean gradient decreases to 20 mm Hg, and the valve area increases to 0.7 cm^2. A 23-mm-diameter larger balloon is used, and after inflations, the mean gradient is decreased to 9 mm Hg and the valve area increases to 1.0 cm^2, despite a decrease in cardiac output to 2.84 L/min.

A prototypic procedure involves a test inflation, a second "boosted" inflation, and a third inflation during which the balloon may rupture. It is critical to recognize that only those inflations in which the balloon locks into position in the valve should be considered effective. If the balloon is undersized, it will continue to "watermelon seed" or squirt back and forth in the valve when it is fully inflated. Either an inflation with a larger inflation volume or a larger balloon is necessary in this instance. It is important not to exceed the echocardiographically determined anulus diameter when choosing larger-sized balloons. The vast majority of patients can be successfully treated with a 20-mm-diameter nominal balloon size. Occasional smaller patients may require an 18-mm-diameter balloon. Ten to twenty percent of patients require a 23-mm-diameter balloon for successful single-balloon retrograde dilatation. The risk of aortic cusp avulsion and aortic insufficiency is significantly greater when a 23-mm-diameter balloon is used. A balloon size up to 20 mm in diameter will usually be accommodated by a 12.5 French arterial sheath. The 23-mm-diameter balloon size requires a 14 French arterial sheath. If the balloon is ruptured during balloon inflations, it is unlikely to come back out through the same sheath through which it was introduced. The balloon can be pulled back until it wedges into the sheath, and the sheath and balloon removed as a single unit. A new sheath is then necessary to replace the old one, because the initial sheath will accordion or become deformed by the balloon withdrawal process.

After the balloon is removed, a diagnostic catheter is placed over the existing extra-stiff wire into the left ventricle, the wire removed, and the pressure gradient reassessed. It is typical to have reductions in gradient of about 50%. Gradient reductions may also be caused by depression of left ventricular contractility caused by interference with aortic outflow during the balloon inflations. Occasional patients will develop a low-output state as a consequence. It may take 24–48 h for ventricular function to return to baseline. Thus, a reassessment of cardiac output and recalculation of the Gorlin estimated valve area is the best measure of adequacy of dilatation. Increases in valve area are typically modest. Overall, the valve area will increase from 0.6 cm^2 up to 0.9 or 1.0 cm^2 (Fig. 3).

Retrograde BAV may also be accomplished using a double-balloon technique. Bilateral femoral arterial access is necessary. The aortic valve must be crossed independently from each femoral arterial access site. This allows smaller sheaths on either side. Two balloons can be inflated simultaneously across the aortic valve. There is less difficulty with balloon slippage. There are no clear guidelines for balloon sizing in this setting. Exceeding the aortic annulus diameter measured by echocardiography with the combined diameter of the two balloons may be risky.

At the completion of the procedure, the arterial sheath is removed. If preclosure with a suture device has been placed, a wire should be passed back into the sheath and the initial knots tied over the wire as the sheath is withdrawn, so that if hemostasis is not successful, the sheath can be replaced. In the event that manual compression is chosen for sheath removal, prolonged compression is typically necessary. A FemoStop is especially useful to accomplish hemostasis in this setting. More rigid mechanical clamps may result in arterial conclusion. Prolonged FemoStop compression may result in deep venous thrombosis, so careful monitoring of the FemoStop is essential.

ANTEGRADE TECHNIQUE FOR BALLOON AORTIC VALVULOPLASTY

The antegrade technique is performed via a femoral venous access and transseptal puncture (Figs. 4–7 and videos 1–3 on the CD). Compared to the retrograde technique, it provides the advantage of avoiding a large-caliber arterial puncture and has the disadvantages of necessitating transseptal puncture and being a more complex overall technical approach *(9,19–21)*.

The antegrade technique involves establishing transseptal access. Especially for patients with atrial fibrillation, transesophageal echocardiography prior to the procedure is important to rule out the potential for left atrial thrombus. Obtaining vascular access at the outset of the procedure via the left femoral artery, via the left femoral vein for a pulmonary artery catheter for measurement of cardiac output, and via the right femoral vein for transseptal puncture is usual. The right femoral venous access can initially be obtained with a 6 or 8 French sheath, and a suture closure is used to preclose the venous puncture. After a 14 French sheath is placed for passage of the transseptal equipment, the sutures are left outside of the puncture site.

After transseptal puncture, a Mullins sheath is placed in the left atrium. Antegrade passage into to the left ventricle is obtained with a single-lumen balloon catheter. A 7 French single-lumen balloon catheter will ordinarily accommodate a wide variety of guide-wire sizes and make the establishment of left ventricular access fairly easy. This catheter can be used for left ventricular pressure measurement to compare to a retrograde transarterial central aortic pressure for gradient measurement. The need to cross the valve retrograde is eliminated, which can save a great deal of time in patients with severely deformed or very tight valves. After the gradient and valve area are confirmed, the single-lumen balloon catheter is advanced into the left ventricular apex via the Mullins sheath and looped in the apex. Further advancement will usually force the balloon catheter to cross the stenotic aortic valve antegrade (Fig. 4). It is sometimes necessary to partially deflate the balloon. In cases when the balloon will not advance around the apex, a curved guide wire can be used to facilitate this step. A straight floppy guide wire such as a Wholey wire is often useful to help advance the balloon tip catheter antegrade across the aortic valve. When the balloon catheter is in the aortic arch, a large-curve guide wire can be used to pass it over the arch into the descending aorta. Simply advancing the balloon catheter will usually result in the catheter becoming lodged in one of the arch vessels. The large-curve guide wire eliminates this entanglement. When the balloon catheter is in the descending aorta, a 0.032-in. extra-stiff guide wire is

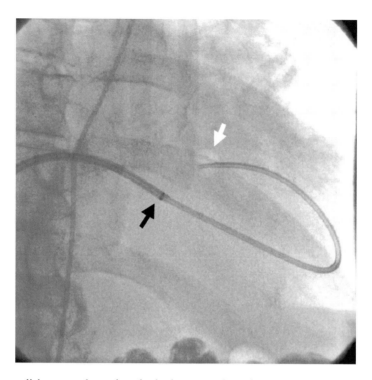

Fig. 4. To accomplish antegrade aortic valvuloplasty, a catheter is passed via the transseptal route into the left ventricle. A single lumen balloon catheter is looped through the Mullins sheath into the left ventricular apex and passed toward the aortic valve. The aortic valve is then crossed antegrade, and a wire is passed via the venous access through the right atrium, left atrium, left ventricular apex, and into the aorta. The wire can then be snared in the descending aorta and stabilized for antegrade passage of the balloon. The black arrow shows the tip of the Mullins sheath in the left ventricle. The white arrow shows the tip of a single lumen balloon catheter approaching the aortic valve.

passed from the femoral venous access point through the balloon catheter into the descending aorta (Fig. 5). A 10-mm gooseneck snare can then be passed retrograde from the femoral arterial sheath into the descending aorta to snare and fix the guide wire (Fig. 6 and video 1 on the CD). The snare may be withdrawn and the guide wire exteriorized and clamped outside of the femoral arterial sheath. This provides even more support. Advancement of the balloon through the left atrium, traversing the left ventricular apex, and crossing the aortic valve requires this degree of support. Simply parking the 0.032-in. guide wire in the descending aorta is inadequate. Snaring the wire in the descending aorta and leaving the snare is usually adequate, although in some cases the wire will pull out of the snare. It is this latter situation that necessitates exteriorizing the guide wire via the femoral sheath (see video 2 on the CD). Once the wire is looped through the circulation, either advancing or withdrawing it will cause substantial friction. It is critical to advance or withdraw the wire only when it is covered by a catheter. The bare wire may cause enough friction to lacerate the mitral leaflets if it is withdrawn without first covering it with a catheter.

After access is obtained and the wire looped into the descending aorta and snared, a balloon catheter can be passed antegrade via a 14 French right femoral venous sheath through the inferior vena cava, across the transseptal puncture, via the mitral valve and left ventricular apex into the ventricular outflow, and then across the aortic valve. A con-

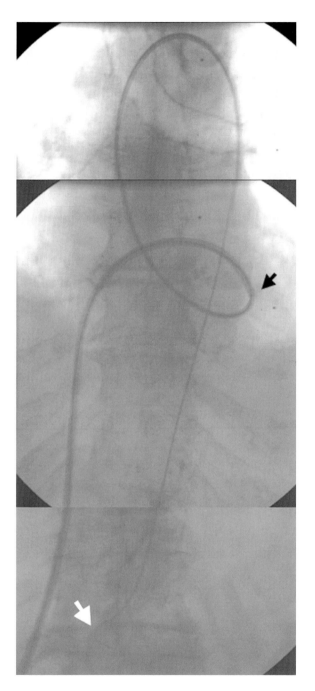

Fig. 5. A wire loop can be seen throughout the circulation. In the bottom left-hand corner of the picture, via femoral venous access a Mullins sheath is passed up to the right atrium, through the left atrium, and into the left ventricle. The black arrow denotes the tip of the Mullins sheath near the left ventricular apex. A single-lumen balloon catheter has been passed through the Mullins sheath around the left ventricular apex, across the stenotic aortic valve, and through the aortic arch. A guide wire has been passed through the catheter into the descending aorta and, in this case, into the right femoral artery. The white arrow at the bottom of the picture shows the J-tip of the wire in the right femoral artery. Thus, the wire traverses the entire circulation, beginning in the right femoral vein, coursing through the heart and central aorta, and ending in the femoral artery on the same side.

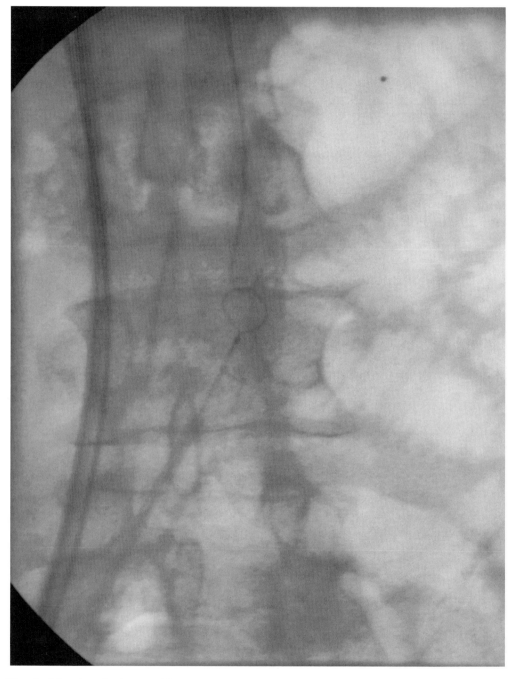

Fig. 6. After the wire is placed in the descending aorta, a gooseneck snare can be passed retrograde through an arterial sheath and used to fix the wire in position. The snare can be left in place to stabilize the wire in the descending aorta or the wire may be pulled through the sheath and exteriorized.

ventional balloon may be used. Twenty-millimeter or 23-mm-diameter balloons will be reasonably accommodated by the 14 French venous sheath. Once the wire is passed through the arterial system and exteriorized on the arterial side, it is also possible to place a large-caliber arterial sheath and use this route for retrograde aortic valvuloplasty. The

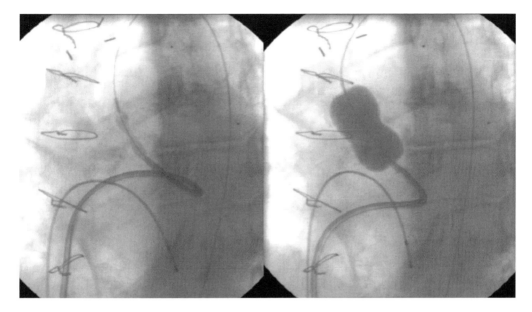

Fig. 7. After the wire loop has been passed through the circulation, a balloon catheter can be passed antegrade across the aortic valve. In the left-hand panel, an Inoue balloon traverses the left ventricular apex and is straddling the aortic valve. In the right-hand panel, the balloon is fully inflated. Some of the loop in the left ventricular apex has been pulled back to engage the balloon in the valve. As soon as the balloon is deflated, the catheter shaft is advanced to re-establish the wire loop in the left ventricular apex.

problem of balloon "watermelon seeding" in the aortic valve is eliminated with this degree of transcirculatory wire support.

The antegrade approach usually uses an Inoue balloon antegrade via the transseptal venous puncture (Fig. 7 and video 3 on the CD). The balloon tracks well over a 0.032-in. guide wire. When the balloon is inflated across the aortic valve and pulled back, there is no difficulty in controlling its position. The inflate–deflate cycle is much more rapid than a conventional balloon with a much briefer period of hypotension. The size and shape of the balloon conform well to the sinuses of Valsalva. Because the balloon is a volume rather than a pressure balloon, sizing is different than for retrograde aortic valvuloplasty. A 26-mm-diameter balloon is currently the smallest nominal size available in the United States. This balloon can be initially inflated to 22 mm in diameter. If this is tolerated well, 23-, 24-, or even 26-mm-diameter inflations will be well tolerated by most patients. Preprocedure assessment of the annular diameter by echocardiography is helpful in guiding balloon inflation size. After an initial inflation, the balloon may be removed while the wire is left in place. A Mullins sheath can then be passed over the wire into the left ventricle for gradient assessment and further decision-making.

The transcirculatory wire may cause hypotension in some patients. If a loop is not maintained in the left ventricular apex, the wire may prop open the mitral and/or aortic valves and the resulting valvular insufficiency can result in a steady decline in systemic blood pressure. Occasional patients will not tolerate this wire pathway under any circumstances, and the procedure cannot be performed in this manner in that group of patients. If the wire has to be removed, it is important to pass any catheter over it through the left ventricle and aortic arch to reduce friction as the wire is pulled back. A 5F pigtail or multipurpose catheter can be used, and left in the left ventriculor (LV) apex after the wire has been removed to preserve transseptal access and for LV pressure measurement.

At the conclusion of the procedure, the wire must be removed using a catheter to cover it. Simply pulling the bare wire through the circulation will generate a tremendous amount of friction and the wire cannot be easily or safely removed in this manner. A 7F balloon flotation catheter or a 5F diagnostic catheter is passed over the wire via the right femoral vein and into, at least, the ascending aorta. This will allow the snare to be removed. With gentle traction, removal of the wire can be accomplished relatively easily. When the wire has been pulled back into a diagnostic catheter, the catheter may be withdrawn until it is in the left ventricle. This will maintain the antegrade transseptal access and leave a catheter in a good position for measurement of a final gradient without interference from the wire. Assessment of the final transaortic valve gradient with the wire completely removed is necessary, because the wire will often cause a false diminution of the transaortic valve pressure gradient, sometimes with the appearance of no gradient whatsoever, even in the face of significant residual aortic stenosis.

Initial experience with this antegrade approach has yielded larger valve areas than can be obtained with the single-balloon retrograde technique *(19)*. The potential mechanism for this finding is the distention of the distal end of the Inoue balloon, which conforms well to the sinus of Valsalva. The aortic leaflets are distended into the sinus by the distal end of the Inoue balloon. In contrast, a conventional balloon has straight sides and will achieve no more than a diameter smaller than the inner diameter of the anulus and, substantially, less than the sinus of Valsalva.

COMPLICATIONS OF BALLOON AORTIC VALVULOPLASTY

A number of management problems are common during BAV (Table 3). Predominant among them is hypotension. This could result from left ventricular depression from balloon occlusion of the outflow tract, bleeding from the large caliber femoral access site, perforation of the left ventricle as a result of wire passage or the sharp tip of the balloon catheter, and aortic insufficiency resulting from damage to the leaflets or anulus during the course of balloon inflations. During balloon inflations, blood pressure drops precipitately and it is important to withdraw the balloon from the valve orifice before the balloon is fully deflated to allow forward cardiac output to be restored. At the same time, it is important to be cognizant that the large size of the balloon may obstruct the arch vessels if it is left overlying the brachiocephalic or carotid origins. In cases where the hemoglobin is low prior to the initiation of the procedure, transfusion so that a reasonable starting level of hemoglobin is present is important, as is a type and screen so that blood can be readily available in the event of bleeding.

Bradycardia is also relatively common. This may result from abrasion of the septum by catheters or conducting system injury as the rigid aortic anulus is distended against the atrioventricular conducting system during balloon inflations. In patients with underlying bundle branch block or atrioventricular block, placement of a temporary pacemaker is important so that bradycardia can be managed rapidly. Occasionally, patients will develop heart block and ultimately require a permanent pacemaker. Major complications are encountered as a consequence of the severity of illness and multiple comorbid conditions typical in the BAV population. Death in the hospital occurs in 5–8% of patients *(22)*. The majority of these deaths occur outside of the cardiac catheterization laboratory as a consequence of other complications of the procedure. One or two percent of patients will expire

Table 3
Common Management Problems

Bradycardia
 Conducting system injury
 Vagal
 Perforation
Hypotension
 LV depression
 Bleeding
 Perforation
 Aortic insufficiency
 Sheath injury

in the catheterization laboratory because of LV power failure after balloon inflations and failure to recover left ventricular function or from mechanical complications related to trauma from balloons. Bleeding is the most common complication. As many as one-fourth of patients require transfusion, and, in some reports, 5–7% require surgical vascular repair for femoral access complications (23). The use of suture closure has resulted in less frequent transfusions and shorter lengths of stay. The preclosure technique of placing a small 6 or 8 French sheath, then preloading percutaneous suture closure and not tying knots, followed by placement of the large sheath, and, ultimately, removal of the sheath and closing of the suture knots at the end of the procedure is well described. In one report, this technique completely eliminated the need for transfusions and surgical vascular repair (16).

Cardiac perforation from wires or balloons is an important complication that must be considered whenever hypotension occurs in the periprocedure timeframe. Liberal use of echocardiography in the catheterization laboratory or recovery area is critical to recognize and treat pericardial effusion and tamponade at the earliest possible juncture (Table 4).

RESULTS OF BALLOON AORTIC VALVULOPLASTY

The acute hemodynamic results of BAV are often modest. The cardiac output increases a small but statistically significant amount. Decreases in transvalvular pressure gradient range from 30% to 50%. Using the single-balloon retrograde technique, it is uncommon to have residual gradients of less than 10 mm Hg in patients with preserved cardiac output. Increases in valve area typically are from preprocedure levels of 0.6 cm^2 to postprocedure levels of 0.9 cm^2 using the retrograde single-balloon approach. With the antegrade Inoue balloon approach, a mean postprocedure valve area of 1.2–1.4 cm^3 is common, and postprocedure transvalvular pressure gradients less than 10 mm are frequent. Most patients are clinically improved for 12–18 mo (24).

The long-term results of BAV have been described. Comparisons of survival in this patient group with untreated patients with severe aortic stenosis suggest that there are no survival benefits attributable to the procedure (25–27). Patients who achieve good hemodynamic results typically will be clinically improved, sometimes with minimal improvements in Gorlin valve area. Most patients have sustained clinical improvement for 1–1.5 yr. The major goal of this procedure is palliation of symptoms. It is unwise to offer BAV to patients with severe aortic stenosis who are only mildly symptomatic, because the procedure has significant risks and offers only symptomatic benefits. For

Table 4
In-Hospital Complications of Aortic Valvuloplasty

Cardiac death	5–8%
Noncardiac death	1–2%
Embolism	2–5%
Myocardiac infarction	1–2%
Tamponade	<1%
Shock	1–3%
Cardiac surgery	1%
Transfusion	23%
Vascular repair	5–7%

those patients who are severely debilitated, the procedure improves quality of life tremendously. Patients are often made relatively functional at a time when this is all that can be offered to them.

LIMITATIONS OF BALLOON AORTIC VALVULOPLASTY

A number of technical and procedural issues limit the utility of this procedure. The retrograde approach requires crossing the aortic valve retrograde, which may not be possible in some patients. Large-caliber balloons necessitate large-size vascular access for either the antegrade or retrograde routes. Improvements in balloon technology have been slower for valvuloplasty than for coronary equipment because of the smaller patient population served by these devices.

Restenosis remains the major limitation of the utility of this procedure. Histopathologic studies have demonstrated the mechanism of successful BAV to be fracture of the calcific nodules seen in the aortic valve leaflets *(28)*. The nodules are typically amorphous calcium encased in a fibrotic capsule on the superior or aortic arch side of the leaflets. The pressure of balloon inflation, which causes cracks or hinge points in these nodules, allows greater mobility of the valve leaflets. These nodules refibrose, and the cracks or hinge points are obliterated by this healing process. Animal studies have demonstrated less rapid calcification of valve leaflets in a setting where calcium blockers are used *(29)*. More recently, the inflammatory lesion thought to contribute to the progression of aortic stenosis has responded to therapy with statin drugs *(30)*. It remains to be seen whether medical therapy might slow the occurrence of restenosis after BAV.

The most promising light on the horizon that would overcome these severe limitations is the development of percutaneous aortic valve replacement. The basic techniques necessary to accomplish this procedure are similar to those used in BAV and many create a new emphasis on BAV as a predilatation strategy. Initial human results are encouraging *(31)*. This latter development would also overcome the obvious limitation imposed on balloon catheter therapy by regurgitant lesions (Table 5). Regurgitant lesions make the utility of BAV impossible in a significant number of patients. Percutaneous valve replacement would be an ideal therapy in this setting.

BALLOON PULMONIC VALVULOPLASTY

Pulmonic stenosis is synonymous with a congenital etiology. The pulmonic valve is unlikely to be affected by acquired cardiovascular diseases. Most patients present in

Table 5
Limitations of Balloon Aortic Valvuloplasty

Retrograde access to LV
Hemodynamic assessment
    Low gradient/low output
Large-caliber ballons
    Slow inflate–deflate cycle
    12 to 14 French femorial arterial access
Restenosis
    Fibrosis of cracks/fissures made by balloon
Regurgitant lesions

Table 6
Intervention for Pulmonic Stenosis

Class I
    Exertional dyspnea, angina, syncope, presyncope
    Asymptomatic, normal cardiac output, peak gradient >50 mm
Class IIa
    Asymptomatic, normal cardiac output, peak gradient 40–49 mm
Class IIb
    Asymptomatic, normal cardiac output, peak gradient 30–39 mm
Class III
    Asymptomatic, normal cardiac output, peak gradient <30 mm

childhood. Symptoms are unusual until adolescence or adulthood. Adults usually present with symptoms of fatigue or dyspnea.

Balloon pulmonic valvuloplasty (BPV) is the treatment of choice for these adult patients and has excellent long-term results. The approach can be considered curative. The AHA/ACC Task Force recognizes valvuloplasty for pulmonic stenosis as a Class I indication for symptomatic patients with dyspnea, angina, syncope, or presyncope, as well as those who are asymptomatic with peak transpulmonic gradients over 50 mm Hg (Table 6) *(6)*.

Long-term studies of the results of valvotomy for pulmonic stenosis in children, adolescents, and adults have shown excellent results. In a large study on the natural history of congenital heart defects, patients were followed for up to 25 yr after BPV *(32)*. The probability of survival was similar to that of the general population and the vast majority of patients remained asymptomatic. Reoperation was rarely necessary for those treated in childhood. Patients with gradients less than 25 mm did not experience an increase in gradient. Patients with gradients greater than 50 mm clearly required therapy. For children in the intermediate zone, there was some uncertainty regarding a best recommendation for treatment. The probability of 25-yr survival was 96%. The probability of survival was less than 80% in a subgroup of patients more than 12 yr old with cardiomegaly. Less than 20% of the patients managed medically for low gradients required a valvotomy.

Balloon pulmonic valvuloplasty for pulmonic stenosis in adolescents and adults has also been well described. In one study with a mean follow-up of 7 yr, the vast majority

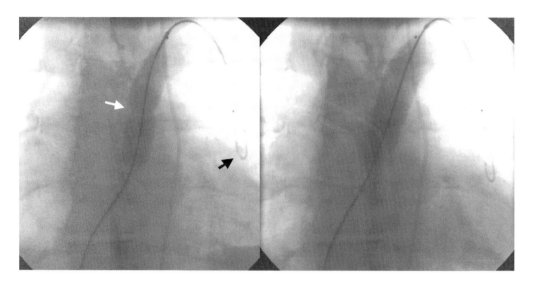

Fig. 8. Balloon pulmonic valvuloplasty is accomplished by antegrade transvenous passage of a wire across the stenotic pulmonary valve into the left pulmonary artery. In the left panel, a balloon catheter is inflated across the stenotic pulmonic valve. The white arrow shows an indentation in the balloon caused by the stenosis. The black arrow shows the tip of the guide wire anchored in the left distal pulmonary artery. In the right-hand panel, the indentation in the center of the balloon has been relieved as the balloon is fully inflated to treat the stenotic pulmonic valve.

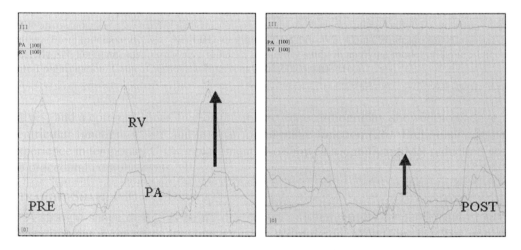

Fig. 9. Hemodynamics with pulmonic valvuloplasty. Before valvuloplasty, the right ventricular pressure is 80 mm Hg. The black arrow denotes the large gradient between the pulmonary artery and the right ventricle across the stenotic pulmonic valve. After valvuloplasty, the gradient is dramatically diminished, again shown by the black arrow. Although the pulmonic pressure has remained relatively constant, the right ventricular pressure has fallen dramatically. Both panels are shown on a 100-mm Hg scale.

of patients remained free of symptoms throughout the study period *(33)*. Incompetence of the pulmonic valve was noted in 7 of 53 (13%) after balloon valvuloplasty, but had disappeared at follow-up in all of these patients. The gradient decreased on average from over 90 mm Hg to less than 40 mm Hg at the time of the procedures. At late follow-up, there was a further decrease in the gradient, probably as a result of regression of right ventricular infundibular hypertrophy.

The technique of BPV involves the passage of a conventional or Inoue balloon catheter via the femoral route antegrade through the right atrium and right ventricle, and across the pulmonic valve (Fig. 8). The wire may be "anchored" in the left pulmonary circulation. Echocardiography to assess the pulmonary valve annular diameter prior to BPV is an important part of planning the procedure. A balloon-to-annulus ratio between 1.1 and 1.3 is usually selected. One or two balloon inflations are usually sufficient to result in elimination of the stenosis. Typical hemodynamic results are shown in Fig. 9.

REFERENCES

1. Safian RD, Berman AD, Diver DJ, et al. Balloon aortic valvuloplasty in 170 consecutive patients: N Engl J Med 1988;319:125–130.
2. Otto CM, Mickel MC, Kennedy JW, et al. Three-year outcome after balloon aortic valvuloplasty. Insights into prognosis of valvular aortic stenosis. Circulation 1994;89:642–650.
3. Kuntz RE, Tosteson AN, Berman AD, et al. Predictors of event-free survival after balloon aortic valvuloplasty. N Engl J Med 1991;325(1):17–23.
4. O'Neill WW. Predictors of long-term survival after percutaneous aortic valvuloplasty: report of the Mansfield Scientific Balloon Aortic Valvuloplasty Registry. J Am Coll Cardiol 1991;17(1):193–198.
5. Kolh P, Lahaye L, Gerard P, Limet R. Aortic valve replacement in the octogenarians: perioperative outcome and clinical follow-up. Eur J Cardio-Thorac Surg 1999;16(1):68–73.
6. Task Force on Practice Guidelines (Committee on Management of Patients with Valvular Heart Disease). ACC/AHA guidelines for the management of patients with valvular heart disease. A report of the American College of Cardiology/American Heart Association. J Am Coll Cardiol 1998; 32:1486–1588.
7. Fusman B, Faxon D, Feldman T. Hemodynamic rounds: transvalvular pressure gradient measurement. Cathet Cardiovasc Intervent 2001;53:553–561.
8. Feldman T, Laskey W. Alchemy in the cath lab: creating a gold standard for the evaluation of aortic stenosis. Cathet Cardiovasc Diag 1998;44:14–15.
9. Feldman T. Transseptal antegrade access for aortic valvuloplasty. Cathet Cardiovasc Intervent 2000; 50:492–494.
10. Omran H, Schmidt H, Hackenbroch M, et al. Silent and apparent cerebral embolism after retrograde catheterisation of the aortic valve in valvular stenosis: a prospective, randomised study. Lancet 2003; 361(9365):1241–1246.
11. Ford LE, Feldman T, Chiu YC, Carroll JD. Hemodynamic resistance as a measure of functional impairment in aortic valvular stenosis. Circ Res 1990;66: 1–7.
12. Feldman T, Ford LE, Chiu YC, Carroll JC. Changes in valvular resistance, power dissipation, and myocardial reserve with aortic valvuloplasty. J Heart Valve Dis 1992;1:55–64.
13. O'Toole MF, Feldman T, Chiu YC, Carroll JD. Turbulence intensity in aortic stenosis: frequency characteristics and effect of alterations in left ventricular function. J Heart Valve Dis 1993;2:94–102.
14. Feldman T, Carroll JD, Chiu YC: An improved catheter for crossing stenosed aortic valves. Cathet Cardiovasc Diag 1989;16:279–283.
15. Feldman T. Core curriculum for interventional cardiology: percutaneous valvuloplasty. Cathet Cardiovasc Intervent 2003;60:48–56.
16. Solomon LW, Fusman B, Jolly N, et al. Percutaneous suture closure for management of large French size arerial puncture in aortic valvuloplasty. J Invas Cardiol 2001;13:592–596.
17. Feldman T. Percutaneous suture closure for management of large French size arterial and venous puncture. J Intervent Cardiol 2000;13:237–242.
18. Feldman T, Chiu YC, Carroll JD. Single balloon aortic valvuloplasty: increased valve areas with improved technique. J Invas Cardiol 1989;1:295–300.
19. Eisenhauer AC, Hadjipetrou P, Piemonte TC. Balloon aortic valvuloplasty revisited: the role of the inoue balloon and transseptal antegrade approach. Cathet Cardiovasc Intervent 2000;50(4):484–491.
20. Bahl VK, Chandra S, Goswami KC, Manchanda SC. Balloon aortic valvuloplasty in young adults by antegrade, transseptal approach using Inoue balloon. Cathet Cardiovasc Diagn 1998;44(3): 297–301.

21. Bhargava B, Agarwal R, Yadav R, et al. Percutaneous balloon aortic valvuloplasty during pregnancy: use of the Inoue balloon and the physiologic antegrade approach. Cathet Cardiovasc Diagn 1998;45(4):422–425.
22. Percutaneous balloon aortic valvuloplasty. Acute and 30-day follow-up results in 674 patients from the NHLBI Balloon Valvuloplasty Registry. Circulation 1991;84:2383–2397.
23. Anwar A, Vallabhan R, Dalton R, et al. Percutaneous vascular surgery after aortic valvuloplasty: initial clinical experience. J Invas Cardiol 2000;12(4):218–220.
24. Agarusl A, Attani S, Astiani R, et al. Survival after balloon aortic valvuloplasty in elderly patients without surgical options. Circulation, in press.
25. Kastrup J, Wennevold A, Thuesen L, et al. Short- and long-term survival after aortic balloon valvuloplasty for calcified aortic stenosis in 137 elderly patients. Dan Med Bull. 1994;41(3):362–365.
26. Eltchaninoff H, Cribier A, Tron C, et al. Balloon aortic valvuloplasty in elderly patients at high risk for surgery, or inoperable. Immediate and mid-term results. Eur Heart J 1995;16(8):1079–1084.
27. Lieberman EB, Bashore TM, Hermiller JB, et al. Balloon aortic valvuloplasty in adults: failure of procedure to improve long-term survival. J Am Coll Cardiol 1995;26(6):1522–1528.
28. Feldman T, Glagov S, Carroll JD. Restenosis following successful balloon valvuloplasty: bone formation in aortic valve leaflets. Cathet Cardiovasc Diagn 1993;29:1–7.
29. Thompson SA, Smith GB, Cobb SM, et al. Effects of calcium channel blockers on calcium uptake in rat aortic valve allografts. Circulation 1992;86(6):1973–1976.
30. Novaro GM, Tiong IY, Pearce GL, Lauer MS, Sprecher DL, Griffin BP. Effect of hydroxymethylglutaryl coenzyme a reductase inhibitors on the progression of calcific aortic stenosis. Circulation 2001;104(18):2205–2209.
31. Cribier A, Eltchaninoff H, Bash A, et al. Percutaneous transcatheter implantation of an aortic valve prosthesis for calcific aortic stenosis: first human case description. Circulation 2002;106(24):3006–3008.
32. Hayes CJ, Gersony WM, Driscoll DJ, et al. Second natural history study of congenital heart defects. Results of treatment of patients with pulmonary valvar stenosis. Circulation 1993;87(2 Suppl):I28–137.
33. Chen CR, Cheng TO, Huang T, et al. Percutaneous balloon valvuloplasty for pulmonic stenosis in adolescents and adults. N Engl J Med 1996;335:21–25.

3

Pathophysiology and Percutaneous Coronary Sinus Repair of Mitral Regurgitation

Nicholas Valettas, MD
Joseph H. Gorman III, MD,
and Robert C. Gorman, MD

CONTENTS

INTRODUCTION

Consisting of an anterior and posterior leaflet, a fibromuscular annulus, multiple chordae tendinae, and two papillary muscles, the mitral valve complex (Fig. 1) protects the left atrium and the pulmonary vascular bed from exposure to left ventricular pressures during systole and directs the entire left ventricular stroke volume into the systemic circulation. Structural abnormalities or dysfunction of any of the components of the valvular complex, or of the adjacent ventricular (or atrial) musculature that helps anchor the valve, can result in valvular incompetence. By definition, primary mitral regurgitation (MR) describes valvular incompetence caused by abnormalities in one or more of the components of the mitral valve complex alone, whereas functional (secondary) MR refers to valvular incompetence, secondary to abnormalities of the left ventricle that distort the anatomy of the mitral valve complex and render the valve incompetent. This distinction is of more than just semantic importance, for it carries significant therapeutic implications. Management of MR also depends on the acuity with which valvular incompetence develops. In acute MR, a significant portion of the stroke volume is ejected into a left atrium that is unaccustomed to this regurgitant volume, resulting in a rapid elevation of left atrial and pulmonary pressures and the rapid onset of symptoms. In chronic MR, however, left

From: *Contemporary Cardiology: Interventional Cardiology:*
Percutaneous Noncoronary Intervention
Edited by: H. C. Herrmann © Humana Press Inc., Totowa, NJ

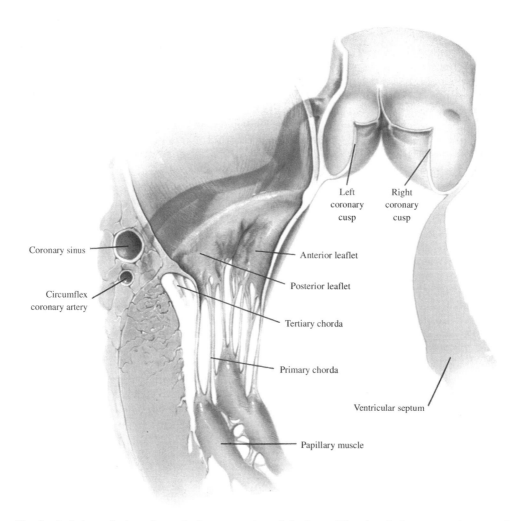

Fig. 1. Artist's rendering of a sagittal cross-section of the heart. The view is from posterior commissure to anterior commissure. Note the close association of the mural annulus with the coronary sinus. The anterior annulus is in continuity with the aortic valve. (From Harlan, Star, and Harwin. Manual of cardiac surgery. Volume II. Reprinted with permission.)

ventricular and atrial enlargement often can accommodate the regurgitant volume and allow the patient to remain completely asymptomatic for an extended period of time.

Definitive therapy for MR has, historically, been limited to surgical correction of the underlying lesion. Recent advances in percutaneous techniques now provide the opportunity for percutaneous therapy of MR. Two strategies have emerged as the most promising therapeutic modalities: (1) percutaneous mitral valve annuloplasty and (2) the percutaneous Alfieri procedure. This chapter will focus on the first of these two strategies. A detailed review of the anatomy of the mitral valve complex will provide the anatomic background for the procedure and will be followed by a discussion of the pathophysiology of acute and chronic MR with an emphasis on functional MR, because it is this subgroup that is most suitable for therapeutic percutaneous mitral valve annuloplasty. The chapter will end with a review of the clinical and laboratory studies assessing the efficacy and safety of this new therapeutic technique.

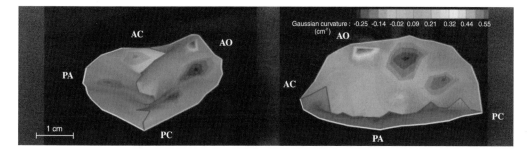

Fig. 2. Image of a human mitral valve annulus and leaflets created with real-time three dimensional echocardiography. Note the nonplanar "saddle" shape of the annulus. The color scale represents leaflet curvature; The red end of the scale represents concavity of the leaflets toward the ventricle. Blue represents convexity toward the ventricle. In sheep experiments, the "blue" areas have been found to be consistent with "strut" chord insertion points. AC = anterior commissure; PC = posterior commissure; PA = posterior annulus. AO represents the position of the aortic valve. (Color illustration is printed in insert following p. 236.)

ANATOMY OF THE MITRAL VALVE COMPLEX

Mitral Annulus

The mitral valve sits obliquely in the heart, in close apposition to the left ventricular outflow tract and aortic valve, with its major cross-sectional axis running in a postero-medial to anterolateral direction. The mitral annulus defines the atrioventricular "plane" and consists of a three-dimensional saddle-shaped ring *(1)* of fibromuscular tissue to which the leaflets are attached. This saddle-shape is extremely well conserved across mammalian species. It has been proposed that this distinctive shape acts to impose an added degree of leaflet curvature above and beyond leaflet bulging, and in doing so, it diminishes leaflet stress (Fig. 2) *(2)*. The anterior portion of the annulus is in direct continuity with the aortic valve, spanning the left coronary and noncoronary sinuses (Fig. 3). At either end of this area of mitral–aortic continuity are the left and right trigones. The right trigone together with the membranous septum form the central fibrous body through which the His bundle courses. Extending from the left and right trigones, respectively, the anterior and posterior fila coronaria are fibrous subendocardial cords that partly encircle the annulus. A less distinct sheet of fibroelastic tissue connects the tips of the fila coronaria, thus completing the annular ring. This heterogeneity in the consistency of the annulus is of great functional significance, imparting a degree of flexibility to the valve that optimizes its function throughout all phases of the cardiac cycle *(3)*.

Mitral Leaflets and Subvalvular Apparatus

Unlike the tricuspid valve and both semilunar valves, the mitral valve has only two leaflets that, when open and viewed *en face* from their left ventricular aspect, resemble a bishop's miter. The anterior (or aortic) leaflet covers one-third of the annular circumference with its base in direct continuity with the aortic valve. In the open position, the leaflet hangs into the left ventricular outflow tract opposite the interventricular septum. When closed, the leaflet forms part of the floor of the left atrium; its free edge defines the lesser curvature of a crescent-shaped closure line formed by apposition of the free edges of both leaflets. The posterior (mural) leaflet covers the remaining two-thirds of the annular circumference, with its free edge forming the greater curvature of the valvular closure line. Pleats in the free edge of the posterior leaflet divide the leaflet into three segments

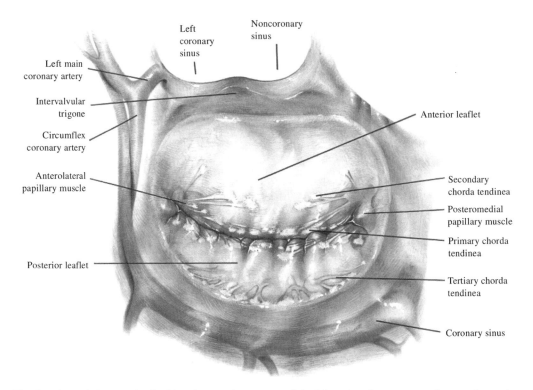

Left
coronary
sinus

Noncoronary
sinus

Left main
coronary artery

Intervalvular
trigone

Circumflex
coronary artery

Anterolateral
papillary muscle

Posterior leaflet

Anterior leaflet

Secondary
chorda tendinea

Posteromedial
papillary muscle

Primary chorda
tendinea

Tertiary chorda
tendinea

Coronary sinus

Fig. 3. View of the annulus looking from atrium to ventricle. Note that the coronary sinus and associated venous structures "encircle" the mural annulus almost from commissure to commissure. Also demonstrated is the aortic–mitral continuity. (From Harlan, Star, and Harwin. Manual of cardiac surgery. Volume II. Reprinted with permission.)

or scallops: P1, P2, and P3. The middle scallop (P2) is typically the largest of the three and is the scallop most commonly involved in mitral valve prolapse *(3)*.

The ventricular surface of the anterior leaflet has two distinct zones: a crescent-shaped peripheral rough zone that contains the leaflets chordal attachments and a central clear zone devoid of any chordal anchors *(4)*. The ventricular surface of the posterior leaflet, on the other hand, has three distinguishable zones: a peripheral rough zone, a central clear zone, and a basal zone. The basal zone is 2–3 mm thick and receives chordal attachments (Fig. 4). The free edges of the anterior and posterior rough zones demarcate the valve's closure line. When viewed in profile and with the leaflets closed, the closure line lies below the annular plane, rising to the level of the plane at each commissure and giving the valve its classic saddle-shaped appearance. This ventricular displacement of the closure line is a direct result of the 1.5–2.1 ratio of leaflet surface area to annular area *(5)*.

Anchoring the mitral valve leaflets and providing the valve with the tensile strength required to withstand the high pressures generated during ventricular systole, the chordae tendinae extend from both papillary muscles and attach to the ventricular surface of the leaflets (Fig. 5). Anatomically, the chordae are subdivided into leaflet and inter-leaflet, or commissural, chordae. Leaflet chordae are further subdivided depending on which leaflet they are attached. All chordae attached to the anterior leaflet are classified as rough zone chordae, whereas the posterior leaflet also contains cleft chordae and basal chordae in addition to rough zone chordae. The rough zone chordae can be further subdivided into first-order (primary) and second-order (secondary) chords. Primary chords are numerous thin chords that insert only on the free edge of the mitral

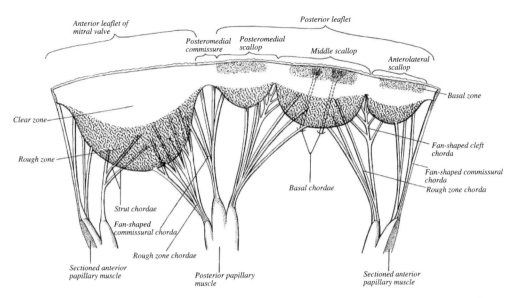

Fig. 4. Schematic of the ventricular surface of the mitral valve opened by cutting the annulus and anterior (anteromedial) papillary muscle and showing the zones of the leaflets and the respective chordae tendinae. (Reprinted from ref. *4* with permission.)

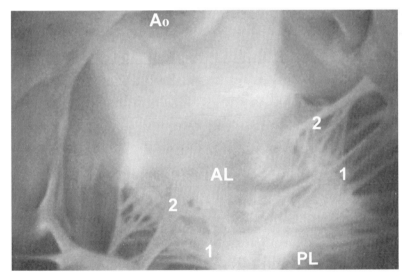

Fig. 5. Videoscopic photograph of the ventricular surface of the mitral valve showing the primary (1) and secondary (2) chordae tendinae. Obvious differences in the thickness between the chords are easily seen. Other labeled structures include the aortic valve (Ao), the anterior mitral leaflet (AL), and the posterior mitral leaflet (PL). (Reprinted from ref. *6* with permission.)

leaflets, whereas secondary chords are thicker structures that insert in the rough zone and have no attachment with the free edge of the valve leaflet (Fig. 4). This morphological difference appears to be functionally important, as suggested by Obadia et al. *(6)* in their study using an isolated pig heart model in which they assessed the effect of disruption of the primary or secondary chords on valvular integrity and ventricular function. Sectioning of the primary chords resulted in severe acute MR as a result of mitral leaflet incompetence. However, when only the secondary chords were sectioned, the mitral

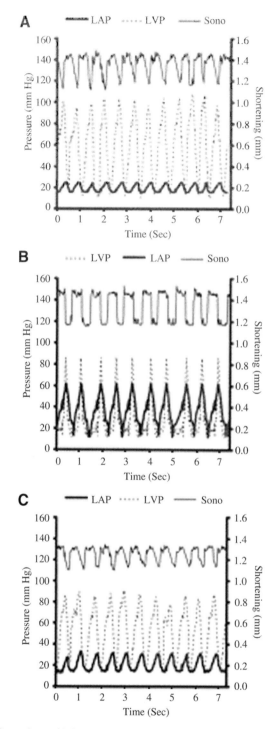

Fig. 6. Hemodynamic tracings of left ventricular (LVP) and left atrial pressures (LAP) in the control group (**A**), primary chord group (**B**), and secondary chord group (**C**). Large v waves representing MR are only seen in group B, suggesting that the primary chordae are essential to maintaining mitral valve competence. In group C, despite disruption of the secondary chords, mitral competence is preserved although shortening fraction is reduced (Sono), reflecting impaired contractility. (Reprinted from ref. 6 with permission.)

valve remained competent, although there was a statistically significant deterioration in left ventricular function as assessed by sonomicrometric measurements of fractional shortening (Fig. 6).

Two papillary muscles tether the chords to the left ventricle and contribute to the tensile strength of the mitral valve complex. They typically arise from the distal third of the left ventricular myocardium, and when viewed in a short-axis projection, they occupy antero-lateral and posteromedial positions (Fig. 7). A degree of variability often exists in the number and location of the papillary muscles. In a study of 200 normal hearts, Rusted et al. *(7)* found that the anterolateral papillary muscle was single in 70% of cases, where-as in 60% of cases, the posteromedial papillary muscle consisted of a group of two or three papillary muscles or of a single belly with two or three heads. Less variable is the arterial supply to the papillary muscles. The posteromedial papillary muscle is supplied by the right coronary artery in isolation and is more prone to ischemic dysfunction, whereas the anterolateral papillary muscle typically has a dual arterial supply (from an obtuse marginal branch of the left circumflex artery and a diagonal branch of the left anterior descending artery) and is usually protected from ischemic damage *(8)*.

Coronary Sinus

Although technically not part of the mitral valvar complex, the coronary sinus is nonetheless an important structure because of its close proximity to the posterior mitral annulus (Figs. 1 and 3). Lying posterior in the left atrioventricular groove, the coronary sinus measures 2–3 cm in length and drains the majority of cardiac veins into the right atrium. Its orifice lies between the opening of inferior vena cava as it enters the atrium and the tricuspid annulus and can be easily cannulated via a percutaneous venous approach. The main tributary emptying into the coronary sinus is the great cardiac vein, which orig-inates at the cardiac apex and runs in the anterior interventricular groove parallel to the left anterior descending artery. As discussed below, this close relationship between the mitral annulus and the coronary sinus provides a percutaneous transcatheter approach to the mitral annulus and is the foundation for percutaneous mitral valve annuloplasty for the treatment of MR *(9,10)*.

PATHOPHYSIOLOGY OF MITRAL REGURGITATION

Mitral regurgitation is often characterized as acute or chronic, depending on the rapidity of onset *(11)*. Additionally, both acute and chronic MR can be primary, if they result from structural abnormalities of the valvar complex, or functional, if the regurgitation is secondary to diseases affecting the left ventricle that result in leaflet malcoaptation and incompetence *(12)*. Because treatment of mitral regurgitation by percutaneous mitral valve annuloplasty is tailored for patients with functional MR, it is this subgroup that will be reviewed here. Attention will be focused on the pathophysiology of MR as a result of nonischemic (dilated) and ischemic cardiomyopathies because these two clinical entities account for the majority of patients with MR that will be suitable for percutaneous therapy.

Functional MR Associated with Nonischemic Dilated Cardiomyopathy

Mitral regurgitation in dilated cardiomyopathy is, in the majority of cases, a chronic process that carries a poor prognosis *(13)*. As in the normal heart, volume overload of the failing heart eventually leads to further systolic dysfunction in a ventricle with little reserve. In a canine model of mitral regurgitation, Urabe et al. *(14)* showed that the

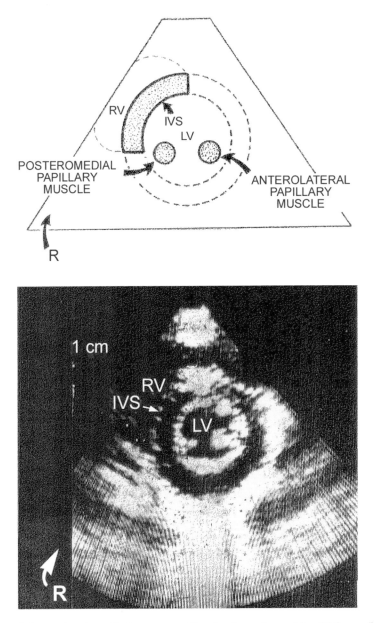

Fig. 7. Parasternal short-axis schematic **(upper panel)** and echocardiographic still frame **(lower panel)** showing the anterolateral and posteromedial papillary muscles. RV = rigt ventricle, IVS = interventricular septum, LV = left ventricle, R = reference mark. (From Weyman AE. Standard plane positions—standard imaging planes. In: Weyman AE, ed. Principles and practice of echocardiography, 2nd ed. Philadelphia: Lippincott Williams and Wilkins, 1994:98–123. Reprinted with permission.)

predominant mechanism of systolic dysfunction in MR is contractile dysfunction of cardiomyocytes due to a loss of myofibrils. Chronic mitral regurgitation eventually results in progressive left ventricular dilatation and eccentric hypertrophy, with a concomitant increase in left ventricular (LV) end diastolic volume and wall stress (afterload) *(15)*. As ventricular dimensions and afterload increase, the afterload reduction provided by the

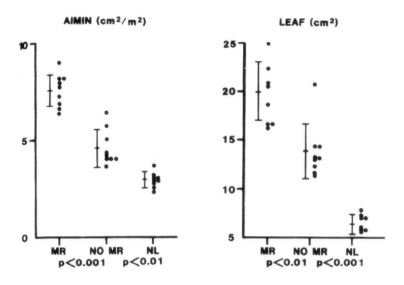

Fig. 8. Plots of annular area index (AIMIN) and leaflet occlusional area (LEAF) in patients with dilated cardiomyopathy and MR (MR), dilated cardiomyopathy and no MR (NO MR), and controls (NL). See text for details. (Reprinted from ref. *14* with permission.)

low-pressure sink in the left atrium is eventually overcome and left ventricular ejection performance is further impaired *(16)*.

The exact mechanism of functional MR in patients with nonischemic cardiomyopathy remains open to debate. Several hypotheses have been advanced as the primary pathogenic mechanisms, including alterations in mitral annular size *(17,18)*, papillary muscle displacement accompanying LV dilatation *(19,20)*, and alterations in the transmitral pressure gradient acting to close the leaflets *(21)*. Using quantitative echocardiography, Boltwood et al. *(17)* compared leaflet occlusional area, mitral annular area index, left ventricular volume, and left atrial volume as well as chordal length and tethering length in nine patients with dilated cardiomyopathy and MR, nine patients with dilated cardiomyopathy and no MR, and nine control subjects. The MR group displayed a significantly increased leaflet occlusional area and annular area index (Fig. 8) when compared to the no MR group and the control group. There was no significant difference, however, in chordal length, tethering length, or ventricular volumes among the three groups. Furthermore, stepwise linear regression analysis showed that leaflet occlusional area strongly correlated with annular area, suggesting that the degree of leaflet coaptation is chiefly determined by annular size, and as the size of the annulus increases, more and more leaflet tissue is needed simply to occlude the orifice. This leaves less leaflet tissue available for the coaptation zone, compromising the integrity of the valvular seal.

A central role for annular dilatation in the pathogenesis of functional MR was also proposed by Timek et al. *(18)* in an ovine model of LV dysfunction and MR. Surgically implanted myocardial markers in the left ventricle, mitral annulus, and mitral leaflets were used to record three-dimensional alterations in ventricular and valvular geometry associated with the development of a pacing-induced, tachycardia-mediated cardiomyopathy. All nine sheep developed MR after pacing. This was associated with annular dilatation and a significant increase in systolic leaflet edge separation, suggesting decreased leaflet coaptation (Fig. 9). The left ventricular chamber

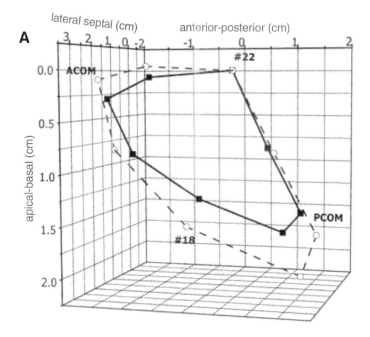

Fig. 9. Changes in annular size with the development of tachycardia-mediated cardiomyopathy (**A**) and associated changes in leaflet edge separation (**B**) as measured by surgically implanted myocardial markers. (Reprinted from ref. *17* with permission.)

became more spherical as it dilated and the distance between the two papillary muscles increased, but this was not associated with apical displacement of the mitral valve leaflet coaptation point, implying that the MR was the result of annular dilatation rather than papillary muscle displacement.

An alternative theory on the pathogenesis of MR in dilated cardiomyopathy, focusing on the effects of altered leaflet tethering geometry on the integrity of leaflet coaptation, was proposed by Otsuji et al. *(19)* in a canine model of heart failure. Left ventricular dysfunction was induced by infusions of esmolol and phenylephrine, and ventricular dilatation was controlled by surgically altering the degree of pericardial constraint. Three-dimensional (3D) echocardiography was used for reconstruction of the cardiac chambers and mitral apparatus from which the geometric relations between the papillary muscles and mitral valve were obtained. The degree of MR increased from none at baseline to trace when global ventricular dysfunction without cavity dilatation occurred and then to moderate when the pericardium was opened and the ventricle was permitted to dilate (Fig. 10). LV dilatation was accompanied by annular dilatation as well as apical displacement of the papillary muscles, resulting in an increase in the tethering length, defined as the distance between the papillary muscle tips and the anterior mitral annulus. Although both mitral annular area and tethering length were predictors of MR in univariate analysis, only tethering length remained an independent predictor of MR by multiple regression analysis, implying that the geometric changes of the mitral valve attachments at the papillary muscle level, rather than the size of the annulus, determine the development of MR (Fig. 11).

Geometric changes in vivo, however, do not occur independent of altered myocardial dynamics, which may also contribute to the development of mitral regurgitation *(22)*,

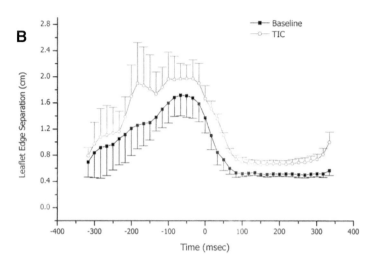

Fig. 9. *(Continued)*

making it difficult to isolate the effect of each parameter independently. In an elegant study using an in vitro left ventricular model, He et al. *(21)* tested the integrated hypothesis that functional mitral regurgitation represented an imbalance between the forces acting to close the mitral leaflets and the restraining forces tenting the leaflets open (Fig. 12). Porcine mitral valves with intact subvalvular structures were tested in the mechanical model under physiological pulsatile flow conditions using normal saline as the rheologic fluid. This model provided three degrees of freedom such that papillary muscle position, annular size, and myocardial contractility could each be altered independently. Transmitral pressure gradients were measured directly and regurgitant fraction (representing the degree of MR) was calculated as the ratio of the regurgitant flow rate to the forward flow rate. Mitral regurgitation was greatest with apical and posterolateral papillary muscle displacement and with annular dilatation, although annular dilatation was required to generate clinically significant levels of MR, as defined by a regurgitant fraction >20%. A lower transmitral pressure also significantly increased the regurgitant fraction but was not the dominant factor.

The results of the above studies into the pathogenesis of mitral regurgitation carry important therapeutic implications because the most effective therapies will be those targeting the primary underlying mechanisms of MR. The success of surgical mitral valve annuloplasty *(23)* clearly implicates annular dilatation in the mechanism of functional MR. Surgical annuloplasty, however, is associated with significant morbidity and mortality in this high-risk group of patients, making a percutaneous approach to mitral valve annuloplasty an attractive alternative.

Mechanism of Ischemic Mitral Regurgitation

The pathogenesis of both acute ischemic mitral regurgitation (IMR) in the absence of papillary muscle rupture and chronic IMR is complex. Experimental analysis of clinically relevant ovine models using tantalum marker imaging, sonomicrometry array localization, and three-dimensional echocardiography *(24–29)*, as well as detailed clinical echocardiographic studies have more clearly elucidated the mechanism of the complex geometric and temporal perturbations that cause a structurally normal mitral valve to leak, often massively, early or late after a myocardial infarction.

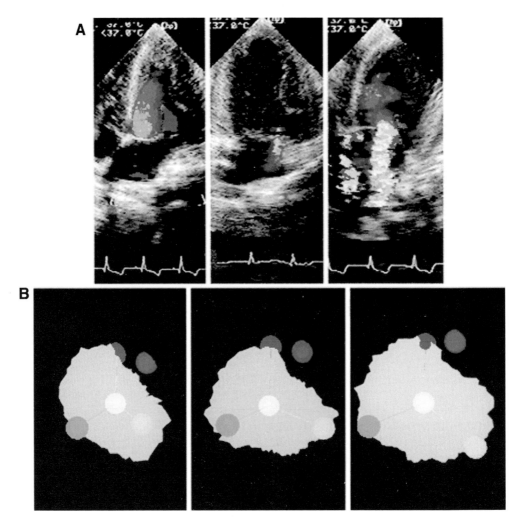

Fig. 10. **(A)** Apical two-chamber echocardiographic images with color-flow mapping showing the development of MR with progressive LV dysfunction and ventricular dilatation. At baseline (left), there is no MR. Trace MR is seen with LV dysfunction pericardial restraint (middle), whereas moderate MR develops when the LV is dilate with the pericardium cut open (right). **(B)** Annular dilatation and relatio papillary muscles to mitral annulus at baseline (left), LV dysfunction without (middle), and LV dysfunction with dilatation (right). Mitral annulus is shown with the papillary muscle tips as yellow and green balls. The red ball is the anterior reference point located in medial trigone. (Color illustration is printed in insert following p. 236.) (Reprinted from ref. *18* with permission.)

ACUTE IMR

Numerous studies have conclusively demonstrated that loss of papillary muscle shortening alone as result of acute ischemia does not cause MR. *(5,22,30–33)*. The term "papillary muscle dysfunction" is, therefore, erroneous and should be avoided. With ischemia or infarction, the posterior papillary muscle elongates 2–4 mm in sheep and dogs *(34,35)*; the tip moves 1.5–3 mm closer to the annulus *(35)*. These are very small changes and echocardiographic studies in dogs, sheep, and humans uniformly fail to show mitral valve prolapse with acute IMR in the absence of papillary muscle rupture *(36–39)*. In the sheep model of acute IMR, the uninfarcted anterior papillary muscle contracts earlier and more vigorously than before infarction. This moves the tip 4–5

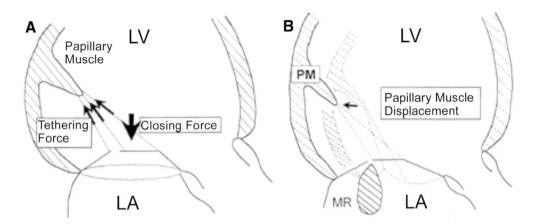

Fig. 11. Schematic representation of the pathogenesis of MR resulting from to papillary muscle displacement and alterations in the tethering distance between the papillary muscle tips and the mitral annulus. (Reprinted from ref. *19* with permission.)

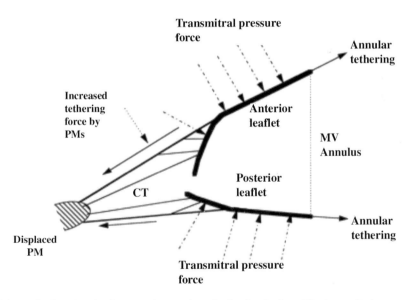

Fig. 12. Schematic showing the forces acting on the mitral valve leaflets. The transmitral pressure force is generated by ventricular systole and is proportional to the contractile state of the ventricle. Tension in the chordae tendinae (CT) and papillary muscle (PM) determines the tethering force. Apical displacement of the PM stretches the chordae and increases the tethering force. (Reprinted from ref. *19* with permission.)

mm further away from the annular plane at mid-systole than before infarction *(24)*. This discoordination of normal synchronous papillary muscle contraction has a complex effect on leaflet coaptation that has been meticulously characterized by Miller and his colleagues *(27,28)* using tantalum marker technology. It is sufficient to say that the interaction of these rather small changes in papillary muscle contraction dynamics and location cause subtle distortions of valvular leaflet coaptation that are not simply leaflet prolapse and tethering. Annular dilatation is at best mild (10–15%) and located primarily along the posterior annulus in the ovine model of acute IMR *(24–26,40)*. This degree of dilatation is within the physiologic range achieved by varying loading conditions in sheep *(41)*. Leaflet area in sheep exceeds maximum annular area by 50–100% *(40)*. These data suggest that acute IMR results from a complex interaction of very small geometric and temporal changes that, for the most part, are not demonstrable by standard imaging techniques and are not discernible in a flaccid heart at the time of surgery.

Chronic IMR

Ovine experiments using sonomicrometry array localization to study postinfarction MR that evolves during the first 8 wk after infarction have added insight relevant to the pathogenesis of chronic IMR. In this model, a combination of asymmetric annular dilatation and leaflet tethering by both papillary muscles occur to produce chronic IMR. The annular area dilates by at least 70% at all time-points during systolic ejection. The dilatation involves the entire annulus, even the fibrous portion between the trigones of the heart. The posterior or mural portion of the annulus directly adjacent to the infarct moves away from the relatively fixed anterior commissure (at the anterior fibrous trigone) and stretches the anterior portion of the mural annulus and the posterior portion of the aortic-based annulus, which are remote from the infarct. This finding illustrates how a moderately sized (21% of the LV mass) localized infarct remodels and distorts remote, uninfarcted myocardium including the mitral valve annulus (Fig. 13) *(42)*.

Interestingly, the posterior papillary muscle tip to posterior commissure relationship does not change significantly. Both these points are displaced *together*, away from the anterior commissure as a result of the remodeling process (Fig. 14). This indicates that the posterior papillary muscle tethering is more pronounced at its most anterior connection with both leaflets near the center of the coaptation line and not at the commissure. The anterior papillary muscle tip is displaced significantly from both commissures but further from the posterior commissure. This indicates the tethering effect of the anterior papillary muscle is greatest along both leaflets from the anterior commissure to the middle of the coaptation line. Together, these findings suggest that in this model, the postinfarction ventricular remodeling process tethers the anterior portion of both leaflets.

The concept of leaflet tethering as a contributing factor in the pathogenesis of chronic IMR is not new *(19,21,43)*. Two recent echocardiographic reports, one studying the same sheep model presented here and one human study, demonstrated findings very consistent with the above-cited experimental results. Otsuji and colleagues applied a very effective three-dimensional echocardiographic technique to quantify leaflet tethering in the same ovine mode *(19)*. These authors also reported mid-systolic distortions between both papillary muscle tips and the anterior commissure, but did not observe changes between papillary muscle tips and the posterior commissure or annular dilatation. Yiu et al., using quantitative two-dimensional echocardiography, corroborated these findings clinically by comparing normal controls with a cohort of patients with varying degrees of chronic IMR *(43)*. They found that ventricular distortions, which most closely correlated with the degree of MR occurred between the posterior papillary muscle tip and anterior commissure ($R = 0.55$) and posterior displacement of the anterior papillary muscle tip ($R = 0.65$).

To summarize, the geometric changes that lead to acute IMR are multiple but extremely subtle (<5 mm) and are not reliably imaged by currently available clinical modalities. Chronic IMR involves larger changes (1–2 cm) that cause moderate to severe annular dilatation and complex leaflet tethering along the anterior and mid-leaflet coaptation line.

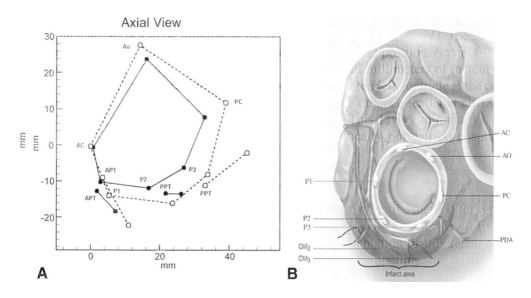

Fig. 13. (A) An end systolic axial view of the mitral valve annulus and papillary muscle as imaged by sonomicrometry before (solid) and 8 wk after infarction in an ovine model of chronic ischemic mitral regurgitation. **(B)** Artist's drawing of how the transducers are placed in relation to the mitral annulus and the location of the infarct. Note the stretching of both the posterior part of the aortic portion of the annulus (Ao to PC) and the anterior part of the mural portion of the annulus (AC to P1 to P2). Also, note how the portion of the annulus between P2 and PC along with the posterior papillary muscle tip (PPT) pulls away form the relatively fixed anterior commissure. This animal had a competent valve prior to infarction and developed 3+ MR at 8 wk postinfarction. (From ref. *19*.)

CORONARY SINUS-BASED PERCUTANEOUS MITRAL VALVE REPAIR

It has been show that surgical placement of an undersize annuloplasty ring, either partial or complete, can improve valve competence in patients with dilated nonischemic MR and chronic ischemic MR. Although such procedures can ameliorate symptoms, they historically have an operative mortality that ranges from 3% to 29.4% *(17,44–48)* and a rate of reoperation up to 14.7% *(47,49,50)*. In addition, there is still no evidence that reduction annuloplasty increases survival in heart failure patients with MR *(51)*.

For these reasons, widespread interest has arisen in developing less invasive percutaneous methods for annular reduction to diminish MR in symptomatic patients with heart failure. As can be seen from Fig. 3, the coronary sinus provides an almost direct approach to the entire posterior mitral annulus using standard venous access approaches. Several devices exploiting this anatomy are in early phases of development (Table 1). Most have been tested for proof of principle in animals; some have been tested for short-term safety and efficacy in patients; none have received Food and Drug Administration (FDA) approval. No reports have been presented for any device regarding chronic implantation in a heart failure model. As a result, concerns regarding repair durability, coronary artery kinking, coronary sinus thrombosis, and cardiac perforation exist. Because of the competitive nature of the intellectual property rights surrounding this technology, only vague descriptions of the latest generation devices are publicly available and are summarized below and in Table 1.

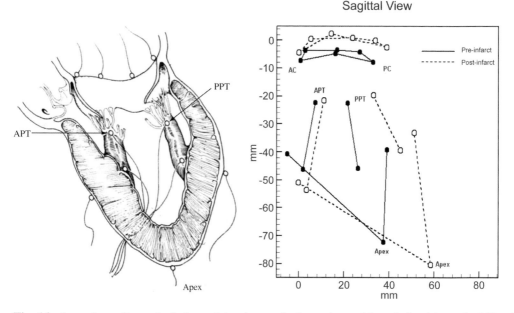

Fig. 14. An end systolic sagittal view of the sheep mitral annulus and its relationship to the LV and papillary muscles before and 8 wk postinfarction. An artist drawing is provided for orientation of the sonomicrometry transducers. Note how the posterior papillary muscle tip (PPT) and the posterior annulus are retracted away form the anterior commissure. Of interest is the fact the anterior papillary muscle tip (APT) also moves away from the annular plane after infarction even though it is not directly affected by the infarct. The heart shown in this figure is the same one shown in Fig. 13. (From ref. *21*.)

Viacor

Viacor's Percutaneous Transvenous Mitral Annuloplasty™ (PTMA) technology originally relied on placement of a Teflon-coated nitinol bar. The bar was substantially straight and rigid and was connected to a flexible push rod to facilitate delivery. The device ranged from 35 to 85 mm in length and was delivered via a 7 French LuMax guiding catheter that had been advanced into the coronary sinus, with the distal tip engaging the anterior interventricular vein. In a recently reported study, this first-generation device was found to be effective in reducing acute IMR in the ovine model previously described in this chapter. Placement of the device in this model reduced the septal–lateral mitral annular dimension from 30 ± 2.1 to 24 ± 1.7 mm *(9)*. Please see videos which demonstrate the ovine results (courtesy of Motoya Hayase and an animation of this technique (courtesy of Viacor, Inc.) in the accompanying CD-ROM.

Although showing proof of principle, the performance of the device in this acute model gave very little information about how it would perform in humans with chronic IMR, where annular dilatation is much more extreme. Subsequently, the Viacor device has been tested extensively for several years using the chronic ovine model of IMR at the University of Pennsylvania. During this time, the device has been evaluated in over 60 animals and the technology has evolved significantly. The latest-generation PTMA device has been placed and evaluated with a combination of fluoroscopy and three-dimensional echocardiography. The current series of animal experiments with this device

Table 1
Coronary Sinus–Based Mitral Valve Repair Technology

Company	Product description	Status
Cardiac Dimensions	Annular repair via the coronary sinus that uses traction with a fixed-length tendon between two anchors	Chronic animal study in pacing model completed
Edwards/Jomed	Jomed technology of annular repair via coronary sinus using two stents with a tensioning member that shortens over time	Estimate human implants to begin in 2004 with market release late 2006/2007
Mitralife/eV3	Percutaneous mitral annular reshaping via the coronary sinus ("C-Cure")	Seven patients implanted in Venezuela
QuantumCor Medical	Transcatheter mitral valve repair using annular heating that results in collagen shrinking	Conducting animal studies
Viacor	Reshaping of the mitral annulus via the coronary sinus utilizing a "straightening bar" that can be sized and easily removed	Food and Drug Administration feasibility study for 10 patients to temporarily place device in patients prior to surgery

has been very successful, with MR being reduced from 3+ to 0 or 1+ acutely. Chronic device studies have not yet been reported.

A clinical safety study is currently underway at the Cleveland Clinic. In this study, the first-generation device is placed in patients undergoing surgery for "open" repair for functional MR. To maximize safety, the device is placed after the sternotomy is performed. Mitral regurgitation is assessed by transesophageal echocardiography. The device is then removed and the operation performed.

Cardiac Dimensions

This device is constructed of nitinol wire with distal and proximal anchors connected by an intervening cable. It is placed via an 8 F catheter positioned in the coronary sinus with its tip at the orifice of the anterior interventricular vein. The distal anchor is first deployed from the guide sheath into the distal great cardiac vein and locked in position. Tension is then applied to the device to reduce the underlying mitral annulus. The tension is maintained while the proximal anchor is deployed into the body of the coronary sinus and locked in position.

Studies using this technology have been carried out in an ovine rapid-pacing model of heart failure. Nine animals were paced until they developed at least moderate MR. The device was successfully placed in all animals. Before device placement, the mitral regurgitant jet area exceeded 20% of the left atrial area in all animals. After device positioning, there was a significant reduction in the mitral annular dimension and in the extent of MR. Mitral regurgitation was completely eliminated in seven of the nine animals, with only trivial MR in the remaining two animals. During placement, there were no atrial or ventricular arrhythmias, blood pressure remained unchanged, and there were no episodes of coronary sinus perforation or dissection *(10)*.

This company is now making plans to test their device in more clinically applicable models of IMR. No human studies have been reported to date.

eV3/Mitralife/C-Curve

This device is placed in the coronary sinus via a 10 F catheter using fluoroscopy and intracardiac echocardiography. Like the two previous devices, it is designed to shorten the posterior annulus.

This is the only device on which chronic implantation studies are reported—albeit only in normal animals. Eight normal sheep have had chronic C-Cure implantation and survived for 180 d with no postprocedural complications. All devices in the acute evaluations study tracked quickly and easily into position. The average baseline mitral annular diameter was 2.55 cm and average postactuation diameter was 1.83 cm—a 28% reduction in size. Angiography confirmed the integrity of the left coronary arteries. At 6 mo follow-up in the chronic pathology study, angiography showed normal coronary arteries and a patent coronary sinus. Echocardiography indicated no change in ventricular function or size and normal mitral valve function. Gross pathology findings also presented normal valves and a coronary sinus free of thrombus *(52)*.

The clinical evaluation of the C-Cure device system was initiated in September 2001 in Caracas, Venezuela. This initial human evaluation established that the MitraLife device could be safely delivered to and deployed within the coronary sinus. No arrhythmias, AV blocks, or hemodynamic compromise were observed. Furthermore, the human-use evaluations demonstrated that cinching the device within the coronary sinus caused a decrease in MR and mitral annular diameter. Further description and discussion of this device is given in Chapter 4.

QuantumCor

This technology is based on the hypothesis that application of controlled, noncoagulating heat, generated by radiofrequency energy, can be used to reduce the posterior mitral annulus by shrinkage of collagen. This shrinkage is proposed to alter the geometry of the posterior annulus and improve the coaptation of the mitral leaflets and correct mitral regurgitation that results from ischemic heart disease. The effects of shrinkage are immediate and the shrinkage does not regress over time because the collagen, heated to a selected level, retains its intrinsic strength. Additionally, the fibrotic healing response to the annular heating can add strength and possibly enhance the initial shrinkage of the annulus. QuantumCor's strategy for device development includes both surgical and percutaneous approaches to mitral heating.

CONCLUSION

Coronary sinus-based mitral valve repair is still very early in its development but enough preliminary work has been done to a least provide proof of principle. Although the technology is promising, there are still both safety and efficacy issues that need to be assessed in appropriate animal models before this technology is appropriate for routine use in humans.

REFERENCES

1. Levine RA, Handschumacher MD, Sanfilippo AJ, et al. Threedimensional echocardiographic recon-struction of the mitral valve, with implications for the diagnosis of mitral valve prolapse. Circulation 1989;80:589–598.
2. Salgo IS, Gorman III JH, Gorman RC, et al. The effect of annular shape on leaflet curvature in reduc-ing mitral leaflet stress. Circulation 2002;106(6):711–717.
3. Ho SY. Anatomy of the mitral valve. Heart 2002;88(Suppl IV):iv5–iv10.
4. Williams PL, Warwick R, Dyson M, Bannister LH. Gray's anatomy, 37th ed. London: Churchill Livingston, 1989:709–711.
5. Perloff JK, Roberts WC. The mitral apparatus: functional anatomy of mitral regurgitation. Circulation 1972;46:227–239.
6. Obadia JF, Casali C, Chassignolle JF, Janier M. Mitral subvalvular apparatus: different functions of pri-mary and secondary chordae. Circulation 1997;96:3124–3128.
7. Rusted IE, Scheifley CH, Edwards JE, et al. Guides to the commisures in operations upon the mitral valve. Proc Staff Meet Mayo Clin 1951;26:297–305.
8. McQuillan BM, Weyman AE. Severe mitral regurgitation secondary to partial papillary muscle rupture following myocardial infarction. Rev Cardiovasc Med 2000;1(1):57–60.
9. Liddicoat JR, MacNeil BD, Gillinov AM, et al. Percutaneous mitral valve repair: a feasibility study in an ovine model of acute ischemic mitral regurgitation. Catheter Cardiovasc Intervent 2003;60: 410–416.
10. Kaye DM, Byrne M, Alferness C, Power J. Feasibiltiy and short-term efficacy of percutaneous mitral annular reduction for the therapy of heart failure–induced mitral regurgitation. Circulation 2003;108:1795–1797.
11. Carabello BA, Crawford FA. Valvular heart disease. N Engl J Med 1997;337:32–41.
12. Carabello BA. Mitral valve regurgitation. Curr Probl Cardiol 1998;199–241.
13. Junker A, Thayssen P, Nielsen B, Andersen PE. The hemodynamic and prognostic significance of echo-Doppler-proven mitral regurgitation in patients with dilated cardiomyopathy. Cardiology 1993;83(1–2):14–20.
14. Urabe Y, Mann DL, Kent RL, et al. Cellular and ventricular contractile dysfunction in experimental canine mitral regurgitation. Circ Res 1992;70:131–47.
15. Carabello BA. Mitral regurgitation: basic pathophysiologic principles. Mod Concepts Cardiovasc Dis 1988;57:53–58.
16. Corin W, Monrad ES, Murakami T, et al. The relationship of afterload to ejection performance in chronic mitral regurgitation. Circulation 1987;76:59–67.
17. Boltwood CM, Tei C, Wong M, Shah PM. Quantitative echocardiography of the mitral complex in dilated cardiomyopathy: the mechanism of functional mitral regurgitation. Circulation 1983;68:498–508.
18. Timek TA, Dagum P, Lai DT, et al. Pathogenesis of mitral regurgitation in tachycardia-mediated car-diomyopathy. Circulation 2001;104[Suppl I]:I47–I53.
19. Otsuji Y, Handschumacher MD, Schwammenthal E, et al. Insights from three-dimensional echocardio-graphy into the mechanism of functional mitral regurgitation: direct in vivo demonstration of altered leaflet tethering geometry. Circulation 1997;96:1999–2008.
20. Sabbah H, Kono T, Rosman H, et al. Left ventricular shape is the primary determinant of functional mitral regurgitation in heart failure. J Am Coll Cardiol 1992;20:1594–1598.
21. He S, Fontaine AA, Schwammenthal E, et al. Integrated mechanism for functional mitral regurgitation. Circulation 1997;96:1826–1834.
22. Kaul S, Spontnitz WD, Glasheen Wp, Touchstone DA. Mechanism of ischemic mitral regurgitation: an experimental evaluation. Circulation 1992;84:2167–2180.
23. Bach DS, Bolling SF. Improvement following correction of secondary mitral regurgitation in end-stage cardiomyopathy with mitral annuloplasty. Am J Cardiol 1996;78:966–969.
24. Gorman JH III, Gorman RC, Jackson BM, et al. Papillary muscle discoordination rather than increased annular area facilitates mitral regurgitation after acute posterior infarction. Circulation 1997;96(Suppl II):124–127.
25. Gorman JH III, Gorman RC, Jackson BM, et al. Three-dimensional annular changes in acute ischemic mitral regurgitation. Surg Forum 1996;47:288–290.
26. Gorman RC, McCaughan J, Ratcliffe MB, et al. Pathogenesis of acute ischemic mitral regurgitation in three dimensions. J Thorac Cardiovasc Surg 1995;109:684–693.

27. Glasson JR, Komeda M, Daughters GT, et al. Early systolic mitral leaflet "loitering" during acute ischemic mitral regurgitation. J Thorac Cardiovasc Surg 1998;116(2):193–205.

28. Komeda M, Glasson JR, Bolger AF, et al. Geometric determinants of ischemic mitral regurgitation. Circulation 1997;96(Suppl): II-128–II-33.

29. Otsuji Y, Handschumacher MD, Liel-Cohen N, et al. Mechanism of ischemic mitral regurgitation with segmental left ventricular dysfunction: three-dimensional echocardiographic studies in models of acute and chronic progressive regurgitation. J Am Coll Cardiol, 2001;37(2):641.

30. Llaneras MR, Nance ML, Streicher JT, et al. A large animal model of ischemic mitral regurgitation. Ann Thorac Surg 1994;57:432.

31. Godley RW, Wann LS, Rogers EW, et al. Incomplete mitral leaflet closure in patients with papillary muscle dysfunction. Circulation 1981;63:565.

32. Mittal AK, Langston M Jr, Cohn KE, et al. Combined papillary muscle and left ventricular wall dysfunction as a cause of mitral regurgitation. Circulation 1971;44:174.

33. Tsakiris AG, Rastelli GC, Amorim DD, et al. Effect of experimental papillary muscle damage on mitral valve closure in intact anesthetized dogs. Mayo Clin Proc 1970;45:275.

34. Hirakawa S, Sasayama S, Tomoike H, et al. In situ measurement of papillary muscle dynamics in the dog left ventricle. Am J Physiol: Heart Circ Physiol 1977;2:H384.

35. Gorman RC, McCaughan JS, Ratcliffe MB, et al. A three-dimensional analysis of papillary muscle spatial relationships in acute postinfarction mitral insufficiency. Surg Forum 1994;45:330.

36. Sharma SK, Seckler J, Israel DH, et al. Clinical, angiographic and anatomic findings in acute severe ischemic mitral regurgitation. Am J Cardiol 1992;70:277.

37. Kono T, Sabbah HN, Stein PD, et al. Left ventricular shape as a determinant of functional mitral regurgitation in patients with severe heart failure secondary to either coronary artery disease or idiopathic dilated cardiomyopathy. Am J Cardiol 1991;68:355.

38. Kono T, Sabbah HN, Rosman H, et al. Mechanism of functional mitral regurgitation during acute myocardial ischemia. J Am Coll Cardiol 1992;19:1101.

39. Kinney EL, Frangi MJ. Value of two-dimensional echocardiographic detection of incomplete mitral leaflet closure. Am Heart J 1985;109:87.

40. Gorman JH 3rd, Gorman RC, Jackson BM, et al. Distortions of the mitral valve in acute ischemic mitral regurgitation. Ann Thorac Surg 1997;64(4):1026–1031.

41. Gorman III JH, Gorman RC, Jackson BM, et al. The effect of inotropic state on the size of the mitral annulus. J Am Coll Cardiol 2001;37(324A):1087–1101.

42. Jackson BM, Gorman JH 3rd, Moainie SL, et al. Extension of borderzone myocardium in postinfarction dilated cardiomyopathy. J Am Coll Cardiol 2002;40:1160–1167. (in press).

43. Yiu SF, Enriquez-Sarano M, Tribouilloy C, et al. Determinants of the degree of functional mitral regurgitation in patients with systolic left ventricular dysfunction: a quantitative clinical study. Circulation 2000;102(12):1400–1406.

44. Bulkley BH, Roberts WC. Dilatation of the mitral annulus. Am J Med 1975;59:457.

45. Siniawski H, Weng Y, Hetzer R. Decision-making aspects in the surgical treatment of ischemic mitral incompetence. In: Ischemic Mitral incompetence, Vetter HO, Hetzer R, Schmutzler H., eds. New York: Springer-Verlag, 1991:137.

46. Dion R. Ischemic mitral regurgitation: when and how should it be corrected. J Heart Valve Dis 1993;2:536.

47. Cohn LH. Surgical treatment of ischemic mitral regurgitation by repair and replacement. In: Ischemic mitral incompetence. Vetter HO, Hetzer R, Schmutzler H, eds. New York: Springer-Verlag, 1991:179.

48. David TE, Ho WC. The effect of preservation of chordae tendineae on mitral valve replacement for postinfarction mitral regurgitation. Circulation 1986;74(Suppl I):I–116.

49. Oury JH, Cleveland, JC, Duran CG, Angell WW. Ischemic mitral valve disease: classification and systemic approach to management. J Cardiac Surg 1994;9:262.

50. Angell WW, Oury JH. A comparison of replacement and reconstruction in patients with mitral regurgitation. J Thorac Cardiovasc Surg 1987;93:665.

51. Gillinov AM, Wierup PN, Blackstone EH, et al. Is repair preferable to replacement for ischemic mitral regurgitation? J Thorac Cardiovasc Surg 2001;122(6):1125–1141.

52. Bailey LR, Luna-Guerra J, Sheahan B, et al. A percutaneous approach for the treatment of mitral regurgitation evaluated in the healthy bovine model. Am J Cardiol 2002;90:39H.

4

Percutaneous Coronary Sinus Approach to the Treatment of Mitral Regurgitation

Fumiaki Ikeno, MD, Yasuhiro Honda, MD, Heidi N. Bonneau, RN, MS, Ali H.M. Hassan, MD, and Peter J. Fitzgerald, MD, PhD

CONTENTS

INTRODUCTION

Mitral valve regurgitation (MR) is a common disease involving multiple etiologies. Whereas the structural causes include myxomatous degeneration, rheumatic changes, calcified annulus, infective endocarditis, and chordal rupture, functional MR is primarily the result of incomplete coaptation of normal mitral leaflets as a result of progressive mitral annular dilation, alteration in left ventricular (LV) geometry, and/or papillary muscle dysfunction *(1–4)*. This secondary MR frequently accompanies acute ischemic or chronic heart failure *(5)* and triggers a vicious cycle of continuing volume overload, ventricular dilation, progression of annular dilation, and increased LV wall tension, thus further worsening MR and heart failure *(6,7)*. In addition, this functional disorder can eventually lead to loss of systolic sphincteric contraction of mitral annulus and chordae tendinae retraction with fibrosis.

Functional MR secondary to LV dysfunction is a significant clinical problem, representing an independent or strong predictor of mortality in patients with both ischemic and nonischemic heart failure *(5,8–10)*. Although medical therapies play a leading role

From: *Contemporary Cardiology: Interventional Cardiology:*
Percutaneous Noncoronary Intervention
Edited by: H. C. Herrmann © Humana Press Inc., Totowa, NJ

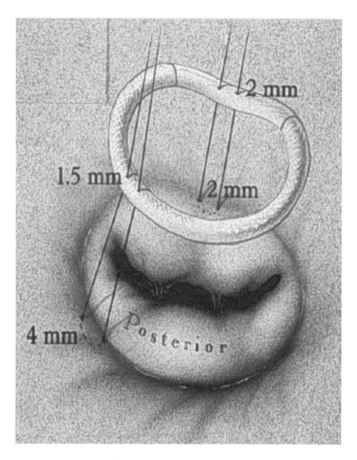

Fig. 1. Surgical annuloplasty.

in alleviating this complication, recent data suggest that mitral valve repair also appears promising *(11)*. In the absence of structural mitral valve abnormalities, the dimension of the mitral annulus is the most significant determinant of mitral leaflet coaptation, regurgitant orifice area, and subsequent MR. Hence, the dominant modality of current surgical approach is insertion of a mitral annuloplasty ring that reduces annular circumference and pushes the posterior leaflet forward for better coaptation, thereby decreasing MR *(1,4)* (Fig. 1). Maintaining the mitral valve and subvalvar apparatus by this approach is of paramount importance to the preservation of overall LV function, offering a critical advantage over the conventional valve replacement technique in heart failure patients with MR.

Nevertheless, a relatively high hospital morbidity and mortality may render surgical treatment prohibitive in the majority of heart failure patients *(11,12)*. This limitation led to a demand for substantially less invasive approaches that can be applied to patients even with severely compromised LV function. Recently, several percutaneous treatment modalities via the coronary sinus have become the target of clinical research *(13–16)*. The anatomic proximity of the coronary sinus to the posterior mitral annulus, coupled with ease of percutaneous access to this large vein, offers a basis for the development of less invasive, catheter-based mitral annuloplasty *(17,18)*. This chapter provides an overview of the rationale for using the coronary sinus for percutaneous mitral annuloplasty, as well as other percutaneous approaches to directly address mitral valvular pathology.

A   **B**

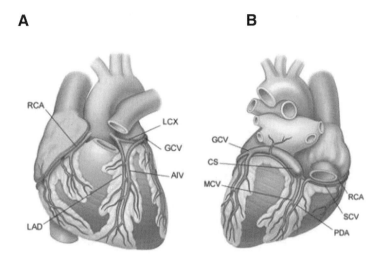

Fig. 2. Anatomy of epicardial vascular system. (**A**) Anterior view of the heart. RCA = right coronary artery; LAD = left anterior descending artery; CFX = circumflex coronary artery; GCV = great cardiac vein; AIV = anterior interventricular vein. (**B**) Posterior view of the heart. CS = coronary sinus; MCV = middle cardiac vein; PDA = posterior descending artery; SCV = small cardiac vein. (From Oesterle SN, Reifart N, Hauptmann E, Hayase M, Yeung AC. Percutaneous in situ coronary venous arterialization: report of the first human catheter-based coronary artery bypass. Circulation 2001;103(21):2539–2543.)

ANATOMY OF CORONARY SINUS

Location and Major Tributaries

The coronary sinus runs along the circumflex coronary artery in the atrioventricular groove parallel to the posterior mitral annulus. It courses from the origin of the anterior interventricular vein, which runs adjacent to the left anterior descending coronary artery on the anterior surface of the heart (Fig. 2). As the main drainage channel of venous blood from the myocardium, the coronary sinus drains a number of smaller veins: typically, from left to right along its course, great cardiac vein, oblique vein of Marshal, posterior vein of the left ventricle, posterior interventricular vein, middle cardiac vein, and small cardiac veins (Figs. 2 and 3A) The coronary sinus orifice, the aperture through which most of the venous drainage of the heart is returned to the circulation, lies anteroinferiorly of the tricuspid orifice in the right atrium.

Size, Length, and Shape

There are numerous variations in size, length, and shape of the coronary sinus. The diameter of the atrial ostium ranges between 7 and 16 mm (9.7); the cross-sectional area of the coronary sinus is between 0.67 and 2.09 mm^2 *(19,20)* (Fig. 4). The average length is between 15 and 70 (37.0) mm *(21)*. A short coronary sinus has the length of a phalanx of a finger (7% of cases); a coronary sinus of medium length with its cylindrical form corresponds to two phalanges in 74% of cases; and an elongated coronary sinus has the length of three phalanges and exhibits a tubular, extended form in 18% of cases.

Venous Valves

The entrance of the coronary sinus into the right atrium is guarded by a more or less complete and sufficient fold, the Thebesian valve *(22)*. The valve drops across the coronary

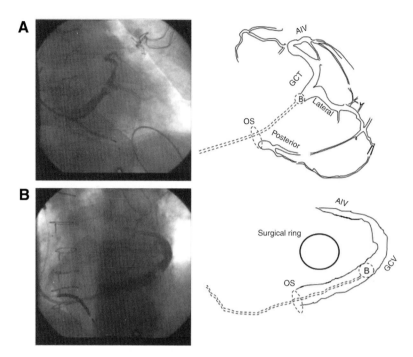

Fig. 3. Coronary sinus venography by retrograde contrast injection with proximal balloon occlusion. **(A)** Coronary sinus and its major tributaries; **(B)** relationship between the coronary sinus/great cardiac vein and a surgically implanted mitral annular ring. AIV = anterior interventricular vein; GCV = great cardiac vein; OS = ostium of coronary sinus; B = balloon; Lateral = lateral vein of left ventricle; Posterior = posterior vein of left ventricle.

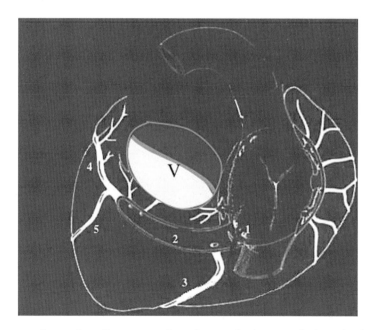

Fig. 4. 1: Coronary sinus ostium; 2: coronary sinus; 3: posterior interventricular vein; 4: anterior interventricular vein; 5: left marginal vein; V: mitral valve.

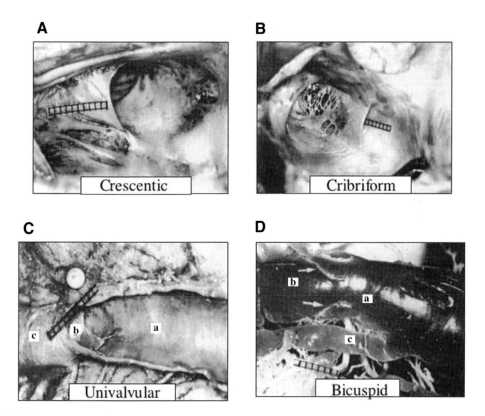

Fig. 5. (A) Seminlunar valve at the artrial ostium of the coronary sinus (CS), the valve of Thebesius; view from the right atrium. **(B)** Cribrate valve at the atrial ostium of the CS, the valve of Thebesius; view from the right atrium. **(C)** Univalvular Viessenian valve: (a) marked by a scale, at the transition of the CS (b) into the great cardiac vein (c). **(D)** Corrosion cast of the cardiac veins; at the entrance of the CS, there are impressions of two endothelial folds; bicuspid formation of the ostial valves (arrows) of the great cardiac vein (Vieussenian valve): (a) coroanry sinus, (b) great cardiac vein, (c) posterior left ventricular vein. (Courtesy of from LANDES Bioscience, Texas, USA.)

sinus orifice whenever the pressure in the right atrium exceeds that in the vein (i.e., during atrial contraction). The types of valve shape have several patterns: incomplete (50%), crescentic (34%), cribriform (7%), semiannular (7%), and thread (2%). Whereas 31% of hearts have a complete valve, the ostium is valveless in 19% *(23–25)* (Figs. 5A and 5B).

The anatomic marker dictating the site where the great cardiac vein widens to become the coronary sinus is the Vieussens valve, which presents in 65–87% of hearts *(22)*. Several morphological types can be distinguished: unicuspid (62%), bicuspid (25%), tricuspid (<1%), and multiple valves <1% *(24)* (Figs. 5C and 5D).

STRATEGIC IMAGING PRIOR TO CATHETER-BASED MITRAL ANNULOPLASTY

Because anatomic variation can be remarkable in the human, prior assessment of the venous anatomy as well as its adjacent structures is crucial for both patient triage and successful catheter-based mitral annuloplasty. First, the location, size, length,

A   **B**

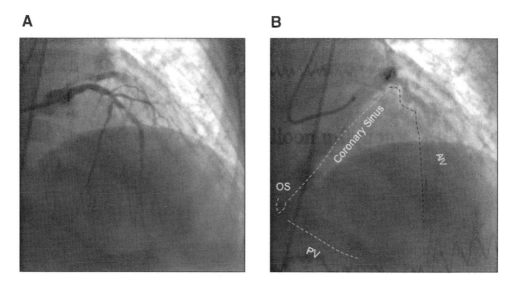

Fig. 6. Coronary angiography with the venous followthrough phase. (**A**) Left anterior descending coronary artery angiogram in the right anterior oblique projection; (**B**) contrast washout phase elucidative of coronary vein. AIV = anterior interventricular vein; OS = ostium of coronary sinus; PV = posterior vein of left ventricle.

shape, and valves of the coronary sinus can directly influence the feasibility and efficacy of coronary sinus annuloplasty devices. In particular, the relative position of the coronary sinus to the mitral annulus holds the key to successful results. Second, close proximity of the coronary sinus to the circumflex coronary artery may introduce the potential risk of distortion or damage to the artery by placement of an annuloplasty device in the coronary sinus. Thus, significant atherosclerotic lesions or previously implanted stents in the circumflex coronary artery should be pre-evaluated. Third, the presence and degree of mitral annular calcification are also important because whether the device can effectively modify the annular dimension partly depends on the rigidity of the mitral annulus.

Coronary angiography is the gold standard for the assessment of coronary artery lesions. With enough contrast for the venous followthrough phase, this conventional method can also provide a venous road map as well as a visual correlation between the arterial and venous anatomies (Fig. 6). In humans, the great cardiac vein generally crosses over the circumflex coronary artery in its distal portion at the transition into the coronary sinus. Pinching of the circumflex coronary artery by the coronary sinus annuloplasty device must be avoided. Direct venography by a retrograde injection into the coronary sinus with proximal balloon occlusion can offer the best method for the venous anatomy evaluation, allowing more precise morphologic and morphometric assessment of the coronary sinus (Fig. 3). Currently, advanced noninvasive imaging techniques using computerized tomography or magnetic resonance imaging technologies have been rapidly developed (Figs. 7 and 8). Three-dimensional images of the heart are particularly useful for evaluating the geographic relationship between the coronary sinus and mitral valve.

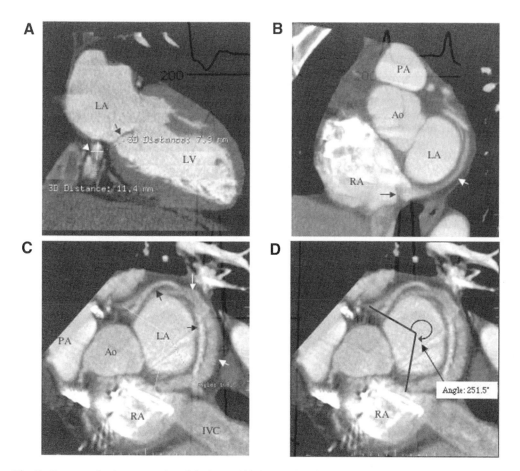

Fig. 7. Computerized tomography of the heart. (**A**) A two-chamber view of the apical–basal position of the greater cardiac vein (GCV) in relation to the mitral valve. Black arrow indicates the posterior leaflet of the mitral valve; white arrow indicates the GCV. (**B**) A short-axis view of the coronary sinus with a prominent Thebesian valve at its entrance (black arrow). White arrow indicates the GCV. (**C**) The intertwined relationship between the GCV (white arrow) and the left circumflex artery (black arrow). (**D**) The same picture with an angular measurement of how much the mitral annulus is covered by the GCV. (16-slice MDCT, retrospective EKG gating, 1.25-mm detector width, 0.5-s gantry rotation, 135-cm³ Omnipaque-300 infused intravenously at a rate of 3 cm³/s. Scanning commence at 50-s delay from the start of contrast infusion.) Ao = aorta; RA = right atrium; LA = left atrium; PA = pulmonary artery; IVC = inferior vena cava. (Courtesy of Dr. Frandics P. Chan, Department of Radiology, Stanford University.)

DEVICES ADDRESSING ANNULAR PATHOLOGY

Percutaneous Mitral Annuloplasty Devices

Several investigators are developing percutaneous catheter-based annuloplasty devices, the majority of which are a "ringlike" implant for insertion into the coronary sinus. By surrounding the anterolateral and posterior portion of the mitral valve annulus, these prototypes are designed to push the dislocated posterior annulus anteriorly for improved leaflet coaptation. One other approach uses no implant device but, rather, heat energy to shrink the mitral annulus, thereby generating a similar effect. In animal

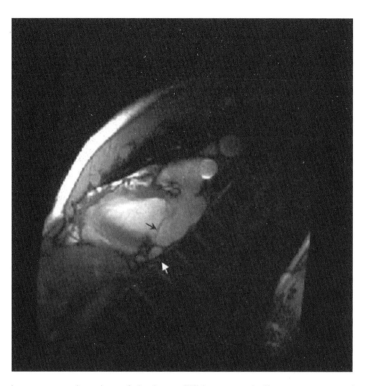

Fig. 8. Magnetic resonance imaging of the heart. White arrow indicates coronary sinus; black arrow indicates posterior leaflet of mitral valve. (Courtesy of Dr. Phillip C. Yeung, Division of Cardiolovascular Medicine, Stanford University.)

studies, each device has shown promising acute results; some investigators have also reported chronic animal data or preliminary human experience.

STENTLIKE IMPLANT DEVICE

A stent-based approach is being tested as a partial annular ring implant device (Edwards Lifesciences, Irvine, CA). The 8F prototype consists of three elements: two anchor stents to be deployed into the great cardiac vein and the coronary sinus, respectively, and the middle stent foreshortening to reshape the coronary sinus (Fig. 9). In an animal model, the average reduction in anterior–posterior distance of the mitral annulus was 24% at 9 wk, resulting in significantly improved MR. Further animal studies are underway, and a clinical study is expected in 2004.

C-SHAPE IMPLANT DEVICE

A C-shape annular ring implant device is being developed and has been tested in healthy ovine models (C-Cure; ev3, Plymouth, MN) (Fig. 10). The implant device is preloaded in a 10F delivery catheter and is actuated via a handle on the catheter. For acute evaluations, a prototype device was delivered via a 12F jugular vein sheath into the coronary sinus under fluoroscopic guidance. Intracardiac echocardiography was also used to guide the correct placement and amount of actuation to obtain optimal results. The average mitral annular diameter was 25.5 mm at baseline and 18.3 mm at postactuation (28% reduction, $p = 0.004$). In a separate study of chronic pathology, healthy ovine underwent chronic C-Cure implantation and survived for 180 d with no postprocedural complications. At 6 mo follow-up, pathologic evaluation revealed a patent coronary sinus, normal

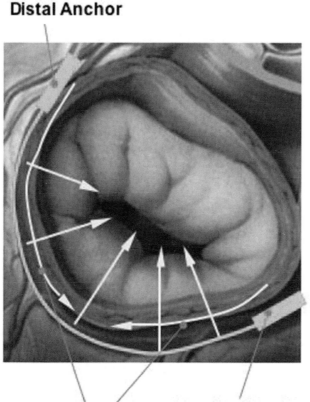

Distal Anchor

Foreshortening **Proximal Anchor**

Fig. 9. A concept of the stent-based percutaneous mitral annuloplasty device. The device (indicated in green) consists of three elements: two anchor stents (gray arrow) to be deployed into the great cardiac vein and the coronary sinus, respectively, and the middle stent foreshortening to make the posterior leaflet attached to the anterior leaflet (yellow arrow). (Courtesy of Edwards Lifesciences, Irvine, CA.)

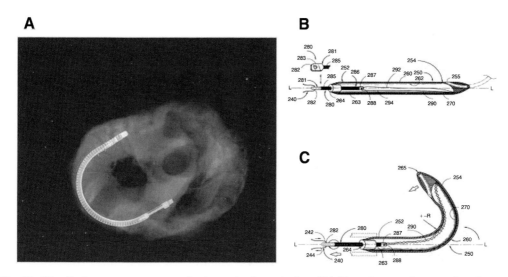

Fig. 10. The C-shape percutaneous mitral annuloplasty device: **(A)** X-ray image of an ex vivo sheep heart with the implanted device; **(B, C)** schematic drawings of the prototype annuloplasty system. (Courtesy of C-Cure, eV3, Plymouth, MN.)

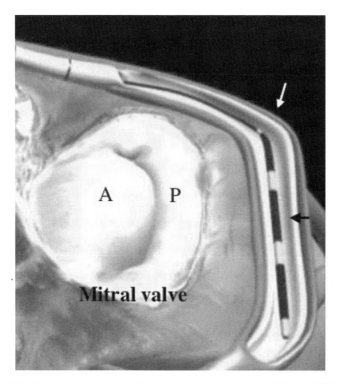

Fig. 11. The straight-shape percutaneous mitral annuloplasty device. (Viacor, Wilmington, MA) The device (black arrow) pushes forward the posterior annulus, thereby increasing leaflet coaptation. The white arrow indicates great cardiac vein and coronary sinus. A = anterior mitral leaflet; P = posterior mitral leaflet. (From Liddicoat JR, Mac Neill BD, Gillinov AM, Cohn WE, Chin CH, Prado AD, Pandian NG, Oesterle SN. Percutaneous mitral valve repair: a feasibility study in an ovine model of acute ischemic mitral regurgitation. Cathet Cardiovasc Intervent 2003;60(3):410–416.)

valves, and a coronary sinus free of thrombus. Echocardiography showed no change in ventricular function or size and normal mitral valve function *(26)*. Preliminary human experience in temporary C-Cure placement also showed a significant MR reduction with no procedural complications.

STRAIGHT-SHAPE IMPLANT DEVICE

A straight-shape device is being developed as a temporally or permanent annuloplasty implant in the coronary sinus (Viacor, Wilmington, MA) (Fig. 11). The implant device consists of a composite nitinol and stainless-steel construct, coated with medical-grade Teflon and polyethylene plastic. It is comprised of a substantially straight and rigid element, available in lengths ranging from 35 to 85 mm, that maintains its shape in the coronary sinus. This causes conformational changes in the mitral annulus, pushing forward the posterior annulus with outward counterforce on coronary sinus near the commissures. In a feasibility study using an ovine model of acute ischemic MR, a 7F sheath was placed in the right internal jugular vein and the coronary sinus was selected by a balloon-tipped catheter *(17)*. The annuloplasty device was delivered through a 7F guiding catheter placed in the coronary sinus under fluoroscopic guidance. The septal–lateral mitral annular diameter decreased from 30 ± 2.1 to 24 ± 1.7 mm ($p = 0.03$). The MR grade was reduced from 3–4 to 0–1 in all animals, and the MR jet area sig-

A   **B**

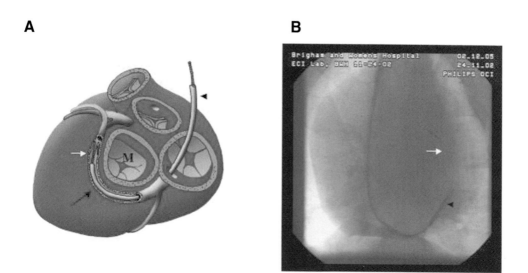

Fig. 12. The wire-based percutaneous mitral annuloplasty device. **(A)** Positioning of the wire-based mitral annular constraint device in the coronary sinus in relation to the posterior aspect of the mitral valve. M = mitral valve; black arrow = the coronary sinus and great cardiac vein; white arrow = the constraint device and distal anchor; black arrowhead = 8F guide sheath. **(B)** Fluoroscopic device image in animal model. White arrow = the constraint device and distal anchor; black arrow head = 8F guide sheath. (Courtesy of Cardiac Dimensions, Kirkland, WA.)

nificantly decreased from 6.5 ± 2.2 to 0.4 ± 0.5 cm^2 ($p < 0.03$). As preliminary human experience, several patients underwent temporary device placement immediately prior to the mitral valve repair surgery, confirming the feasibility of this technique in humans as well.

WIRE-BASED IMPLANT DEVICE

A wire-based implantable device is being developed and has been tested in an animal model of heart-failure-induced MR (Cardiac Dimensions, Kirkland, WA) (Fig. 12). The device is constructed of nitinol wire with distal and proximal anchors connected by an intervening cable. In a feasibility study using a tachycardia-paced chronic heart failure MR model of sheep, an 8F guide sheath containing the device was placed in the coronary sinus/great cardiac vein via a 9F right internal jugular vein sheath *(18)*. The distal anchor was first deployed into the distal great cardiac vein and locked in position. Tension was then applied to the device and maintained while the proximal anchor was deployed into the body of the coronary sinus and locked in position. After the device insertion, the mitral annular septal–lateral dimension was reduced by $25 \pm 2.5\%$, resulting in a substantial reduction in heart-failure-induced MR (MR/left atrium area ratio: $42 \pm 6\%$ to $4 \pm 3\%$; $p = 0.003$). This was accompanied by significant improvement in pulmonary capillary wedge pressure (26 ± 3 to 18 ± 3 mm Hg; $p < 0.01$) and cardiac output (3.4 ± 0.3 to 4.3 ± 0.4 L/min, $p = 0.01$).

HEAT ENERGY APPROACH

A heat energy approach could be a unique alternative to the implantable coronary sinus annuloplasty devices (QuantumCor, Lake Forese, CA). The principle mechanism is to shrink annular collagen by the heat generated with a coronary sinus probe, improving

A **B**

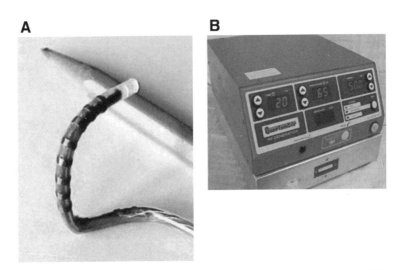

Fig. 13. The heart energy annuloplasty device: **(A)** experimental heart energy probe; **(B)** prototype RF energy generator. (Courtesy of Quantumcor, Lake Forese, CA.)

mitral competence without implanted materials. The prototype catheter has eight electrodes (approx 1.5×2 mm), and the tip of the probe is malleable to conform to the annulus shape (Fig. 13). Delivery of radio-frequency (RF) energy to the electrodes is computer controlled by maximum temperatures sensed by adjacent thermocouples. In a preliminary sheep study, variable degrees of acute annular contraction could be achieved: The reduction in A-P distance of the mitral annulus was 0% (sham) to 26%. At necropsy, there was no evidence of thrombosis or damage to coronary arteries or cardiac vein. Long-term animal studies are ongoing.

Potential Limitations

There are several potential issues particular to percutaneous coronary sinus repair of MR. As described previously, the relative position of the coronary sinus to the mitral annulus can significantly affect the effectiveness of this technique (Fig. 14). In a study by von Ludinghausen, based on detailed dissections of 350 human cadaveric hearts, the widely postulated location of the coronary sinus in the left posterior coronary sulcus was found in only 12% of the cases studied. In most specimens, the coronary sinus was in a displaced position toward the posterior wall of the left atrium. The displacement or elevation was slight (1–3 mm) in 16% of the cases, moderate (4–7 mm) in 50%, and extreme (8–15 mm) in 22% *(24)*. Acceptable degrees of coronary sinus displacement for this technique remain to be investigated.

Other possible issues include the following: the venous valves that might make direct catheter cannulation difficult in some patients; potential damage, pinching, or stent deformation of the adjacent circumflex coronary artery; and significant mitral annular calcification that might limit the annuloplasty effect (Fig. 15), as also discussed previously. Additionally, the congested coronary sinus space as a result of the implant device inside might affect the hemodynamics of cardiac circulation in the short or long term. The risks of coronary sinus thrombosis/occlusion and erosion/perforation over the long term need to be determined as well.

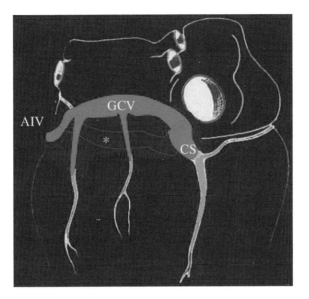

Fig. 14. Elevation of the CS from the posterior coronary sulcus (atrio-ventricular grove) to the posterior wall of the left atrium. AIV = anterior interventricular vein; GCV = great cardiac vein; CS = coronary sinus; the asterisk indicates the left atrio-ventricular grove. (Courtesy of LANDES Bioscience, Texas, USA.)

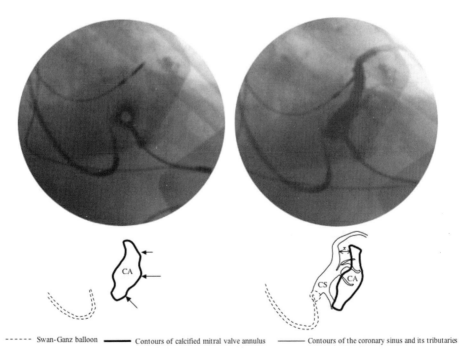

Fig. 15. Mitral annular calcification and coronary sinus venography by retrograde contrast injection with proximal balloon occlusion: **(A)** significant mitral annular calcification (black arrow); **(B)** relationship between the coronary sinus/great cardiac vein and mitral annular calcification. The coronary sinus/great cardiac vein were in a displaced position toward the posterior wall of the left atrium. X = the gap between great cardiac vein and mitral annulus; CS = coronary sinus; CA = calcification of annulus.

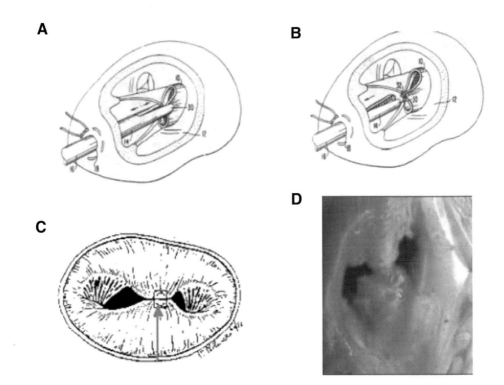

Fig. 16. Surgical edge-to-edge repair method: **(A, B)** Schematic representation of Affieri edge-to-edge repair with central leaflet edge approximation resulting in a double-orfice valve; **(C)** a suture (red arrow) apposes the middle scallop of the posterior (top) and anterior leaflets (bottom); **(D)** animal valve after surgical edge-to-edge repair.

DEVICES ADDRESSING VALVULAR PATHOLOGY

Although mitral annuloplasty is effective for functional MR secondary to heart failure, coexistence of primary valvular pathology, including structural leaflet changes and severely calcified annulus, can limit the number of candidates for this technique. To circumvent this limitation, several surgical methods addressing the valvular pathology have been developed, one of which is the edge-to-edge or Alfieri technique, that creates a so-called double orifice mitral valve with central leaflet suturing (Fig. 16). The simplicity of this technique as well as its clinical success *(27–29)* have encouraged the development of less invasive, catheter-based, edge-to-edge repair technologies. The initial results in a short-term animal model appear promising. Combined use of this method with a percutaneous annuloplasty device could offer further clinical benefit, particularly in high-risk patients with complex MR *(30)*.

Percutaneous Edge-to-Edge Mitral Valve Repair Devices

One prototype system of the percutaneous edge-to-edge repair consists of an implantable V-shaped clip attached to a delivery catheter, and a guide catheter with a bidirectional steering mechanism at the distal tip (Evalve, Redwood City, CA) (Fig. 17). The clip, constructed of implant-grade metals and covered with polyester, is a two-armed, soft tissue approximation device that has an outside diameter of 15F catheter in a closed state with a grasping span of 20 mm. It is designed to vertically coapt up to 8 mm

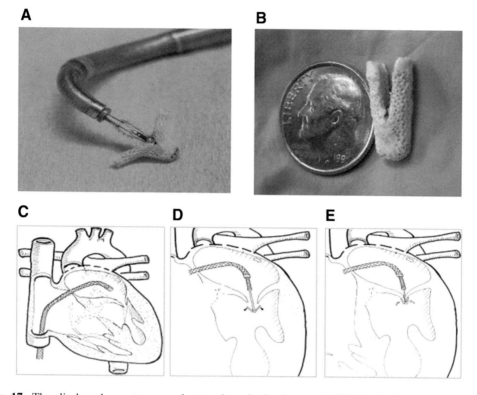

Fig. 17. The clip-based percutaneous edge-to-edge mitral valve repair: **(A)** the distal end of the delivery system and the polyester-covered clip shown in the open position; **(B)** the clip shown in the closed position; **(C)** Schematic of the guide catheter across the atrial septum; **(D)** the tip of the catheter crosses the mitral valve and the clip is opened (black arrow); **(E)** the clip is closed and both leaflets are attached (gray arrow). (Courtesy of Evalve, Redwood City, CA.)

of leaflet height and to promote leaflet-to-leaflet healing around and into the device to maintain a point of permanent leaflet approximation.

The device is placed transseptally into the left atrium using femoral vein access. The implantable clip attached to the delivery catheter is opened, advanced through the mitral orifice, and then retracted to grasp the middle scallops of the anterior and posterior mitral leaflets during systole. If needed, the clip can be opened and repositioned. After a functional double orifice is confirmed by echocardiography, the clip is locked and detached from the delivery system. These manipulations of the clip are all controlled by the delivery catheter handle mechanisms.

In a feasibility study with 14 healthy adult pigs *(31)*, all animals demonstrated a successful double orifice before the final clip detachment (a single grasp, 57%; two attempts, 29%; three attempts, 7%; five attempts, 7%). Immediate postmortem examination revealed that the clip successfully approximated the middle scallops of the anterior and posterior leaflets in all animals, except for two studies in which an incomplete grasp had caused a clip release from the anterior mitral leaflet.

Another percutaneous edge-to-edge repair system is also being developed and is under preclinical testing (Edwards Lifesciences, Irvine, CA). The prototype is delivered using a similar transseptal technique to the above system but utilizes a vacuum mechanism to capture the anterior and posterior mitral leaflets. A double orifice is created with needle stitches of the mitral leaflets, and the suture is fastened with a nitinol clip (Fig. 18). Results of animal studies using this device are pending.

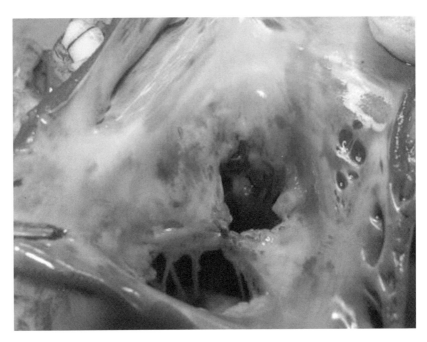

Fig. 18. The suture-based percutaneous edge-to-edge mitral valve repair. Postmortem examination (viewed from the left atrium) in animal model shows well-apposed anterior (right) and posterior (left) mitral valve leaflets.

Potential Limitations

Potential issues particular to percutaneous edge-to-edge repair of MR include large device size (a 24F guide catheter), technically demanding procedures, long-term durability, risk of endocarditis, and leaflet degeneration and stress. In addition, the feasibility and efficacy of this technique might be limited in subsets of patients with extreme pathology including rheumatic disease or a ruptured papillary muscle. Extended animal data are being analyzed, and further technological improvements are ongoing.

THE FUTURE AND POTENTIAL CLINICAL APPLICATIONS

Chronic heart failure is a significant public health problem in the United States, affecting nearly 5 million people, with an estimate of 550,000 new cases diagnosed annually *(32)*. Despite the mounting evidence that surgical correction of secondary MR would provide long-term clinical benefits, patients with severe LV dysfunction are often considered poor operative candidates because of their high perioperative morbidity and mortality. With the advent of novel catheter-based procedures, an exciting new era for percutaneous management of high-risk heart failure patients with functional MR might evolve. In combination with percutaneous devices to address valvular pathology, catheter-based annuloplasty might also offer a therapeutic option for a certain subset of primary MR patients with concurrent comorbidities, such as advanced age, renal failure, cerebral infarction, or respiratory diseases. Furthermore, ischemic MR that is considered reversible might be successfully managed with temporary device placement. Although the experience described in this chapter is derived from first-generation devices, the promising results of preliminary animal studies encourage our future endeavor toward the establishment of safety and efficacy of these technologies in humans.

REFERENCES

1. Miller DC. Ischemic mitral regurgitation redux—to repair or to replace? J Thorac Cardiovasc Surg 2001;122:1059–1062.
2. Gillinov AM, Wierup PN, Blackstone EH, et al. Is repair preferable to replacement for ischemic mitral regurgitation? J Thorac Cardiovasc Surg 2001;122:1125–1141.
3. Bolling SF, Pagani FD, Deeb GM, Bach DS. Intermediate-term outcome of mitral reconstruction in cardiomyopathy. J Thorac Cardiovasc Surg 1998;115:381–386; discussion 387–388.
4. Boltwood CM, Tei C, Wong M, Shah PM. Quantitative echocardiography of the mitral complex in dilated cardiomyopathy: the mechanism of functional mitral regurgitation. Circulation 1983;68:498–508.
5. Trichon BH, Felker GM, Shaw LK, et al. Relation of frequency and severity of mitral regurgitation to survival among patients with left ventricular systolic dysfunction and heart failure. Am J Cardiol 2003;91:538–543.
6. Lamas GA, Mitchell GF, Flaker GC, et al. Clinical significance of mitral regurgitation after acute myocardial infarction. Survival and Ventricular Enlargement Investigators. Circulation 1997;96: 827–833.
7. Trichon BH, O'Connor CM. Secondary mitral and tricuspid regurgitation accompanying left ventricular systolic dysfunction: is it important, and how is it treated? Am Heart J 2002;144:373–376.
8. Robbins JD, Maniar PB, Cotts W, et al. Prevalence and severity of mitral regurgitation in chronic systolic heart failure. Am J Cardiol 2003;91:360–362.
9. Conti JB, Mills RM, Jr. Mitral regurgitation and death while awaiting cardiac transplantation. Am J Cardiol 1993;71:617–618.
10. Blondheim DS, Jacobs LE, Kotler MN, et al. Dilated cardiomyopathy with mitral regurgitation: decreased survival despite a low frequency of left ventricular thrombus. Am Heart J 1991;122:763–771.
11. Harris KM, Sundt TM, 3rd, Aeppli D, et al. Can late survival of patients with moderate ischemic mitral regurgitation be impacted by intervention on the valve? Ann Thorac Surg 2002;74:1468–1475.
12. Bolling SF. Mitral reconstruction in cardiomyopathy. J Heart Valve Dis 2002;11(Suppl 1):S26–S31.
13. Cazeau S, Leclercq C, Lavergne T, et al. Effects of multisite biventricular pacing in patients with heart failure and intraventricular conduction delay. N Engl J Med 2001;344:873–880.
14. Oesterle SN, Reifart N, Hauptmann E, et al. Percutaneous in situ coronary venous arterialization: report of the first human catheter-based coronary artery bypass. Circulation 2001;103:2539–2543.
15. Thompson CA, Nasseri BA, Makower J, et al. Percutaneous transvenous cellular cardiomyoplasty. A novel nonsurgical approach for myocardial cell transplantation. J Am Coll Cardiol 2003;41:1964–1971.
16. Herity NA, Lo ST, Oei F, et al. Selective regional myocardial infiltration by the percutaneous coronary venous route: a novel technique for local drug delivery. Cathet Cardiovasc Intervent 2000;51: 358–363.
17. Liddicoat JR, Mac Neill BD, Gillinov AM, et al. Percutaneous mitral valve repair: a feasibility study in an ovine model of acute ischemic mitral regurgitation. Cathet Cardiovasc Intervent 2003;60:410–416.
18. Kaye DM, Byrne M, Alferness C, Power J. Feasibility and short-term efficacy of percutaneous mitral annular reduction for the therapy of heart failure-induced mitral regurgitation. Circulation 2003;108:1795–1797.
19. Mohl W. Pressure controlled intermittent coronary sinus occlusion—an alternative to retrograde perfusion of arterial blood. In: Mohl W, Wonlner E, Glogar D, eds. The coronary sinus. Darmastadt: Steinkopff 1984;418–423.
20. Platzer W. Atlas der topographischen anatomie. Stuttgart 1982:108–109.
21. Mohl W. Coronary sinus interventions in cardiac surgery. 2000.
22. Thebesius AC. De circulo sanuinis in corde. Lugduni Batavorum 1708.
23. Hellerestein HK, Orbison JL. Anatomic variations of the orfice of the human coronary sinus. Circulation 1961;3:1–35.
24. v. Ludinghausen M, Schott C. Microanatomy of the human coronary sinus and its major tributaries. Darmastadt: Steinkopff 1990:93–122.
25. Marshall J. On the development of the great anterior veins in man and mammalia; including and account of certain remnants of foetal structure found in the adult, a comparative view of these grate veins in the different mammalia, and an analysis of their occasional perculiaritis in the hehuman subject. Philos Trans R Soc Lond 1950;140:133–170.
26. Bailey LR, Luna-Guerra J, Sheahan B, et al. A percutaneous approach for the treatment of mitral regurgitation evaluated in the healthy bovine model. Am J Cardiol 2002;90(6A).

27. Maisano F, Torracca L, Oppizzi M, et al. The edge-to-edge technique: a simplified method to correct mitral insufficiency. Eur J Cardiothorac Surg 1998;13:240–245; discussion 245–246.
28. Maisano F, Schreuder JJ, Oppizzi M, et al. The double-orifice technique as a standardized approach to treat mitral regurgitation due to severe myxomatous disease: surgical technique. Eur J Cardiothorac Surg 2000;17:201–205.
29. Totaro P, Tulumello E, Fellini P, et al. Mitral valve repair for isolated prolapse of the anterior leaflet: an 11-year follow-up. Eur J Cardiothorac Surg 1999;15:119–126.
30. Alfieri O, Maisano F, De Bonis M, et al. The double-orifice technique in mitral valve repair: a simple solution for complex problems. J Thorac Cardiovasc Surg 2001;122:674–681.
31. St Goar FG, Fann JI, Komtebedde J, et al. Endovascular edge-to-edge mitral valve repair: short-term results in a porcine model. Circulation 2003;108:1990–1993.
32. O'Connell JB, Bristow MR. Economic impact of heart failure in the United States: time for a different approach. J Heart Lung Transplant 1994;13:S107–S112.

5

Percutaneous Mitral Valve Repair with the Edge-to-Edge Technique

Frederick G. St. Goar, MD, James I. Fann, MD, Ted E. Feldman, MD, Peter C. Block, MD, and Howard C. Herrmann, MD

CONTENTS

INTRODUCTION
SURGICAL MANAGEMENT
DEVELOPMENT OF PERCUTANEOUS TECHNOLOGY
DESCRIPTION OF THE EVALVE™ REPAIR SYSTEM
PRECLINICAL RESULTS
EARLY HUMAN EXPERIENCE
THE FUTURE
CONCLUSIONS
REFERENCES

INTRODUCTION

Mitral regurgitation (MR), a common finding, is clinically significant, in part the result of its detrimental effect on left ventricular function. Patients with mild MR can remain asymptomatic for many years. However, moderate to severe MR gradually produces ventricular contractile dysfunction and dilation. Although left ventricular filling pressures are initially maintained in the near-normal range, ultimately left ventricular failure occurs and clinical symptoms develop. Because MR causes volume overload of the left ventricle, a vicious cycle develops. Volume overload leads to remodeling with left ventricular dilation and consequent left ventricular dysfunction. Left ventricular dilation also produces abnormalities of mitral valve support and enlargement of the mitral annulus. These changes lead to progressive worsening of MR *(1)*.

When MR is caused by pathology specific to the valve leaflets such as myxomatous degeneration it is referred to as degenerative MR. Mitral regurgitation that is a consequence of ventricular or annular abnormalities, including cardiomyopathy or left ventricular or papillary dysfunction as a result of ischemia, is referred to as functional MR. In patients with symptomatic moderate to severe, or severe MR (i.e., greater than grade 2), surgical

From: *Contemporary Cardiology: Interventional Cardiology:*
Percutaneous Noncoronary Intervention
Edited by: H. C. Herrmann © Humana Press Inc., Totowa, NJ

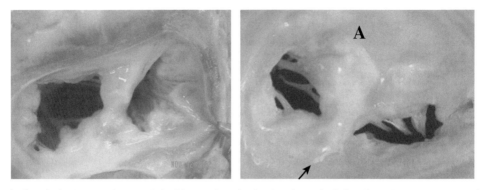

Fig. 1. Surgical edge-to-edge repair looking at the mitral valve from the left atrium. A suture apposes the middle scallop of the posterior **(top)** and anterior **(bottom)** leaflets creating a double-orifice valve **(right)**. On the left is shown the 6-mo healing response of the clip in a porcine model.

intervention is recommended. Surgery is also recommended for asymptomatic patients with severe MR who have evidence of left ventricular dysfunction, atrial fibrillation, or pulmonary hypertension *(2)*.

SURGICAL MANAGEMENT

The preferred technique for the surgical management of mitral regurgitation is a repair procedure *(3,4)*. Patients undergoing mitral valve repair have consistently demonstrated improved- short and long-term outcomes when compared to patients who receive a mitral valve prosthesis *(5)*. In spite of these favorable results, mitral valve repair is still performed in less than half of patients undergoing mitral valve surgery *(6)*. Valve replacement is selected based on anatomic limitations, including leaflet pathology and/or a severely calcified annulus, patient comorbidities, and surgeon experience and preference. Complex valvular pathology potentially compromises the outcome of a repair *(7)*. In order to expand the number of potential candidates for repair, surgeons have developed novel techniques, including chordal shortening and transposition, sliding leaflet repair, and the edge-to-edge, or Alfieri, technique *(8)*. First described for repair of anterior leaflet prolapse in 1991, the edge-to-edge technique involves apposing the middle scallops of the anterior and posterior leaflet with a stitch creating a so-called "dual" or "double-orifice" mitral valve (Fig. 1, right). This approach has been successfully used to treat MR resulting from prolapse of either one or both leaflets, as well as for functional regurgitation secondary to ischemia or cardiomyopathy *(9,10)*.

In a recent report from Alfieri's group, central double-orifice repair was performed in 260 patients followed for up to 7 yr *(11)*. The majority (81%) of the patients had degenerative etiology. At 5 yr, survival was 94% and freedom from reoperation was 90%. Freedom from reoperation was lower (72% vs 92%) in patients who did not undergo a concomitant annuloplasty procedure; however, annuloplasty was not a multivariable predictor of freedom from reoperation *(11)*. A subpopulation evaluation of Alfieri's extensive experience revealed a 97% 3-yr freedom from reoperation in a group of 29 patients who underwent an intention-to-treat isolated edge-to-edge repair *(12)*. The clinical success and simplicity of this technique has thus prompted interest in the development of a catheter-based technology that would enable the interventional cardiologist to perform a percutaneous, endovascular valve repair in the cardiac catheterization laboratory.

DEVELOPMENT OF PERCUTANEOUS TECHNOLOGY

Initial attempts at developing a technology that could be used to perform an edge-to-edge repair on a beating heart were reported by Oz and colleagues *(13)*. They described their experience with a mitral valve "grasper" placed through a left ventriculotomy to appose the center of the anterior and posterior leaflets with a graduated spiral screw. Experimentally, explanted adult human mitral valves were mounted in a mock circulatory loop, which could simulate various hemodynamic conditions. In vitro, the mitral screw remained attached to the valve leaflets during durability testing of over 6.8 million cycles. Percent regurgitant flow was decreased from $72 \pm 7\%$ to $34 \pm 17\%$ ($p = 0.0025$). In vivo, seven dogs had the grasper/coil placed under direct vision via a ventriculotomy or atriotomy. At 48 h, coaptation of the mitral leaflets was demonstrated and with no evidence of MR. Two animals were followed to 12 wk, at which time the device was integrated into the tissue of both leaflets.

Alfieri et al. reported experience with a suture-based edge-to-edge approach delivered via a thoracotomy and placed via the left atrium *(14)*. In eight adult sheep, using suction to stabilize the leaflets, a single suture was successfully placed across the center of the two mitral leaflets. A specially designed knot pusher with integrated cutter was used to tie and cut the suture. The authors proposed that their technique may be applicable to the surgical treatment of ischemic MR in conjunction with revascularization procedures or MR in heart failure patients.

Another group of investigators initially also pursued an endovascular edge-to-edge repair technique using a suture-based approach. The system evolved into a catheter-delivered, steerable, and repositionable clip that grasps the leaflets from the ventricular aspect and then immobilizes them from the atrial aspect, each in a reversible fashion. This technology is now used for endovascular percutaneous cardiovascular valve repair (CVRS, Evalve™, Redwood City, CA) *(15)*.

DESCRIPTION OF THE EVALVE™ REPAIR SYSTEM

The system consists of a steerable guide catheter, a separately steerable clip delivery system, and an implantable clip. The system is inserted percutaneously and advanced to the mitral valve via a transseptal approach. The clip is advanced through the mitral valve orifice and, under echocardiographic guidance, is used to grasps the leaflets from the ventricular side. The clip is detached from the delivery system after MR has been satisfactorily reduced. The specific components of the system are described in more detail below.

Evalve Clip

Mounted on the distal end of the CVRS, the Evalve Clip, is a two-armed, soft tissue grasping and approximating device that, when closed, has an outside diameter of 15F, and in its grasping position, it spans 20 mm. It is designed to vertically coapt up to 8 mm of leaflet height and 4 mm of width to replicate the Alfieri surgical approach in length and width of tissue apposition. It is constructed of implant-grade metals and the clip is covered with polyester (Fig. 2). On the atrial side of the clip are "grippers," which are small, flexible, multipronged friction elements that appose and stabilize tissue against the clip arms. After leaflet tissue is captured between the arm and gripping components, the clip is closed and deployed in a locked position. The clip is designed to promote leaflet-to-leaflet healing around and into the device in order to allow the development of a point of tissue-supported permanent leaflet approximation. The clip can be repositioned using real-time echo assessment to attain the best possible result before final deployment.

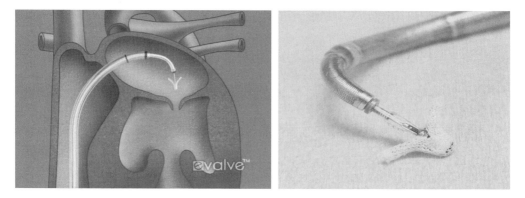

Fig. 2. Distal end of the delivery system and polyester-covered clip shown in the open position (**left**: schematic; **right**: actual).

Device Overview

The CVRS consists of a 24F steerable guide catheter with a 22F distal end, which is introduced via the femoral vein and placed across the atrial septum using standard transseptal techniques. The distal end of the guide catheter has a multidirectional steering mechanism. Once in the left atrium, the tip of the guide is positioned over the mitral valve using handle torque and steering. The repositionable clip attached to the delivery catheter is then introduced through the guide catheter in a closed position. The two arms of the clip are opened in the left atrium once the clip is aligned with the long axis of the heart near the origin of the MR jet. Under echocardiographic guidance, the arms are rotated until they are perpendicular to the line of leaflet coaptation. The open, aligned clip is advanced across the mitral orifice and then retracted to grasp the leaflets during systole (Fig. 3). The atrial grippers with frictional elements are lowered onto the atrial side of the leaflets, approximating (capturing) and stabilizing leaflet tissue against the arms on the ventricular side of the leaflet. When a double orifice has been demonstrated by echocardiography, the clip arms are closed in a locked position. If needed, the grippers can be raised, the clip can be reopened, and the system repositioned. Opening, closing, locking, and deployment of the clip are all controlled by delivery catheter handle mechanisms. Once a functional double orifice has been confirmed and MR sufficiently reduced, the clip is detached from the delivery system.

PRECLINICAL RESULTS

The clip system was tested in a physiologic bench model of MR. The model was created by removing the left atrium of an isolated pig heart and transsecting primary chordae of the middle scallop of the posterior leaflet. With the heart immersed in a warm water bath, a tube was placed through the left ventricular apex, and the ventricular pressure varied to mimic the cardiac cycle and create physiologic mitral leaflet motion. The clip was positioned in the left atrium over the line of leaflet coaptation, then advanced through the mitral orifice, pulled back to grasp the leaflets, and closed to coapt tissue. When the clip resolved turbulent regurgitation through the valve (i.e., MR), it was detached from the delivery catheter.

The CVRS was refined for percutaneous endovascular delivery in an acute porcine model. This included development of a steerable guide catheter, delivered transseptally into the left atrium via femoral vein access. In a recently reported study, a double orifice

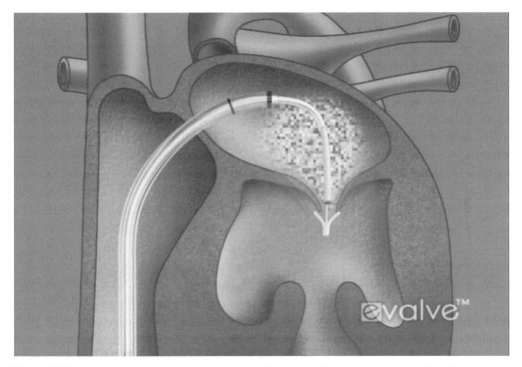

Fig. 3. CVRS guide catheter across atrial septum. The clip delivery system is positioned through the guide. The clip is in the open position in the left ventricle, ready to be retracted to grasp mitral leaflets.

was created in 14 anesthetized normal adult pigs. Direct epicardial echocardiographic guidance was used to place the clip *(15)*. A double orifice was created in all 14 animals, sometimes requiring several grasps. There was no MR or echocardiographic evidence of mitral stenosis after clip deployment. In two animals, the clip released from the anterior leaflet, retrospectively determined to be related to an improper grasping technique with the clip not fully opened. Acute postmortem analysis confirmed a double orifice in 12 pigs with clip deployment perpendicular to the line of coaptation.

Separate chronic animal studies were conducted to evaluate the healing response of the clip with extended follow-up *(16)*. At 4 wk, the entire clip was encapsulated in a layer of tissue. There was evidence of tissue deposition and leaflet-to-leaflet healing. At 12 wk, tissue encapsulation was further developed with leaflet-to-leaflet bridging between the arms of the clip. At 24 wk, development of mature solid tissue bridging was present (Fig. 4). Scanning electron microscopy of three mitral valves (one each at 4 wk, 12 wk, and 24 wk) showed complete tissue encapsulation of the clip with endothelial cells on the surface. In summary, the clip became well incorporated into the valve leaflets, with no significant tissue growth beyond the sides of the clip or evidence of tissue necrosis between the clip arms. Privitera et al. recently reported surgical pathological findings of a patient who received isolated edge-to-edge repair and then 4 yr later underwent cardiac transplantation for progressive heart failure in spite of a competent mitral valve *(17)*. The point of suture apposition of the leading edge of the anterior and posterior mitral leaflets was shown to be encapsulated with endothelial tissue with a functional fibrous bridge. The pathological findings demonstrated at 6 and 12 mo follow-up in the Evalve porcine model are remarkably similar to the pathology of the 4-yr surgical result.

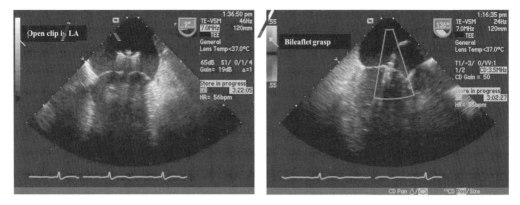

Fig. 4. Still-frame transesophageal images of the open clip positioned in the left atrium before advancement through the mitral valve **(left)** and after grasping of both leaflets prior to release from the clip delivery system **(right)**.

The efficacy of the clip was evaluated in an acute in vivo model of MR. Regurgitation was created by transecting primary chordae of the middle posterior leaflet scallop. After successful placement of the clip, serial echocardiography demonstrated durable resolution of MR in animals with chordal transaction. In addition, in one animal with moderate intrinsic (i.e., functional MR), the regurgitation resolved with clip placement and the animal remained free of MR at midterm follow-up. Subsequent pathological examination confirmed a double-orifice valve and full tissue encapsulation of the clip.

EARLY HUMAN EXPERIENCE

Investigational Device Exemption (IDE) approval was obtained by Evalve, Inc. to proceed with a human Phase I safety and feasibility trial (EVEREST 1). The results for the first 27 patients treated in this trial were recently reported (*23*). Mean patient age was 69 years, 59% were male, 44% were New York Heart Association class III or IV, and 41% were in atrial fibrillation. The mitral regurgitation etiology was degenerative in 93% of patients, and ishemic in 2 patients (7%).

A clip was implanted in 24 of 27 patients. The 3 patients in whom a clip was not was placed were among the first 7 patients treated and represent an important part of the early learning curve. Successful edge-to-edge leaflet coaptation with creation of a double orifice could be performed in all 27 patients. Of the 24 in whom a clip was deployed, 67% had resultant 2+ or less mitral regurgitation at discharge.

The primary endpoint of major adverse events was noted in only four patients. One patient had a neurologic deficit classified as a stroke, with full recovery later. A clip detached from one of the two mitral leaflets in three patients, without embolization in any cases. There were no cases of cardiac surgery for failed clip, myocardial infarction, cardiac tamponade. or septicemia. The echocardiography core lab evaluation of mitral regurgitation in post roll-in patients showed a decrease of MR severity from 3.7 at baseline to 1.6 at 30 d.

Among patients who required surgery after clip placement, a repair was performed in 83%. One patient underwent late valve replacement. It is of critical importance that the option for surgical repair was preserved in all patients, even when surgery was performed for inadequate control of the mitral regurgitation greater than 30 d after clip implantation.

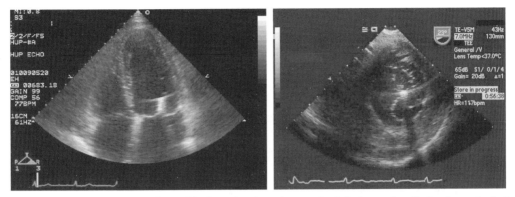

Fig. 5. Transthoracic echocardiographic four-chamber view on the left shows the clip in place attached to the ventricular side of both mitral leaflets 24 h postprocedure. On the right, a gastric short-axis TEE view of a clip not yet released in a different patient documents the double inlet opening of the mitral valve (see video 2 for real-time movie).

For purposes of illustration, we describe the technique and results in the first patient (worldwide case number 3) treated at the Hospital of the University of Pennsylvania. This 55-yr-old man had a remote history of cardiomyopathy, with predominant resolution of his left ventricular dysfunction (ejection fraction about 50%). Other medical problems included a history of mitral valve prolapse with mild MR, mild chronic obstructive pulmonary disease (COPD) secondary to smoking, and insignificant coronary artery disease. Three months prior to admission, the patient presented in respiratory distress with new-onset, rapid atrial fibrillation. Echocardiography demonstrated moderate to severe (3+) MR. After medical stabilization, anticoagulation, and rate control and having met EVEREST I eligibility requirements, the patient was offered percutaneous edge-to-edge valve repair and signed informed consent.

On the day of his procedure, the patient underwent right and left heart catheterization, transesophageal echocardiogram (TEE) evaluation, and DC cardioversion prior to percutaneous valve repair. Baseline hemodynamic data were notable for a mean pulmonary capillary wedge pressure of 20 mm Hg, and echocardiography confirmed the presence of moderate–severe MR (Fig. 5). The vena contracta diameter was 0.58 cm and the peak systolic pulmonary venous flow was reduced to 30 cm/s.

The procedure was performed as described above utilizing a combination of echocardiographic and fluoroscopic imaging. Most of the initial positioning was done using TEE with final clip orientation in a short-axis view from transthoracic echocardiogram (TTE). In some patients, TTE short-axis views might be limited, requiring transgastric TEE or intracardiac echocardiographic views. Multiple leaflet grasps were made before a final position was deemed successful. The clip was then deployed, catheters removed, and hemostasis obtained by manual compression.

Clinical follow-up, including transthoracic (TTE) echocardiography, is required prior to hospital discharge and at 1 and 6 mo per protocol. The quantitative echocardiographic measurements were improved at 1 mo, with an increase in peak systolic pulmonary venous flow to 46 cm/s, mild to moderate MR by color-flow jet, and the patient remains in NYHA class II. The patient remains improved with no change in the final grade of MR at 6 mo follow-up. Representative images from this patient are shown in Figs. 4–6. Videos depicting a grasp both angiographically (video 1) and on transesophageal echocardiography (video 2) are shown on the accompanying CD-ROM.

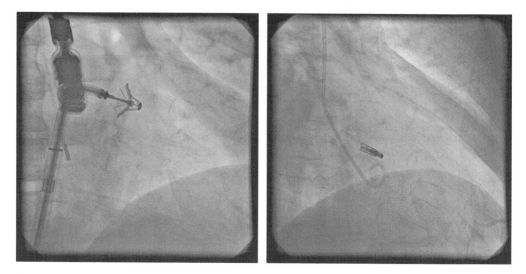

Fig. 6. Angiographic still frames depict the open clip **(left)** with the grippers down after a grasp just before clip closure. The mitral leaflets are held between the grippers and the clip. On the right is shown the final clip placement after closure and release.

THE FUTURE

The Endovascular Valve Edge-to-Edge Repair Study (EVEREST I) is currently underway in the United States and will provide initial information on safety and feasibility of the procedure. The EVEREST I trial inclusion criteria include symptomatic moderate to severe or severe MR or asymptomatic subjects with compromised left ventricular function. All patients must be candidates for mitral valve surgery. Based on the early clinical experience in this ongoing trial, percutaneous edge-to-edge mitral valve repair appears safe, and the degree of mitral regurgitation can be significantly reduced in the majority of treated patients. In several patients, MR was not sufficiently reduced. In these patients, it was elected not to deploy a clip and it was safely removed. These patients subsequently received mitral valve surgery on an elective basis. A future option for patients in whom a single clip does not adequately resolve the MR would be the use of a second clip.

The clinical success and durability of the surgical edge-to-edge repair, both with and without an annuloplasty ring, has been well documented *(18,19)*. Although a free-standing, intention-to-treat edge-to-edge technique is rarely performed at the time of surgical repair, the extensive Alfieri experience supports a clinical potential for this approach *(12)*. Multiple endovascular indirect annuloplasty ("sinoplasty") systems are in preclinical development and could also offer adjunctive technology in situations of extreme pathology *(20)*. A technique that facilitates valve repair without adjunctive annuloplasty potentially allows for more physiologic ventricular contraction, as annular motion contributes significantly to ventricular dynamics. By fastening the leaflets together, the edge-to-edge repair ensures a fixed area of effective coaptation. With this technique, the remainder of the coaptation line closes physiologically without disturbing subvalvular or annular architecture and function. This might significantly impact left ventricular hemodynamics and avoid the compromise in cardiac output frequently seen in patients after mitral valve replacement.

Improved postoperative functional status and overall freedom from reoperation for surgical edge-to-edge repair has been reported to be 95% at 6 yr *(9)*. Durability of the repair technique is supported by a mathematical model of mitral valve stresses and net force, which are shown to be minimal at the point of leaflet coaptation *(21)*. The greatest stress on the leading edge of the leaflets, which is the point of apposition, occurs in diastole when the transvalvular gradient is typically only several millimeters of mercury. In this theoretical model, systolic forces applied to the valve by the left ventricle at the coaptation site are not only parallel to the annulus but the force on each leaflet is also symmetrical and opposite the force on the opposing leaflet. This favors minimal systolic stress a the site of the edge-to-edge repair where theoretically normalized coaptation occurs *(22)*.

CONCLUSIONS

The surgical edge-to-edge repair has been shown to be an effective method for repairing either structurally or functionally deficient mitral valves. The catheter-based Evalve CVRS is the first successful percutaneous endovascular adaptation of this repair technique. While the initial data from the EVEREST I trial are compelling, the strategy for application and indications for this procedure clearly remain to be determined. Based on the success of the feasibility trial for the Evalve clip, the FDA has approved proceeding with a pivotal Phase II trial. This will be a randomized comparison by intention to treat of percutaneous mitral valve repair using the Evalve clip to standard surgical repair with an estimated enrollment of over 250 patients. This and other future studies should help to refine the technique and technology, and establish its clinical applicability. Future studies are also indicated to evaluate the potential for adjunctive catheter-based annuloplasty systems. Given the significant potential for improvement in patient morbidity and mortality, by avoidance of an open-chest incision, cardiac arrest, and cardiopulmonary bypass, it is imperative to develop this and other catheter-based interventions for the management of valvular heart disease. Future studies are also indicated to evaluate the potential for adjunctive catheter-based annuloplasty systems. Given the significant potential for improvement in patient morbidity and mortality, by avoidance of an open-chest incision, cardiac arrest, and cardiopulmonary bypass, it is imperative to develop this and other catheter-based interventions for the management of valvular heart disease.

REFERENCES

1. Enriquez-Sarano M, Nkomo V, Mohty D, Avierinos JF, Chaliki H. Mitral regurgitation: predictors of outcome and natural history. Adv Cardiol 2002;39:133–143.
2. Bonow RO, Carabello B, de Leon AC Jr, et al. Guidelines for management of patients with valvular heart disease: executive summary. Circulation 1998;98:1949–1984.
3. Miller DC. Ischemic mitral regurgitation redux—to repair or to replace? J Thorac Cardiovasc Surg 2001;122(6):1059–1062.
4. Lawrie GM. Mitral valve repair vs replacement: current recommendations and long-term results. Cardiol Clin 1998;16(3):437–448.
5. Enriquez-Sarano M, Schaff HV, Orszulak TA. Valve repair improves the outcome of surgery for mitral regurgitation: a multivariate analysis. Circulation 1995;91(4):1022–1028.
6. STS U.S. Cardiac Surgery Database. Mitral valve repair and replacement patients: incidence of complications summary. www.sts.org (accessed 2002).
7. Fann JI, Ingels NB, Miller C. Pathophysiology of mitral valve disease and operative indications. In: Cardiac surgery in the adult. 15. LH Edmunds, ed. McGraw-New York: 1997:959–987.
8. Galloway AC, Grossi EA, Bizekis CE, et al. Evolving techniques for mitral valve reconstruction. Ann Surg 2002;3:288–294.
9. Umana JP, Salehizadeh B, DeRose JJ, et al. "Bow-tie" mitral valve repair: an adjuvant technique for ischemic mitral regurgitation. Ann Thorac Surg 1998;66:1640–1646.

10. Maisano F, Schreuder JJ, Oppizzi M, et al. The double orifice technique as a standardized approach to treat mitral regurgitation due to severe myxomatous disease: surgical technique, Eur J Cardiothorac Surg 2000;17:201–215.
11. Alfieri O, Maisano F, DeBonis M, et al. The edge-to-edge technique in mitral valve repair: a simple solution for complex problems. J Thorac Cardiovasc Surg 2001;122:674–681.
12. Alfieri O, Maisano F. Intent to treat isolated edge-to-edge mitral valve repair without annuloplasty: clinical proof of principal for an endovascular percutaneous approach. Eur Heart J (In press.)
13. Morales DLS, Madigan JD, Choudhri AF, et al. Development of an off bypass mitral valve repair. Heart Surg Forum 1999;2:115–120.
14. Alfieri O, Elefteriades JA, Chapolini RJ, et al. Novel suture device for beating-heart mitral leaflet approximation. Ann Thorac Surg 2002;74:1488–1493.
15. St. Goar FG, Fann JI, Komtebedde J, et al. Endovascular edge-to-edge mitral valve repair: acute results in a porcine model. Circulation 2003;108:1990–1993.
16. Fann J, St. Goar F, Komtebedde J, et al. Off pump edge-to-edge mitral valve technique using a mechanical clip in a chronic model. Circulation 2003;108:17:IV-493.
17. Privitera S, Butany J, Cusimano RJ, et al. Alfieri mitral valve repair: clinical outcome and pathology. Circulation 2002;106:e173–e174.
18. Gatti G, Crane G, Trane R, et al. The edge-to-edge technique as a trick to rescue an imperfect mitral valve repair. Eur J Cardiothorac Surg 2002;22:817–820.
19. Maisano F, Caldarola A, Blasio A. Midterm results of edge-to-edge mitral valve repair without annuloplasty. J Thorac Cardiovasc Surg 2003;126(6):1987–1997.
20. Herrmann HC. Percutaneous valve repair and replacement. Journal of Invasive Cardiology 2004;16: 59S-64S.
21. Arts T, Meerbaum S, Reneman R, et al. Stresses in the closed mitral valve: a model study. J Biomech 1983; 16:539–527.
22. Votta E, Maisano F, Soncini M, et al. 3-D computational analysis of the stress distribution on the leaflets after edge-to-edge repair of mitral regurgitation. J Heart Valve Dis 2002;11:810–822.
23. Herrmann HC. Wasserman HS, Whitlow PL, Block PC, Gray WA, Foster E, Feldman TE. Percutaneous edge-to-edge mitral valve repair; preliminary results of the EVEREST-I study. Circulation 2004; 10: III-438.

6

Percutaneous Valve Insertion for the Treatment of Calcific Aortic Valve Stenosis

Alain Cribier, MD, *Helene Eltchaninoff,* MD, *Christophe Tron,* MD, *Fabrice Bauer,* MD, *and Martin B. Leon,* MD

CONTENTS

INTRODUCTION

In acquired aortic valve stenosis, aortic valve replacement (AVR) is the treatment of choice, offering symptomatic relief and improving long-term survival of patients. Whereas the rate of operative mortality ranges from 3% to 8% in the majority of cases *(1–3)*, the operative risk is much higher in patients with emergency operation, very old age, advanced NYHA functional classification, associated coronary bypass surgery, or severe left ventricular dysfunction *(4–8)*. However, even in these complicated settings, surgery is known to improve survival over no intervention *(9–12)*. Prolonged life expectancy has resulted in an aging population and, consequently, in an increased number of patients requiring AVR. Balloon aortic valvuloplasty (BAV), introduced in 1986 *(13)*, has been shown to provide a temporary improvement of valvular function and relief of symptoms in patients in whom surgery is considered too high risk or contraindicated *(14–19)*. As a palliative treatment, its use is currently limited to patients who are declined for AVR because of poor clinical condition or severe comorbidities, mainly elderly patients. Given the limited therapeutic options in this subset of patients, there has been interest in the development of a percutaneous delivered aortic valve.

Recently, the development of catheter-based heart valves has become a challenging and fascinating area for research in interventional cardiology. From as early as 1965, several

From: *Contemporary Cardiology: Interventional Cardiology:*
Percutaneous Noncoronary Intervention
Edited by: H. C. Herrmann © Humana Press Inc., Totowa, NJ

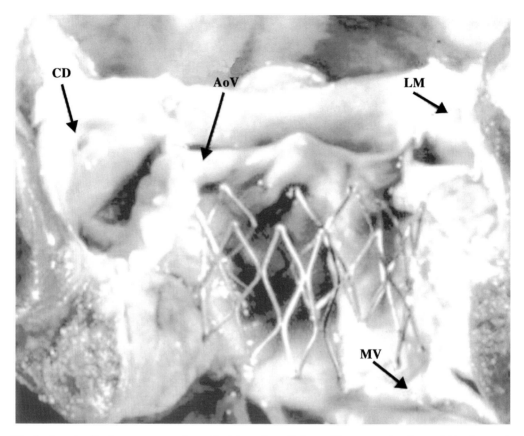

Fig. 1. Longitudinal postmortem view of a 14-cm-long Palmaz–Shatz stent in place within the aortic annulus of a severely calcific aortic valve. In this position, the stent does not impede the coronary ostia or the mitral valve insertion. CD = right coronary artery ostium; LM = left main coronary ostium; AoV = aortic valve; MV = mitral valve insertion.

authors *(20–23)* have reported various catheter-based systems for the treatment of aortic regurgitation that, however, could never lead to human application. Recent advances in stent technology have opened a new way to the development of implantable balloon-expandable valvular prosthesis. In 1992, Andersen et al. *(24)* reported the first animal trial in which a porcine bioprosthesis attached to a wire-based stent was evaluated. This model of percutaneous implantable valve could be successfully delivered at various aortic sites, but despite encouraging experimental results, here again, technical limitations precluded human application. Eight years later, in 2000, Bonhoeffer et al., using a prosthetic heart valve made from bovine jugular vein mounted into a platinum–iridium stent, reported their successful experience of percutaneous implantation into the native pulmonary valve of a lamb *(25)*, followed by the first human implantations of the device in right ventricle to pulmonary artery conduits *(26)*, with satisfactory short-term and midterm results.

In our group, the concept of percutaneous valve replacement emerged in the early 1990s, as a potential option for the treatment of nonsurgical patients with end-stage calcific aortic stenosis for whom BAV was the only therapeutic option. The goal was to improve the results of BAV and to overcome the high restenosis rate associated with this technique *(27–31)*. Personal unpublished autopsy observations on fresh cadavers of patients with calcific aortic stenosis showed that a stent, 23 mm in diameter, could effectively open the native diseased valve, regardless of the amount of calcification, and strongly adhere within it, without impairing the coronary ostia and the mitral valve insertion (Fig. 1). A company interested in the project was identified in 1999 (Percutaneous Valve Technologies, Fort, Lee, NJ, USA). An original percutaneous heart valve (PHV) was developed, which was extensively tested ex vivo and in more than 100 animals *(32)* before being successfully implanted for the first time in a human in April 2002 *(33)*. Since then, several improvements to the PHV device have been made, and the clinical experience was enriched by seven additional patients with end-stage aortic stenosis and multiple comorbidities, in whom the technique was applied on a compassionate basis. The technique used for PHV implantation will be described, followed by an overview of our early clinical experience.

TECHNIQUE OF PERCUTANEOUS VALVE IMPLANTATION

Device Description

The device consists of a PHV, a crimping tool, and a commercially available percutaneous valvuloplasty balloon catheter used for PHV delivery.

THE PHV

The PHV (Fig. 2) is a radio-opaque stainless-steel balloon-expandable stent with an integrated unidirectional trileaflet tissue valve. Initially made of bovine pericardium, the tissue valve is currently made of three equal sections of equine pericardium, preserved in a low-concentration solution of glutaraldeyhyde. The valve is firmly attached by sutures to the stent frame. The stent is 14 mm in length, with a maximal diameter of 22 mm. The PHV durability of this equine pericardial bioprosthesis passed 200 million cycles (5 yr) in bench testing.

CRIMPING TOOL

The crimping tool (Fig. 3) is a reusable compression device that symmetrically reduces the overall diameter of the PHV from its expanded size to its collapsed size. The compression mechanism is manually closed by means of a rotary knob located on the housing. The crimper comprises a check gage used to verify that the balloon assembly is suitable to allow unimpeded introduction via a 24F sheath.

DELIVERY TRANSLUMINAL VALVULOPLASTY BALLOON CATHETER

This catheter is a Z-MED II (NuMed, Inc., Hopkinton, NY, USA) with a shaft size of 9F, a length of 120 cm, with a balloon size of 30 mm in length and 22 mm in diameter at full inflation.

Preprocedural Evaluation

Within a week preceding PHV implantation, baseline transthoracic (TTE) and transesophageal (TEE) echocardiography, cardiac catheterization with hemodynamic measurements, left ventricular and aortic angiograms, and coronary arteriography are obtained to assess the type and severity of aortic stenosis, the amount and distribution of valvular calcification, the aortic annulus diameter, the left ventricular function, and the association of other valvular, coronary, and peripheral artery diseases. These data, together with the patient's clinical status, are crucial for the therapeutic decision.

Procedure of PHV Implantation

The technique is performed under local anesthesia and mild sedation. Aspirin (160 mg) and clopidogrel (300 mg) are administered 24 h before the procedure. The PHV is implanted using the antegrade transseptal approach.

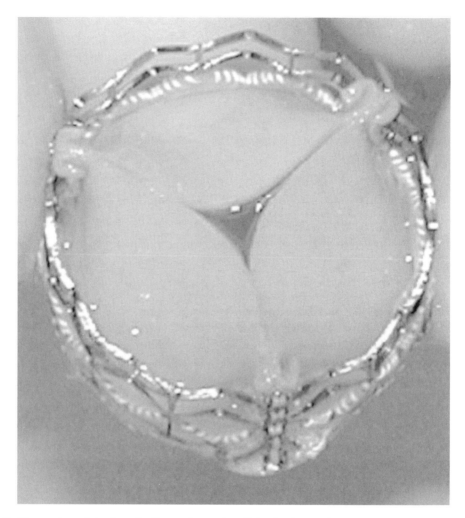

Fig. 2. Upper view of the three-leaflet equine pericardial valve inserted within the stainless-steel stent.

BASELINE MEASUREMENTS

The procedure of PHV implantation starts with a reassessment of some baseline parameters. Through an 8F sheath in the left femoral vein, a 7F Swan–Ganz catheter is advanced to the pulmonary artery and used to measure the right-side pressures and the cardiac output by thermodilution. Through a 6F sheath in the right femoral artery, a 6F pigtail catheter is advanced in the ascending aorta. One or several supraaortic angiograms are performed in order to select the optimal view on which the aortic valvular apparatus projects perpendicular to the screen and the coronary ostia are clearly visible. The antero-posterior view is generally selected and a frame, frozen on another screen, will be used as one marker at the time of PHV implantation. This pigtail catheter will be left in place in the ascending aorta during the entire procedure and used for continuous aortic blood pressure monitoring and post-PHV implantation angiographies. Blood samples are obtained from the aorta and the right cardiac cavities for measurement of oxygen saturation. Finally, through a 6F sheath in the left femoral vein, a 5F pacemaker lead is advanced into the right ventricle. The stimulation parameters are controlled and the pacemaker set on demand at 80 beats/min.

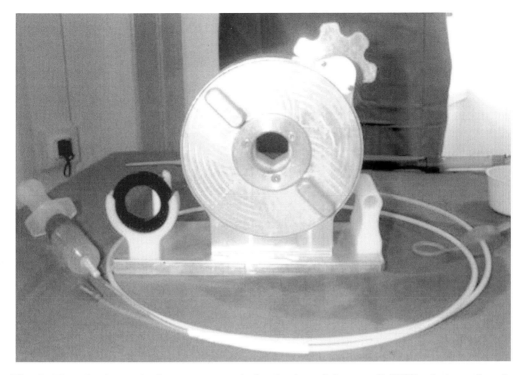

Fig. 3. The crimping tool allows a symmetrical reduction of the overall PHV's diameter from its expanded size to its collapsed size.

TRANSSEPTAL CATHETERIZATION

The regular technique of transseptal catheterization is required, using an 8F Mullins sheath and Brockenbrough needle through the right femoral vein (RFV). We prefer crossing the septum in the 90° left lateral view, at the distal third of a virtual line connecting the aortic valve (showed by the valvular calcification and the distal tip of the pigtail catheter) to the posterior border of the heart (Fig. 4). After completion of the transseptal puncture, heparin, 5000 IU, is administered intravenously.

Through the Mullins sheath in the left atrium, in the right anterior oblique (RAO) 40° position, a 7F Swan–Ganz catheter (Edwards Lifesciences, Irvine, CA, USA) is advanced and used to cross the mitral valve. The transaortic valvular gradient is recorded, using the pressures obtained with the Swan–Ganz catheter and the pigtail catheter in the aorta. The aortic valve area is calculated using the Gorlin formula.

GUIDE WIRE PLACEMENT

The Swan–Ganz catheter with its balloon inflated is advanced inside the left ventricle in such a way that its distal tip faces the native aortic valve. A 0.035-in. straight guide wire is advanced through it and used to cross the aortic valve (Fig. 5A). The Swan–Ganz catheter with its balloon deflated is pushed over the wire into the ascending aorta and the balloon reinflated. The guide wire is then removed.

A 0.035-in. 360-cm-long stiff guide wire (Amplatz, Extra Stiff, COOK, Bjaeverskov, Denmark) is advanced through the Swan–Ganz catheter within the descending aorta (Fig. 5B) and its distal tip positioned at the level of the onset of iliac arteries. The Swan–Ganz catheter with its balloon deflated is then removed, leaving the guide wire in place.

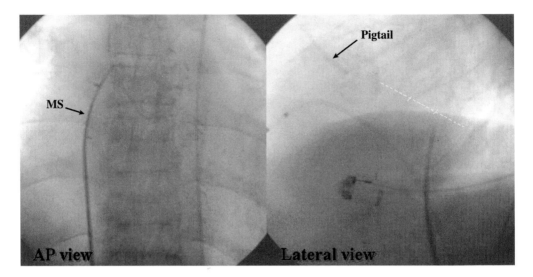

Fig. 4. Technique of transseptal puncture. In the lateral view, the septum is crossed at the distal third of a virtual line traced between the aortic valve and the edge of the heart. MS = Mullins sheath.

Through an 8F sheath in the left femoral artery, a catheter snare (Microvena, Amplatz Goose Neck, GN 2500, White Bear Lake, MN, USA) is used to externalize the long guide wire through the femoral artery (Fig. 5C). During this maneuver, attention must be given to maintain a large guide-wire loop inside the left ventricle in order to avoid any traction of the anterior mitral valve leaflet with the guide wire. Straightening the guide-wire between the mitral valve and the aortic valve might lead to severe mitral regurgitation and subsequent hemodynamic collapse. Thus, the second investigator must push forward the wire from the right femoral vein while the first investigator pulls it out from the left femoral artery. This maneuver should be performed with continuous fluoroscopic control of the intraventricular guide wire loop. The externalized parts of the wire should be equivalent on both sides (about 100 cm).

DILATATION OF THE INTERATRIAL SEPTUM

A 10-mm balloon septostomy catheter (Owens, Boston-Scientific Scimed, Inc, Maple Grove, MN, USA) is advanced over the stiff guide wire through a 10F sheath in the right femoral vein and positioned within the interatrial septum. A 30 : 70 contrast media/saline solution in a 10-mL syringe is used for balloon inflation (Fig. 5D). At least two balloon inflations are performed and held for 30 s. The balloon catheter is then removed.

BALLOON AORTIC PREDILATATION

In the 40° right anterior oblique view, a 23-mm balloon valvuloplasty catheter (Z-Med II; NuMED Canada, Inc, Cornwall, Ontario, Canada) is prepared, purged of air, and advanced over the stiff guide wire through a 14F sheath (COOK, Bjaeverskov, Denmark) in the right femoral vein and positioned across the native aortic valve. During this maneuver, the intraventricular guide wire loop has to be maintained.

With the aortic blood pressure monitored and using a 10 : 90 contrast media/saline solution in a 20-mL syringe, the balloon is fully inflated and deflated (Fig. 6). Two to three balloon inflations are generally performed. The balloon is then deflated and

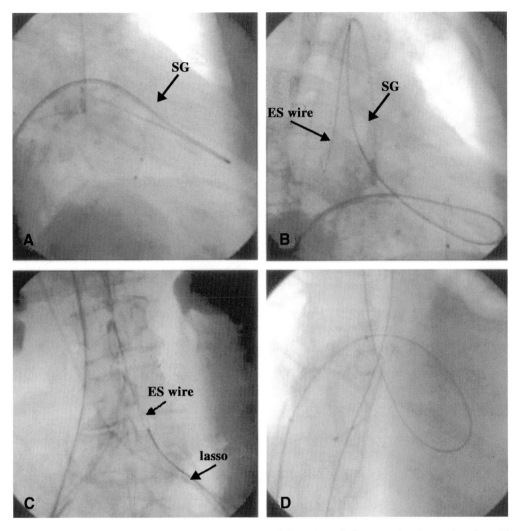

Fig. 5. (A) Position of the distal tip of the Swan–Ganz (SG) catheter before crossing the aortic valve with the 0.035-in. straight guidewire. (B) The 0.035-in. extra-stiff 360-cm-long guidewire is pushed through the Swan–Ganz catheter in the descending aorta. (C) The extra-stiff guide wire (ES wire) is externalized through the left femoral artery using a lasso. (D) Transatrial septum dilatation using a 10-cm-diameter balloon dilatation catheter.

withdrawn. While withdrawing the catheter, the coinvestigator must push forward the guide wire from the right femoral artery in order to maintain the guide-wire loop unchanged in the left ventricle. Of note, the persistence of a notable waist at full balloon inflation would be an exclusion criteria for PHV implantation.

PHV IMPLANTATION

After a meticulous rinsing procedure, the PHV is crimped over the delivery balloon catheter. The balloon is inflated with a 10 : 90 contrast media/saline solution and carefully purged of air. Using a 20-mL syringe, the amount of solution able to obtain a 22-mm balloon diameter at full inflation is determined, using a specially designed 22-mm measuring ring. The balloon is then totally deflated and the PHV crimped over it.

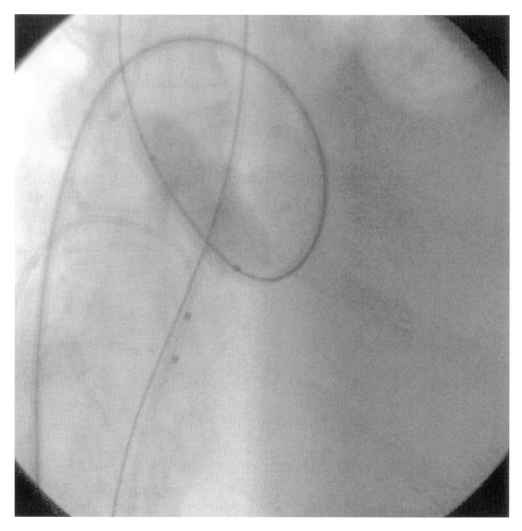

Fig. 6. Predilatation of the native aortic valve using a 23-mm-diameter balloon catheter advanced over the extra-stiff guide wire through the right femoral vein.

Before use, it is checked that the PHV–balloon assembly slides smoothly inside the 24F measuring gage.

From the left femoral artery, A 7F Sones (B-type) catheter is advanced over the stiff 360-cm-long, 0.035-in. guide wire until its distal tip is positioned in the aortic arch, about 2 cm above the aortic valve. The 14F introducer is removed from the right femoral vein and replaced by a 24F introducer (COOK, Bjaeverskov, Denmark). The PHV–balloon assembly is then introduced inside the 24F catheter over the guide wire and advanced across the interatrial septum, through the left atrium, across the mitral valve, and into the left ventricle until its distal tip faces the native aortic valve.

The PHV–balloon assembly is carefully positioned across the native diseased valve. Accurate positioning is facilitated by the use of the Sones catheter inserted on the same wire through the left femoral artery and in contact with the distal end of the delivery balloon catheter. The Sones catheter prevents any uncontrolled ejection of the device in the ascending aorta and is used to push the device backward if necessary (pulling

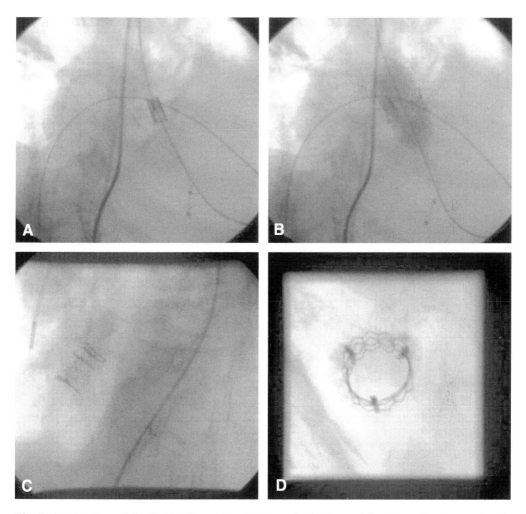

Fig. 7. (**A**) Position of the PHV at the mid-part of the calcifications of the diseased native aortic valve before delivery; (**B**) balloon inflation for PHV delivery; (**C**) the PHV in place within the native aortic valve in the antero-posterior view; (**D**) right anterior oblique cranial view of the PHV confirming the circular shape of the stent frame.

back the device by a traction exerted on the delivery balloon catheter could lead to loss of the large catheter loop in the left ventricle, with the subsequent risk of massive mitral regurgitation and collapse). Using the calcification of the native valve on fluoroscopy and the frozen selected frame of the supra-aortic angiogram as markers, the PHV is accurately positioned at the mid-part of the native valve (Fig. 7A).

Immediately prior to balloon inflation for PHV delivery, rapid (220 beats/min) right ventricular pacing is initiated (Fig. 8). The marked decrease in cardiac output/transaortic blood flow induced by the tachycardia allows for stable balloon inflation across the aortic valve. This fast pacing is interrupted immediately after PHV release and its total duration does not exceed a few seconds. PHV deployment is obtained by balloon inflation using the entire amount of contrast media solution prepared in the syringe and immediately deflated (Fig. 7B). After PHV delivery, the deflated balloon is withdrawn, leaving the guide wire in place across the PHV. A 6F pigtail catheter is pushed over the

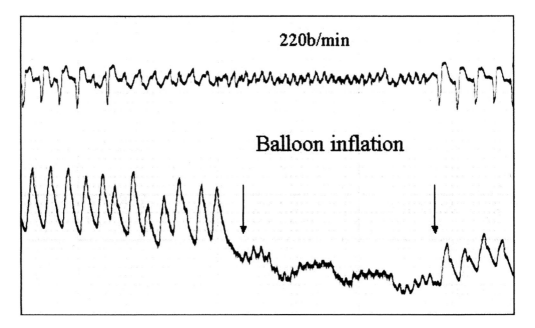

Fig. 8. Aortic blood pressure recording during the PHV delivery phase showing the effect of a 220-beats/min fast right ventricular pacing. The transitory fast-pacing-induced decrease in blood flow allows optimal balloon stabilization at the time of PHV delivery.

guide wire, through the 24F introducer in the right femoral vein and advanced to mid-left ventricle. The 360-cm-long guide wire is then removed by traction from the left femoral vein (Figs. 7C and 7D). The goal of the pigtail catheter is to prevent any injury to the mitral valve apparatus (leaflets and chordaes) by the stiff wire at the time of withdrawal.

ASSESSMENT OF VALVULAR FUNCTION AFTER PHV IMPLANTATION

Using the pigtail catheter in the left ventricle and one of the two catheters in place in the ascending aorta (pigtail or Sones catheters), the trans-PHV systolic pressure gradient is measured (Fig. 9). A Swan–Ganz catheter is advanced through the 24F sheath and used for cardiac output measurement and calculation of the PHV aortic valve area by the Gorlin formula. A supra-aortic angiogram is performed to assess any residual aortic regurgitation (Fig. 10A). A left ventricular angiogram is performed using the pigtail catheter in the left ventricle to assess the ventricular function and the degree of any mitral regurgitation.

The Sones catheter is removed and replaced sequentially by a left and a right coronary Judkins catheter to perform a selective coronary arteriography and assess the patency of the coronary arteries and the position of the coronary ostia with regard to the PHV's upper limits (Fig. 10B and 10C).

END OF PROCEDURE

Before removing all of the catheters, blood samples are obtained from the right and left cavities for measurement of oxygen saturation and assessment of transatrial shunting. All of the catheters are removed. The arterial entry sites are closed with puncture closing devices (Angio-Seal; St. Jude Medical Europe, Zaventem, Belgium). The venous entry sites are closed by manual compression.

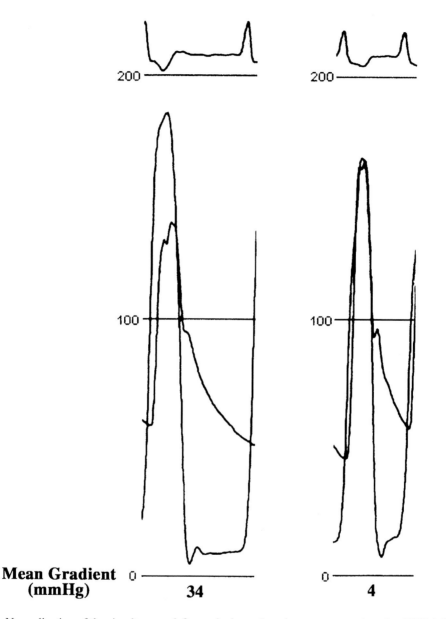

Fig. 9. Normalization of the simultaneous left ventricular and aortic pressures tracing after PHV delivery. The absence of any residual gradient after PHV implantation was observed in all cases.

Clinical and Echocardiographic Follow-up

The patients are closely monitored during follow-up, with clinical assessment and TTE, TEE and Doppler examinations at d1. TTE and Doppler will be repeated at d7 and every month thereafter. Postprocedural treatment includes aspirin (160 mg) and clopidogrel (75 mg) daily. Subcutaneous low-molecular-weight heparin is administered during the hospitalization stay. Oral anticoagulants are given only in patients with chronic atrial fibrillation and started 2d before discharge.

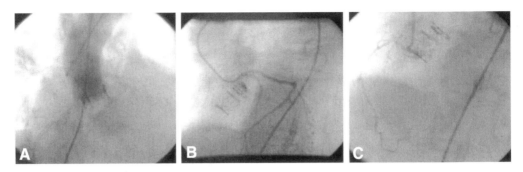

Fig. 10. Post-PHV implantation supra-aortic angiogram showing mild residual aortic regurgitation. **(B,C)** The selective left and right coronary angiographies, respectively, performed after PHV delivery, confirming the patency of the coronary ostia.

CLINICAL EXPERIENCE

Patients

The patients were highly selected on the basis of severely symptomatic calcific aortic stenosis that could benefit from aortic valve replacement, but with an extremely high risk for open heart surgery, and declined by cardiac surgeons. The operative risk was assessed on the association of cardiac and noncardiac factors, including advanced age, severe left ventricular dysfunction, severe associated coronary artery disease, recent stroke or myocardial infarction, and coexisting conditions, including chronic obstructive pulmonary disease, renal failure, cancer, prior cardiac surgery, or other severe comorbidities. The operative risk was also scored according to standard surgical practice and/or surgical risk scoring systems such as the Parsonnet's Score *(34)*.

Exclusion criteria included native aortic annulus <19 mm and >25 mm on baseline echocardiography, patients in whom a 23-mm-balloon inflation could not be fully inflated or displayed a notable waist during the native aortic valve predilatation procedure, thrombus in the left atrium or the left ventricle, pre-existing mitral prosthetic heart valve, evidence of endocarditis, unstented left main coronary artery disease, severe vascular disease preventing vascular access, and severe coagulopathy.

Approval of our Ethical Committee for compassionate PHV was obtained for each case and all patients and their relatives gave informed consent.

Results

Our early experience is based on eight patients, mean age 77 ± 12 yr (57–91 yr) five males and three females, with end-stage severely symptomatic calcific aortic stenosis and multiple potentially lethal comorbidities. Three of these patients were in cardiogenic shock and all were in NYHA functional Class IV. The aortic valve was tricuspid in all but one patient on TEE. Aortic insufficiency was associated with aortic stenosis in three patients, moderate in two, and massive in one. Two patients had associated coronary artery disease with previous stent implantation. Seven patients had previously been treated with BAV, but either restenosed or had a procedure-related complication.

The PHV could be successfully implanted in all but one patient who presented in cardiogenic shock with recurrent aortic stenosis and massive aortic regurgitation 1 mo after a failed BAV complicated by aortic valve rupture and stroke. In this case, the PHV–balloon assembly was ejected in the ascending aorta at full balloon inflation and the patient died shortly thereafter. In all other cases, the PHV could be accurately delivered within the native aortic valve and remained securely anchored. Hemodynamic collapse occurred during the procedure in three patients, requiring temporary cardiac massage and assisted ventilation in two. This complication was consistently associated with the loss of the large catheter loop in the left ventricle with subsequent massive mitral regurgitation. In all three cases, hemodynamics normalized immediately after PHV implantation. There was no other complication. No residual gradient was observed after PHV implantation on hemodynamic recordings. A post-PHV implantation supra-aortic angiogram demonstrated severe aortic regurgitation in two patients and mild regurgitation in six. In all cases, the coronary ostia were above the upper margin of the PHV. PHV function was dramatically improved on postprocedure echocardiographic evaluation with an increase in mean valve area from 0.52 ± 0.09 to 1.69 ± 0.07 cm^2 ($p < 0.028$) and a decrease in mean transvalvular gradient from 44 ± 13 to 5 ± 3 mm Hg ($p < 0.002$). These results remained unchanged during follow-up with thin and flexible leaflets and cylindrical frame shape (Fig. 7D). Aortic regurgitation was paravalvular in all cases and remained unchanged on sequential echocardiographic controls. Mild transatrial shunting was observed in all cases. The mean duration of the procedure was 138 ± 24 min and the mean fluoroscopy time was 29 ± 16 min.

An immediate and dramatic clinical improvement was observed in all patients following PHV implantation with marked reduction of signs of heart failure. This clinical improvement was associated with a clear-cut increase in left ventricular ejection fraction, which improved from 35 ± 21 to 47 ± 17 ($p = 0.03$), from baseline to last echocardiographic control performed 15 d to 2 mo after PHV implantation.

Two patients with pre-existing chronic renal failure developed acute renal failure after the procedure and required short-term (few than three sessions) hemodialysis with recovery of the baseline renal status. The first three patients died at 18, 2, and 4 wk, respectively, of noncardiac causes. The other patients are alive with no sign of heart failure at 8 wk (two patients) and 4 wk (two patients).

The anticoagulant regimen was limited in these patients to antiplatelet therapy, with aspirin (life-long) and clopidogrel (for 1 mo). This treatment was given in order to limit the risk of platelet aggregation on the bioprosthesis stent frame. No oral anticoagulant was prescribed during the hospitalization stay but prophylactic anticoagulation with heparin in the first two cases or subcutaneous heparin thereafter. However, in addition to antiplatelet treatment, oral anticoagulation was administered after discharge in patients with chronic atrial fibrillation.

TECHNICAL CONSIDERATIONS

In this first series of patients, the transseptal antegrade approach was used to reach the aortic valve and deliver the PHV because it seemed to offer several advantages over the more commonly used retrograde route. The antegrade approach allows the large 24F-size sheath to be introduced and removed without surgery, under local anesthesia. Insertion of the introducer in the femoral vein eliminates the risks of arterial complications that might be feared in elderly patients with fragile and often diseased femoro-iliac arteries. The PHV crosses the native aortic valve through the less diseased surface of the aortic leaflets and in a direction coincident with blood flow, offering more predictable valve delivery. The transatrial puncture site dilatation with a 10-mm-diameter balloon did not result in any significant residual shunting. However, the retrograde route might be used in the future in patients with suitable femoral arteries and might be faster and easier to manage. The retrograde approach would also eliminate the risk of periprocedural collapse because of the traction exerted on the mitral valve by the stiff guide wire or the delivery catheter, in the case of loss of the intraventricular loop during the catheterization maneuvers.

Accurate PHV positioning within the native diseased aortic valve, in the subcoronary position, could be obtained in all cases. The aortic valvular calcifications in the antero-posterior view were used as the primordial marker for positioning the device. PHV was delivered with the calcification located at the midpart of the stent frame. The Sones catheter advanced retrogradely from the left femoral artery over the same guide wire appeared very useful to accurately deliver the PHV at the desired site. Furthermore, the brief period of rapid cardiac pacing and subsequent impairment of cardiac output considerably facilitated PHV delivery by optimal stabilization of the PHV–balloon assembly across the aortic valve. This technique is routinely used in our center for BAV and found to be safe and efficient.

In all cases but one, some degree of paravalvular regurgitation was noted after PHV implantation. The paravalvular leak was mild in six patients and severe in two. Even in these two last cases, regurgitation did not prevent improvement of left ventricular function and clinical status. However, severe paravalvular regurgitation might impair the long-term results after PHV implantation. As assessed by TEE, and confirmed on one postmortem observation of a patient with severe aortic regurgitation who died of noncardiac cause (acute abdominal syndrome), the regurgitation is related to imperfect apposition of the stent frame against the native valvular structures, more particularly at the site of valvular commissures or of calcific nodules. Ongoing refinements in stent design and use of a larger stent diameter might decrease the incidence and severity of paravalvular leaks in the future.

FUTURE OF THE PROCEDURE

This preliminary clinical experience confirms the feasibility of implanting a percutaneous bioprosthesis within the native valve of patients with end-stage severely calcific aortic stenosis, using conventional cardiac catheterization techniques, under local anesthesia and sedation, even under life-threatening circumstances. Satisfactory valvular function was achieved, which remained unchanged during follow-up, and was associated with striking clinical and hemodynamic improvement. The superiority of PHV implantation over BAV—the only available palliative therapeutic option in this subset of patients—is already confirmed. With PHV implantation, an orifice valve area of approx 1.7 cm^2 is consistently obtained, with minimal residual transvalvular gradient, which represents a more than threefold increase from baseline valve area. This instantaneous valvular function improvement is associated with marked early and lasting clinical benefit. In comparison, the valve area obtained with balloon valvuloplasty is rarely over 0.8 cm^2 (35) and early restenosis is frequently observed (36–39). If the stability of PHV function is confirmed on midterm and long-term follow-up, as might be expected from ex vivo studies that indicate several years of valve durability, PHV implantation might become an optimal therapeutic option for this subset of patients.

An ongoing pilot study in our center (I-REVIVE study) has been designed to further assess the technical aspects of the procedure and the long-term outcome. Other pilot trials are expected to start in the near future in European and American centers. If the beneficial effect of PHV implantation is confirmed in long-term follow-up, pivotal multicenter trials would be required to determine the role of this promising new therapeutic approach in patients with aortic stenosis and not amenable for surgical valve replacement.

REFERENCES

1. Kvidal P, Bergström R, Hörte L-G, Stahle E. Observed and relative survival after aortic valve replacement. J Am Cardiol. 2000;35:747–756.
2. Culliford AT, Galloway AC, Colvin SB, et al. Aortic valve replacement for aortic stenosis in persons aged 80 years and over. Am J Cardiol 1991;67:1256–1260.
3. Lytle BW, Cosgrove DM, Taylor PC, et al. Primary isolated aortic valve replacement. Early and late results. J Thorac Cardiovasc Surg 1989;97:675–694.
4. Morris JJ, Schaff HV, Mullany CJ, et al. Determinants of survival and recovery of left ventricular function after aortic replacement. Ann Thorac Surg 1993;56:22–29.
5. Connolly HM, Oh JK, Schaff HV, et al. Severe aortic stenosis with low transvalvular gradient and severe left ventricular dysfunction. Results of aortic valve replacement in 52 patients. Circulation 2000;101:1940–1946.
6. Logeais Y, Langanay T, Roussin R, et al. Surgery for aortic stenosis en elderly patients. A study of surgical risk and predictive factors. Circulation 1994;90:2891–2898.
7. Levinson JR, Akins CW, Mortimer JB, et al. Octogenarians with aortic stenosis. Outcome after aortic valve replacement. Circulation 1989;80(Suppl I):I-49–I-56.
8. Sharony R, Grossi EA, Saunders PC, et al. Aortic valve replacement in patients with impaired ventricular function. Ann Thorac Surg 2003;75:1808–1814.
9. Pereira JJ, Lauer MS, Bashir M, et al. Survival after aortic valve replacement for severe aortic stenosis with low transvalvular gradients and severe left ventricular dysfunction. J Am Coll Cardiol 2002;39:1356–1365.
10. Natsuaki M, Itoh T, Tomita S, Naito K. Reversibility of cardiac dysfunction after valve replacement in elderly patients with severe aortic stenosis. Ann Thorac Surg 1998;65:1634–1638.
11. Lund O, Magnussen K, Knudsen M, et al. The potential for normal long term survival and morbidity rates after valve replacement for aortic stenosis. J Heart Valve Dis 1996;5:258–267.
12. Brogan WC 3rd, Grayburn PA, Lange RA, Hillis LD. Prognosis after valve replacement in patients with severe aortic stenosis and low transvalvular pressure gradient. J Am Coll Cardiol 1993;21:1657–1660.
13. Cribier A, Savin T, Saoudi N, et al. Percutaneous transluminal valvuloplasy of acquired aortic stenosis in elderly patients: an alternative to valve replacement? Lancet 1986;1:63–67.
14. Isner JM, Salem DN, Desnoyer MR, et al. Treatment of calcific aortic stenosis by balloon valvuloplasty. Am J Cardiol 1987;59:313–317.
15. Cribier A, Savin T, Berland J, et al. Percutaneous transluminal balloon valvuloplasty of adult aortic stenosis: report of 92 cases. Am J Cardiol 1987;9:381–386.
16. Safian RD, Berman AD, Diver DJ, et al. Balloon aortic valvuloplasty in 170 consecutive patients. N Engl J Med 1988;319:125–130.
17. Letac B, Cribier A, Koning R, Bellefleur JP. Results of percutaneous transluminal valvuloplasty in 218 adults with valvular aortic stenosis. Am J Cardiol 1988;62:598–605.
18. Eltchaninoff H, Cribier A, Tron C, et al. Balloon aortic valvuloplasty in elderly patients at high risk for surgery, or inoperable. Immediate and mid-term results. Eur Heart J 1995;16:1079–1084.
19. Letac B, Cribier A. Aortic balloon dilatation as a treatment of aortic stenosis: what are the indications? J Interv Cardiol 1993;6:1–6.
20. Davies H. Catheter mounted valve for temporary relief of aortic insufficiency. Lancet 1965;1:250.
21. Moulopoulos SD, Anthopoulos L, Stamanetopoulos S, Stefadorous M. Catheter mounted aortic valves. Ann Thorac Surg 1971;11:423–430.
22. Phillips SJ, Ciborski M, Freed PS, et al. A temporary catheter tip aortic valve: hemodynamic effects on experimental acute aortic insufficiency. Ann Thorac Surg 1976;21:134–137.
23. Matsubara T, Yamazoe M, Tamura Y, et al. Balloon catheter with check valves for experimental relief of acute aortic regurgitation. Am Heart J 1992;124:1002–1008.
24. Andersen HR, Knudsen LL, Hasemkam JM. Transluminal implantation of artificial heart valves: description of a new expandable aortic valve and initial results with implantation by catheter techniques in closed chest pigs. Eur Heart J 1992;13:704–708.
25. Bonhoeffer P, Boudjemline Y, Saliba Z, et al. Percutaneous replacement of pulmonary valve in a right-ventricle to pulmonary-artery conduit with valve dysfunction. Lancet 2000;356:1403–1405.
26. Bonhoeffer P, Boudjemline Y, Saliba Z, et al. Percutaneous replacement of pulmonary valve in a right-ventricle to pulmonary-artery conduit with valve dysfunction. Lancet 2000;356:1403–1405.
27. Block PC, Palacios IF. Clinical and hemodynamic follow up after percutaneous aortic valvuloplasty in the elderly. Am J Cardiol 1988;62:760–763.

28. Bernard Y, Etievent J, Mourand JL, et al. Long-term results of percutaneous aortic valvuloplasty compared with aortic valve replacement in patients more than 75 years old. J Am Coll Cardiol 1992;20:796–801.
29. Otto CM, Mickel MS, Kennedy W, et al. Three-year outcome after balloon aortic valvuloplasty. Insights into prognosis of valvular aortic stenosis. Circulation 1994;89:642–650.
30. Berland J, Cribier A, Savin T, et al. Percutaneous balloon valvuloplasty in patients with severe aortic stenosis and low ejection fraction. Immediate results and 1 year follow up. Circulation 1989;79:1189–1196.
31. Del Cuore MG, Nair CK, Peetz D Jr, et al. Early restenosis following successful percutaneous balloon valvuloplasty for calcific valvular aortic stenosis. Am Heart J 1989;118:181–182.
32. Cribier A, Eltchaninoff H, Borenstein N, et al. Transcatheter implantation of balloon expandable prosthetic heart valves: early results in an animal model. Circulation 2001;104(Suppl II):II-552 (abstract).
33. Cribier A, Eltchaninoff H, Bash A, et al. Percutaneous transcatheter implantation of an aortic valve prosthesis for calcific aortic stenosis: first human description. Circulation 2002;106:3006–3008.
34. Parsonnet V, Dean D, Bernstein AD. A method of uniform stratification of risk for evaluating the results of surgery in acquired adult heart disease. Circulation 1989;79(Suppl I):I-3–I-12.
35. Percutaneous balloon aortic valvuloplasty. Acute and 30-day follow-up results in 674 patients from the NHLBI Balloon Valvuloplasty Registry. Circulation 1991;84:2383–2397.
36. Wang A, Harrison JK, Bashore TM. Balloon aortic valvuloplasty. Prog Cardiovasc Dis 1997;40:27–36.
37. Soyer R, Bouchart F, Bessou JP, et al. Aortic valve replacement after aortic valvuloplasty for calcified aortic stenosis. Eur J Cardiothorac Surg 1996;10:977–982.
38. Lieberman EB, Bashore TM, Hermiller JB, et al. Balloon aortic valvuloplasty in adults: failure of procedure to improve long term survival. J Am Coll Cardiol 1995;26:1522–1528.
39. Letac B, Cribier A, Eltchaninoff H, et al. Evaluation of restenosis after balloon dilatation in adult aortic stenosis by repeat catheterization. Am Heart J 1991;122:55–60.

II   SEPTAL DEFECTS

7

Patent Foramen Ovale
Neurological Considerations

Steven R. Messé, MD, Scott E. Kasner, MD, and Anthony Furlan, MD

CONTENTS

INTRODUCTION

Patent foramen ovale (PFO) and atrial-septal aneurysm (ASA) are congenital cardiac abnormalities that are highly prevalent in the general population. Observational studies have found an association between these anomalies and several neurologic diseases, including stroke, decompression sickness from SCUBA diving, migraine, and others. In this chapter, we will discuss the diagnosis of PFO and ASA, review the data that implicate them as causes of neurologic disorders—particularly cryptogenic stroke in the young—and assess the available treatment options.

BACKGROUND

The foramen ovale, first described in 1564 by Italian surgeon Leonardi Botali, is an opening in the fossa ovalis created by the overlap of the atrial septum primum and secundum. During fetal development, resistance in the pulmonary circulation leads to higher pressure in the right atrium relative to the left, allowing oxygenated blood arriving from the

From: *Contemporary Cardiology: Interventional Cardiology:*
Percutaneous Noncoronary Intervention
Edited by: H. C. Herrmann © Humana Press Inc., Totowa, NJ

umbilical vein to cross through the foramen ovale into the systemic circulation. Following birth, increased blood flow through the pulmonary circulation leads to a relative increase in left atrial pressure pushing the septum primum against the septum secundum and functionally closing the foramen ovale. In most cases, fibrous adhesions result in a permanent anatomical closure of the flap. However, in a significant proportion of the population, adhesions fail to seal the septum, allowing the persistence of the communication between the right and left atria of the heart.

Patent foramen ovale is a common finding in the general population: three autopsy series have reported an overall prevalence of 17%, 27%, and 29%, respectively (1–3). One of the studies observed that the prevalence of PFO declines as the age of the population sampled increases, implying that anatomical closure can occur in adulthood as well (1). Most echocardiographic studies have demonstrated lower prevalences for PFO (3.2–18%), reflecting the difficulty of detecting a shunt that is potentially but not continuously open (4–7). However, the SPARC (Stroke Prevention: Assessment of Risk in a Community) study, a population-based prospective study of stroke risk factors, evaluated 581 patients by transesophageal echocardiography and agitated saline contrast and found a PFO prevalence of 25.6%, comparable to the autopsy studies (8).

An ASA is present when redundant tissue in the region of the fossa ovalis results in excessive septal wall motion during respiration. ASA is not commonly found in isolation; 71–83% also have a PFO present (9–11). The prevalence of ASA has been estimated to be 1–8% in unselected populations (12,13). The SPARC study reported a prevalence of 2.2% (8).

DIAGNOSIS OF PFO AND ASA

Atrial-septal abnormalities are most often diagnosed by transthoracic echocardiogram (TTE) or transesophageal echocardiogram (TEE) with agitated saline contrast injected into an antecubital vein. TEE is considered the standard for PFO diagnosis, as it permits optimal visualization of the interatrial septum and maximal sensitivity for detection of saline contrast in the left atrium if a shunt is present (14,15). A study of 100 patients undergoing endovascular closure found that two-dimensional TEE measurements were strongly correlated with direct invasive balloon sizing ($r^2 = 0.8$; $p < 0.0001$) (16). Although the antecubital vein is preferable for injection of saline contrast because of its ease of access, femoral injection might be a more reliable method. The degree of right to left shunting after injecting agitated saline into the femoral vein has been highly correlated with balloon sizing ($r^2 = 0.7$; $p < 0.0001$), whereas there was no correlation when the injection was given through an antecubital vein (16). Provocative maneuvers have also been shown to increase the sensitivity of these studies. The Valsalva maneuver was the most reliable way to produce a significant right-to-left pressure gradient compared to inspiration, expiration, or cough (17).

Diagnosis of ASA is made by measuring the total excursion of the septal wall into the left and right atrium throughout the respiratory cycle. There is no clear consensus on the degree of motion that is considered excessive, although most studies have chosen a cut-off of 10–15 mm. As noted, visualization of the interatrial septum is best accomplished with TEE.

There is significant variability in the identification of atrial abnormalities on echocardiogram. Two blinded sonographers reviewed 581 TEEs that were performed for the French PFO/ASA study, a large prospective analysis of cryptogenic stroke patients. They disagreed on the presence of PFO in 14% of cases and on the degree of right-to-left shunt in 26% of cases (18). There was slightly better concordance for the detection of ASA, with disagreement on its presence in 6.6% of cases and on the size of the ASA in 10% of cases. In addition, three sonographers reviewed the first 100 TEEs twice and found a meaningful degree of variability in determining the degree of right-to-left shunting (interobserver $\kappa = 0.77$, intraobserver $\kappa = 0.82$) (19).

Transcranial Doppler (TCD) also has a role in the diagnosis and quantification of right-to-left intracardiac shunting. TCD can monitor blood flow through one or both middle cerebral arteries to identify and quantify high-intensity transient signals (HITS) when agitated saline is injected into a vein during a Valsalva maneuver. A study of 308 patients found that a shower pattern of HITS (defined as bubbles too numerous to count) was more likely to be seen by contrast TCD in patients with a stroke compared to controls (odds ratio [OR] = 3.5; 95% confidence interval [CI] = 1.29–9.87). There was an even stronger association with cryptogenic stroke patients (OR = 12.4; 95% CI = 4.08–38.09) (20). Compared with contrast-enhanced TEE, TCD had a sensitivity of 91% and a specificity of 88% (21). TCD complements TEE. TCD cannot differentiate a PFO from an atrial-septal defect (ASD) nor can it characterize the specific morphologic or functional features of a PFO, such as an associated ASA.

PFO, STROKE, AND TRANSIENT ISCHEMIC ATTACK

In 1877, Cohnheim proposed that venous thromboemboli could paradoxically cross through a PFO and result in arterial stroke (22). There is some evidence to support alternative potential mechanisms of stroke in PFO patients including cardiac *in situ* thrombus formation and atrial arrhythmias (10,12,23–27). However, Cohnheim's original hypothesis of paradoxical emboli is generally thought to be the most likely mechanism by which PFO could be linked to stroke.

Numerous studies have found epidemiological associations between cryptogenic stroke and PFO in young patients. The etiology of a cerebrovascular event is considered to be cryptogenic if the diagnostic evaluation is negative, with no identified high-risk cardioembolic or large-vessel source, and the stroke is in a distribution not consistent with small-vessel disease. Among patients less than 55 yr of age, as many as 40% of strokes are cryptogenic (28,29). Recent series, which have relied more heavily upon magnetic resonance imaging (MRI) and TEE, report a cryptogenic stroke rate of about 34% for patients under the age of 45 (30,31).

Lechat and colleagues were the first to demonstrate that PFO was more prevalent in a cohort of young stroke patients (with a mean age of 36 ± 10 yr) than in control patients (40% vs 10%, $p < 0.001$) (5). Soon after, there was another report of ischemic stroke patients under the age of 40 who had a significantly increased prevalence of PFO compared to age-matched controls (50% vs 15%, $p < 0.001$) (32). It was also reported that patients with cryptogenic stroke were significantly more likely to have PFO than patients with a known stroke etiology (33). This finding was true for patients who were less than 55 yr of age as well as for those patients who were greater than 55 yr of age. However, in another study with a relatively older population (mean age = 66 yr), the incidence of PFO was not significantly higher than age-matched controls for either cryptogenic or noncryptogenic strokes, implying that the stroke risk related to the presence of a PFO might not be as high in the elderly population (34). As seen in Table 1, compared to both normal healthy volunteers (3.2–18%) and to patients who have had stroke resulting from known

Table 1
Prevalence of PFO in Stroke Patients

Study	Controls	Stroke of known etiology	Stroke of unknown etiology
Steiner et al., 1998 (36)	—	19/42 (23%)	12/53 (45%)
Cabanes et al., 1993 (24)	9/50 (18%)	43/100 (43%)	36/64 (56%)
Lechat et al., 1988 (5)	10/100 (10%)	4/19 (21%)	20/41 (49%)
Petty et al., 1997 (35)	—	15/61 (25%)	22/55 (40%)
Lamy et al., 2002 (18)	—	—	267/581 (46%)
Cujec et al., 1999 (37)	—	—	52/90 (58%)
Homma et al., 1994 (38)	—	7/38 (18%)	16/36 (44%)

etiology (21–43%), the prevalence of PFO is higher in patients who have had stroke of unknown origin (40–56%) (9,18,28,35–38). Finally, a comprehensive meta-analysis of case-control studies comparing ischemic stroke patients under 55 yr of age to control groups of nonstroke patients reported an increased prevalence of PFO (OR = 3.1; 95% CI = 2.3–4.2) (39).

Many retrospective case-control studies were able to define specific morphologic and functional characteristics of PFO that were associated with an increased risk of stroke. Both increased PFO size (measured as the separation between the septum primum and secundum) and greater degree of right-to-left shunt (usually determined by quantification of microbubbles seen in the two-dimensional imaging plane during provocative maneuvers) have been associated with increased risk of stroke (20,36,40–42). A prospective cohort trial found that right-to-left shunt at rest (in the absence of any provocative maneuvers) in combination with increased septal wall motion (defined as >6.5 mm) was associated with higher risk of recurrent stroke (43). In this cohort of patients with PFO and cryptogenic stroke, the risk of stroke or transient ischemic attack (TIA) recurrence at 3 yr of follow-up was 4.3% (95% CI = 0–10.2) for those with only one or neither of the two high-risk characteristics and 12.5% (95% CI = 0–26.1) for those with both high-risk characteristics (p = 0.05).

A similar association has been found between ASA and the risk of stroke. There was a significantly higher prevalence of ASA in patients referred for TEE to determine the source of a cerebral or systemic embolism than in patients referred for other reasons (15% vs 4%) (11). Table 2 demonstrates the increased prevalence of ASA in patients with a cryptogenic stroke (11–39%) when compared to either patients who have had an ischemic event with a known etiology (6–28%) or to patients who did not have an antecedent event (2–11%). Finally, as in PFO, a meta-analysis of case-control studies comparing stroke patients less than 55 yr of age to control groups of nonstroke patients found an increased likelihood of finding an ASA (OR = 6.1; 95% CI = 2.5–15.2) (39).

Taken together, these observational studies implicate PFO and ASA as a risk factor for stroke. However, there are very little prospective data regarding the risk of a first stroke in people with one of these atrial-septal abnormalities. A single study has described a prospective population-based cohort of people with PFO. In the study, 1102 stroke-free patients underwent TTE with agitated saline contrast and 164 (14.9%) were found to have a PFO. They were followed for a mean of 54.0 ± 22.1 mo during which time the incidence of ischemic stroke was 1.10/100 person-years in subjects with PFO and 0.97/100 person-years

Table 2
Prevalence of ASA in Stroke Patients

Study	Controls	Stroke of known etiology	Stroke of unknown etiology
Cabanes et al., 1993 (24)	4/50 (8%)	28/100 (28%)	25/64 (39%)
Hanna et al., 1994 (6)	3/35 (8%)	2/23 (10%)	6/16 (38%)
Agmon et al., 1999 (13)	8/363 (2%)	—	—
Lamy et al., 2002 (18)	—	—	61/581 (11%)
Mattioli et al., 2001 (44)	36/316 (11%)	68/245 (28%)	—
Lucas et al., 1994 (45)	—	6/100 (6%)	10/48 (21%)

in those without PFO (7). In patients less than 60 yr of age, the incidence of stroke was only 0.52% over the entire follow-up period. Given these low rates, asymptomatic patients are unlikely to benefit from primary prevention.

The clinical problem most often faced by physicians is how to manage patients who are found to have a PFO after they have had an otherwise cryptogenic stroke or TIA. No randomized clinical trial has addressed this issue to date and only three studies have prospectively evaluated the long-term prognosis of PFO patients following a stroke or TIA. All three studies found that medically treated patients with a PFO were not at increased risk of recurrent stroke or death when compared to other cryptogenic stroke patients (43,46,47). The average annual risk of stroke in these studies for patients with cryptogenic stroke and PFO ranged from 1.5% to 7.2%. Combining these three studies results in a pooled relative risk of 0.95 (95% CI = 0.62–1.44) when comparing cryptogenic stroke patients with PFO to those without. Thus, among patients who have had a cryptogenic stroke, PFO alone does not appear to portend an increased risk of subsequent stroke or death.

There are inadequate data in any of these studies to make conclusions about patients with isolated ASA. However, the combination of PFO and ASA bears a much more compelling relationship with stroke. Although the interaction between PFO and ASA is not well understood, the presence of ASA is associated with a larger separation between the septum primum and secundum, a prominent eustachian valve, right atrial fibrous strands, and a larger right-to-left shunt in association with PFO, providing an anatomical substrate for an increased risk of stroke recurrence (46,48,49). In general, the data do suggest an increased risk of stroke recurrence for patients with both PFO and ASA, although an increased risk has not been found across all studies. The French PFO/ASA study demonstrated that cryptogenic stroke patients had increased risk of stroke recurrence if they have both PFO and ASA (3.8% vs 1.1% per year; relative risk [RR] = 2.98; 95% CI = 1.17–7.58), although there was only a trend for combined stroke and death (3.8% vs 1.8% per year; RR = 2.10; 95% CI = 0.86–5.06) (46). In contrast, the PFO in the cryptogenic stroke study (PICSS) did not show an increased risk of stroke or death in patients with both PFO and ASA in the *overall* cohort (8.0% vs 7.7%; RR = 1.04; 95% CI = 0.51–2.12). Unfortunately, PICSS did not provide separate data for the cyptogenic stroke population (47).

The conflicting findings in these two studies regarding patients with both PFO and ASA might be because they were evaluating disparate patient populations. Compared to patients in the French PFO/ASA study, patients in the PICSS study were older (59.0 yr vs 42.5 yr) and, consequently, they had a higher stroke recurrence rate (7.6 vs 1.6%).

Although both studies found that patients with PFO were less likely to have traditional stroke risk factors than other cryptogenic stroke patients, the patients in PICSS had higher rates of hypertension and diabetes compared to the French PFO/ASA study. Thus, atrial abnormalities are less likely to have been responsible for the primary event and also less likely to result in an increased risk of recurrence.

STROKE PREVENTION IN PATIENTS WITH CRYPTOGENIC STROKE AND PFO

Although it appears that PFO alone is not associated with an increased risk of stroke recurrence or death compared to other cryptogenic stroke patients, it might still be possible to lower the recurrent stroke risk in this group. There are no natural history studies that have followed cryptogenic stroke patients with PFO or ASA, because all have received some form of treatment. However, multiple studies have followed these patients after initiating medical therapy with antiplatelet agents or anticoagulation with or without PFO closure either via surgery or an endovascular device. The annual risk of recurrent stroke or TIA has varied widely in these reports, from 0% to 19% (37,46,50–58). Furthermore, there have been very few studies that have compared different therapies and no randomized controlled trials have demonstrated superior efficacy of any therapy. Thus, despite a multitude of reports the optimal management of PFO patients with cryptogenic TIA or stroke remains controversial.

Medical Management of PFO

A combined meta-analysis of five retrospective cohort studies comparing at least two different treatment options found that warfarin was superior to antiplatelet therapy in preventing recurrent stroke or TIA among patients with PFO (OR = 0.37; 95% CI = 0.23–0.60) (59). Further, a meta-analysis of four retrospective cohort studies found that surgical PFO closure was comparable to warfarin treatment (OR = 1.19; 95% CI = 0.62–2.27) (59). However, it is important to emphasize that retrospective or nonrandomized treatment studies have tremendous potential for selection bias that significantly degrades their validity. For example, it is likely that the largest PFOs would be considered for closure or warfarin therapy, whereas the smallest PFOs would be treated with aspirin, resulting in confounding by indication.

Although warfarin might be considered by some to be a conventional medical therapy for patients with PFO and TIA or stroke, there are little prospective data to support its routine use and associated risk of bleeding. The PFO in Cryptogenic Stroke Study (PICSS) is the only prospective randomized trial that evaluated therapy in cryptogenic stroke patients with PFO (47). Patients were randomized to aspirin or warfarin and followed for 2 yr. The average annual rate of stroke or death for those given warfarin compared to those who received aspirin was 4.75% vs 8.95% (RR = 0.53; 95% CI = 0.18–1.58). Although the point estimate of the relative risk suggests that warfarin might be superior, the confidence interval was extremely wide and does not rule out the opposite conclusion of a net benefit for aspirin. Thus, PICSS was unable to conclude that warfarin or aspirin is the superior medication. However, PICSS was primarily designed as a prognostic study and was inadequately powered to find a difference between the treatments. Nonetheless, PICSS has raised questions about the routine use of warfarin in patients with PFO and cryptogenic TIA or stroke.

There are situations in which anticoagulation is clearly indicated for cryptogenic stroke patients with PFO. In the setting of concomitant deep-vein thrombosis (DVT) or pulmonary embolism (PE), current anticoagulation recommendations for venous thromboembolism should guide therapy. The American College of Chest Physicians (ACCP) guidelines recommend at least 3 mo of oral anticoagulation therapy for DVT or PE *(60)*. Of 140 consecutive patients with stroke and PFO in the Lausanne Stroke Registry, only 6 patients (5.5%) had clinical evidence of a DVT *(61)*. The question of whether to screen all cryptogenic stroke patients for DVT is controversial as the yield has been variable, ranging from 10% to 57% using a highly sensitive nuclear medicine scan *(62,63)*.

PFO Closure

Many physicians have advocated permanently closing the PFO with surgery or, increasingly, a transcatheter occlusion device in order to prevent recurrent paradoxical emboli. A number of case series have presented outcome data for patients who have had surgical PFO closure. A series of 30 patients with stroke and PFO who were considered to be at high risk for recurrence underwent surgical closure and then were followed for recurrent events *(64)*. There were no reported significant complications from the surgery and there were no reported recurrent TIAs or strokes at a mean of 2 yr of follow-up. Two patients did have a residual right-to-left shunt when TEE was performed at a mean of 8 mo after the surgery. Another series of 28 cryptogenic stroke patients who received open thoracotomy for PFO closure were followed for a mean duration of 19 mo *(53)*. There were six surgical complications reported, including five patients with postpericardiotomy syndrome and one patient with transient atrial fibrillation. During the follow-up period, there were one stroke and three TIAs, resulting in an average annual risk of recurrence of 9.1%. Of note, all recurrent cerebrovascular events were seen in the group of patients who were greater than 45 yr of age (4/11 patients vs 0/17 patients; $p < 0.02$) implying that their initial stroke might have been the result of another, more traditional cause of stroke and that their risk of stroke recurrence was not reduced by PFO closure. In another series, 91 patients who underwent open thoracotomy for PFO closure were followed for a mean duration of 2 yr *(54)*. There were no perioperative deaths, although transient atrial fibrillation occurred in 11 patients, pericardial effusion requiring drainage in 5, reoperation for bleeding in 3, and a superficial wound infection in 1 patient. There were no recurrent strokes and eight TIAs (one of which was attributed to concomitant giant cell arteritis). In this series, the average annual risk of recurrent cerebrovascular events was 4.5%. See Table 3 for a summary of reported rates of recurrent events in patients who have undergone PFO closure.

Introduced in 1989, transcatheter occlusion devices have increasingly replaced surgery for PFO closure (see Chapters 8–10 for a description of these devices). The placement of the occlusion device is generally well tolerated, with complication rates up to 10%, compared with up to 22% for surgical case series *(54–56,66)*. However, complication rates are difficult to compare between various devices and surgery, as the outcomes have been neither standardized nor validated. In the largest series of 276 patients, device complications were generally minor and included transient ST-segment elevation on electrocardiogram (EKG) in 1.8%, transient atrial fibrillation in 0.8%, and TIA in 0.8%. In addition, two patients (0.8%) had embolization or dislodgement of the device; one was removed by a snare and the other patient required a thoracotomy *(69)*. There were no procedure-related strokes, myocardial infarctions (MIs), or deaths. A residual shunt was seen on TEE in only 1% of patients after 1 yr. During a mean follow-up period of 15.1 mo, the average annual recurrence rate for TIA was 1.7%, and no strokes or peripheral emboli

Table 3

Average Annual Risk of Recurrence, Rate of Peri-procedural Complications, and Rate of Residual Shunting Following Surgical or Transcatheter PFO Closure

Series	No. of patients	Mean follow-up (mo)	Annual risk of TIA	Annual risk of stroke	Annual risk of peripheral emboli	No. of complications	Residual shunt at 1 mo	Residual shunt at 6 mo	Residual shunt at 1 yr
Surgical closure									
Homma et al., 1997 (55)	28	19	6.8%	2.3%	0	6 (21%)	NA	NA	NA
Dearani et al., 1999 (54)	91	24	4.5%	0	0	20 (22%)	NA	NA	NA
Devuyst et al., 1996 (64)	30	24	0	0	0	0	NA	2 (6.7%)	NA
Transcatheter closure									
Bridges et al., 1992 (65)	36	8.4	NA	0	0	0	NA	NA	18%
Ende et al., 1996 (66)	10	32	0	0	0	1 (10%)	4 (44.4%)	2 (22.2%)	0
Sievert et al., 1998 (67)	46	13.2	2%	0	0	NA	NA	NA	NA
Windecker et al., 2000 (56)	80	19.2 ± 16.8	2.5%	0	0.9%	8 (10%)	21 (27%)	NA	NA
Hung et al., 2000 (57)	63	31.2 ± 28.8	2.4%	0.8%	0	3 (4.8%)	NA	NA	14%
Wahl et al., 2001 (68)	152	20.4 ± 19.2	2.4%	0.4%	0.8%	10 (7%)	NA	21%	NA
Braun et al., 2002 (69)	276	15.1	1.7%	0	0	11 (4%)	17%	4%	1%
Martin et al., 2002 (58)	110	27.6 ± 20.4	0.4%	0.4%	0	5 (4.5%)	NA	49%	34%
Onorato et al., 2003 (70)	256	19	0	0	0	23 (8.9%)	NA	NA	2%

were observed. In another series of 124 patients who underwent transcatheter closure of a PFO or atrial–septal defect (ASD), 10 (8%) required subsequent surgery, 2 to repair a femoral artery injury and 8 to remove a misplaced closure device and suture the defect *(71)*. The high surgery rate in this series was probably the result of the inherently increased difficulty of ASD repair compared to PFO closure. Table 3 summarizes rates of complications and residual shunting following surgical or device PFO closure.

Selection of Treatment for Patients with PFO and TIA or Stroke

The advent of percutaneous devices has made PFO closure an increasingly attractive alternative option *(37,56,66)*. Open heart surgery is now done infrequently for simple PFO closure. About 10,000 PFOs have been closed percutaneously worldwide. As noted, percutaneous PFO closure has a very low serious complication rate (<1%) and long-term durability of available devices also appears excellent, with a 5-yr failure rate of <1%.

One of the persuasive arguments for PFO closure is the avoidance of long-term warfarin. Warfarin carries a 1–4% per year risk of significant hemorrhage—no small consideration especially in younger patients. Of course, the issue of long-term warfarin risk becomes moot if aspirin works just as well. Following percutaneous PFO closure, patients are treated with aspirin indefinitely and with clopidogrel usually for 6 mo.

In the United States, percutaneous PFO closure is permitted under a Food and Drug Administration (FDA) Humanitarian Device Exemption (HDE). Importantly, the HDE is based on demonstration of device safety and not efficacy for stroke prevention. The specific HDE wording for the CardioSEAL device is instructive:

> *The CardioSEAL Septal Occlusion System is indicated for the closure of a patent foramen ovale (PFO) in patients with recurrent cryptogenic stroke due to presumed paradoxical embolism through a patent foramen ovale and who have failed conventional drug therapy. Cryptogenic stroke is defined as a stroke occurring in the absence of potential phanerogenic cardiac, pulmonary, vascular or neurological sources. Conventional drug therapy is defined as a therapeutic INR on oral anticoagulants (72).*

Certainly, patients who meet the HDE criteria should be strongly considered for percutaneous PFO closure. However, the HDE poses at least two dilemmas: first, how to define "recurrent cryptogenic stroke," and, second, defining warfarin as the "conventional drug therapy." Both concepts might be outdated. Recurrent cerebrovascular events should include both stroke and TIA—as many as 75% of clinical TIAs lasting more than 1 h result in abnormal diffusion-weighted magnetic resonance imaging (DWMRI) of the brain *(73)*. Thus, the HDE definition of "recurrent stroke" should include MR-positive TIAs.

Not surprisingly, the rate of strict compliance with the HDE requirements for percutaneous PFO closure is unclear. For many clinicians, closing a PFO for a definite recurrent clinical TIA on medical therapy also seems reasonable. Percutaneous PFO closure should also be considered as the initial treatment in patients with cryptogenic stroke or TIA who appear to be at highest risk, such as those with a brisk right-to-left shunt and patients with an atrialseptal aneurysm. In addition, closure should be considered for patients who are unwilling or unable to tolerate or be compliant with medical therapy. Finally, many patients with a single event are psychologically crippled by their PFO and prefer simply to have it closed. Unfortunately, whether percutaneous PFO closure is worse than, equivalent to, or superior to warfarin or aspirin alone (to say nothing of combination therapy or other agents) in patients with cryptogenic stroke and PFO is unknown. That is why two FDA-approved randomized multicenter trials of percutaneous PFO closure vs medical therapy alone are underway (CLOSURE and RESPECT). For patients with first TIA or first stroke presumably as a result of PFO, we recommend percutaneous PFO closure only if the patient is randomized to the device arm within one of these clinical trials.

Timing of Closure

The timing of intervention after acute ischemic stroke is a controversial subject. Studies of carotid endarterectomy have demonstrated that in acute stroke patients, early carotid revascularization has the potential to cause reperfusion injury and hemorrhagic conversion *(74)*. Depending on factors such as the size of the infarct, degree of brain swelling, and level of consciousness, surgeons will frequently wait between 2 and 6 weeks after the stroke to perform carotid endarterectomy. Although PFO closure does not necessarily result in altered cerebral blood flow, the use of heparin, and the possibility of hemodynamic fluctuations during the procedure might warrant a similar caution, particularly if the initial stroke is large. Patients who have had transient neurologic symptoms consistent with TIA are not likely to develop a hemorrhagic complication and, thus, should not have any restrictions on the timing of closure.

PFO AND MIGRAINE

Migraine and PFO are highly prevalent in the same young patient populations. A number of observational cohort studies have found a correlation between PFO and migraine with aura (migrainous headache preceded or accompanied by neurologic symptoms that might include scintillating scotoma, numbness, or weakness). One of the first case-control studies to look at PFO and migraine reported findings from TCD studies with agitated saline contrast in 43 patients with migraine with aura, 73 patients less than 50 yr of age with cerebral ischemia, and a control group of 50 healthy subjects *(75)*. The rate of right-to-left shunt in the migraine patients was 41%, compared to 16% of controls and 35% of patients with stroke ($p < 0.005$). A series of 113 patients with migraine with aura were evaluated for right-to-left shunt using TCD with agitated saline contrast and compared to 53 patients with migraine without aura and 25 healthy age-matched controls *(76)*. The prevalence of PFO was 48% (54/113) in patients with migraine with aura, 23% (12/53) in patients with migraine without aura, and 20% (5/25) in control subjects. The difference between migraineurs with aura and those without aura was significant (OR = 3.13; 95% CI = 1.41–7.04; $p = 0.002$), as was the difference between migraineurs with aura and controls (OR = 3.66; 95% CI = 1.21–13.25; $p = 0.01$), whereas migraineurs without aura did not differ from controls (OR = 1.17; 95% CI = 0.32–4.45). Table 4 summarizes the findings from these case-control trials. Another study evaluated 74 consecutive patients with cryptogenic stroke for atrial abnormalities and migraine history and found PFO in 44 (59%). Of the patients with PFO, 16 (36%) had migraine with aura compared to 4 out of 30 (13%) of the patients without PFO ($p = 0.03$) *(77)*. Similarly, the French PFO/ASA study evaluated a series of 581 cryptogenic stroke patients and found that migraine was more common in patients with PFO (27.3%) than in those without PFO (14.0%). This association was significant after adjustment for age and sex (OR = 1.75; 95% CI = 1.08–2.82), and there was an even stronger association when ASA was also present (OR = 2.71; 95% CI= 1.36–5.41) *(18)*. Finally, in a prospective stroke registry that evaluated 419 ischemic stroke patients less than 45 yr of age, migraine was significantly correlated with the presence of PFO in multivariate analysis (OR = 4.8; 95% CI = 2–11.2; $p < 0.0001$) *(78)*.

Patent foramen ovale closure has been reported to reduce the frequency and severity of migraines *(79)*. A series of 17 patients who had a history of both stroke and migraine

Table 4
Prevalence of PFO in Migraineurs

Study	Controls	Migraine NOS	Migraine with aura	Migraine without aura
Del Sette et al., 1998 (74)	8/50 (16%)	18/44 (41%)	—	—
Anzola et al., 1999 (76)	5/25 (20%)	—	54/113 (48%)	12/53 (23%)

[a]NOS, not otherwise specified.

underwent endovascular closure of a PFO for recurrent stroke prevention and were followed for 6 mo after the procedure. They reported a significant reduction in a composite headache score that reflected frequency, severity, and duration of migraine attacks. Another series found that 16 of 37 patients (43%) who underwent PFO closure for presumed paradoxical embolism or decompression illness had a history of migraine with aura (80). Following closure, 15 of the 16 patients with migraine with aura reported no further headaches or a reduction in the frequency of headaches during a follow-up period of 18.9 mo. Other case series have suggested that migraine with aura might be an indication for PFO closure (70). However, the mechanism whereby PFO might trigger migraine must be elucidated. Speculation has centered around the shunting of venous blood containing higher concentrations of vasoactive substances or multiple microemboli, but evidence for either mechanism is lacking. In addition, the benefit-to-risk ratio of this intervention needs to be rigorously tested in a randomized controlled trial before migraine with aura can be accepted as an indication for closure.

PFO AND DECOMPRESSION SICKNESS

Decompression sickness occurs when the partial pressure of nitrogen in the blood exceeds the ambient pressure during a diver's ascent, forming bubbles that are thought to cause venous microembolic ischemia. Symptoms of decompression sickness range from musculoskeletal pain to cardiopulmonary symptoms and neurologic symptoms. Two studies initially demonstrated a correlation between PFO and unexplained decompression sickness (81,82). Subsequently, a study of divers using TCD and MRI found that multiple unexplained lesions seen on MRI occurred exclusively in divers who had a large right-to-left shunt (although single lesions were seen in some divers who did not have a right-to-left shunt and there were divers with large right-to-left shunts who had no MRI lesions) (83). Another study polled 52 sport divers on their experience with decompression sickness and then performed contrast TEEs to look for PFO (84). The incidence of decompression sickness was 4.5 times higher in those divers with PFO (95% CI = 1.2–18.0; $p = 0.03$). MRI was performed on the divers and 52 nondiving controls. In the cohort of divers, there were 1.23 ± 2.0 brain lesions per person if a PFO was present and 0.64 ± 1.22 lesions if there was no PFO ($p = 0.07$). Among nondiving controls, there were 0.22 ± 0.44 lesions if there was a PFO and 0.12 ± 0.63 lesions if there was no PFO ($p < 0.001$). Table 5 represents a summary of the case-control trials looking at PFO in divers. A similar association between PFO and decompression sickness has been reported in high-altitude aviators and astronauts (87,88). The increased incidence of decompression sickness and increased number of unexplained brain lesions on MRI in patients with PFO suggests that closure of the right-to-left shunt might be beneficial. Unfortunately, no studies have addressed this question and a less invasive approach might

Table 5
Prevalence of PFO in Divers with Decompression Sickness

Study	Divers with DCS	Divers without DCS
Cartoni et al., 1998 (85)	14/22 (63%)	5/19 (26%)
Cantais et al., 2003 (86)	59/101 (58.4%)	25/101 (24.8%)

Note: DCS = decompression sickness.

be to recommend that the patient stop diving. If patients are unwilling to accept this restriction, the potential benefit of closure must be weighed against the risk of the procedure.

PFO AND OTHER NEUROLOGIC DISORDERS

Patent foramen ovale might be more prevalent in patients with transient global amnesia (TGA) (89). Fifty-three consecutive patients with TGA and 100 controls were evaluated with contrast TCD. Right-to-left shunt was observed in 55% of patients with TGA, compared with only 27% of the controls ($p < 0.01$). This finding is controversial however, as another contrast TCD study of 48 TGA patients and 48 controls found no difference in the prevalence of PFO (18.8% vs 16.6%) (90). Given that TGA is unlikely to recur, it is probably not an indication for warfarin or closure of the PFO.

Patent foramen ovale has been implicated in the pathogenesis of some brain abscesses. In children with congenital heart disease causing a right-to-left shunt, brain abscess is a well-known complication (91). Although this is less commonly seen in adults, two patients with dental infections and brain abscesses with a PFO and a significant right-to-left shunt have been reported (92). Overall, approximately 15–60% of brain abscesses are considered to be cryptogenic, with no known predisposing cause. Thus, it is plausible that PFO could contribute to the development of some brain abscesses. Prophylactic antibiotics for dental procedures are controversial in this group of patients but should be strongly considered if the patient has a PFO and has already had a systemic infection or brain abscess without any other obvious etiology.

BEHAVIORAL CONSIDERATIONS IN PATIENTS WITH PFO

Given that the neurologic complications of PFO are most likely the result of right-to-left shunting, it is reasonable to recommend behavioral modifications that might preclude transient elevations in right atrial pressure. Heavy weight lifting should be discouraged and stool softeners should be considered in order to avoid Valsalva-like conditions. Patients who are undertaking prolonged travel should be advised to mobilize frequently to avoid lower extremity venous clot formation.

CONCLUSIONS

Patent foramen ovale and atrialseptal aneurysm are common structural cardiac abnormalities that have been implicated in multiple neurologic diseases, including migraine, decompression sickness in divers, and, most importantly, stroke. It has been estimated that up to 100,000 people each year might be candidates for PFO closure to prevent recurrent paradoxical embolism (15). This number could grow even higher if closure is proven to benefit the other PFO-related neurologic conditions such as migraine. For younger patients with cryptogenic stroke and PFO (with or without ASA), medical treatment options currently include antiplatelet agents or anticoagulation; current data do not demonstrate which is superior. Percutaneous or surgical closure is a more aggressive option, although there is no definitive evidence of superiority to medical therapy in any PFO subgroup. In the subset of patients who appear to have "high-risk" PFO (i.e., shunting at rest, large shunt, associated ASA, or multiple embolic events), closure is a reasonable consideration. In those patients who have failed medical therapy or who are unwilling or unable to comply with long-term warfarin, closure provides another alternative. Transcatheter closure cannot be recommended as first-line therapy for all patients with PFO and an initial cryptogenic cerebrovascular event until randomized controlled trials demonstrate a benefit over medical therapy.

REFERENCES

1. Hagen PT, Scholz DG, Edwards WD. Incidence and size of patent foramen ovale during the first 10 decades of life: an autopsy study of 965 normal hearts. Mayo Clin Proc 1984;59:17–20.
2. Seib G. Incidence of the patent foramen ovale cordis in adult american whites and american negroes. Am J Anat 1934;55:511–525.
3. Thompson T, Evans W. Paradoxical embolism. Q J Med 1930;23:135–152.
4. de Belder MA, Tourikis L, Leech G, Camm AJ. Risk of patent foramen ovale for thromboembolic events in all age groups. Am J Cardiol 1992;69:1316–1320.
5. Lechat P, Mas JL, Lascault G, et al. Prevalence of patent foramen ovale in patients with stroke. N Engl J Med 1988;318:1148–1152.
6. Hanna JP, Sun JP, Furlan AJ, et al. Patent foramen ovale and brain infarct. Echocardiographic predictors, recurrence, and prevention. Stroke 1994;25:782–786.
7. Di Tullio MR, Sacco RL, Sciacca RR, et al. Patent foramen ovale and risk of ischemic stroke in a community—the northern manhattan study. Stroke 2003;34 (abstract).
8. Meissner I, Whisnant JP, Khandheria BK, et al. Prevalence of potential risk factors for stroke assessed by transesophageal echocardiography and carotid ultrasonography: the SPARC study. Stroke prevention: assessment of risk in a community. Mayo Clin Proc 1999;74:862–869.
9. Cabanes L, Mas JL, Cohen A, et al. Atrial septal aneurysm and patent foramen ovale as risk factors for cryptogenic stroke in patients less than 55 years of age. A study using transesophageal echocardiography. Stroke 1993;24:1865–1873.
10. Schneider B, Harath P, Vogel P, Meinertz T. Improved morphologic characterization of atrial septal aneurysm by tranesophageal echocardiography: relation to cerebrovascular events. J Am Coll Cardiol 1990;16:1000–1009.
11. Pearson AC, Nagelhout D, Castello R, et al. Atrial septal aneurysm and stroke: a transesophageal echocardiographic study. J Am Coll Cardiol 1991;18:1223–1229.
12. Silver MD, Dorsey JS. Aneurysms of the septum primum in adults. Arch Pathol Lab Med 1978;102:62–65.
13. Agmon Y, Khandheria BK, Meissner I, et al. Frequency of atrial septal aneurysms in patients with cerebral ischemic events. Circulation 1999;99:1942–1944.
14. Kerut EK, Norfleet WT, Plotnick GD, Giles TD. Patent foramen ovale: a review of associated conditions and the impact of physiological size. J Am Coll Cardiol 2001;38:613–623.
15. Meier B, Lock JE. Contemporary management of patent foramen ovale. Circulation 2003;107:5–9.
16. Schuchlenz HW, Weihs W, Beitzke A, et al. Transesophageal echocardiography for quantifying size of patent foramen ovale in patients with cryptogenic cerebrovascular events. Stroke 2002;33:293–296.
17. Pfleger S, Konstantin Haase K, et al. Haemodynamic quantification of different provocation manoeuvres by simultaneous measurement of right and left atrial pressure: implications for the echocardiographic detection of persistent foramen ovale. Eur J Echocardiogr 2001;2:88–93.
18. Lamy C, Giannesini C, Zuber M, et al. Clinical and imaging findings in cryptogenic stroke patients with and without patent foramen ovale: The PFO–ASA study. Stroke. 2002;33:706–711.
19. Cabanes L, Coste J, Derumeaux G, et al. Interobserver and intraobserver variability in detection of patent foramen ovale and atrial septal aneurysm with transesophageal echocardiography. J Am Soc Echocardiogr 2002;15:441–446.
20. Serena J, Segura T, Perez-Ayuso MJ, et al. The need to quantify right-to-left shunt in acute ischemic stroke: a case-control study. Stroke 1998;29:1322–1328.

21. Blersch WK, Draganski BM, Holmer SR, et al. Transcranial duplex sonography in the detection of patent foramen ovale. Radiology 2002;225:693–699.
22. Cohnheim J. Thrombose und embolie: vorlesung uber allgemeine pathologie. Berlin, 1877:134.
23. Rice MJ, McDonald RW, Reller MD. Fetal atrial septal aneurysm: a cause of fetal atrial arrhythmias. J Am Coll Cardiol 1988;12:1292–1297.
24. Cabanes L, Mas JL, Cohen A, et al. Atrial septal aneurysm and patent foramen ovale as risk factors for cryptogenic stroke in patients less than 55 years of age. A study using transesophageal echocardiography. Stroke 1993;24:1865–1873.
25. Mugge A, Daniel WG, Angermann C, et al. Atrial septal aneurysm in adult patients. Circulation 1995;91:2785–2792.
26. Berthet K, Lavergne T, Cohen A, et al. Significant association of atrial vulnerability with atrial septal abnormalities in young patients with ischemic stroke of unknown cause. Stroke 2000;31:398.
27. Somody E, Albucher JF, Casteignau G, et al. Anomalies of the interatrial septum and latent atrial vulnerability in unexplained ischemic stroke in young adults. Arch Mal Coeur Vaisseaux 2000;93:1495–1500.
28. Lechat P, Mas JL, Lascault G, et al. Prevalence of patent foramen ovale in patients with stroke. N Engl J Med 1988;318:1148–1152.
29. Sacco RL, Ellenberg JH, Mohr JP, et al. Infarcts of undetermined cause: the NINCDS stroke data bank. Ann Neurol 1989;25:382–390.
30. Kittner SJ, Stern BJ, Wozniak M, et al. Cerebral infarction in young adults: the Baltimore–Washington cooperative young stroke study. Neurology 1998;50:890–894.
31. Adams HP Jr, Kappelle LJ, Biller J, et al. Ischemic stroke in young adults. Experience in 329 patients enrolled in the Iowa Registry of stroke in young adults. Arch Neurol 1995;52:491–495.
32. Webster MW, Chancellor AM, Smith HJ, et al. Patent foramen ovale in young stroke patients. Lancet 1988;2:11–12.
33. Di Tullio MR, Sacco RL, Gopal A, et al. Patent foramen ovale as a risk factor for cryptogenic stroke. Ann Intern Med 1992;117:461–465.
34. Jones EF, Calafiore P, Donnan GA, Tonkin AM. Evidence that patent foramen ovale is not a risk factor for cerebral ischemia in the elderly. Am J Cardiol 1994;74:596–599.
35. Petty GW, Khandheria BK, Chu CP, et al. Patent foramen ovale in patients with cerebral infarction. A transesophageal echocardiographic study. Arch Neurol 1997;54:819–822.
36. Steiner MM, Di Tullio MR, Rundek T, et al. Patent foramen ovale size and embolic brain imaging findings among patients with ischemic stroke. Stroke 1998;29:944–948.
37. Cujec B, Mainra R, Johnson DH. Prevention of recurrent cerebral ischemic events in patients with patent foramen ovale and cryptogenic strokes or transient ischemic attacks. Can J Cardiol 1999;15:57–64.
38. Homma S, Di Tullio MR, Sacco RL, et al. Characteristics of patent foramen ovale associated with cryptogenic stroke. A biplane transesophageal echocardiographic study. Stroke 1994;25:582–586.
39. Overell JR, Bone I, Lees KR. Interatrial septal abnormalities and stroke: a meta-analysis of case-control studies. Neurology 2000;55:1172–1179.
40. Van Camp G, Schulze D, Cosyns B, Vandenbossche JL. Relation between patent foramen ovale and unexplained stroke. Am J Cardiol 1993;71:596–598.
41. Hausmann D, Mugge A, Daniel WG. Identification of patent foramen ovale pemitting paradoxic embolism. J Am Coll Cardiol 1995;26:1030–1038.
42. Stone DA, Godard J, Corretti MC, et al. Patent foramen ovale: association between the degree of shunt by contrast transesophageal echocardiography and the risk of future ischemic neurologic events. Am Heart J 1996;131:158–161.
43. De Castro S, Cartoni D, Fiorelli M, et al. Morphological and functional characteristics of patent foramen ovale and their embolic implications. Stroke 2000;31:2407–2413.
44. Mattioli AV, Aquilina M, Oldani A, et al. Atrial septal aneurysm as a cardioembolic source in adult patients with stroke and normal carotid arteries. A multicentre study. Eur Heart J 2001;22:261–268.
45. Lucas C, Goullard L, Marchau M Jr, et al. Higher prevalence of atrial septal aneurysms in patients with ischemic stroke of unknown cause. Acta Neurol Scand 1994;89:210–213.
46. Mas JL, Arquizan C, Lamy C, et al. Recurrent cerebrovascular events associated with patent foramen ovale, atrial septal aneurysm, or both. N Engl J Med 2001;345:1740–1746.
47. Homma S, Sacco RL, Di Tullio MR, et al. Effect of medical treatment in stroke patients with patent foramen ovale: patent foramen ovale in cryptogenic stroke study. Circulation 2002;105:2625–2631.
48. Homma S, Sacco RL, Di Tullio MR, Sciacca RR, PICSS Investigators. Relationship of atrial septal anuerysm with patent foramen ovale: insights from pfo in cryptogenic stroke study (PICSS). Circulation 2001;104(Suppl):II-670 (abstract).

49. Homma S, Sacco RL, Di Tullio MR, et al. Atrial anatomy in non-cardioembolic stroke patients: effect of medical therapy. J Am Coll Cardiol 2003;42:1066–1072.

50. Hanna JP, Sun JP, Furlan AJ, et al. Patent foramen ovale and brain infarct. Echocardiographic predictors, recurrence, and prevention. Stroke 1994;25:782–786.

51. Mas JL, Zuber M. Recurrent cerebrovascular events in patients with patent foramen ovale, atrial septal aneurysm, or both and cryptogenic stroke or transient ischemic attack. French study group on patent foramen ovale and atrial septal aneurysm. Am Heart J 1995;130:1083–1088.

52. Bogousslavsky J, Garazi S, Jeanrenaud X, et al. Stroke recurrence in patients with patent foramen ovale: the Lausanne study. Lausanne stroke with paradoxal embolism study group. Neurology 1996;46:1301–1305.

53. De Castro S, Cartoni D, Fiorelli M, et al. Patent foramen ovale and its embolic implications. Am J Cardiol 2000;86:51G–52G.

54. Dearani JA, Baran US, Danielson GK, et al. Surgical patent foramen ovale closure for prevention of paradoxical embolism-related cerebrovascular ischemic events. Circulation 1999;100(Suppl II):II171–II175.

55. Homma S, Di Tullio MR, Sacco RL, et al. Surgical closure of patent foramen ovale in cryptogenic stroke patients. Stroke 1997;28:2376–2381.

56. Windecker S, Wahl A, Chatterjee T. Percutaneous closure of patent formaen ovale in patients with paradoxical embolism: long-term risk of recurrent thromboembolic events. Circulation 2000;101:893–898.

57. Hung J, Landzberg MJ, Jenkins KJ, et al. Closure of patent foramen ovale for paradoxical emboli: intermediate-term risk of recurrent neurological events following transcatheter device placement. J Am Coll Cardiol 2000;35:1311–1316.

58. Martin F, Sanchez PL, Doherty E, et al. Percutaneous transcatheter closure of patent foramen ovale in patients with paradoxical embolism. Circulation 2002;106:1121–1126.

59. Orgera MA, O'Malley PG, Taylor AJ. Secondary prevention of cerebral ischemia in patent foramen ovale: systematic review and meta-analysis. South Med J 2001;94:699–703.

60. Hyers TM, Agnelli G, Hull RD, et al. Antithrombotic therapy for venous thromboembolic disease. Chest 1998;114:561S–578S.

61. Bogousslavsky J, Garazi S, Jeanrenaud X, Aebischer N, Van Melle G. Stroke recurrence in patients with patent foramen ovale: the Lausanne study. Neurology 1996;46:1301–1305.

62. Lethen H, Flachskampf FA, Schneider R, et al. Frequency of deep vein thrombosis in patients with patent foramen ovale and ischemic stroke or transient ischemic attack. Am J Cardiol 1997;80:1066–1069.

63. Stollberger C, Slany J, Schuster I, et al. The prevalence of deep venous thrombosis in patients with suspected paradoxical embolism. Ann Intern Med 1993;119:461–465.

64. Devuyst G, Bogousslavsky J, Ruchat P, et al. Prognosis after stroke followed by surgical closure of patent foramen ovale: a prospective follow-up study with brain MRI and simultaneous transesophageal and transcranial Doppler ultrasound. Neurology 1996;47:1162–1166.

65. Bridges ND, Hellenbrand W, Latson L, et al. Transcatheter closure of patent foramen ovale after presumed paradoxical embolism. Circulation 1992;86:1902–1908.

66. Ende DJ, Chopra PS, Rao PS. Transcatheter closure of atrial septal defect or patent foramen ovale with the buttoned device for prevention of recurrence of paradoxic embolism. Am J Cardiol 1996;78:233–236.

67. Sievert H, Babic UU, Hausdorf G, et al. Transcatheter closure of atrial septal defect and patent foramen ovale with ASDOS device (a multi-institutional European trial). Am J Cardiol 1998;82:1405–1413.

68. Wahl A, Meier B, Haxel B, et al. Prognosis after percutaneous closure of patent foramen ovale for paradoxical embolism. Neurology 2001;57:1330–1332.

69. Braun MU, Fassbender D, Schoen SP, et al. Transcatheter closure of patent foramen ovale in patients with cerebral ischemia. J Am Coll Cardiol 2002;39:2019–2025.

70. Onorato E, Melzi G, Casilli F, et al. Patent foramen ovale with paradoxical embolism: mid-term results of transcatheter closure in 256 patients. J Intervent Cardiol 2003;16:43–50.

71. Berdat PA, Chatterjee T, Pfammatter J-P, et al. Surgical management of complications after transcatheter closure of an atrial septal defect or patent foramen ovale. J Thorac Cardiovasc Surg 2000;120:1034–1039.

72. USA Food and Drug Administration. HDE #H990011. Washington, DC: FDA, 2000.

73. Albers GW, Caplan LR, Easton JD, et al. Transient ischemic attack—proposal for a new definition. N Engl J Med 2002;347:1713–1716.

74. Pritz MB. Timing of carotid endarterectomy after stroke. Stroke 1997;28:2563–2567.

75. Del Sette M, Angeli S, Leandri M, et al. Migraine with aura and right-to-left shunt on transcranial Doppler: a case-control study. Cerebrovasc Dis 1998;8:327–330.

76. Anzola GP, Magoni M, Guindani M, et al. Potential source of cerebral embolism in migraine with aura: a transcranial Doppler study. Neurology 1999;52:1622–1625.

77. Sztajzel R, Genoud D, Roth S, et al. Patent foramen ovale, a possible cause of symptomatic migraine: a study of 74 patients with acute ischemic stroke. Cerebrovasc Dis 2003;13:102–106.

78. Milhaud D, Bogousslavsky J, van Melle G, Liot P. Ischemic stroke and active migraine. Neurology 2001;57:1805–1811.

79. Morandi E, Anzola GP, Angeli S, et al. Transcatheter closure of patent foramen ovale: a new migraine treatment? J Intervent Cardiol 2003;16:39–42.

80. Wilmshurst PT, Nightingale S, Walsh KP, Morrison WL. Effect on migraine of closure of cardiac right-to-left shunts to prevent recurrence of decompression illness or stroke or for haemodynamic reasons. Lancet 2000;356:1648–1651.

81. Moon RE, Camporesi EM, Kisslo JA. Patent foramen ovale and decompression sickness in divers. Lancet 1989;1:513–514.

82. Wilmshurst PT, Byrne JC, Webb-Peploe MM. Relation between interatrial shunts and decompression sickness in divers. Lancet 1989;2:1302–1306.

83. Knauth M, Ries S, Pohimann S, et al. Cohort study of multiple brain lesions in sport divers: role of a patent foramen ovale. Br Med J 1997;314:701.

84. Schwerzmann M, Seiler C, Lipp E, et al. Relation between directly detected patent foramen ovale and ischemic brain lesions in sport divers. Ann Intern Med 2001;134:21–24.

85. Cartoni D, DeCastro S, Valente G, et al. Identification of scuba divers with patent foramen ovale at risk for decompression sickness. J Am Coll Cardiol 1998;31:515.

86. Cantais E, Louge P, Suppini A, et al. Right-to-left shunt and risk of decompression illness with cochleovestibular and cerebral symptoms in divers: case control study in 101 consecutive dive accidents. Crit Care Med 2003;31:84–88.

87. Bendrick GA, Ainscough MJ, Pilmanis AA, Bisson RU. Prevalence of decompression sickness among U-2 pilots. Aviat Space Environ Med 1996;67:199–206.

88. Gallagher DL, Hopkins EW, Clark JB, Hawley TA. US Navy experience with type II decompression sickness and the association with patent foramen ovale. Aviat Space Environ Med 1996;67:712.

89. Klotzsch C, Sliwka U, Berlit P, Noth J. An increased frequency of patent foramen ovale in patients with transient global amnesia. Analysis of 53 consecutive patients. Arch Neurol 1996;53:504–508.

90. Akkawi NM, Agosti C, Anzola GP, et al. Transient global amnesia: a clinical and sonographic study. Eur Neurol 2003;49:67–71.

91. Aebi C, Kaufmann F, Schaad UB. Brain abscess in childhood—long-term experiences. Eur J Pediatr 1991;150:282–286.

92. Kawamata T, Takeshita M, Ishizuka N, Hori T. Patent foramen ovale as a possible risk factor for cryptogenic brain abscess: report of two cases. Neurosurgery 2001;49:204–206; discussion 206–207.

8

CardioSEAL®, CardioSEAL–STARFlex®, and PFO-Star® Closure of PFO

Michael J. Landzberg, MD

CONTENTS

INTRODUCTION

Post utero, persistence of the patent foramen ovale (PFO) carries mischievous potential, as it appears to have no physiologic or survival benefit for normal individuals. In states of abnormal right-sided cardiac capacitance, PFO has been implicated in worsening hypoxemia resulting from right to left intracardiac passage of deoxygenated blood. Association and causative roles of PFO in much more commonly occurring syndromes, including cerebral and cutaneous decompression disease, migraine with aura, and embolic ischemic stroke, have been suggested.

Percutaneous PFO closure was first reported in 1989 *(1)*, utilizing double-umbrella devices. Double-umbrella devices appeared particularly appealing for the following reasons: (1) versatility and conformability to the atrial surface and defect shape, with minimal device–septal distortion, (2) low profile and minimal distortion of blood-flow patterns, and (3) low metal content, minimizing corrosive and erosive potential. The initial Bard Clamshell Septal Occluder® (Fig. 1) was constructed as a double umbrella with four steel-alloy arms, each with a single springed hinge, on each side, covered in a Dacron meshwork. Opposing umbrellas were offset so as to (1) enable maximal flow profiles so that malposition and embolization would have least potential for adversity and (2) to maximize device arm recognition during deployment. In contrast to the older investigational Rashkind Ductal Occluder® umbrellas, "Clamshell" was designed to improve reliability of seating, as well as to promote more rapid and complete endothelialization and defect closure. Clinically silent stress-mediated device arm fractures, seen with increased frequency in the largest sized devices (33 mm and 40 mm, as measured diagonally), led to withdrawal

From: *Contemporary Cardiology: Interventional Cardiology:*
Percutaneous Noncoronary Intervention
Edited by: H. C. Herrmann © Humana Press Inc., Totowa, NJ

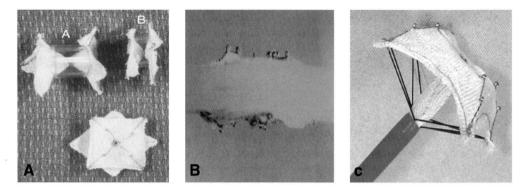

Fig. 1. Double-umbrella devices: **(A)** Bard Septal Clamshell Occluder®; **(B)** CardioSEAL®; **(C)** CardioSEAL–STARFlex®. Device design has emphasized (1) versatility and conformability to the atrial surface and defect shape, with minimal device–septal distortion, and reduction of radial and external stress, (2) low profile and minimal distortion of blood-flow patterns, and (3) low metal content, minimizing corrosive and erosive potential.

of Clamshell from clinical trials and advancement of device design. CardioSEAL® (NMT Medical, Boston, MA, USA) (Fig. 1) modification of Clamshell incorporated two springed hinges on each arm, decreasing mechanical stress. Metal alloy was changed to ferromagnetically inert MP35N, allowing for increased magnetic resonance imaging (MRI) compatibility. The retractive nature of the double-hinged umbrella arms not only improved the "spring-back" potential of CardioSEAL, allowing it to retain its original shape, but also continued to improve conformability to the atrial surface, minimizing device–septal distortion and allowing for most rapid complete closure and endothelialization. "Front-loading" delivery systems with decreased sizes of guiding sheaths were designed, allowing for a 10 French venous deployment systems. Size options increased, including 17-mm, 23-mm, 28-mm, 33-mm and 40-mm diagonal arm length choices. CardioSEAL's most recent STARFlex® (Fig. 1) modification includes internal nitinol microsprings sutured with polyester along the circumference of the umbrellas, attaching each arm to the corresponding two arms on the opposing umbrella. This internal buttressing meshwork allows for autoadjustment within a defect and for greater retraction of opposing umbrella arms toward the septum. This, in turn, allows for least device–septal distortion, radial stiffness, abrasiveness, and erosive stress, a low profile with greatest device contact with atrial surfaces, and smallest device/defect sizing. The previously existing pin–pin locking mechanism of the device to its delivery system, and internal core wire dimensions were modified to allow for even greater flexibility and least tension on, and distortion of, the atrial surface (witnessed during device release from delivery system, with least postrelease device mobility). The 17-mm and 40-mm sizes were eliminated. Newer delivery systems, allowing for easier retrieval of the intact device–delivery system not only after LA umbrella deployment but also after RA umbrella deployment are currently under investigation.

PROCEDURAL ASPECTS: CardioSEAL/CardioSEAL-STARFlex

Technical aspects of PFO closure are similar for all double-umbrella devices, with occasional device- or operator-specific variance. Key goals include (1) optimal PFO access, (2) imaging of the foramen and contiguous structures, (3) engagement of the left atrial umbrella flush with the left atrial–septal surface, and (4) engagement of the right atrial umbrella flush with the right atrial–septal surface. We recommend echocardiographic procedural guidance,

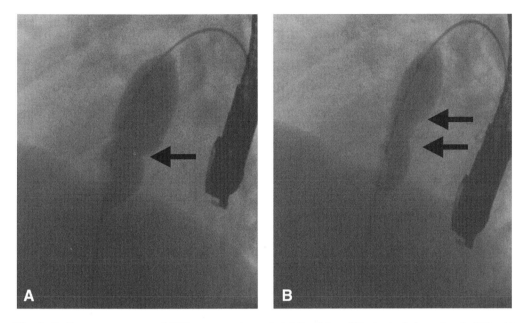

Fig. 2. Balloon assessment of PFO anatomy/tunnel rigidity. Note **(A)** single indentation in FO with "compliant" anatomy and **(B)** double indentation in FO with longer tunnel, potentially with less "compliant" anatomy.

with assessment of the foramen ovale (FO) and contiguous structure anatomy, for all implantation procedures.

After sedation and individualized pain control, venous access is obtained, typically via the right femoral vein. An entry catheter is placed via the IVC and right atrium across the PFO and a guide wire is anchored either within the left atrium or (typically left) pulmonary veins, and the entry catheter is removed. Many implanters utilize a compliant "sizing balloon" (to approximate the anatomy of the PFO), which is placed over the guide wire into the FO, where, upon expansion, its shape mimics the opening of the FO. Tunnel-type FO typically appear with a double-balloon indentation (Fig. 2). Some centers utilize a balloon eversion technique (exchange of the "sizing balloon with a smaller balloon endhole catheter, inflated within the left atrium and firmly retracted to the FO, in theory everting the overlap portion of septum primum) for all FO, particularly those with tunnel anatomy (Fig. 3). The transseptal technique, puncturing septum primum near septum secundum's lower "hinge" point of the tunnel, and implantation of a device to close this newly formed hole, is favored by some implanters in an attempt to avoid device–septal distortion whenever tunnel lengths exceed certain distances specific for that institution *(2)*. In one center's experience, transseptal puncture closure with the CardioSEAL device in patients with long tunnels provided better initial results, as assessed by contrast echocardiography that were not sustained at 6 mo *(3)*.

The utility of these techniques are unclear, although registries and randomized controlled trials could yield further evidence regarding their appropriateness. Some interventionalists place a pigtail angiographic catheter over the guide wire and inject 5–10 cm^3 of contrast directly into the FO, confirming all of the anatomic features of the FO (Fig. 4). After any or all these maneuvers, the device size is chosen. Guidelines for choice of device size classically have had little to do with understanding of septal and FO anatomy; little data exist substantiating a particular rationale. In general, a device

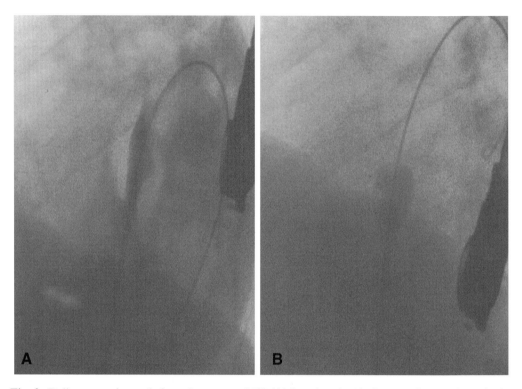

Fig. 3. Balloon eversion technique. Long tunnel FO (**A**) is reduced as balloon endhole catheter in the left atrium is dragged over a wire to and through the FO tunnel (**B**), retracting septum primum.

sufficiently (1) large enough to grasp overlapping primum tissue on the LA side without distortion, (2) large enough to grasp the thickness of septum secundum on the RA side without distortion, or (3) small enough to not distort the atrial septum or contiguous atrial walls, systemic or pulmonary venous inflow, or atrioventricular valve outflow is chosen, with individualization of choice. Anecdotal experience for CardioSEAL and CardioSEAL-STARFlex suggests working from a "23-mm" size model, with extension in uncommon circumstances to larger or smaller sizes based on individualized concerns.

Upon removal of the angiographic or balloon catheter, a 10F 75-cm-long delivery sheath is implanted across the FO, and the guide wire and sheath dilator are removed. The CardioSEAL/CardioSEAL–STARFlex device to be implanted is loaded onto a delivery catheter, and the catheter–device system is placed through the delivery sheath to its distal end within the left atrium. Fluoroscopic guidance is typically utilized, with camera angulation maximizing visualization of tunnel anatomy and contiguous structures (approx 30° up from true lateral and 15° cranial, with adjustment for individual cardiopulmonary anatomy). Guide catheters with radio-opaque tips are particularly useful in assisting in the maintenance of posterior guide angulation on approaching the septal surface, which could reduce device–septal distortion.

Air embolism remains a procedural complication, although rarely serious *(3)*. It is essential to remove air from the guide sheath in a meticulous fashion during dilator or device removal. In this regard, it is important to ensure that the guide tip is free in the left atrium and to use either very slow withdrawal or, alternatively, a positive flushing technique through both the guide and dilator when using a guide catheter with a valve.

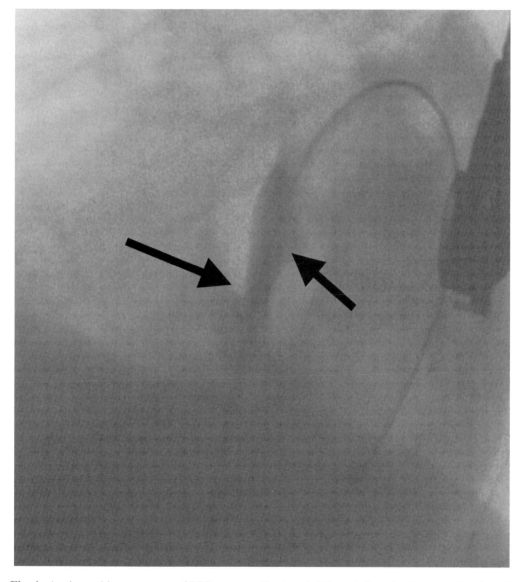

Fig. 4. Angiographic assessment of PFO anatomy. Contrast is injected via a pigtail over a wire directly within the FO. Straight arrow points to septum secundum's "hinge point" of FO tunnel. Hatched arrow notes mobile septum primum within the FO tunnel.

The distal device arms are then extruded or, more typically, the delivery sheath is retracted over the device, delivering the distal arms within the LA. A 10–2 side-facing clockarm configuration of the superior LA arms tends to minimize potential for interference with contiguous structures or distortion within the FO. Arm positioning can be confirmed by transesophageal endocardiography (TEE) or ICE. After confirmation of appropriate arm placement, the delivery sheath and catheter are both retracted allowing these distal, or left atrial, arms to become flush against the septal surface of the FO. Once this occurs, the delivery sheath is further retracted, allowing the proximal, or right atrial, arms to be delivered. Again, arm positioning can be confirmed by TEE or ICE, and upon confirmation of appropriate placement, the device is released from the delivery catheter.

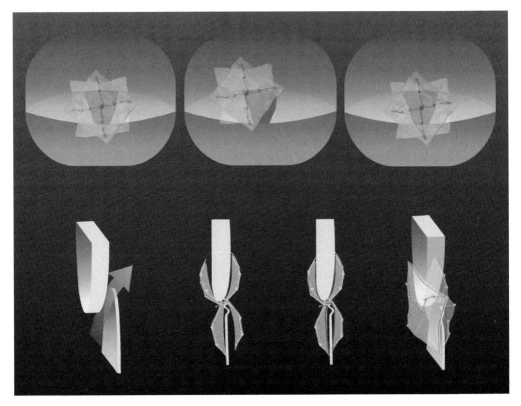

Fig. 5. The internal autoadjusting spring mechanism unique to the CardioSEAL-STARFlex system forces the device to find, and seat within, the central portion of the FO, Theoretically forcing maximal compliant traction against the septal surfaces and promoting more rapid and complete closure.Color (Ilustration is printed in insert following page 236)

An adversity inherent in nearly all transcatheter PFO closure devices is the inability of the interventionalist to personally manipulate the delivery system so as to anatomically center the device, allowing for the most minimal folding and septal distortion and most reliable complete FO closure. The internal autoadjusting spring mechanism unique to the CardioSEAL–STARFlex system, however, forces the device to find, and seat within, the central portion of the FO, theoretically forcing maximal compliant traction back toward the septum, allowing for minimal septal distortion and maximal complete closure (Fig. 5). Right atrial angiography can be used to confirm appropriate device placement and complete closure, although it is not a requisite.

All sheaths and catheters are removed from the body, hemostasis is achieved, and the patient is allowed to convalesce. No reversal of anticoagulation is suggested, and, in fact, might be contraindicated. Skin-to-skin procedural times are typically 15–45 min, dependent on operator experience, patient complexity, and teaching nature of the implanting institution. Recommendations for a specific peri-implantation antiplatelet strategy is unsubstantiated, and we await results of registries and randomized controlled trials in progress for further clues until more specific trials are undertaken. Strategies maximizing immediacy of complete platelet inhibition, usually with a combination of aspirin and clopidogrel for 2–6 mo are typical. Hospital discharge typically occurs within 24 h of implantation.

Device-Related Safety and Efficacy: CardioSEAL/CardioSEAL-STARFlex

Percutaneous PFO closure is now possible with up to seven different devices depending on availability during various phases of investigational development. In the United States, PFO can be closed percutaneously under Food and Drug Administration (FDA)-mandated HDE guidelines in limited specific circumstances both with CardioSEAL (HDE granted 2000) and the Amplatzer PFO Occluder (HDE granted 2002), and with sporadic usage of CardioSEAL in an "off-label" indication given its regulatory approval for closure of other intracardiac defects. Current HDE implantation potential exists for only those persons with recurrent documented stroke despite adequate anticoagulation. PFO closure with all other devices remains limited to investigational trials. Currently, no device has FDA premarket approval (PMA) for this indication.

Assessing efficacy of percutaneous PFO closure for each device has been troublesome given the case-series nature of existing studies, lack of randomized controlled trials, as well as a lack of defined and clinically meaningful endpoints for comparison. The Clamshell–CardioSEAL database has suggested that, for progressive generations of double-umbrella devices, culminating in CardioSEAL and its modifications, annual recurrent combined stroke/TIA (transient ischemic attack) event rate following percutaneous closure has been consistently less than 4%, and, in systematic review, could approach <2% *(1,4–8)*. Device-related adversity has been documented with each occlusion device system, with most notable occurrences including device embolization, cardiac and contiguous structure erosion, pericardial inflammation, device-related thrombosis, infection, device mechanical fracture or dislodgement, and stroke. Other less serious complications could include device-related early and late arrhythmia, transfusion requirement, and precipitation of migraine and chest pain. Although exact incidences of such adversity are difficult to cull from limited available published series, clinically meaningful adversity appears to occur in less than 1–3% of all patients undergoing percutaneous PFO closure with double-umbrella devices *(4–7,9)*. The incidence and clinical relevance of device-related thrombosis and early and late postimplant atrial arrhythmias has yet to be defined and compared to other therapeutic modalities. Of note, given differences in populations studied, procedural technique, periprocedural antiplatelet and anticoagulant strategies, and rigor of follow-up, the precise incidence of device-specific complications and comparative data between devices cannot be currently determined.

Systematic Review and Pooled Analysis

In an attempt to generate meaningful data (to guide construction of sufficiently powered randomized controlled trials) from the disparate and uncontrolled results of series of both medical treatments and percutaneous PFO closure, we recently estimated the relative benefit of transcatheter device closure compared to medical therapy via a systematic review and pooled analysis *(8)*. Analyses were grouped for all devices, including CardioSEAL, CardioSEAL–STARFlex, and PFO-Star, as device-specific data were not presented in the original studies. Relevant studies (1985–2002) were required to report ≥10 patients, followed for ≥1 yr with sufficient data collected and reported to allow for assessment of recurrent neurologic thromboembolic events at 1 yr of follow-up. Analysis of nine articles ($n = 1107$) of transcatheter closure was performed. Percutaneous PFO closure resulted in annualized incidence of 1.9% for stroke or TIA recurrence compared to 5.4% in medical therapy trials, relative risk [RR] = 0.346, 95% confidence interval [CI] = (0.209–0.573, $p < 0.0001$). The actuarial risk of recurrent TIA or stroke at 1-yr follow-up was 64.3% less in patients

Effect Name	Event	Event-free	Effect	Lower	Upper	PValue
Annualized rate of stroke	5/1107	28/895	0.144	0.056	0.372	0.000
Annualized rate of TIA	16/1107	23/895	0.562	0.299	1.058	0.070
Annualized rate of stroke or TIA	21/1107	52/895	0.327	0.198	0.538	0.000
Actuarial rate of stroke or TIA at 1-year	30/1107	68/895	0.357	0.234	0.543	0.000

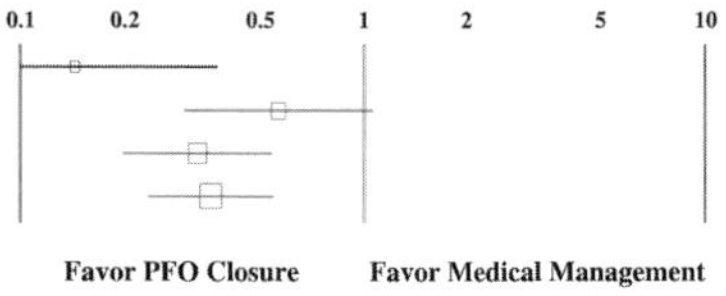

Favor PFO Closure   Favor Medical Management

Fig. 6. Systematic review: stroke and TIA following transcatheter PFO closure compared to medically treated patients.

with percutaneous closure of PFOs compared to medically treated patients (RR = 0.357, 95% CI = 0.234–0.543, $p < 0.0001$). Otherwise expressed, after the first year of follow-up, for every 23 patients who had their PFO closed percutaneuously, 1 stroke or TIA was prevented compared to use of medical therapy (Fig. 6).

CardioSEAL and CardioSEAL-STARFlex: Summary

At present, no comparative data suggest superiority of one PFO closure device compared to another. However, theoretic benefits of double-umbrella devices continue to include lowest device–septal distortion, radial stiffness, abrasiveness and erosive stress, versatility in conformation to varied defect and septal anatomy (allowing for near-universal application within FO), and very low profile, contributing to rapid and complete closure with minimal recognized adversity. Future design strategies incorporate use of an intestinal collagen overlay replacing the Dacron meshwork, allowing for >90% device resorption, en route to designs that ultimately aim for complete bioresorption.

PFO-STAR

PFO-Star is a double "sail" device, designed and tested in Europe in the late 1990s, and similar in appearance to double-umbrella devices but with sentinel differences (Fig. 7). Like Clamshell and its subsequent modifications, PFO-Star has gone through several generations of design modifications.

First-generation PFO-Star (Cardia, Burnsville, MN, USA) was comprised of two opposing "sails," offset from each other, each sail separated from the other by four blunted nitinol wire arms covered in 2-mm-thick polyvinyl alcohol (Ivalon). Sails, covering 22-, 26-, or 30-mm nitinol wires with titanium protective end caps, were connected by a 2-mm center post. Device deployment occurred with a modified biopsy forceps via standard 11–13 French transseptal sheaths in a fashion similar to that with double-umbrella devices. Device fixation within the FO is passive as a result of countertension of the relatively low profile device sails, but does not have a centering mechanism. Device arm fractures seen with first-generation PFO-Star devices were addressed by modification of 26- and 30-mm wire lengths to improve flexibility while retaining retractive potential. Additional changes to the second-generation PFO-Star devices included thinner Ivalon sails, allowing use of 10–12 French transeptal delivery sheaths, as well as modification of the center post to 3- and 5-mm variants, to allow for improved conformation to varied FO tunnel lengths and anatomies. Newer "third-generation" devices include a larger 35-mm device (theoretically for use in patients with PFO with hypermobile septum primum), change in wire tension in an attempt to equate stress on all size devices, movement of the LA Ivalon sail to the external surface of the device wires (theoretically to reduce thrombus promotion), and reduction of the thickness of the Ivalon covering by reinforcement, allowing downsizing of the deployment sheaths to 9–11F.

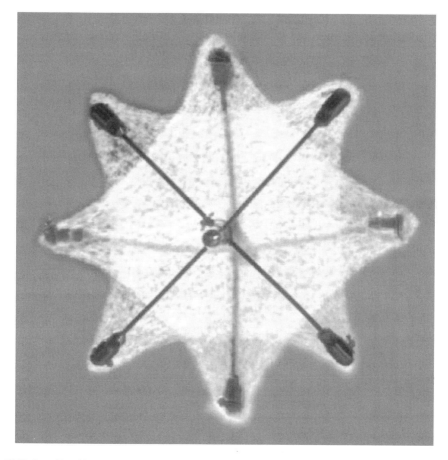

Fig. 7. PFO-Star. Double-umbrellas seen in CardioSEAL and its modifications have turned into double "sails". The PFO-Star device has yet to overcome early investigational suggestions of increased device- and procedure-related adversity.

Device deployment is similar in nature to that of CardioSEAL and CardioSEAL-STARFlex. A modified bioptome replaces the delivery–cable system of the double umbrellas. Of note, the wires of the PFO-Star are designed to allow for complete device retraction and removal if attached to the delivery bioptome.

Device-Related Safety and Efficacy: PFO-Star

PFO-Star currently is available in Europe only, as an investigational implant. As with the double-umbrella devices, assessing efficacy of this more recently introduced "double-sail" device is troublesome given the case-series nature of existing studies, lack of randomized controlled trials, as well as a lack of defined and clinically meaningful end points for comparison.

Databases exist in a number of centers *(9–13)*, with limited follow-up. Device-related adversity has been documented at each center, with most notable occurrences, including device embolization, cardiac and contiguous structure erosion, pericardial inflammation and effusion, device-related thrombosis, device mechanical fracture or dislodgement, stroke, and unusually high incidence of air embolization with ST-segment electrocardiographic changes during implantation; exact incidences of such adversities are difficult to cull from limited available published series *(9–14)*. Less critical, although important other complications have included device-related early and late atrial arrhythmias.

PFO-Star: Summary

PFO-Star appears to be a late-model spin-off of double-umbrella devices, with fewer device and delivery system parts and mechanics. However, at present, there appears to be no theoretic improvement in device–septal distortion, radial stiffness, abrasiveness, erosive stress, versatility in conformation to varied defect and septal anatomy, or profile, when compared to CardioSEAL and its STARFlex modification. Study of this device remains in relatively early, single- or related-center nonrandomized trials with nonstandard design, although with potentially meaningful adversity (erosions, effusions, embolizations, thrombus formation, high incidence of air embolization). The significance of these findings, as well as the potential impact of this device, at such early stages of development and study remains unclear.

RANDOMIZED CONTROLLED TRIALS: THE TIME HAS ARRIVED FOR COMPARISONS

Relative risks and benefits of therapies aimed at controlling or eliminating syndromes associated with PFO hinge upon study of the mechanisms of these diseases, the effects of specific planned therapies, and randomized controlled comparison treatment trials to guide individual and population recommendations. The data allowing for construction of randomized controlled trials (RCTs) with (1) well-defined enrollment criteria and outcomes measures and (2) statistical powering to allow for trial completion, assessment of superiority of individual treatments, and the answering of necessary scientific and clinical questions to allow for improved patient care exist. The largest such trial, CLOSURE-1, is a more than 1600-patient RCT currently ongoing in more than 80 participating centers. The study utilizes neurologists as principal investigators to evaluate CardioSEAL-STARFlex versus best medical therapy and is sufficiently powered to test superiority of percutaneous PFO closure versus medical therapy in persons with imaging-confirmed index stroke, evaluating similar hard neurologic end points as primary outcome. As clinicians dedicated to the care of patients with PFO-associated syndromes, we feel compelled to begin to answer the questions that could lead to improved care for those affected with such syndromes. This can best be accomplished through organizing institutional and regional care teams, and enrolling patients, whenever possible, into existing or new RCTs testing therapies and devices designed to limit PFO-associated risk.

REFERENCES

1. Bridges ND, Hellendbrand W, Latson L, et al. Transcatheter closure of patent foramen ovale after presumed paradoxical embolism. Circulation 1992;86:1902–1908.
2. Ruiz LE, Alboliras ET, Pophal SG. The puncture technique: a new method for transcatheter closure of patent foramen ovale. Cathet Cardiovasc Intervent 2001;53:369–372.
3. Herrmann HC, Silvestry FE, Glaser R, et al. Percutaneous PFO and ASD closure in adults: results and device comparison in 100 consecutive implants at a single center. Cathet Cardiovasc Intervent 2004, in press.
4. Windecker S, Wahl A, Chatterjee T, et al. Percutaneous closure of patent foramen ovale in patients with paradoxical enmbolism: long-term risk of recurrent thromboembolic events. Circulation 2000:101:892–898.

5. Hung J, Landzberg MJ, Jenkins JK, et al. Closure of patent foramen ovale for paradoxical emboli: intermediate-term risk of recurrent neurological events following tanscatheter device placement. J Am Coll Cardiol 2000;35:131.
6. Butera G, Bini MR, Chessa M, et al. Transcatheter closure of patent foramen ovale in patients with cryptogenic stroke. Ital Heart J 2001;2:115–118.
7. Martin F, Sanchez PL, Doherty E, et al. Percutaneous transcatheter closure of patent foramen ovale in patients with paradoxical embolism. Circulation 2002;106:1121–1126.
8. Khairy P, O'Donnell CP, Landzberg MJ. Transcatheter closure versus medical therapy of patent foramen ovale and presumed paradoxical thromboembolism: a systematic review. Ann Intern Med 2003;139:753–760.
9. Braun MU, Fassbender D, Schoen S, et al. Transcatheter closure of patent foramen ovale in patients with cerebral ischemia. J Am Coll Cardiol 2002;39:2019–2025.
10. La Rosee K, Krause D, Becker M, et al. Transcatheter closure of atrial septal defects in adults: practicality and safety of four different closure devices used in 102 patients. Dtsch Med Wochenschr 2001;126:1030–1036.
11. Sievert H, Horvath K, Zadan E, et al. Patent foramen ovale closure in patients with transient ischemic attack/ stroke. J Intervent Cardiol 2001;14:261–266.
12. Stauffier JC, Serra M, Juillard JM, et al. Percutaneous closure of patent foramen ovale: preliminary experience with PFO-Star. Arch Mal Coeur Vaiss 2004;97:37–41.
13. Schwerzmann M, Windecker S, Wahl A, et al. Percutaneous closure of patent foramen ovale: impact of device design on safety and efficacy. Heart 2004;90:186–190.
14. Krumsdorf U, Ostermayer S, Billinger K, et al. Incidence and clinical course of thrombus formation on atrial septal defect and patent foramen ovale closure devices in one thousand consecutive patients. J Am Coll Cardiol 2004;43:302–309.

9

Percutaneous Closure of Patent Foramen Ovale with the Amplatzer PFO Occluder

European Experience

Andreas Wahl, MD, Stephan Windecker, MD, and Bernhard Meier, MD

INTRODUCTION

The foramen ovale, which remains probe-patent throughout adulthood in approximately one-fourth of the general population *(1)*, has increasingly been recognized as potential mediator of several disease manifestations, including paradoxical embolism, refractory hypoxemia as a result of right-to-left shunt in patients with right ventricular infarction or severe pulmonary disease, orthostatic desaturation in the setting of the rare platypnea–orthodeoxia syndrome, neurological decompression illness in divers, and, more recently, migraine with aura. Percutaneous closure of the patent foramen ovale (PFO) has been shown safe and feasible using a variety of transseptal occlusion devices in previous reports *(2–10)*. Initial device-related complications inflicted by large delivery systems, device dislodgment and embolization, structural failure, thrombus formation,

From: *Contemporary Cardiology: Interventional Cardiology:
Percutaneous Noncoronary Intervention*
Edited by: H. C. Herrmann © Humana Press Inc., Totowa, NJ

and inability to reposition or remove the device have been reduced by recent improvements in device design. In particular, the appreciation of anatomic and physiologic differences between PFOs and atrial–septal defects (ASDs), led to the development of devices specifically designed for percutaneous PFO closure. The Amplatzer PFO Occluder® (AGA Medical, Golden Valley, MN, USA) is a self-expanding device manufactured from nitinol wire with polyester fabric, which is fully removable and repositionable as long as it remains screwed to the delivery cable *(11,12)*. In particular, the differences in design in contrast to the Amplatzer ASD Occluder are a smaller left than right atrial disk (except for the smallest model) and a slightly elongated, thin, and flexible waist connecting the two retention disks. In this chapter, the anatomy of the PFO, the currently available diagnostic techniques, the rationale for PFO closure, and the technique and the results of PFO closure using the Amplatzer PFO Occluder will be reviewed.

ANATOMY

The interatrial septum consists of two overlapping embryological structures: the left-sided partially fibrous septum primum and the right-sided muscular septum secundum. After having grown from the periphery to the center, these structures leave a central opening located infero-posteriorly, called the foramen ovale, with the septum primum serving as a one-way slit valve for physiologic right-to-left shunt during *in utero* development. The blood flow from the umbilical vein entering through the inferior vena cava keeps the foramen ovale open until after birth. From then on, the postnatal establishment of the pulmonary circulation, with subsequent increase in left atrial pressure to a level slightly above right atrial pressure, results in functional closure of the foramen ovale by apposition of the septum primum against the septum secundum. In most individuals, this is followed by anatomical closure in the ensuing months, through fusion of the caudal portion of the septum primum on the left side with the cranial portion of the septum secundum on the right side. In a large minority of the general population, however, this fusion does not take place, and the foramen ovale remains able to be opened. Indeed, autopsy studies revealed that the foramen ovale remains patent in approximately one-fourth of the general population *(1)*. This is called patent foramen ovale (PFO) and represents the most common persistent abnormality of fetal origin. In these individuals, the PFO permits intracardiac shunting during those periods when right atrial exceeds left atrial pressure. The prevalence of PFO appears to decline in older age groups, from 34% during the first three decades to 25% for the fourth to eighth decade, and to 20% in the ninth decade and beyond. Together with the tendency of an increasing PFO size with increasing age, from a mean of 3.4 mm in the 1st decade to 5.8 mm in the 10th decade of life, and unless selective mortality is operative, this suggests that smaller PFOs could spontaneously close even late in life. There is no gender preference, but recently a family trait has been reported, at least in females *(13)*.

Atrial–septal aneurysm (ASA) is a congenital abnormality of the atrial septum characterized by a redundant, amuscular membrane in the region of the fossa ovalis. The prevalence of ASA in the general population varies from 1% in autopsy series *(14–16)* to 2.2% in a recent population-based transesophageal echocardiographic study *(17)*. ASA is associated with a PFO in 50–85% of cases.

Atrial–septal dysmorphogenesis, evident as increased frequency of PFO and ASA, has recently been correlated with heterozygous mutations of the cardiac homeodomain transcription factor NKX2-5 in mice *(18)*. This observation provides the first evidence that the incidence of PFO might be related to genetic factors and that the PFO represents an index of septal dysmorphogenesis encompassing other defects such as ASA and ASDs.

DIAGNOSIS

A PFO cannot be detected on clinical grounds, but requires either noninvasive imaging modalities (i.e., transthoracic or transesophageal echocardiography) or invasive right heart catheterization with catheter passage of the defect. Indirect proof of a PFO can be derived with transcranial Doppler ultrasound, with a sensitivity and specificity approaching that of transesophageal echocardiography *(19)*. Likewise, indicator dilution and pulse oxymetry techniques have been validated and found to have a sensitivity of 85% and 76%, respectively, whereas both have a specificity of 100% *(20)*. However, none of these latter techniques can distinguish between a shunt at the level of the PFO or elsewhere, nor do they give information on the presence or absence of an associated ASA. Thus, multiplane transesophageal contrast echocardiography with Valsalva maneuver remains the most sensitive and specific method for the noninvasive detection of a PFO. It allows for the precise anatomical definition of the opening, with demonstration of a right-to-left shunt either by color Doppler mapping or bubble contrast injection. Using aerated saline or colloid solution injected into an antecubital vein *(21,22)*, the severity of the shunt can be semiquantitatively graded according to the amount of bubbles crossing the septum: grade 0 = no shunt, grade 1 = minimal shunt (1–5 bubbles), grade 2 = moderate shunt (6–20 bubbles), and grade 3 = severe shunt (>20 bubbles) *(21)*. In addition, transesophageal echocardiography allows for reliable exclusion of other potential cardiac sources of embolism.

The criteria for distinction between a floppy interatrial septum and ASA vary among autopsy, transthoracic, and transesophageal echocardiography studies. ASA is generally diagnosed if the diameter of the base of the flimsy portion of the interatrial septum exceeds 15 mm, if the excursion of the aneurysmal membrane exceeds 10 mm in either the left or right atrium, or if the sum of the total excursion is greater or equal to 10 mm *(16)*.

PATHOPHYSIOLOGY AND RATIONALE FOR PFO CLOSURE

Since the initial description of a stroke in a young woman with a PFO by Cohnheim in 1877 and besides its physiologic role in the fetal circulation, the pathophysiological aspects of the PFO have been increasingly appreciated giving rise to disease manifestations such the following:

- Paradoxical embolism *(23)* allowing for embolization of thrombus *(24,25)*, air, or fat *(26)*. In this respect, the rationale for PFO closure in cryptogenic stroke patients will be discussed in detail below. The risk of a PFO in the perioperative period has not been investigated systematically. However, the increased presence of potential emboli (air, venous clots, or fat) in association with unphysiological intrathoracic pressures is of concern. It has been suggested that high-risk patients should be screened for the presence of a PFO before elective susceptible surgical procedures *(27)*.
- Refractory hypoxemia resulting from right-to-left shunt in patients with right ventricular infarction *(28)* or severe pulmonary disease. In the presence of a PFO, right ventricular infarction can be complicated by hypoxemia as a result of to right-to-left shunt. This occurrence should be suspected in the case of hypoxemia not responsive to the administration of oxygen. Percutaneous PFO closure allows for rapid and effective elimination

of this complication and should be considered the procedure of choice in such cases. The PFO has also been identified as an independent risk factor for mortality (odds ratio [OR] = 11) and a complicated in-hospital course (OR = 5) in patients with a major pulmonary embolism *(29)*. This has been related to the PFO-mediated right-to-left shunt in the presence of elevated pulmonary artery pressures predisposing to arterial hypoxemia and paradoxical embolism with cerebral and vascular embolic complications, including death. The PFO gains similar importance in patients with elevated pulmonary artery pressures as a result of chronic pulmonary parenchymal or vascular disease and in patients with elevated right atrial pressures resulting from congenital heart disease.

- Orthostatic desaturation in the setting of the platypnea–orthodeoxia syndrome *(30,31)*, a rare clinical entity with unusual complaint of dyspnea related to arterial oxygen desaturation induced by the upright position and relieved by recumbency. The clinical recognition of this syndrome is established by arterial blood gas analysis both in the upright and supine position revealing orthostatic desaturation. The etiologic classification of the platypnea–orthodeoxia syndrome is based on the site of the right-to-left shunt into intracardiac (PFO, ASD), pulmonary vascular, and pulmonary parenchymal shunts (in areas with low ventilation–perfusion ratio). Several clinical conditions have been associated with the platypnea–orthodeoxia syndrome, including chronic liver disease with position-dependent ventilation–perfusion mismatch, amiodarone pulmonary toxicity, and patients with interatrial communications in conjunction with pneumonectomy, pulmonary embolism, loculated pericardial effusion, constrictive pericarditis, and enlargement of the ascending aorta. The therapeutic approach to patients with the platypnea–orthodeoxia syndrome is directed at the elimination of the underlying source of vascular shunting. Because the most common aetiologic association of the platypnea–orthodeoxia syndrome is with an interatrial communication established via a PFO, both surgical and percutaneous PFO closure have been shown feasible and effective in small uncontrolled studies. This procedure is curative by elimination of the right-to-left shunt with resolution of pulmonal arterial oxygen desaturation and, thereby, relief of symptoms. In light of the minimal invasive nature of percutaneous PFO closure and the severity of the frequently associated comorbid conditions, we believe that percutaneous PFO closure should be considered the therapy of choice in this patient population.

- Neurological decompression illness in divers *(32–34)* is caused by regional gas nucleation in predominantly fat-containing tissue as well as by arterial gas embolism, with both conditions being related to ischemic brain lesions. It has been hypothesized that a right-to-left shunt in divers with PFO allows for systemic embolization of venous gas bubbles and, therefore, increases the risk of decompression illness. Although divers with PFO are more likely to suffer from decompression illness and appear to have more ischemic brain lesions compared with divers without PFO, diving is associated with a higher incidence of ischemic brain lesions regardless of the presence of a PFO *(35)*. A preventive role of PFO closure in such individuals is intriguing but not yet defined.

- Migraine headache with aura. Using transcranial contrast Doppler ultrasound, two studies *(36–37)* reported an association between migraine with aura and presence of a right-to-left shunt presumably resulting from PFO. The prevalence of right-to-left shunt was similar to the prevalence of PFO in cryptogenic stroke patients *(36)*. This observation has prompted speculations about the role of PFO in patients with migraine complicated by aura. Changes in arterial oxygenation mediated by the right-to-left shunt via PFO have been implicated as a trigger for migraine with aura. Similarly, PFO-mediated paradoxical embolism of triggering substances or particulate matter has been suggested to explain migraine attacks and the increased risk of stroke in young patients with migraine and aura. Along this line, a recent study reported a significant improvement following percutaneous closure of various atrial–septal defects, suggesting a causal link between migraine with aura and presence of a right-to-shunt *(38)*. In our experience *(39)*, among 215 patients undergoing percutaneous PFO closure, 48 (22%) had suffered from migraine in the year prior to PFO closure, which is twice the expected prevalence of 10–12% in the general population. In patients with migraine with aura (*n* = 37), percutaneous PFO closure reduced the frequency of migraine attacks by 54%, and in patients with migraine without aura (*n*=11), the reduction was by 62%; however, it had no effect on headache frequency in patients suffering from nonmigraine headaches (*n* = 23). At this point in time, it has to be cautioned that the relation of migraine with aura and PFO requires further study in larger patient populations using transesophageal contrast echocardiography rather than transcranial Doppler ultrasound to identify the anatomic correlate. Only if this association is truly related to the presence of a PFO and not to a surrogate marker such as right-to-left shunt should therapeutic interventions aimed at elimination of the defect be contemplated.

The mechanism for right-to-left shunting via PFO in patients with paradoxical embolism, right ventricular infarction, or severe pulmonary disease is related to a transient (phase after Valsalva maneuver, during coughing, defecation, etc.) or permanent pressure gradient (decreased right ventricular compliance following right ventricular infarction or increased pulmonary artery pressure in the case of severe pulmonary disease). In contrast, the mechanism for right-to-left shunting with the platypnea–orthodeoxia syndrome remains unknown, as the right-sided pressures are typically normal and without measurable changes when assuming an upright posture during cardiac catheterization. Hypothetical explanations for right-to-left shunting in the upright position have been related to redistribution of blood flow, unequal compliance between diseased right and left heart chambers, subtle changes in pulmonary vascular resistance, and right ventricular output, or mechanical distortion of the fossa ovalis and the atria.

PFO AND PARADOXICAL EMBOLISM

Paradoxical embolism occurs when venous thrombotic material crosses through the PFO into the arterial circulation. Rarely, a thrombus caught within the PFO could be documented. Although large thrombi may occasionally pass through the PFO, this is more common for smaller clots of a few millimeters that would normally embolize to the lungs and spontaneously lyze in the lung filter without clinical sequelae. These paradoxical emboli will only be recognized clinically if they embolize to a sensitive organ such as the brain, the eye, or the heart via the coronary arteries. The source of these clots cannot be established in most patients. Thus, systematic screening for venous thrombosis is not warranted because of the insufficient sensitivity and specificity of venous Doppler examinations and venography for detection of small thrombi. In addition, the embolized thrombus might not have left thrombotic material behind. Although coagulation disorders and prothrombotic genetic polymorphisms such as factor V Leiden mutation, anticardiolipin antibodies, protein C and S deficiency, and prothrombin G20210A mutation have an increased prevalence in patients with deep venous thrombosis, their role in patients with paradoxical embolism remains poorly defined. Although most emboli presumably arise from systemic veins, the PFO itself has been suspected to be a source of thrombus. However, the fact that, to our knowledge, dislodging of such thrombi has not been reported during percutaneous PFO closure argues against this hypothesis.

Thus, the clinical diagnosis of paradoxical embolism remains presumptive in the majority of cases, because direct confirmation of a thrombus caught in the PFO is only rarely available. It should be entertained in patients with ischemic stroke or systemic embolism (1) without identifiable left-sided thromboembolic source, (2) with the potential for right-to-left shunt via PFO demonstrated by transesophageal echocardiography, and (3) with the presence of thrombotic material in the venous system or right heart chambers. The third criterion is optional, as the small thrombi frequently involved are difficult to document.

PFO AND ASA IN CRYPTOGENIC STROKE PATIENTS

Stroke is the third leading cause of mortality, and the leading cause of both serious morbidity and serious neurologic disease in Western societies. In younger patients, the etiology of ischemic stroke remains unknown in up to 40% despite an extensive diagnostic evaluation and is referred to as cryptogenic (40–42). Several case-control studies using contrast echocardiography revealed a strong relation between the presence of PFO and cryptogenic stroke in young adults aged <55 yr (21,43–47), whereas this relationship has been controversial in older age groups (44–46,48). Overell et al. (49) recently summarized the currently available evidence in a meta-analysis of case-control studies and confirmed a significant association between ischemic stroke and PFO. In patients younger than 55 yr, the PFO conferred a relative risk (RR) of 3 (95% confidence interval [CI] = 2–4) comparing ischemic stroke with nonstroke control subjects, and a RR of 6 (95% CI = 4–10) comparing cryptogenic stroke versus known-stroke-cause control subjects. These findings were more recently confirmed in the prospective PFO in Cryptogenic Stroke Study (PICCS) (50). In addition, patients with cryptogenic stroke related to PFO are at risk for recurrence despite medical treatment (50–54), a risk that is particularly pronounced in patients with PFO and associated ASA (17,52,53). In these patients, paradoxical embolism via a PFO has been implied as the most likely stroke mechanism (23) and, therefore, therapeutic measures for secondary prevention intend to eliminate thrombus formation, paradoxical embolization, or both.

Certain morphologic characteristics of PFO appear to predispose patients for paradoxical embolism. Both, larger PFO size (22,42,55,56) and a greater degree of right-to-left shunt as assessed by crossing microbubbles (22,55,57) signify a higher risk for suffering paradoxical embolism in the presence of PFO. The combination of PFO with an ASA constitutes a particularly high-risk situation with a RR of 16 (95% CI = 3–86) comparing ischemic stroke with nonstroke control subjects, and a RR of 17.1 (95% CI = 2–134) comparing cryptogenic stroke versus known-stroke-cause control subjects (age <55 yr) (49).

Atrial–septal aneurysm has been associated with cerebral ischemic events in numerous case-control studies (16,17,47,49,52,53,58–60). Of note, patients with PFO associated with ASA appear at higher risk for stroke as well as stroke recurrence compared to patients with PFO alone (47,52,53,60,61). Accordingly, ASA may act as a facilitator for paradoxical embolism via the following mechanisms: (1) The presence of ASA might increase the PFO diameter as a result of the highly mobile atrial–septal tissue, leading to a more frequent and wider opening of the otherwise small channel (22). (2) ASA might promote a right-to-left shunt by redirecting flow from the inferior vena cava toward the PFO (62). (3) ASA has been considered a nidus for local thrombus formation with subsequent embolization, but the data presented do not support this theory (14,58,63).

Although emboli from the ASA, itself, were considered, paradoxical embolism has been suggested as the principal mechanism for ASA-related embolic events *(17,61)*. Patients with both PFO and ASA constitute a high-risk population with a three fold to five fold increased risk for recurrent embolic events compared with patients with PFO alone *(49)*. Furthermore, secondary prevention with acetylsalicylic acid has been found insufficient for protection against recurrent cerebrovascular events in patients with both PFO and ASA *(52,53)*. Assuming paradoxical embolism as the most likely stroke mechanism in these patients, surgical or transcatheter treatment of PFO associated with ASA constitute alternative treatment options.

THERAPEUTIC OPTIONS FOR SECONDARY PREVENTION

Despite the growing recognition of the PFO, particularly when associated with an ASA, as a risk factor for paradoxical embolism, the optimal treatment strategy for symptomatic patients remains undefined. Most patients with presumed paradoxical embolism are treated medically with antithrombotic medications, with a paucity of data concerning the efficacy of oral anticoagulantion as opposed to antiplatelet therapy. Surgical PFO closure has proved feasible, but the procedure is associated with the well-known complications of cardiac surgery *(64,65)*, and the results have been mixed with respect to stroke prevention *(64–66)*. Percutaneous PFO closure is a catheter-based technique using atrial–septal occlusion devices. It has been initially advocated for prevention of recurrent stroke in 1992 *(2)* and safety and feasibility have been addressed in several studies *(2–10)*.

Medical Treatment

Comess et al. *(67)* described 33 patients with PFO and paradoxical embolism, mostly treated with acetylsalicylic acid or warfarin, who were followed for 18 mo and had a recurrent event rate of 14.4% per year (combined end point of transient ischemic attack and stroke). Mas et al. *(52)* retrospectively analyzed the risk of recurrence in 132 patients (mean age 40 yr) with cryptogenic stroke associated with isolated PFO (69 patients), ASA (25 patients) or both (38 patients) treated with either acetylsalicylic acid (250–500 mg/d) or oral anticoagulation (target international randomized ratio values [INR]: 2–3) during a mean follow-up period of 23 mo. The average annual rate of recurrence was 1.2% for ischemic stroke and 3.4% for the combined end point of transient ischemic attack and ischemic stroke. Patients with both a PFO and an ASA had an average annual rate of recurrent ischemic stroke of 4.4%, and of recurrent ischemic stroke or transient ischemic attack of 11.7%. Similar recurrence rates in patients (mean age = 44 yr) with PFO and cryptogenic stroke on medical treatment were reported from the Lausanne Stroke Registry *(51)*. Ninety-two patients were treated with acetylsalicylic acid (250 mg daily), and 37 patients were treated with oral anticoagulation (target INR = 3.5). The average annual recurrence rate was 1.9% for ischemic stroke and 3.8% for the combined end point of transient ischemic attack and ischemic stroke, with an annual vascular death (stroke) rate of 0.7% during a follow-up period of 3 yr. There were no statistically significant differences between the two antithrombotic drug regimens.

Mas et al. *(53)* also recently reported on the clinical outcome of 581 patients (mean age = 42 yr) with cryptogenic stroke, who were treated with acetylsalicylic acid 300 mg/d and followed prospectively for up to 4 yr. The risk of recurrent stroke or transient ischemic attack at 4 yr was 5.6% in patients with PFO alone ($n = 216$), 19.2% in patients with both PFO and ASA (n=51), 0% in patients with ASA alone ($n = 10$), and 6.2% in patients without atrial–septal abnormality (n=304). The authors concluded that patients with both PFO and ASA are at substantial risk for recurrence requiring additional preventive strategies beyond treatment with acetylsalicylic acid alone, whereas patients with a PFO alone are at low risk for recurrence comparable to those patients without atrial–septal abnormality. It has been hypothesized, however, that a large PFO rather than the associated ASA was responsible for the high recurrence rate in this study (68). Despite the low recurrence rate in patients with PFO alone, it cannot be excluded that percutaneous PFO closure reduces further events even in these patients. Notably, patients without atrial–septal abnormalities had significantly more competing stroke risk factors, such as arterial hypertension, smoking, or hypercholesterolemia, than PFO patients, possibly camouflaging the PFO risk.

In the prospective PFO in Cryptogenic Stroke Study (PICCS) (50), the presence of PFO was reported not to adversely impact on recurrent cerebrovascular events regardless of PFO size and presence of an ASA. However, only 42% of patients included in this study had suffered a cryptogenic stroke as opposed to stroke of known etiology (i.e., large vessel [11%], lacunar [39%], other determined cause [4%], or conflicting mechanism [4%]). Therefore, it comes as no surprise that PFO was only an innocent bystander in the majority of patients. Notwithstanding, the investigators were able to reproduce the previously documented association of PFO with cryptogenic stroke as well as a higher prevalence of large PFOs in cryptogenic stroke patients compared with controls of known stroke cause. Furthermore, the recurrent stroke and death rates at 2 yr were 9.5% or 17.9% for cryptogenic stroke patients with PFO receiving warfarin or acetylsalicylic acid, respectively (RR = 0.52, 95% CI = 0.16–1.67, $p = 0.3$). Although not significant, this corresponds to a 48% event reduction in favor of warfarin and contrasts with the event rates of 16.5% or 13.2% for warfarin- or acetylsalicylic acid-treated patients, respectively, in the entire PICCS cohort of PFO patients. Given the relatively low level of anticoagulation achieved with warfarin (mean INR = 2.0), a therapeutic benefit of oral anticoagulation over acetylsalicylic acid cannot be excluded.

Surgical PFO Closure

Homma et al. (64) reported on surgical PFO closure in 28 patients (mean age = 41 yr) with presumed paradoxical embolism. The open thoracotomy procedure was complicated by postpericardiotomy syndrome in five patients (18%) and transient atrial fibrillation in one patient (4%). During follow-up, one recurrent ischemic stroke and three recurrent transient ischemic attacks were observed, amounting to an actuarial recurrence rate of 20% at 13 mo. In contrast, Ruchat et al. (66) observed only 1 perioperative transient ischemic attack with no further recurrent embolic events during a mean follow-up of 3 yr in 32 patients (mean age = 40 yr). Of note, a residual shunt as assessed by transesophageal echocardiography was noted in three patients (9%) after surgery. In the largest surgical series from the Mayo Clinic (65), 91 consecutive patients (mean age = 44 yr) with at least 1 prior cerebrovascular ischemic event underwent surgical PFO closure by direct suture or patch closure. An intraoperative transesophageal echocardiography documented complete closure in all but one patient. There was no operative mortality, but a 21% morbidity consisting of atrial fibrillation in 12%, pericardial drainage for effusion in 4%, exploration for bleeding in 3%, and superficial wound infection in 1% of patients. During follow-up (mean = 1.9±2.2 yr, 176 patient-yr), the actuarial freedom from recurrent cerebral events was 93% at 1 yr and 83% at 4 yr.

Percutaneous PFO Closure

Initial techniques of percutaneous ASD closure were documented by King et al. in the 1970s (69), Rashkind in the 1980s (70), and Sideris et al. in the 1990s (71). After Bridges et al. first proposed that percutaneous PFO closure would reduce the incidence of recurrent strokes (2), percutaneous PFO closure has been shown to be safe and feasible in numerous studies, using a variety of devices, according to historical availability. In these studies, the reported success rates varied between 98% and 100%, with complication rates between 0% and 10%. Complete PFO closure was achieved in 51–100% of patients (2,4–10) and the reported yearly recurrence rates varied between 0% and 3.4%. Thus, the clinical efficacy of percutaneous PFO closure with respect to secondary prevention of recurrent embolic events compares favorably with previous studies of medical (51,52,67) and surgical (64–66) therapy.

However, it has to be emphasized that the true therapeutic efficacy of percutaneous PFO closure as adjunct or alternative to medical treatment in cryptogenic stroke patients is unknown, as a randomized study comparing the efficacy of percutaneous PFO closure versus medical treatment alone has yet to be completed. Unfortunately, given the low expected recurrence rates and the ensuing large patient numbers and long follow-up time required, first results from such studies cannot be expected before 5 yr. We, therefore, analyzed the patient cohort with cryptogenic stroke and PFO seen at our university-hospital-based stroke center and compared the risk of recurrent cerebrovascular events in patients who underwent percutaneous PFO closure or medical treatment alone. The two groups were comparable with respect to age, sex, cardiovascular risk factors, and associated ASA. However, patients undergoing percutaneous PFO closure had a larger right-to-left shunt at baseline and were more likely to have suffered more than one cerebrovascular event. Nonetheless, at 4 yr of follow-up, percutaneous PFO closure resulted in a trend toward risk reduction of death, stroke, or transient ischemic attack combined, and of recurrent stroke or transient ischemic attack compared with medical treatment. Thus, percutaneous PFO closure was at least as effective as medical treatment in the overall population. However, patients in whom complete PFO occlusion was achieved after percutaneous PFO closure had a significantly lower risk of recurrent stroke or transient ischemic attack compared with medically treated patients. Similarly, patients with more than one cerebrovascular event at baseline had a significantly lower risk of recurrent stroke or transient ischemic attack following percutaneous PFO closure compared with medically treated patients. There were no significant differences in the risk of recurrent events between treatment groups with respect to sex, older age, prior stroke, arterial hypertension, smoking, hypercholesterolemia, diabetes, or associated ASA (72).

This superiority of percutaneous PFO closure compared with medical treatment in patients with complete PFO occlusion is in line with our previously reported finding that complete compared with incomplete PFO occlusion results in a significantly lower risk of recurrence in patients undergoing percutaneous PFO closure (4,7). This observation lends further support to paradoxical embolism being the prevalent mechanism for cerebrovascular events in this patient population. Furthermore, it highlights that complete PFO occlusion is desirable for therapeutic efficacy in patients undergoing percutaneous PFO closure, a goal that can be achieved in >90% of patients with the most recent devices *(8,9)*.

The higher efficacy of percutaneous PFO closure compared to medical treatment in patients with more than one cerebrovascular event indicates that these patients represent a high-risk population. Indeed, these patients suffered recurrent cerebrovascular events despite medical treatment, suggesting inadequate protection by medical treatment alone. Of course, the benefits of percutaneous PFO closure in our study were associated with a certain risk of procedural complications, albeit without any long-term sequelae, and with the incremental cost of the procedure and the device. Thus, ultimate proof of paradoxical embolism being the principal stroke mechanism in such patients and of the superiority of percutaneous PFO closure over medical treatment will have to await the results of prospective, randomized trials such as the Percutaneous Closure of Patent Foramen Ovale and Cryptogenic Embolism (PC) trial *(7)*.

AMPLATZER PFO OCCLUDER DEVICE

The Amplatzer PFO Occluder (AGA Medical, Golden Valley, MN, USA) is a self-expanding double-disk device manufactured from 0.005-in. nitinol wire with a polyester fabric patch sewn into both disks (Fig. 1). The device is currently commercially available in three sizes, with the right atrial disc measuring 18, 25, or 35 mm, respectively. Smaller devices appear more snuggly nested in the fossa ovalis and might thus be more likely to secure complete closure of the PFO. On the other hand, they are more likely to be embolized or to incompletely cover a slitlike PFO. The device can be constrained within a 8F (18 or 25-mm device) or 9F (35-mm device) delivery system and reassumes its double disk shape upon delivery into the atria. The design of the Amplatzer PFO Occluder with a dominant right-sided disk pays tribute to the fact that a PFO acts as a one-way valve from right-to-left, thus minimizing the risk for device embolization from left to right. At the same time, it reduces the contact surface of prosthetic, possibly thrombogenic, material in the arterial circulation and reduces the risk of impairing neighboring structures such as the orifices of the pulmonary veins. While the Amplatzer ASD Occluder is self-centering and stents the ASD by means of its short and thick waist, the retention disks of the Amplatzer PFO Occluder are connected by a thin and longer flexible waist, which allows for free parallel movement of both disks. This affords a flexible adaptation of the retention disks to the atrial septum even in an oblique, channel-type PFO structure. The self-centering feature of the thick (ASD commensurate), short neck of the ASD device is not warranted for a PFO. Most importantly, the Amplatzer PFO Occluder is fully retrievable and repositionable as long as it remains screwed onto the 0.038-in. delivery cable. It is released by unscrewing the delivery cable in a counterclockwise fashion. On the other hand, the competing devices require a time-consuming removal from the delivery sheath prior to a new placement attempt, with renewed risk for air entrapment. Therefore, the fully retrievable and repositionable feature of the Amplatzer PFO Occluder without removal from the sheath might be an important safety mechanism in the prevention of procedural complications. Furthermore, the Amplatzer PFO Occluder is compatible with significantly smaller sheaths than its competitors. Because access to the venous circulation in adults is considered innocuous, this may

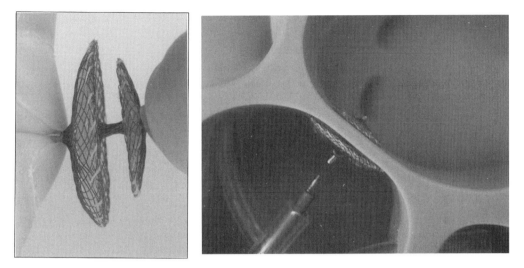

Fig. 1. A 25-mm Amplatzer PFO Occluder with a right-sided disk measuring 25 mm and a left-sided disk of 18 mm. The right panel shows the implantation in a model heart.

seem of little clinical significance at first glance, but might, nevertheless, reduce the incidence of vascular access site complications, such as arterio-venous fistulae.

IMPLANTATION PROCEDURE OF THE AMPLATZER PFO OCCLUDER AND FOLLOW-UP

After venous access is gained following local anesthesia via the right femoral vein, the PFO is crossed under fluoroscopic guidance in the antero-posterior (AP) view using a 6F multipurpose catheter (Fig. 2). We do not use routine transesophageal echocardiographic guidance because it provides little additional information, is poorly tolerated by the supine patients, and comes, therefore, at the cost of sedation or general anesthesia. Using a 0.035-in. wire, the multipurpose catheter is exchanged for the 8–9F Amplatzer delivery system with a distal 45° curve. Because of the risk of periprocedural air embolism, meticulous care has to be taken to ensure thorough evacuation of the air contained within the delivery system. Side arm sheaths of competing devices require four measures to avoid air embolism. First, the obturator of the sheath is pulled back while the guide wire remains in the left atrium or a pulmonary vein. This avoids blockage of the endhole and allows the blood to follow the receding obturator, and thereby blood fills the void rather than air sucked in from the outside. Second, this is carried out while the patient performs a Valsalva maneuver to increase left atrial pressure above outside pressure. Third, the device is introduced into the short loader under water and deployed and pulled back in at least once before leaving the water. Fourth, the loader is connected to the sheath with the device peeking out a few millimeters, again while the patient performs a Valsalva maneuver. Conversely, the Amplatzer introducer can be purged like a normal endhole catheter. Steps 1 and 2 can therefore be skipped. The Amplatzer PFO Occluder is then pushed with the delivery cable to the tip of the sheath positioned in the left atrium. The left atrial disk is deployed and gently pulled back against the atrial septum under fluoroscopic guidance in a left anterior oblique projection. To deploy the right atrial disk, tension is maintained

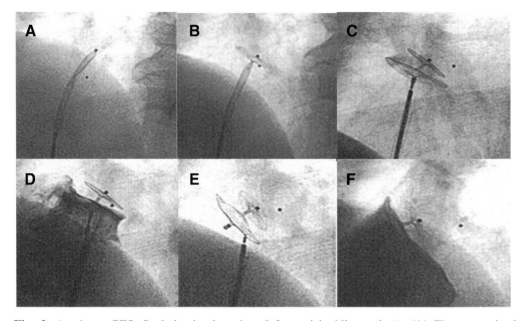

Fig. 2. Amplatzer PFO Occluder implantation (left cranial oblique view). **(A)** The constrained Amplatzer PFO Occluder is advanced within the 8F Amplatzer delivery sheath, which had been advanced across the PFO into the left atrium. **(B)** The left atrial disk is deployed by withdrawing the delivery sheath and then gently pulled against the interatrial septum. **(C)** Further traction of the delivery sheath under tension of the left atrial disk against the interatrial septum allows for release of the right atrial disk. The device has reassumed its double-disk shape connected by a thin waist, passing across the PFO. **(D)** A right atrial contrast injection by hand through the delivery sheath opacifies the right side of the interatrial septum, confirming a correct position of the device. Note the nearly horizontal orientation of the Amplatzer PFO Occluder and the indentation of the septum by the lower part of the disk. This results from the tension of the delivery cable upon the device. **(E)** Release of the device from its delivery cable by counterclockwise rotation. The device assumes the more perpendicular position of the interatrial septum. **(F)** Control right atrial angiography by hand injection through the sheath delineating the right atrial septum and correct device position. The left atrial septum can be visualized during the levo phase.

on the delivery cable while the delivery sheath is further withdrawn (see Video 1 on accompanying CD-ROM). After aspiration of the air from the sheath, a right atrial contrast angiography by a hand injection through the side arm of the delivery sheath serves to delineate the atrial septum (see Video 2 on accompanying CD-ROM). The so-called "Pacman Sign" (Fig. 3) refers to the aspect of the device on fluoroscopy that should be achieved before release. Seen in profile, the cranial halves of the left and right atrial disks should appear like open jaws biting into the thick septum secundum, reminding one of the arcade game figure Pacman about to gobble up a dot *(73)*. Upon verification of a correct position, the device is unscrewed from the delivery cable. The transseptal sheath is then used for a final contrast medium injection (see Video 3 on accompanying CD-ROM). The contrast can be followed to also delineate the left atrial contour and disk placement. Finally, the sheath is removed and hemostasis achieved by manual compression. The procedure, which can be performed on an outpatient basis, typically lasts around 30 min, with a fluoroscopy time of 5 min.

Antibiotics during the intervention are commonplace, and prevention against endocarditis is recommended for a few months until the device is completely covered by tissue.

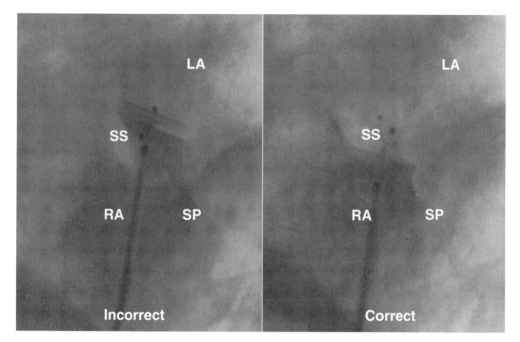

Fig. 3. The so-called "Pacman Sign" referring to the aspect of the device on fluoroscopy that should be achieved before release. Seen in profile, the cranial halves of the left and right atrial disks should appear like open jaws biting into the thick septum secundum, reminding one of the arcade game figure Pacman about to gobble up a dot. The left panel depicts the incorrect position; the right panel the correct position. LA = left atrium; RA = right atrium; SP = septum primum; SS = septum secundum.

Follow-up treatment includes acetylsalicylic acid (80–300 mg daily) for a few months, with the addition of clopidogrel (75 mg qd) or warfarin (INR = 2.5–3.5) at some centers. We perform a transthoracic contrast echocardiographic examination within 24 h of percutaneous PFO closure, in order to confirm correct device position and to look for a residual right-to-left shunt. All of our patients are treated with acetylsalicylic acid 100 mg once daily and Clopidogrel 75 mg once daily for 1–6 mo for antithrombotic protection until full device endothelialization. At 6 mo after percutaneous PFO closure, a contrast transesophageal echocardiographic study with aerated colloid solution injected into an antecubital vein is repeated, to assess for a residual shunt following endothelial overgrowth (Fig. 4). If the PFO proves completely closed, the medication is discontinued, unless required for another indication, such as associated coronary artery disease. In case of persistence of a small residual shunt, we recommend the continuation of acetylsalicylic acid. Small residual shunts might close late. In case of persistence of a moderate or large residual shunt, we recommend implantation of a second device, which results in complete closure in most cases. Of course, surgical PFO closure might also be contemplated at this stage, but an additional percutaneous attempt is preferable.

RESULTS OF PERCUTANEOUS PFO CLOSURE USING THE AMPLATZER PFO OCCLUDER

To our knowledge, there is only one large study reporting midterm results after percutaneous PFO closure using mostly the Amplatzer PFO Occluder *(74)*. In this study, 248

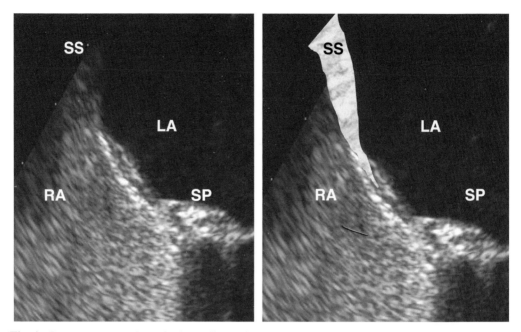

Fig. 4. Contrast transesophageal echocardiography documenting complete closure of the patent foramen ovale 6 mo after implantation of a 25-mm Amplatzer PFO Occluder. The right panel outlines the septum secundum. LA = left atrium; RA = right atrium; SP = septum primum; SS = septum secundum.

out of 256 patients received an Amplatzer PFO Occluder, which was successfully implanted in all cases.

In our experience, based on 350 consecutive patients between November 1998 and November 2003, percutaneous PFO closure using the Amplatzer PFO Occluder proved feasible without echocardiographic guidance with a high success rate (>99%) at first attempt. Failed implantation, resulting from the inability to canulate the PFO, was rare (three cases; <1%). In these patients, we refrained from performing a transseptal puncture for device implantation, as recommended by some authors, because failure to pass either rules out the presence of a PFO or demonstrates a PFO too small to be considered a risk. The only complication encountered was a case of suspected air embolism, with transient symptoms (0.3%; chest pain for 3 min without ECG changes). In order to assess the influence of device design on the risk of procedural complications, the completeness of PFO closure, and the clinical recurrence of embolic events, we prospectively compared 100 consecutive patients with paradoxical cerebrovascular events undergoing percutaneous PFO closure with either the PFO-STAR ($n = 50$) or the Amplatzer PFO Occluder ($n = 50$) *(75)*. Although percutaneous PFO closure was successful in all patients, significantly more placement attempts were required with the PFO-STAR, as compared to the Amplatzer PFO Occluder. In addition, procedure and fluoroscopy times were longer for the PFO-STAR, and procedural complications were more common, as compared with the Amplatzer PFO Occluder. Furthermore, transesophageal contrast echocardiography at 6 mo showed a significantly higher rate of complete closure for the Amplatzer PFO Occluder. There was also a trend for a higher freedom from recurrent cerebrovascular events with the Amplatzer PFO Occluder.

CONCLUSION

It has to be remembered that the diagnosis of PFO-mediated paradoxical embolism remains presumptive and that cryptogenic embolism is not necessarily synonymous with paradoxical embolism. Both a PFO and cryptogenic stroke may coexist without causal relation, and in such patients, PFO closure will not reduce the risk of recurrence, as reflected by the small recurrence rate despite complete PFO closure in our and other series. Percutaneous PFO closure is a procedure that can be performed with a high success and low morbidity rate in patients with presumed paradoxical embolism. The clinical efficacy with respect to secondary prevention of recurrent embolic events compares favorably with previous studies of medical *(51,52,67)* and surgical *(64–66)* therapy.

In patients with cryptogenic stroke and PFO seen at our university-hospital-based stroke center, percutaneous PFO closure resulted in a trend toward risk reduction of death, stroke, or transient ischemic attack combined, and of recurrent stroke or transient ischemic attack compared with medical treatment. Thus, in our experience, percutaneous PFO closure was, overall, at least as effective as medical treatment. Patients in whom complete PFO occlusion was achieved after percutaneous PFO closure had a significantly lower risk of recurrent stroke or transient ischemic attack compared with medically treated patients. Similarly, patients with more than one cerebrovascular event at baseline had a significantly lower risk of recurrent stroke or transient ischemic attack following percutaneous PFO closure compared with medically treated patients *(72)*.

Randomized trials comparing medical treatment with interventional PFO closure are needed to determine the best therapeutic strategy in this patient population *(7)*. Until results from such trials become available, the implantation of PFO occlusion devices will remain feasible, but should be performed only in appropriately selected and fully informed patients. Depending on the results of randomized trials, and in light of the minimal invasive nature of the percutaneous approach, the short procedure duration, and short hospital stay, percutaneous PFO closure could in the near future be considered the procedure of choice in this patient population. In that case, about 50,000 interventions per year would become necessary in the United States alone, representing about 1 per 10 percutaneous coronary interventions.

REFERENCES

1. Hagen PT, Scholz DG, Edwards WD. Incidence and size of patent foramen ovale during the first 10 decades of life: an autopsy study of 965 normal hearts. Mayo Clin Proc 1984;59:17–20.
2. Bridges ND, Hellenbrand W, Latson L, et al. Transcatheter closure of patent foramen ovale after presumed paradoxical embolism. Circulation 1992;86:1902–1908.
3. Ende DJ, Chopra PS, Rao PS. Transcatheter closure of atrial septal defect or patent foramen ovale with the buttoned device for prevention of recurrence of paradoxic embolism. Am J Cardiol 1996;78:233–236.
4. Windecker S, Wahl A, Chatterjee T, et al. Percutaneous closure of patent foramen ovale in patients with paradoxical embolism: long-term risk of recurrent thromboembolic events. Circulation 2000;101:893–898.
5. Hung J, Landzberg MJ, Jenkins KJ, et al. Closure of patent foramen ovale for paradoxical emboli: intermediate-term. J Am Coll Cardiol 2000;35:1311–1316.
6. Wahl A, Windecker S, Eberli FR, et al. Percutaneous closure of patent foramen ovale in symptomatic patients. J Intervent Cardiol 2001;14:203–209.
7. Wahl A, Meier B, Haxel B, et al. Prognosis after percutaneous closure of patent foramen ovale for paradoxical embolism. Neurology 2001;57:1330–1332.
8. Braun MU, Fassbender D, Schoen SP, et al. Transcatheter closure of patent foramen ovale in patients with cerebral ischemia. J Am Coll Cardiol 2002;39:2019–2025.
9. Bruch L, Parsi A, Grad MO, et al. Transcatheter closure of interatrial communications for secondary prevention of paradoxical embolism: single-center experience. Circulation 2002;105:2845–2848.

10. Martin F, Sanchez PL, Doherty E, et al. Percutaneous transcatheter closure of patent foramen ovale in patients with paradoxical embolism. Circulation 2002;106:1121–1126.

11. Sharafuddin MJ, Gu X, Titus JL, et al. Transvenous closure of secundum atrial septal defects: preliminary results with a new self-expanding nitinol prosthesis in a swine model. Circulation 1997;95:2162–2168.

12. Han Y, Gu X, Titus JL, et al. New self expanding patent foramen ovale (PFO) occlusion device. Cathet Cardiovasc Intervent 1999;47:370–376.

13. Arquizan C, Coste J, Touboul PJ, Mas JL. Is patent foramen ovale a family trait? A transcranial doppler sonographic study. Stroke 2001;32:1563–1566.

14. Silver MD, Dorsey JS. Aneurysms of the septum primum in adults. Arch Pathol Lab Med 1978;102:62–65.

15. Hanley PC, Tajik AJ, Hynes JK, et al. Diagnosis and classification of atrial septal aneurysm by two-dimensional echocardiography: report of 80 consecutive cases. J Am Coll Cardiol 1985;6:1370–1382.

16. Pearson AC, Nagelhout D, Castello R, et al. Atrial septal aneurysm and stroke: a transesophageal echocardiographic study. J Am Coll Cardiol 1991;18:1223–1229.

17. Agmon Y, Khandheira BK, Meissner I, et al. Frequency of atrial septal aneurysms in patients with cerebral ischemic events. Circulation 1999;99:1942–1944.

18. Biben C, Weber R, Kesteven S, et al. Cardiac septal and valvular dysmorphogenesis in mice heterozygous for mutations in the homeobox gene Nkx2-5. Circ Res 2000;87:888–895.

19. Di Tullio M, Sacco RL, Venketasubramanian N, et al. Comparison of diagnostic techniques for the detection of a patent foramen ovale in stroke patients. Stroke 1993;24:1020–1024.

20. Karttunen V, Ventila M, Ikaheimo M, Niemela M, Hillbom M. Ear oximetry: a noninvasive method for detection of patent foramen ovale: a study comparing dye dilution method and oximetry with contrast transesophageal echocardiography. Stroke 2001;32:448–453.

21. Webster MW, Chancellor AM, Smith HJ, et al. Patent foramen ovale in young stroke patients. Lancet 1988;2:11–12.

22. Homma S, Di Tullio MR, Sacco RL, et al. Characteristics of patent foramen ovale associated with cryptogenic stroke. A biplane transesophageal echocardiographic study. Stroke 1994;25:582–586.

23. Thompson T, Evans W. Paradoxical embolism. Q J Med 1930;23:135–150.

24. Caes FL, Van Belleghem YV, Missault LH, et al. Surgical treatment of impending paradoxical embolism through patent foramen ovale. Ann Thorac Surg 1995;59:1559–1561.

25. Falk V, Walther T, Krankenberg H, Mohr FW. Trapped thrombus in a patent foramen ovale. Thorac Cardiovasc Surg 1997;45:90–92.

26. Pell AC, Hughes D, Keating J, Christie J, et al. Brief report: fulminating fat embolism syndrome caused by paradoxical embolism through a patent foramen ovale. N Engl J Med 1993;329:926–929.

27. Sukernik MR, Mets B, Bennett-Guerrero E. Patent foramen ovale and its significance in the perioperative period. Anesth Analg 2001;93:1137–1146.

28. Silver MT, Lieberman EH, Thibault GE. Refractory hypoxemia in inferior myocardial infarction from right-to-left shunting through a patent foramen ovale: a case report and review of the literature. Clin Cardiol 1994;17:627–630.

29. Konstantinides S, Geibel A, Kasper W, et al. Patent foramen ovale is an important predictor of adverse outcome in patients with major pulmonary embolism. Circulation 1998;97:1946–1951.

30. Altman M, Robin ED. Platypnea (diffuse zone I phenomenon?). N Engl J Med 1969;281:1347–1348.

31. Seward JB, Hayes DL, Smith HC, et al. Platypnea–orthodeoxia: clinical profile, diagnostic workup, management, and report of seven cases. Mayo Clin Proc 1984;59:221–231.

32. Reul J, Weis J, Jung A, Willmes K, Thron A. Central nervous system lesions and cervical disc herniations in amateur divers. Lancet 1995;345:1403–1405.

33. Knauth M, Ries S, Pohimann S, et al. Cohort study of multiple brain lesions in sport divers: role of a patent foramen ovale. Br. Med J 1997;314:701–705.

34. Germonpre P, Dendale P, Unger P, Balestra C. Patent foramen ovale and decompression sickness in sports divers. J Appl Physiol 1998;84:1622–1626.

35. Schwerzmann M, Seiler C, Lipp E, et al. Relation between directly detected patent foramen ovale and ischemic brain lesions in sport divers. Ann Intern Med 2001;134:21–24.

36. Del Sette M, Angeli S, Leandri M, et al. Migraine with aura and right-to-left shunt on transcranial Doppler: a case-control study. Cerebrovasc Dis 1998;8:327–330.

37. Anzola GP, Magoni M, Guindani M, et al. Potential source of cerebral embolism in migraine with aura: a transcranial Doppler study. Neurology 1999;52:1622–1625.

38. Wilmshurst PT, Nightingale S, Walsh KP, Morrison WL. Effect on migraine of closure of cardiac right-to-left shunts to prevent recurrence of decompression illness or stroke or for haemodynamic reasons. Lancet 2000;356:1648–1651.

39. Schwerzmann M, Wiher S, Nedeltchev K, et al. Percutaneous closure of patent foramen ovale reduces the frequency of migraine attacks. Neurology 2004;62:1399–1401.

40. Hart RG, Miller VT. Cerebral infarction in young adults: a practical approach. Stroke 1983;14:110–114.

41. Sacco RL, Ellenberg JH, Mohr JP, et al. Infarcts of undetermined cause: the NINCDS Stroke Data Bank. Ann Neurol 1989;25:382–390.

42. Steiner MM, Di Tullio MR, Rundek T, et al. Patent foramen ovale size and embolic brain imaging findings among patients with ischemic stroke. Stroke 1998;29:944–948.

43. Lechat P, Mas JL, Lascault G, et al. Prevalence of patent foramen ovale in patients with stroke. N Engl J Med 1988;318:1148–1152.

44. de Belder MA, Tourikis L, Leech G, Camm AJ. Risk of patent foramen ovale for thromboembolic events in all age groups. Am J Cardiol 1992;69:1316–1320.

45. Di Tullio M, Sacco RL, Gopal A, et al. Patent foramen ovale as a risk factor for cryptogenic stroke. Ann Intern Med 1992;117:461–465.

46. Hausmann D, Mugge A, Becht I, Daniel WG. Diagnosis of patent foramen ovale by transesophageal echocardiography and association with cerebral and peripheral embolic events. Am J Cardiol 1992;70:668–672.

47. Cabanes L, Mas JL, Cohen A, et al. Atrial septal aneurysm and patent foramen ovale as risk factors for cryptogenic stroke in patients less than 55 years of age. A study using transesophageal echocardiography. Stroke 1993;24:1865–1873.

48. Jones EF, Calafiore P, Donnan GA, Tonkin AM. Evidence that patent foramen ovale is not a risk factor for cerebral ischemia in the elderly. Am J Cardiol 1994;74:596–599.

49. Overell JR, Bone I, Lees KR. Interatrial septal abnormalities and stroke: a meta-analysis of case-control studies. Neurology 2000;55:1172–1179.

50. Homma S, Sacco RL, Di Tullio MR, et al. Effect of medical treatment in stroke patients with patent foramen ovale: patent foramen ovale in Cryptogenic Stroke Study. Circulation 2002;105:2625–2631.

51. Bogousslavsky J, Garazi S, Jeanrenaud X, et al. Stroke recurrence in patients with patent foramen ovale: the Lausanne Study. Lausanne Stroke with Paradoxal Embolism Study Group. Neurology 1996;46:1301–1305.

52. Mas JL, Zuber M. Recurrent cerebrovascular events in patients with patent foramen ovale, atrial septal aneurysm, or both and cryptogenic stroke or transient ischemic attack. French Study Group on Patent Foramen Ovale and Atrial Septal Aneurysm. Am Heart J 1995;130:1083–1088.

53. Mas JL, Arquizan C, Lamy C, et al. Recurrent cerebrovascular events associated with patent foramen ovale, atrial septal aneurysm, or both. N Engl J Med 2001;345:1740–1746.

54. Nedeltchev K, Arnold M, Wahl A, et al. Outcome of patients with cryptogenic stroke and patent foramen ovale. J Neurol Neurosurg Psychiatry 2002;72:347–350.

55. Hausmann D, Mugge A, Daniel WG. Identification of patent foramen ovale permitting paradoxic embolism. J Am Coll Cardiol 1995;26:1030–1038.

56. Schuchlenz HW, Weihs W, Horner S, Quehenberger F. The association between the diameter of a patent foramen ovale and the risk of embolic cerebrovascular events. Am J Med 2000;109:456–462.

57. Stone DA, Godard J, Corretti MC, et al. Patent foramen ovale: association between the degree of shunt by contrast transesophageal echocardiography and the risk of future ischemic neurologic events. Am Heart J 1996;131:158–161.

58. Mugge A, Daniel WG, Angermann C, et al. Atrial septal aneurysm in adult patients. A multicenter study using transthoracic and transesophageal echocardiography. Circulation 1995;91:2785–2792.

59. Mattioli AV, Aquilina M, Oldani A, et al. Atrial septal aneurysm as a cardioembolic source in adult patients with stroke and normal carotid arteries. A multicentre study. Eur Heart J 2001;22:261–268.

60. Mattioli AV, Bonetti L, Aquilina M, et al. Association between atrial septal aneurysm and patent foramen ovale in young patients with recent stroke and normal carotid arteries. Cerebrovasc Dis 2003;15:4–10.

61. Meier B, Lock JE. Contemporary management of patent foramen ovale. Circulation 2003;107:5–9.

62. De Castro S, Cartoni D, Fiorelli M, et al. Morphological and functional characteristics of patent foramen ovale and their embolic implications. Stroke 2000;31:2407–2413.

63. Schneider B, Hanrath P, Vogel P, Meinertz T. Improved morphologic characterization of atrial septal aneurysm by transesophageal echocardiography: relation to cerebrovascular events. J Am Coll Cardiol 1990;16:1000–1009.

64. Homma S, Di Tullio MR, Sacco RL, et al. Surgical closure of patent foramen ovale in cryptogenic stroke patients. Stroke 1997;28:2376–2381.

65. Dearani JA, Ugurlu BS, Danielson GK, et al. Surgical patent foramen ovale closure for prevention of paradoxical embolism-related cerebrovascular ischemic events. Circulation 1999;100:II171–II175.

66. Ruchat P, Bogousslavsky J, Hurni M, et al. Systematic surgical closure of patent foramen ovale in selected patients with cerebrovascular events due to paradoxical embolism. Early results of a preliminary study. Eur J Cardiothorac Surg 1997;11:824-827.

67. Comess KA, De Rook FA, Beach KW, et al. Transesophageal echocardiography and carotid ultrasound in patients with cerebral ischemia: prevalence of findings and recurrent stroke risk. J Am Coll Cardiol 1994;23:1598–1603.

68. Schuchlenz HW, Weihs W, Beitzke A, et al. Transesophageal echocardiography for quantifying size of patent foramen ovale in patients with cryptogenic cerebrovascular events. Stroke 2002;33:293–296.

69. King TD, Thompson SL, Steiner C, Mills NL. Secundum atrial septal defect. Nonoperative closure during cardiac catheterization. JAMA 1976;235:2506–2509.

70. Rashkind WJ. Transcatheter treatment of congenital heart disease. Circulation 1983;67:711–716.

71. Sideris EB, Sideris SE, Fowlkes JP, et al. Transvenous atrial septal defect occlusion in piglets with a "buttoned" double-disk device. Circulation 1990;81:312–318.

72. Windecker S, Wahl A, Nedeltchev K, et al. Comparison of medical treatment with percutaneous closure of patent foramen ovale in patients with cryptogenic stroke. J Am Coll Cardiol 2004;44:750–758.

73. Meier B. Pacman sign during device closure of the patent foramen ovale. Catheter Cardiovasc Intervent 2003;60:221–223.

74. Onorato E, Melzi G, Casilli F, et al. Patent foramen ovale with paradoxical embolism: mid-term results of transcatheter closure in 256 patients. J Intervent Cardiol 2003;16:43–50.

75. Schwerzmann M, Windecker S, Wahl A, et al. Percutaneous closure of patent foramen ovale: impact of device design on safety and efficacy. Heart 2004;90:186–190.

10

Transcatheter Closure of Atrial–Septal Defects Using the Amplatzer Devices

Hitendra Patel, MD, Ralf Holzer, MD,
Qi-Ling Cao, MD,
and Ziyad M. Hijazi, MD

CONTENTS

INTRODUCTION
PATHOPHYSIOLOGY
CLINICAL PRESENTATION
MANAGEMENT
TRANSCATHETER DEVICE CLOSURE OF SECUNDUM ASD
TRANSCATHETER CLOSURE OF SECUNDUM ASD:
   STEP-BY-STEP TECHNIQUE
TROUBLESHOOTING
RESULTS
COMPLICATIONS
SUMMARY
REFERENCES

INTRODUCTION

An atrial–septal defect (ASD) is defined as an opening or defect in the atrial septum, between the right and left atrium. It excludes the patent foramen ovale. Four types of ASDs are recognized with distinct anatomic and embryological differences:

1. Primum defects arise from abnormal atrial–septal tissue development from the endocardial cushions.
2. Secundum result from defects in the septum primum with incomplete overlap of septum secundum.
3. Sinus venosus (superior vena cava type and inferior vena cava type) are defects in the part of the atrial septum that develops from the embryonic sinus venosus.
4. Coronary sinus septal defect is a defect in septation between the coronary sinus and the left atrium (LA).

From: *Contemporary Cardiology: Interventional Cardiology:*
Percutaneous Noncoronary Intervention
Edited by: H. C. Herrmann © Humana Press Inc., Totowa, NJ

Atrial–septal defects are some of the most common types of congenital heart defect; however, at present, only the secundum type is amenable for transcatheter closure.

Secundum ASD

This is a defect or deficiency in the septum primum and it may be single (90%) or multiple (fenestrated). The defect produces an incomplete overlap of septum primum and septum secundum, leading to a direct communication between the right and left atria *(1,2)*. The defect is, therefore, bordered by the limbus of the fossa ovalis or the C-shaped septum secundum. ASDs comprise 7% of all congenital heart defects and are twice as common in females. Most isolated defects are sporadic with no identifiable genetic marker. However, ASDs are associated with the Holt–Oram syndrome, an autosomal dominant disorder mapped to chromosome 12q and characterized by upper limb skeletal abnormalities: absent or hypoplastic radii and conduction defects. Ellis–van Creveld syndrome, an autosomal recessive skeletal dysplasia mapped to chromosome 4p, is associated with an absence of the atrial septum. Patients with secundum ASDs have a higher incidence of associated mitral valve prolapse, partial anomalous pulmonary venous return, and complex congenital heart defects.

PATHOPHYSIOLOGY

Atrial-level shunts occur in diastole and their direction depends on the differences in the right and left atrial pressures and compliance. The compliance of the atria is determined by their respective ventricular compliance. Ventricular compliance is determined by the ventricular wall thickness and contractility. Ventricular wall thickness is directly proportional to ventricular pressure needed to overcome the resistance to flow, the pulmonary vascular resistance (PVR) in the case of the right ventricle (RV) and systemic vascular resistance for the left ventricle (LV). As RV pressure and PVR increase, the RV wall thickness increases, leading to a fall in RV and right atrial (RA) compliance. Normally, the mean left atrial pressure (LAP) is 6–9 mm Hg and mean right atrial pressure (RAP) is 1–4 mm Hg, favoring a left-to-right (L-R) shunt; however, this is only a real factor in small defects. In large defects with equal atrial pressures, the amount and direction of flow across the ASD is dependent on the difference in compliance of the right and left atria and ventricles. Normally, the RA and RV compliance is much higher than that of the LA and LV, resulting in a L-R shunt across the ASD and its magnitude is dependent on the relative difference between the RV and LV compliance. At birth, the RV and LV wall thickness and the PVR and SVR are similar. Hence, right and left atrial and ventricular compliances are similar and the amount of flow across the ASD is minimal or can be bidirectional. As soon as lung inflation occurs and the PVR starts to fall, the RV compliance begins to increase relative to the LV. This leads to L-R flow across the ASD, which will continue to increase as the PVR continues to fall and the RV compliance continues to increase. LV compliance further decreases with age as the arteriolar elasticity decreases and SVR increases, leading to higher BP (blood pressure). This leads to higher energy expenditure by the LV to overcome increased afterload and subsequent LV hypertrophy. Decreased LV compliance with a subsequent elevation in LA pressure produces an increased L-R atrial-level shunt. The L-R shunt at the atrial level results in right-sided volume overload.

CLINICAL PRESENTATION

History

Small defects, usually less than 5 mm without right-sided volume overload, have no effect on the natural history of the individual. Some of these defects might close spontaneously. The majority of patients with moderate to large defects are usually asymptomatic at the time of diagnosis and remain so until the second decade of life. The physiologic impact of the L-R shunt increases with age. If the diagnosis is missed in the second decade of life, there may be a progressive increase in symptoms and a progressive decrease in exercise tolerance and occasionally overt congestive heart failure may manifest. Some of these patients may present with atrial arrhythmias, including atrial flutter and fibrillation. Unusual symptoms of orthodeoxia and platypnea can occur in the fifth to sixth decade. Pulmonary vascular disease might develop in 5–10% of patients with significant defects usually in the fourth or fifth decade of life. Paradoxical cerebral or systemic emboli rarely occur with true septal defects. They are far more prevalent with patent foramen ovale. Infective endocarditis is very uncommon and prophylaxis for isolated secundum ASD is not recommended.

Physical Examination

An ASD results in an increased volume load on the RA and RV. This can produce a split S1 with a loud second component as a result of forceful and late closure of the tricuspid valve. The classical finding is a wide, fixed splitting of S2. The wide split results from the late closure of the pulmonary valve because of the increased volume load that has to be ejected by the RV. The late closure is accentuated by increased capacitance of the pulmonary bed. In patients with a dilated RV, the time required for depolarization is increased and may manifest by an incomplete right bundle branch block observed on the surface ECG. This further prolongs RV ejection time, delaying pulmonary valve closure. Normal physiologic splitting of S2 results from respiratory variations in loading of the right and left sides of the heart (i.e., increased venous return to the RV with inspiration and increased venous return to the left ventricle with expiration). In the presence of an atrial–septal communication, these changes are transmitted to both sides and respiratory variation in splitting of S2 cannot occur. An ejection systolic murmur, usually grade 2–3/6 results from relative pulmonary valve stenosis produced by increased blood flow across it. Occasionally, mid-diastolic flow murmur can be heard secondary to increased flow across the tricuspid valve.

Laboratory findings

CHEST RADIOGRAPHY

Mild to moderate cardiomegaly can be seen because of enlargement of the RA and RV. There are increased pulmonary vascular markings in patients with large L-R shunts.

ECG

Normal sinus rhythm with right axis deviation, intraventricular conduction delay with deep S-wave in lead 1, and RSR's in V1 and V3R can be observed. Occasionally, a counterclockwise loop can be seen with left-axis deviation and Q-waves in leads 1 and AVL.

ECHOCARDIOGRAPY

Transthoracic echocardiography (TTE) is helpful in delineating the L-R shunt. However, it is not adequate for precisely finding the location and surrounding rims of the ASD. A dilated RA and RV as well as paradoxical ventricular septal motion secondary to a volume-loaded RV are noted. Flow acceleration across the tricuspid and pulmonary valves is seen as a result of the increased volume across these valves. It is important to ensure normal pulmonary venous return. Transesophageal (TEE) or intracardiac echocargiography (ICE) are the imaging tools of choice to delineate the exact location and surrounding rims of the ASD. Furthermore, TEE can evaluate any associated cardiac anomalies and can determine suitability for catheter closure.

CARDIAC CATHETERIZATION

This is not usually required for diagnosis. However, in older patients, a diagnostic cardiac catheterization with full hemodynamic and coronary assessment may be justified.

MANAGEMENT

A hemodynamically significant ASD should be considered an indication for closure irrespective of the age of the patient. Such defects are usually associated with significant L-R shunts, causing the Qp:Qs to exceed 1.5.1 (1). The magnitude of the L-R shunt is mainly dependent on the relative compliances of LV and RV and, therefore, can be diminished in the presence of pulmonary vascular disease and other disorders that are associated with reduced right ventricular compliance (1).

Echocardiographic signs of hemodynamically significant ASDs include right ventricular and right atrial volume overload, or evidence of increased pulmonary artery pressures. These are important findings when considering percutaneous closure of these defects and they can be readily identified using two-dimensional and Doppler echocardiography. The parasternal long-axis view is particularly useful in obtaining standardized measurements of right ventricular dimensions, whereas the apical four-chamber view should be utilized to obtain right atrial dimensions.

Once the diagnosis has been made, there is no advantage in delaying percutaneous closure of these defects. Device closure of hemodynamically significant ASDs should be considered in asymptomatic adults, to prevent subsequent development of atrial arrhythmias, pulmonary vascular disease, and other complications related to the presence of the defect. This approach is even more so justified by the low incidence of complications related to percutaneous closure of the ASD. However, the indication for device closure in asymptomatic adult patients with medium-sized ASDs without evidence of right atrial or right ventricular volume overload and normal distal pulmonary artery pressures is questionable.

Long-standing right atrial and right ventricular volume loading is associated with irreversible arrhythmogenic changes to both the RA and RV. Although symptoms related to an ASD are rare in the first decade of life, they become more common with advancing age. Congestive cardiac failure is common in patients above the age of 40 yr and the incidence of atrial arrhythmias has been found to be as high as 52% in patients aged 60 yr or older (3). Pulmonary vascular disease develops in 5–10% of patients with ASDs with a female preponderance (4), and a pulmonary vascular resistance exceeding 7 Wood units in the presence of 100% inspired oxygen is usually considered a contraindication to ASD closure. The role of medical management is rather limited in the treatment of ASDs and confined to temporary symptomatic treatment until definitive therapy via percutaneous or surgical closure has been initiated. In rare circumstances, a diuretic can be used to decrease pulmonary congestion, and afterload reducing agents have a theoretical role in decreasing systemic relative to pulmonary vascular resistance (thereby decreasing the L-R shunt).

TRANSCATHETER DEVICE CLOSURE OF SECUNDUM ASD

Currently in the United States the only Food and Drug Administration (FDA)-approved device for catheter closure of secundum ASD is the Amplatzer Septal Occulder (ASO) device. It was approved in December 2001 for all age groups, including pediatrics. Under an FDA requirement, operators need to be proctored at their institution prior to independent ordering and implantation. The device is manufactured by AGA Medical Corporation, (Golden Valley, MN, USA; www.amplatzer.com) and general indications for closure of ASDs include the presence of a hemodynamically significant ASD with secondary right heart volume overload in the absence of pulmonary vascular disease.

Contraindications to transcatheter ASD closure include the presence of associated cardiac anomalies requiring cardiac surgery, systemic or local infections or sepsis within 1 mo of the scheduled device placement, bleeding disorders or contraindications to antiplatelet therapy, or the presence of an intracardiac thrombus. Patients allergic to nickel might suffer an allergic reaction. This is a relative contraindication, as most nickel allergies are type 1 hypersensitivity reactions and it is unclear if intracardiac devices will mount a similar reaction. A consultation with an allergist should be sought.

Other technical factors that might preclude successful ASD device closure include anatomical characteristics such as deficient superior, inferior, and posterior rims. Although not being a contraindication, successful closure of these defects with deficient rims does require considerable clinical experience with the ASO device and should, therefore, only be attempted by very experienced operators.

Device Description

The ASO device is constructed from a 0.004- to 0.0075-in. Nitinol (55% nickel and 45% titanium) wire mesh that is tightly woven into two flat disks (Fig. 1). There is a 3- to 4-mm connecting waist between the two disks, corresponding to the thickness of the atrial septum *(5)*. Nitinol has superelastic properties with shape memory. This allows the device to be stretched into an almost linear configuration and placed inside a small sheath for delivery and then reform to its original configuration within the heart when not constrained by the sheath. The device size is determined by the diameter of its waist and is constructed in various sizes ranging from 4 to 40 mm (1-mm increment up to 20 mm; 2-mm increments up to 40 mm). The 40-mm device is currently available under an investigational device exemption (IDE) because of a lack of enough data about safety. The two flat disks extend radially beyond the central waist to provide secure anchorage. Patients with secundum ASD usually have L-R shunt. Therefore, the LA disk is larger than the RA disk. For devices 4–10 mm in size, the LA disk is 12 mm and the RA disk is 8 mm larger than the waist. However, for devices larger than 11 mm and up to 34 mm in size, the LA disk is 14 mm larger than the connecting waist and the RA disk is 10 mm larger than the connecting waist. For devices larger than 34 mm, the LA disk is 16 mm larger than the waist and the RA disk is 10 mm larger than the waist. Both disks are angled slightly toward each other to ensure firm contact of the disks to the atrial septum. There are a total of three Dacron polyester patches sewn securely with polyester thread into each disk and the connecting waist to increase the thrombogenicity of the device. A stainless-steel sleeve with a female thread is laser welded to the center of the atril surface of the

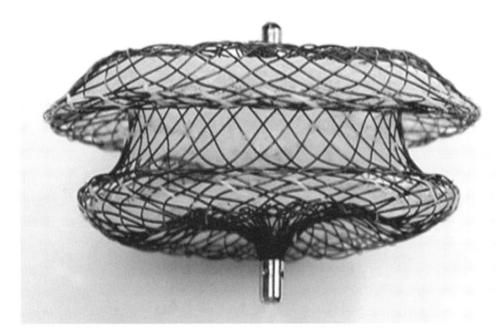

Fig. 1. The Amplatzer Septal Occluder demonstrating the two disks (top is the left atrial disk and bottom is the right atrial disk and the connecting waist.

RA disk. This sleeve is used to screw the delivery cable to the device. For device deployment, we recommend using a 6F delivery system for devices < 10 mm in diameter. A 7F delivery system for devices 10–15 mm in diameter; a 8F sheath for devices 16–20 mm in diameter; a 9F sheath for devices 22–28 mm in diameter; a 10F sheath for devices 30–34 mm in diameter; a 12F sheath for the 36- and 38-mm diameter devices; a 14F sheath for the 40-mm-diameter device. The cost of each device is $3300.

Amplatzer Delivery System

The delivery system is supplied sterilized and separate from the device. It contains all the equipment needed to facilitate device deployment. It consists of the delivery sheath of specified French size and length and appropriate dilator, a loader device used to collapse the device and introduce it into the delivery sheath, a delivery cable (inner diameter = 0.081 in.) where the device is screwed onto its distal end and it allows for loading, placement, and retrieval of the device, a plastic Pin-vice that facilitates unscrewing of the delivery cable from the device during device deployment, and a Touhy–Borst adapter with a side arm for the sheath, to act as a one way stop-bleed valve. All delivery sheaths have a 45° angled tip. The 6F sheath has a length of 60 cm, the 7F is available in lengths of 60 and 80 cm, and the 8F, 9F, 10F, and 12F sheaths are all 80 cm. The cost of the delivery system is $350.

A double-lumen balloon catheter with a 7F shaft and a compliant Nylon balloon is ideal for sizing the secundum ASD by flow occlusion without overstretching of the defect. The balloon catheter is angled at 45° and there are radio-opaque markers for calibration at 2, 5, and 10 mm. The balloon catheters are available in two sizes: 24 mm (maximum volume = 30 cm^3 and used to size defects ≤22 mm) and 34 mm (maximum volume = 90 cm^3 and used to size defects ≤40 mm). Other sizied balloon catheters are made by NuMED Inc. and are available in various sizes (20, 25, 30, and 40 mm).

Table 1
Materials/Equipment Required for Transcatheter Closure of ASD Using the Amplatzer Devices

Item	Sizes	Cost
Amplatzer Septal Occluder	4–40 mm	$3300
Amplatzer delivery system	7F–12F	$350
Amplatzer Supra stiff exchange	0.035 in.	$70
Length guide wire		
Multipurpose catheter	6F–7F	$10
Amplatzer sizing balloons	24 and 34 mm	$195
Amplatzer rescue system	9F, 12F	$350

Table 1 summarizes all necessary materials for ASD closure.

TRANSCATHETER CLOSURE OF SECUNDUM ASD: STEP-BY-STEP TECHNIQUE

Preprocedure

It is the responsibility of the interventional cardiologist to review all pertinent data related to the patient and the defect to be closed. Noninvasive data should be assessed by the echocardiographer. Ensure that appropriate devices and delivery systems are available. The procedure and complications should be explained to the patient prior to the procedure and opportunity given to ask questions and informed consent obtained. Aspirin, 81–325 mg, should be started 48 h prior to the procedure. If allergic to aspirin, clopidogrel (Plavix), 75 mg, can be used; however, nonpublished data suggest more issues with hemostasis at the end of the procedure.

Procedure

Access the right femoral vein with a 7F–8F short sheath. Place another short 11F sheath (preferably 30 cm long) in the same vein or the left femoral vein for the ICE catheter. An arterial monitoring line might also be useful if the patient's condition is unstable, the ASD is too large, or the procedure is performed under general endotracheal anesthesia. If the femoral venous route is not available, we advocate the transhepatic approach (6). Subclavian or internal jugular venous approaches are not recommended because of the sharp angle between the septum and superior vena cava. Heparin is administered to achieve ACT > 200 s at the time of device deployment. Antibiotic coverage for the procedure is recommended, we use cefazolin, 20 mg/kg, up to 1 g intravenously. The first dose is given at the time of procedure and two further doses 6–8 h apart.

Routine right heart catheterization should be performed in all cases to ensure the presence of normal pulmonary vascular resistance. The left-to-right shunt can also be calculated. Echocardiographic assessment of the secundum ASD should be performed simultaneously either by TEE or ICE (5,7). A comprehensive study should be performed looking at all aspects of the ASD anatomy (location, size, presence of additional defects, and adequacy of the various rims). Figure 2 and Video 1 on the accompanying CD-ROM demonstrate full assessment of the defect by ICE and the steps of closure. The important rims to define are the superior/SVC rim, the superior–posterior/right upper pulmonary vein rim, anterior–superior/aortic rim, inferior/IVC and coronary sinus rim, and posterior rim at the crux of the heart. The anterior–superior is the least important and is usually absent in larger defects (>20–22 mm).

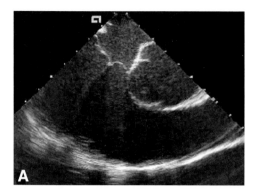

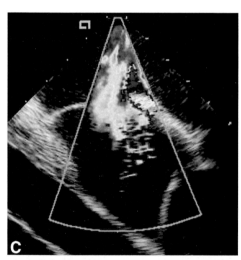

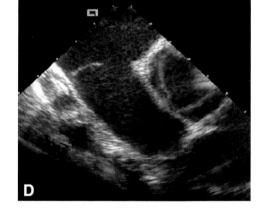

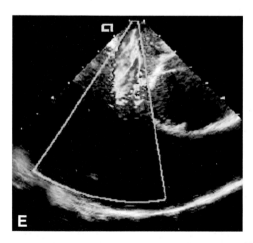

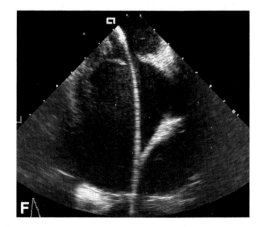

Fig. 2.

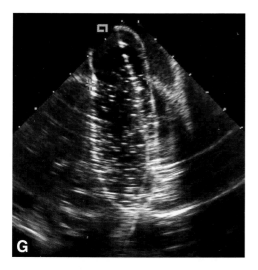

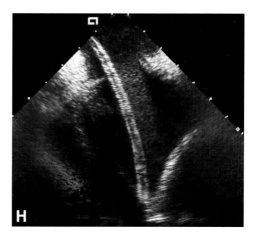

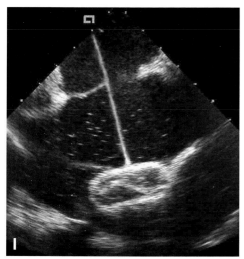

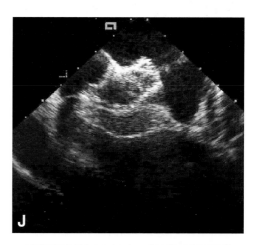

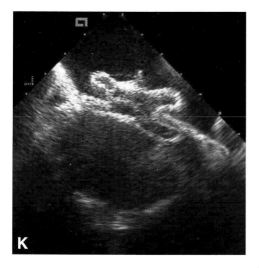

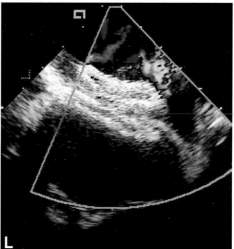

Fig. 2.

How to Cross the ASD

Use a multipurpose catheter, the MP A1 or A2 has the ideal angle. Place the catheter at the IVC/RA junction. The IVC course should guide the catheter toward the atrial septal defect, and keep a clockwise torque on the catheter while advancing it toward the septum (posterior). If unsuccessful, place the catheter in the SVC and slowly pull the catheter into the RA and keep a clockwise posterior torque to orient the catheter along atrial septum until it crosses the defect. TEE/ICE can be very useful for guiding the catheter across difficult defects.

Right Upper Pulmonary Vein Angiogram

It can be useful to perform an angiogram in the right upper pulmonary vein (Fig. 3A) in the hepatoclavicular projection (35° LAO/35° cranial). This delineates the orientation, anatomy, shape, and length of the septum. This can become handy when the device is deployed but not released; the operator can position the image intensifier (I/I) in the same view of the angiogram and compare the position of the device with the septal orientation prior to and after device release (Figs. 3C and 3D).

Defect Sizing

Position the MP catheter in the left upper pulmonary vein. Prepare the appropriate sizing balloon according to the manufacturer's guidelines. We prefer to use the AGA 24- or 34-mm balloons, as they are very compliant and do not distort or overstretch the defect during flow occlusion sizing. The shaft of the balloon catheter also has markers that facilitate calibration and allow orientation of the I/I so that it is perpendicular to the balloon for optimal sizing by fluoroscopy. Pass an extra-stiff floppy/J-tipped 0.035-in. exchange length guide wire (Amplatzer superstiff wire). This gives the best support within the atrium for the balloon, especially in large defects. Remove the MP catheter and the femoral sheath. We advance the sizing balloon catheter over the wire directly without a venous sheath. Most sizing balloons require an 8F or F9 sheath. The balloon catheter is advanced over the wire and placed across the defect under both fluoroscopic and echocardiographic guidance. The balloon is then inflated with diluted contrast until the left to right shunt ceases, as observed by color-flow Doppler TEE/ICE (flow occlusion). The best ECHO view for measurement is to observe the balloon in its long axis (Fig. 2G). In this view, the indentation made by the ASD margins can be visualized and precise measurement made.

Fig. 2. Intracardiac echocardiographic images in a patient with large secundum ASD. (**A**) Home view demonstrating the right atrium, tricuspid valve, right ventricle, aortic root, and pulmonary artery. (**B**) Septal view, demonstrating the large ASD measuring 16–19 mm (arrow), right and left atria and the superior and inferior rims. (**C**) Caval view with color Doppler demonstrating the entire superior rim and the defect (arrow). (**D**) Short-axis view demonstrating the defect (arrow), aortic root, absent anterior rim and good posterior rim, and both atria. (**E**) Same view with color Doppler. (**F**) The exchange wire (arrow) across the defect into the left upper pulmonary vein. (**G**) Sizing balloon occluding the defect. This is the stretched diameter (arrows) of the defect measuring 24 mm. (**H**) Delivery sheath (arrow) across the defect into the left upper pulmonary vein. (**I**) The left atrial disk (arrow) deployed in the left atrium. (**J**) The right atrial disk (arrow) deployed in the right atrium. (**K**) The device released demonstrating good position. (**L**) Color Doppler demonstrating no residual shunt. RA: right atrium; LA: left atrium; RV: right ventricle; AO: aortic root; PA: pulmonary artery; SVC: superior vena cava; AV: aortic valve; LPV: left pulmonary vein. (Color illustrations of C, E and L is printed in insert following page 236.)

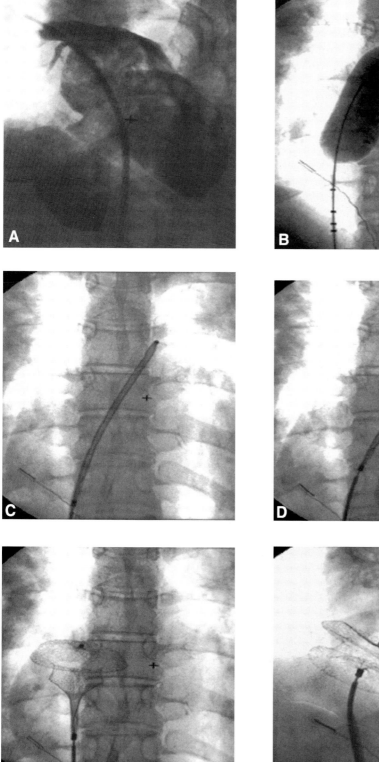
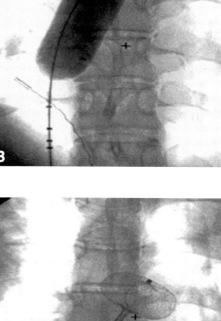

Fig. 3.

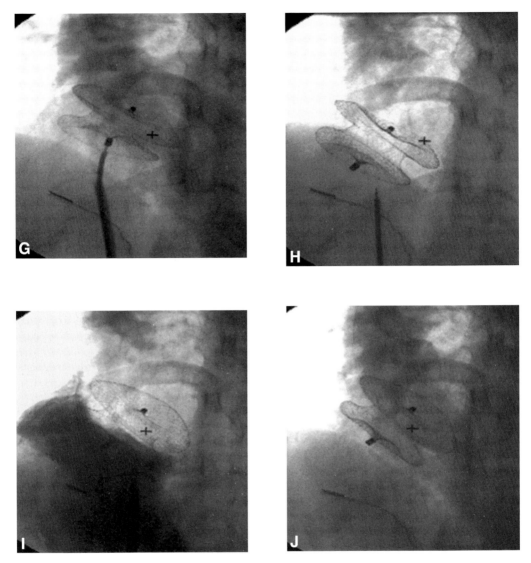

Fig. 3. Cine angiographic images in the same patient as Fig. 2. Black arrow represents the AcuNav catheter for intracardiac echocardiography. (**A**) Angiogram in the right upper pulmonary vein in the hepatoclavicular projection (35° LAO/35° cranial) demonstrating left to right shunt (arrow). (**B**) Cine image during balloon sizing of the defect demonstrating the stretched diameter (white arrows) of the defect. (**C**) Cine fluoroscopy during advancement of the device inside the delivery sheath (white arrow). (**D**) Cine fluoroscopy during deployment of the left atrial disk of the Amplatzer device (white arrow). (**E**) Cine fluoroscopy during deployment of the connecting waist (white arrow) and part of the right atrial disk. (**F**) Cine fluoroscopy after the right atrial disk has been deployed (white arrow). (**G**) Cine angiography of the pulmonary levophase of a right atrial angiogram prior to device release demonstrating good device position. (**H**) Cine fluoroscopy after the device has been released from the cable (white arrow). (**I**) Right atrial angiogram demonstrating good device position. (**J**) The pulmonary levo phase of the right atrial angiogram demonstrating no residual shunt.

Fluoroscopic Measurement

Angulate the X-ray tube so the beam is perpendicular to the balloon. The 2-mm calibration markers on the catheter shaft can help with angulation. They are seen distinctly separate at the appropriate angulation. Measure the balloon diameter at the site of the indentation as per the diagnostic function of the laboratory (see Fig. 3B and Video 2 on the accompanying CD-ROM). If a discrepancy exists between the echocardiographic and the fluoroscopic measurements, we have found that the echocardiographic measurement is usually more accurate. Once the size is determined, deflate the balloon and pull it back into the RA/IVC junction, leaving the wire in the left upper pulmonary vein. This is a good time to recheck the ACT and give the first dose of antibiotics.

Device Selection

If the defect has adequate rims (>5 mm), we usually select a device 0–2 mm larger than the balloon-stretched diameter. However, if the superior/anterior rim is deficient (<5 mm), we select a device 4-mm larger than the balloon-stretched diameter. Once the device size is selected, open the appropriate size delivery system. Flush the sheath and dilator. The proper size delivery sheath is advanced over the guide wire to the left upper pulmonary vein (Fig. 2H). Both dilator and wire are removed, keeping the tip of the sheath inside the left upper pulmonary vein. Extreme care must be exercised not to allow passage of air inside the delivery sheath. An alternative technique to minimize air embolism is passage of the sheath with the dilator over the wire until the inferior vena cava–right atrium junction, remove the dilator, and attach the Touhy–Borst adapter with a side arm to the sheath. Aspirate to "deair" the sheath and flush it using the side arm. Then, advance the sheath over the wire into the left atrium while continuously flushing the side arm of the sheath. Open the selected device and inspect it, ensure that it is the appropriate size, and inspect the wire mesh and the stitch work that secures the polyester disks. Thoroughly wet the device in normal saline. Attach the device on to the tip of the delivery cable by screwing it into the "female" receiver on the right-side disk.

Advance the loading device in the correct orientation from the back of the attaching cable toward the device. Load the device by collapsing it into the loading device by pulling swiftly on the delivery cable and applying forward tension to the loading device. This is performed underwater or under blood to expel air bubbles out of the system. Once the device is loaded, the system can be flushed further with normal saline or with the patient's own blood to ensure that no air is trapped inside. The loader containing the device is attached to the proximal hub of the delivery sheath. The cable with the ASO device is advanced to the distal tip of the sheath, taking care not to rotate the cable while advancing it in the long sheath to prevent premature unscrewing of the device. Both cable and delivery sheath are pulled back as one unit to the middle of the left atrium. Position of the sheath can be verified using cine fluoroscopy or TEE/ICE.

The LA disk is deployed first under fluoroscopic and or echocardiographic guidance by retracting the sheath over the cable (Fig. 2I). Caution should be taken not to interfere with the left atrial appendage and that the left disk not open in the pulmonary vein or the atrial appendage. Part of the connecting waist should be deployed in the left atrium, very close (few millimeters) to the atrial septum (the mechanism of ASD closure using the ASO device is stenting of the defect). While applying constant pulling of the entire assembly and retracting the delivery sheath off the cable, the connecting waist and the right atrial disk are deployed in the ASD itself and in the RA, respectively (Fig. 2J). Proper device position can be verified using different techniques:

1. Fluoroscopy in the same projection as that of the angiogram. Good device position is evident by the presence of two disks that are parallel to each other and separated from each other by the atrial septum. In the same view, the operator can perform the "Minnesota

Wiggle" (the cable is pushed gently forward and pulled backward). Stable device position manifests by the lack of movement of the device in either direction.

2. TEE/ICE. The echocardiographer should look for the two disks. One disk should be in the left atrium and the other in the right atrium. The septum should be seen separating the two disks. Two views are essential for this evaluation: the long axis and the short axis views.

3. The last method to verify device position can be achieved by angiography. This is done with the camera in the same projection as the first angiogram to profile the septum and device using either the side arm of the delivery sheath, or a separate angiographic catheter inserted in the sheath used for ICE, or a separate puncture site. Good device position manifests by opacification of the right atrial disk alone when the contrast is in the right atrium and opacification of the left atrial disk alone on pulmonary levo phase.

If device position is not certain or is questionable after all these maneuvers, the device can be recaptured entirely or partly into the sheath and repositioned following the above steps. Once device position is verified, the device is released by counterclockwise rotation of the delivery cable using a pin vise. There is often a notable change in the angle of the device as it is released from the slight tension of the delivery cable and as it self-centers within the ASD and aligns with the interatrial septum. Reassess the device position with TEE/ICE with color Doppler and angiography once released (Figs. 2 and 3 and Videos 1 and 2 on the accompanying CD-ROM). Once the procedure is complete, recheck the ACT and, if appropriate, remove the sheath and achieve hemostasis. If ACT is above 250 s, we have been reversing the effect of heparin using protamine sulfate.

Technique for Closure of Multiple Secundum ASDs

Often, the fossa ovalis might have more than one defect. If two defects are present and separated by more than 7 mm from each other, we cross each defect separately *(8)*. We size each one and then leave the delivery system in each defect. We initially deploy the smaller device, then the larger device and release sequentially starting with the smaller device.

If there are multiple fenestrations, we use the Amplatzer multifenestrated (cribriform) device (these devices are similar in design to the Amplatzer PFO device except the two disks are equal in size). These devices are still investigational and are available in three sizes: 18, 25, and 35 mm (the size of device is dictated by the size of the disk, not the connecting waist). The device should be deployed in the middle of the septum so that it can cover all fenestrations.

Postprocedure Monitoring

Patients are recovered overnight in a telemetry ward. Some patients might experience an increase in atrial ectopic beats. Rarely, some patients might have sustained atrial tachycardias. Administer two more doses of cefazolin, 20 mg/kg up to 1 g 6–8 h apart. Resume aspirin therapy, 3–5 mg/kg/d, and continue it for 6 mo.

The following day, an ECG, a CXR (PA and lateral), and a TTE with color Doppler should be performed to assess device position and presence of residual shunt. We also recommend repeat CXR 1 wk after the procedure to look for device position.

Recheck ECG, CXR, and a TTE/TEE at 6 mo postprocedure to assess all aspects of device position *(7)* and cardiac function. If device position is good with no residual shunt, follow-up can be annual for the first 2 yr, then every 3–5 yr. We suggest long-term follow-up so that long-term device performance can be assessed and any new information communicated to the patient. The patient is asked not to engage in full activity for 4–5 d to allow healing of the femoral access sites and refrain from contact sports for 1 mo after the procedure. Magnetic resonance imaging (MRI) (if required) can be performed any time after implantation and direct current cardioversion can be done should the need arise at any time after closure.

Postprocedure Medications

Aspirin as described earlier is recommended. Infective endocarditis prophylaxis for 6 months should be given when needed. After 6 mo, if there is no residual shunt, endocarditis prophylaxis and aspirin can be discontinued. If a residual leak exists, aspirin therapy and endocarditis prophylaxis should be continued until complete closure is documented.

TROUBLESHOOTING

Air Embolization

A meticulous technique should be used to prevent air entry. We prefer to place the sheath at the mouth of the left upper pulmonary vein. Doing so allows free flow of blood into the sheath. Forceful negative pressure should not be applied to aspirate the sheath. If a large amount of air is introduced on the left side, it will usually pool in the right coronary sinus and right coronary artery. This might manifest with bradycardia, asystole, or profound hypotension. If this occurs, immediately place a right coronary catheter in the right coronary sinus and forcefully inject saline or contrast to displace the air and hence reperfuse the right coronary system.

Cobra-Head Formation

The left disk maintains a high profile when deployed, mimicking a cobra head. This can occur if the left disk is opened in the pulmonary vein or left atrial appendage or if the left atrium is too small to accommodate the device size. It can also occur if the device is defective or if the device has been loaded with unusual strain on the device. If this occurs, check the site of deployment; if appropriate, recapture the device and remove it and inspect the device. If the "cobra head" forms outside the body, use a different device. If the disk forms normally, try deploying the device again. Do not release a device that has a "cobra-head" appearance.

Device Embolization

If a device embolizes, it has to be removed. This can be done surgically or by transcatheter snare and recapture into a long sheath. The transcatheter technique is difficult and should not be done if the operator is inexperienced in snaring techniques. Furthermore, the catheter laboratory should be equipped with large Mullins-type sheaths (12F–14F) and should have various sized snares. We use the gooseneck snare (Microvena Corp.). The device should not be pulled across valves because it might damage the chordae and leaflets. Always use a long sheath to pull the device outside the body. To snare a device, we usually use a sheath 2F sizes larger than the sheath that was used to deliver the device. On rare occasions, if the left atrial disk cannot be collapsed inside the sheath, we introduce another snare from the right internal jugular vein and snare the stud of the microscrew of the LA disk and stretch it toward the internal jugular vein while the assistant is pulling the device with the snare toward the femoral vein. This allows the device to collapse further and come out the sheath in the femoral vein.

Prolapse of the Left Disc Across the Defect During Deployment

On occasion, especially in patients with large defects with deficient anterior/superior rims, when the left disk is deployed, it opens perpendicular to the plane of the atrial septum and prolapses through the superior anterior part of the defect. To overcome this problem, there are some tips that we can offer: Use a device that is at least 4 mm larger than the measured balloon diameter; if this is not possible or it does not work, change the angle of the deployment by placing the sheath in the right upper pulmonary vein rather than the left. This could change the disk orientation. Another potential solution is to use a long sheath with a sharper curve that is stiffer (Mullins-type sheath) and rotate it posterior in the left atrium. Cook Inc. has developed a new sheath, the "Hausdorf sheath," that has a sine curve that can be quite useful in changing the deployment angle. The last potential method is to place the dilator of the delivery system in the other femoral vein and position it in the left atrium and ask the assistant to hold the LA disk in the LA while the operator is deploying the waist and RA disk in the respective locations. Once the device is deployed, remove the dilator. We have found this technique to work very well *(9)*.

Recapture of the device

To afford the smallest sheath size for device delivery, its wall thickness should small, with a resultant decrease in sheath strength. To recapture a device prior to its release, the operator should hold the sheath at the groin with his/her left hand, and with his/her right hand, pull the delivery cable forcefully inside the sheath. If the sheath is damaged/kinked (accordion effect), use the exchange (rescue) system to change the damaged sheath. First, extend the length of the cable by screwing the tip of the rescue cable to the proximal end of the cable attached to the device. Then, remove the sheath and exchange it with the 9F or 12F exchange sheath. To further strengthen the 9F or 12F sheaths to facilitate device retrieval, introduce the dilator of the rescue system over the cable inside that sheath until it is a few centimeters from the tip of the sheath. The dilator in this position significantly strengthens the sheath, allowing the operator to pull back the device, cable, and the dilator as one unit inside the sheath.

Release of the Device with a Prominent Eustachian Valve

To avoid the possibility of cable entrapment during release, advance the sheath to the hub of the right disk. Then, release the cable and immediately draw back inside the sheath before the position of the sheath is changed.

RESULTS

The results of percutaneous device closure of atrial septal defects using the Amplatzer Septal Occluder have been excellent *(10–12)*. In 2002, Du and colleagues reported a nonrandomized multicenter experience comparing surgical with transcatheter closure of ASDs using the ASO in 442 patients *(10)*. The procedural success rate for patients undergoing transcatheter closure of an ASD was 95.7%, compared to 100% in patients who opted for surgical closure of their intraatrial communication. However, the rate of procedure- or device-related complications has been found to be significantly lower for percutaneous closure when compared to surgical techniques *(10)*, with a complication rate of 7.2% for device closure and a complication rate of 24.0% for surgical closure of ASDs, with 0% mortality for either group. However, patients who underwent device closure were somewhat older than those who underwent open surgical closure.

In the same study, the mean length of hospital stay has been found to be significantly lower in patients undergoing percutaneous device closure of an intraatrial communication (1.0 d) when compared to patients who opted for a surgical approach (3.4 d). The reduced length of hospital stay positively influences the cost-effectiveness of the transcatheter approach to close ASDs. In a study by Kim et al., the mean cost for transcatheter closure was identified at $11,541, which was significantly lower than the costs of surgical closure at $21,780 *(13)*. Data on long-term follow-up has been limited, but, so far, there has been no evidence of any long-term device related complications after percutaneous ASD device closure.

COMPLICATIONS

In the US phase II trial *(10)* comparing device to open surgical closure, the incidence of complications was 7.2% for device closure, far less than what was encountered by open surgical technique (24%). Most complications were related to rhythm disturbance, with very few patients requiring long-term medical therapy. In particular, device embolization was rare with the majority encountered during the early learning curve of the investigators. Other complications included heart block (reported in only one patient), atrial arrhythmia which usually resolves by 6 mo, and headaches reported in about 5% of patients after device placement. We cannot offer any logical explanations to these headaches. However, the headaches resolve within 6 mo.

SUMMARY

The Amplatzer Septal Occluder is a safe versatile device used for closure of secundum ASDs. Patient selection and operator experience are very important for the success of the procedure. Long-term follow-up is needed to ensure long-term safety of the device.

REFERENCES

1. Porter CJ, Feldt RH, Edwards WD, et al. Atrial septal defects. In: Moss and Adams' heart disease in infants, children, and adolescents: including the fetus and young adult, 6th ed. Baltimore, MD: Williams and Wilkins, 2001:603–617.
2. Vick GW. Defects of the atrial septum including atrioventricular septal defects. In: The science and practice of pediatric cardiology, 2nd ed. Garson, Bricker, Fisher, and Neish, eds. Williams and Wilkins, Baltimore, MD: 1998:1141–1180.
3. Murphy JG, Gersh BJ, McGoon MD, et al. Long-term outcome after surgical repair of isolated atrial septal defect. N Engl J Med 1990;323:1645–1650.
4. Steele PM, Fuster V, Cohen M, Ritter DG, et al. Isolated atrial septal defect with pulmonary vascular obstructive disease—long-term follow-up and prediction of outcome after surgical correction. Circulation 1987;76(5):1037–1042.
5. Masura J, Gavora P, Formanek A, Hijazi ZM. Trans-catheter closure of secundum atrial septal defects using the new self-centering Amplatzer septal occluder: initial human experience. Cathet Cardiovasc Diagn 1997;42:388–393.
6. Weeks SM. Unconventional venous access. Tech Vasc Intervent Radiol 2002;5(2):114–120.
7. Hijazi ZM, Cao Q, Patel HT, Rhodes J, et al. Trans-esophageal echocardiographic results of catheter closure of atrial septal defects in children and adults using the Amplatzer device. Am J Cardiol 2000;85: 1387–1390.
8. Cao Q, Radtke W, Berger F, Zhu W, et al. Transcatheter closure of multiple atrial septal defects. Initial results and value of two- and three-dimensional transesophgeal echocardiography. Eur Heart J 2000; 21(11):941–947.

9. Abdul Wahab H, Bairam AR, Cao QL, Hijazi ZM. Novel technique to prevent prolapse of the Amplatzer septal occluder through large atrial septal defect. Catheter Cardiovasc Interv 2003;60:543–545.

10. Du ZD, Hijazi ZM, Kleinman CS, Silverman NH, Larntx K, for the Amplatzer investigators. Comparison between transcatheter and surgical closure of secundum atrial septal defect in children and adults: results of a multi-center non-randomized trial. J Am Coll Cardiol 2000;39:1836–1844.

11. Durongpisitkul K, Soongswang J, Laohaprasitiporn D, et al. Comparison of atrial septal defect closure using amplatzer septal occluder with surgery. Pediatr Cardiol 2002;23(1):36–40.

12. Fischer G, Stieh J, Uebing A, et al. Experience with transcatheter closure of secundum atrial septal defects using the Amplatzer septal occluder: a single centre study in 236 consecutive patients. Heart. 2003;89(2):199–204.

13. Kim JJ, Hijazi ZM. Clinical outcomes and cost of Amplatzer transcatheter closure as compared with surgical closure of ostium secundum atrial septal defects. Med Sci Monit 2002;8(12): CR787–CR791.

11

An Overview of Device Closure of Ventricular Septal Defects Using the Amplatzer Devices

Ralf Holzer, MD, Qi-Ling Cao, MD, and Ziyad M. Hijazi, MD, FACC

CONTENTS

BACKGROUND AND HISTORY
ANATOMY OF THE VENTRICULAR SEPTUM
VENTRICULAR SEPTAL DEFECTS IN THE ADULT POPULATION
PATIENT SELECTION
PREPROCEDURE EVALUATION
AMPLATZER VSD DEVICES
PROCEDURE: PROTOCOL AND TECHNIQUE
SUMMARY
REFERENCES

BACKGROUND AND HISTORY

Ventricular septal defects (VSD) are the most common congenital cardiac anomalies, accounting in isolation for almost 20% of congenital cardiac lesions *(1)*. VSDs have also been reported after myocardial infarction *(2,3)*, trauma *(4,5)*, as well as residual defects after prior attempts at surgical closure.

Depending on size, VSDs can cause variable degrees of left-to-right shunting with or without pulmonary hypertension. Small muscular defects diagnosed in infancy have a high likelihood of spontaneous closure, whereas larger defects tend to persist through adulthood *(6)*. The likelihood of spontaneous closure decreases with advancing age and is less common for defects located within the perimembranous region of the ventricular septum *(6)*. Irrespective of the hemodynamic effects of VSDs, there is an additional risk of developing subacute bacterial endocarditis *(7)*.

Surgical closure has been advocated as the gold standard for treatment of large VSDs. Surgical closure of perimembranous VSDs yields excellent results, with low morbidity and mortality *(8,9)*. However, the outcome is less favorable in patients with increased surgical

From: *Contemporary Cardiology: Interventional Cardiology: Percutaneous Noncoronary Intervention*
Edited by: H. C. Herrmann © Humana Press Inc., Totowa, NJ

Table 1
Reported Series of Transcatheter VSD Device Closure (Including More Than Five Patients)

Year	Author (ref.)	No. of pts.	VSD type	Device	Results
2003	Thanopoulos et al. (43)	10	Perimembranous	Amplatzer MEMBVSD	Procedural success 10/10; residual shunts at 24 h: 1/10; residual shunts at 3 mo: 0/10
2003	Arora et al. (23)	137	Perimembranous (91); muscular (46)	Amplatzer MVSD (90); Amplatzer MEMBVSD (17); detachable coils (1); Rashkind double umbrella (29)	Procedural success 130/137, *1; CHB; residual shunts at 24 h: 9/130; residual shunts at 9 mo: 1/130
2003	Holzer et al. (37)	18	Postinfarct	Amplatzer PIVSD	Procedural success 16/18; residual shunts at F/U: 8/10; mortality 7/18 (2 poss. proc. related)
2003	Holzer et al. (39)	75	Muscular	Amplatzer MVSD	Procedural success 72/83 procedures; residual shunts at 12 mo: 4/26; mortality 3/75 (2 procedure related)
2003	Bass et al. (40)	27	Perimembranous	Amplatzer MEMBVSD	Procedural success 25/27; residual shunts at 1 wk: 2/27;
2003	Szkutnik et al. (28)	7	Postinfarct	Amplatzer MVSD; Amplatzer septal occluder	Procedural success: 5/7; mortality 1/7 (0 procedure related)
2002	Hijazi et al. (42)	6	Perimembranous	Amplatzer MEMBVSD	Procedural success: 6/6, trivial AR 1; residual shunting postprocedure: 0/6
2000	Hijazi et al. (33)	8	Muscular	Amplatzer MVSD	Procedural success 8/8; residual shunts postprocedure: 6/8 residual shunts at 6 mo: 0/8

Year	Author	n	VSD type	Device	Results
1999	Janorkar et al. (44)	16	Muscular	Rashkind double umbrella	Procedural success 14/16; residual shunts at 6 mo: 5/15; mortality 3/16 (2 procedure related)
1999	Thanopoulos et al. (31)	6	Muscular	Amplatzer MVSD	Procedural success: 6/6; residual shunting postprocedure: 0/6
1999	Kalra et al. (45)	30	Perimembranous (28); muscular (2)	Rashkind double-umbrella coil (1)	Procedural success: 26/30; residual shunting on F/U: 8/30; coil embolization: 1
1998	Landzberg and Lock (17)	18	Postinfarct	Rashkind double-umbrella clamshell device	Procedural success 17/18; residual shunting in all; mortality 7/18 (3 procedure related)
1997	Sideris et al. (19)	25	Muscular; perimembranous	Buttoned device	Procedural success 18/25; residual shunts postprocedure: 5/18; surgical device recovery in 2
1994	Rigby and Redington (13)	13	Perimembranous	Rashkind double umbrella	Procedural success 10/13; surgical device recovery in 1
1991	Bridges et al. (46)	21	Muscular	Rashkind double umbrella	Procedural success 21/21; Qp:Qs postprocedure <1.1: 1
1988	Lock et al. (12)	6	Postinfarct; muscular	Rashkind double umbrella	Procedural success: 5/6 procedures; residual shunting at postprocedure: 5/6; mortality 4/6; device embolization: 1

risk factors, multiple previous cardiac surgical interventions, poorly accessible muscular VSDs or "Swiss-cheese" -type VSDs *(10,11)*.

In 1988, Lock and colleagues reported the first experience of transcatheter closure of muscular VSDs in seven patients using the Rashkind double-umbrella device *(12)*. Since then, different devices have been used to close muscular as well as perimembranous *(13)* VSDs with variable success, such as the Clamshell/cardioSEAL device *(14–18)*, the buttoned device *(19)*, as well as detachable coils *(20–23)*. Since 1998, different types of the Amplatzer device have been used to close VSDs *(23–42)*.

Table 1 illustrates all larger series (including more than five patients) of transcatheter VSD device closure reported in the literature to date. Results using the Amplatzer VSD devices were promising, as these devices were specifically designed for closure of VSDs *(37,40)*.

Devices for closure of VSDs have not only been used in the cardiac catheterization laboratory *(47)*. In 1993, Fishberger and colleagues first reported intraoperative VSD device closure using the Rashkind double-umbrella device in 10 patients *(48)*. More recently, Bacha and colleagues reported perventricular device closure of muscular VSDs without cardiopulmonary bypass, using the Amplatzer mVSD device in six patients *(47)*.

ANATOMY OF THE VENTRICULAR SEPTUM

The anatomy and location of VSDs not infrequently causes confusion among adult cardiologists because of the inaccurate use of terminology.

The most common defects are perimembranous VSDs, which are located underneath the aortic valve in the left ventricular outflow tract, with an opening on the right ventricular side incorporating the membranous septum, which is located in mid-superior portion of the septum closely related to the tricuspid valve and crux of the heart. These defects, also termed "infracristal VSDs," account for about 80% of all VSDs and can extend into the inlet or outlet portions of the ventricular septum.

Closely related to these defects are the classical inlet-type VSDs, which account for about 5–8% of all congenital VSDs. These defects are located more posterior underneath the tricuspid valve and, in their classical form, are completely surrounded by muscular septal tissue. However, in practice, the perimembranous and the inlet-type VSD are often confluent and difficult to distinguish.

A rare form of VSDs (5–7%) are those located superior directly underneath the pulmonary valve (subpulmonary) within the conus/infundibular ventricular septum in the outlet portion of the right ventricle. These defects, unless very large, are not related to the tricuspid valve and are associated with fibrous continuity of the aortic and pulmonary valves. They have been termed "supracristal" or "doubly-committed" VSDs and have an increased risk of developing progressive aortic insufficiency.

Muscular VSDs account for 5–20% of all congenital VSDs. Most commonly, these defects are located within the apex or mid-muscular septum, whereas anterior or postero-inferior location as well as a multifenestrated ventricular septum ("Swiss-cheese" VSDs) are rare.

VENTRICULAR SEPTAL DEFECTS IN THE ADULT POPULATION

Ventricular septal defects are rare in the adult population without congenital heart disease. Most frequently, the adult cardiologist encounters this entity after myocardial infarction. Less commonly, the adult cardiologist will encounter these abnormalities as a result of cardiac trauma *(4,5)* or iatrogenic trauma (e.g., after surgical replacement of the aortic valve) *(53)*. These patients are frequently high-risk candidates for surgical closure and the presence of a hemodynamically significant VSD should be considered a relative indication for VSD device closure.

The incidence of post-myocardial-infarction ventricular septal rupture remains as high as 0.2%. Ventricular septal rupture (VSR) is usually observed within 1 wk of the initial myocardial infarction (MI) and still carries a poor prognosis. Without surgical or percutaneous VSD closure, the mortality exceeds 90%, and even with surgical intervention, the reported early mortality ranges between 19% and 46% *(39)*. Cardiogenic shock and inferior myocardial infarcts are poor prognostic factors and the clinical course of postinfarction VSDs is characterized by sudden hemodynamic deterioration, even in patients who appear clinically stable, which does not allow much room for conservative management.

The outcome of transcatheter closure of postinfarct VSDs has been less favorable than reported results of congenital muscular VSDs *(12,17,18,24–26,28,39,54)*. In 2003, Holzer et al. reported a 30-d mortality of 28% in 18 patients in whom transcatheter closure with the Amplatzer postinfarct muscular VSD device was attempted *(39)*. Szkutnik and colleagues reported a series of seven patients in whom device closure using the Amplatzer Septal Occluder (ASO) as well as the Amplatzer muscular VSD device was attempted with one death. However, the procedures were performed in acutely surviving patients between 2 and 10 wk after the initial myocardial infarct. Complicating factors of transcatheter device closure have been identified as the frequently moribund status of these patients as well as VSD enlargement resulting from ongoing necrosis of surrounding tissues. This contributes to the residual VSDs observed in up to 80% of patients *(39)*.

Another group of patients encountered by the adult cardiologist are patients with a small hemodynamically insignificant VSDs and a secondary history of endocarditis. Device closure in these patients should be considered elective after adequate treatment of endocarditis.

PATIENT SELECTION

General Indications for VSD Closure

A nonrestrictive VSD with pulmonary hypertension in the absence of irreversible pulmonary vascular disease is an absolute indication for closure of the defect. Closure is also recommended in asymptomatic older children and adults with a restrictive VSD but a hemodynamically significant left-to-right shunt (usually Qp : Qs > 1.5 : 1), to prevent long-term complications such as pulmonary hypertension, arrhythmias, aortic regurgitation, double-chambered right ventricle endocarditis *(1,55)*. A very sensitive tool to evaluate significant left-to-right shunts is transthoracic echocardiography, demonstrating volume loading of left atrium (LA) and/or left ventricle (LV).

Further indications for VSD closure are the presence of VSD-related complications, such as subacute bacterial endocarditis (SBE) or the development of aortic regurgitation as a result of aortic cusp prolapse into the VSD.

Surgical Closure Versus Percutaneous Device Closure

Large nonrestrictive VSDs in either perimembranous or muscular location in small infants will remain the domain of cardiac surgical intervention for some time. A recent study by Holzer and colleagues, reporting the results of device closure of muscular VSDs in 75 patients, suggests an increased risk of complications and an increased risk of residual shunts in infants of lower weight at the time of the procedure *(37)*.

However, in older children and adults, the results of percutaneous VSD device closure have significantly improved, especially since the introduction of the Amplatzer VSD devices, and this procedure should, therefore, be considered a suitable alternative to surgical intervention. This is specifically true for muscular VSDs, where the overall mortality and frequency of residual VSDs after surgical VSD closure remains higher than for perimembranous VSDs (10,56). These VSDs are frequently hidden within the coarse right ventricular trabeculations, thereby difficult to localize through the standard surgical approach via the right atrium (37). The recent results of percutaneous closure of perimembranous VSDs using the Amplatzer membranous VSD device have also been encouraging, with closure rates of up to 92% within 1 wk of the procedure without any major device-related complications (40,42,43). This procedure could, therefore, be offered as an equivalent alternative to surgical intervention in larger patients.

Percutaneous Approach or Perventricular Approach

Several authors have reported intraoperative device closure of muscular VSDs (47–52). However, many of the reports advocated the use of cardiopulmonary bypass to place the device under direct vision. Recently, Bacha and colleagues reported on the "perventricular" approach to close VSDs in the operating room under transesophageal echocardiography (TEE) guidance without cardiopulmonary bypass, using the Amplatzer mVSD device with excellent results (47). This type of approach is favorable in smaller patients, where the size of delivery sheath might be associated with rhythm disturbances and hemodynamic compromise (37). In addition, patients with concomitant cardiac anomalies requiring surgical correction would benefit from this approach.

PREPROCEDURE EVALUATION

All patients require careful assessment to plan and prepare a successful percutaneous intervention. The indications for VSD device closure need to be reviewed and the patient's pertinent history forms a crucial part of the preprocedure assessment.

Chest X-ray (CXR) and electrocardiogram (EKG) form an important part of the routine assessment. The EKG needs to be analyzed for evidence of ventricular hypertrophy, pre-existing AV block or bundle branch block as well as presence of arrhythmias. The CXR needs to be reviewed for the presence of cardiomegaly, abnormal pulmonary vascular pattern suggestive of pulmonary hypertension, or other pulmonary abnormalities.

Laboratory investigations, such as renal function, complete blood count, or blood grouping, can usually be postponed until the day of catheterization but might need to be performed earlier if there is a suggestion of coexisting renal abnormalities.

The most important component of the preprocedure assessment is transthoracic echocardiography (TTE). Echocardiographic evidence of a reduced Doppler gradient across the VSD (nonrestrictive) in the absence of right ventricular outflow tract obstruction, or evidence of LV volume overload, as suggested by an increased LVEDD above the normal reference range, need to be carefully documented. The size, number, and locations of all VSDs need to be analyzed. Also, the relationship to cardiac valves and chordal attachments of AV valves needs to be documented (57).

All standard views should be utilized to adequately document the morphology of the VSD(s), with parasternal short-axis view, long-axis view, and apical four-chamber view being the most important to evaluate the precise location of the VSD. The parasternal long-axis view demonstrates perimembranous VSDs as well as anterior mid-muscular VSDs. The short-axis view at the level of the aortic valves facilitates differentiation between perimembranous VSDs (7–12 o'clock) and subpulmonary VSDs (1–2 o'clock). The short-axis view at the level near the tip of the mitral valve demonstrates anterior defects between 12 and 1 o'clock, mid-muscular defects between 9 and 12 o'clock, and inlet defects between 7 and 9 o'clock *(1)*. The four-chamber view at the level of the atrioventricular valves can be utilized to demonstrate apical VSDs, mid-muscular VSDs, inlet-type VSDs, as well as perimembranous VSDs. In addition, the five-chamber view demonstrates high anterior subaortic perimembranous VSDs.

For subaortic defects, the margin to the aortic valve needs to be carefully evaluated. A distance of less than 4–5 mm would favor the use of the Amplatzer membranous VSD device, whereas a distance of less the 2 mm would be considered unsuitable for any form of device closure. Supracristal defects are unsuitable for VSD device closure. It is important to document pre-existing valvar regurgitation or Doppler gradients across aortic, pulmonary, or AV valves for comparison with postclosure echocardiograms.

AMPLATZER VSD DEVICES

General Description

The group of Amplatzer VSD devices (AGA Medical Corporation, Golden Valley, MN) are made of nitinol wire (Fig. 1). Nitinol is an alloy of nickel and titanium. The devices are self-expandable, consisting of two flat disks that are linked via a central connecting waist, the diameter of which determines the size of the device. Polyester fabric is incorporated into each disk as well as the waist to enhance thrombosis.

Muscular VSD Device

The Amplatzer muscular VSD device has two disks that exceed the diameter of the connecting waist by 8 mm (Fig. 1). The connecting waist itself has a length of 7 mm. The device is available in sizes from 4 to 18 mm, requiring delivery sheaths size between 6F and 9F.

Postinfarct VSD Device

The Amplatzer postinfarct muscular VSD device is similar in design to the muscular device with two differences: The length of the waist is 10 mm to accommodate the thick septum in adult patients and the disks are 10 mm larger than the connecting waist. The device is available in sizes ranging from 16 to 24 mm, requiring delivery sheaths size between 9F and 12F.

Membranous VSD Device

The Amplatzer Membranous VSD Occluder is the most recent addition to the family of Amplatzer VSD devices (Fig. 1). The two disks are unequal, with the aortic end of the asymmetrical left ventricular disk exceeding the connecting waist (length = 1.5 mm) by only 0.5 mm to avoid impingement on the aortic valve, whereas the apical end is 5.5 mm larger than the waist. The apical end of the left ventricular disk contains a platinum marker. The right ventricular disk in contrast symmetrically exceeds the diameter of the connecting waist by 2 mm. The device is available in sizes from 4 to 18 mm, requiring delivery sheaths size between 7F and 9F.

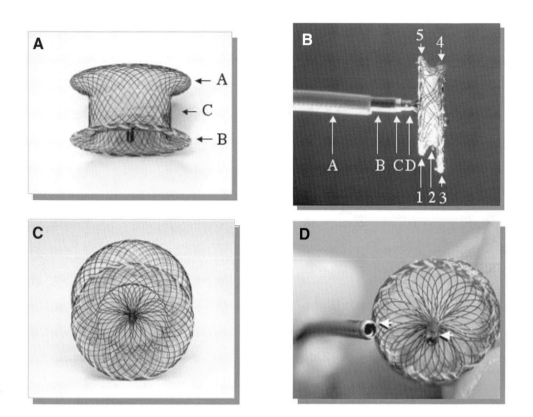

Fig. 1. (A,C) Muscular VSD device. Note, A and B denote the disks of the device and C denotes the connecting waist. For the congenital muscular device, C is 7 mm in length and the size of the device is dictated by diameter of C. A and B exceeds C by 8 mm; however, for the postinfarct VSD device, C is 10 mm in length and A and B exceeds C's diameter by 10 mm. **(B,D)**, Lateral view of the Amplatzer membranous VSD device attached to its delivery system (above) and pusher catheter and microscrew of device (bottom). The left ventricle disk is designated by the numbers 3 and 4. Note that the aortic end of the LV disk (designated by the arrow at 4) is 0.5 mm larger than the waist; the opposite end (designated by the arrow at 3) is 5.5 mm larger than the waist. The right ventricle disk (designated by the numbers 1 and 5) is 2 mm larger than the waist at both sides. The connecting waist (designated by the number 2) is 1.5 mm long. The delivery sheath is designated by A, the pusher catheter is designated by B, the capsule at the end is (designated by O). The screw of the device (designated by D) is screwed into the cable (not seen). Dacron polyester patches are visible within the nitinol mesh of the device.

Delivery Systems

GENERAL

The delivery system for muscular and postinfarct VSDs is identical to that for the Amplatzer septal occluder. It consists of a long Mullins-type sheath with its dilator, a cable, loader, and a pin vise.

MEMBRANOUS VSD DEVICE

The delivery system for the membranous VSD device is similar to that for the ASD, with an additional catheter (pusher) to facilitate correct deployment of the device. The pusher has a metal capsule used to align the flat portion of the screw of the membranous VSD device. This is important for correct orientation of the LV disk *(42)*. The delivery sheath is braided and has a very tight curve to facilitate positioning in the LV apex.

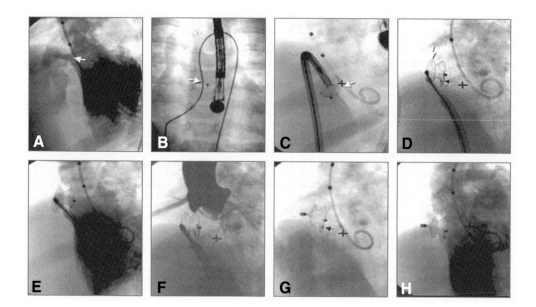

Fig. 2. (A) Angiogram in the LV in the left anterior oblique projection in a 2.5-yr-old male infant with perimembranous VSD measuring 7 mm (arrow) and left ventricle volume overload. **(B)** Cine image of an arteriovenous wire loop. **(C)** Cine image during deployment of the LV disk (arrow) of an 8-mm membranous device in the LV. **(D)** Cine image during deployment of the waist and right ventricular disk (white arrow). Note: the black arrow points to the platinum marker at the left ventricle disk. **(E)** Cine angiogram in the left ventricle prior to device release demonstrating good device position. **(F)** Cine angiogram in the ascending aorta prior to device release demonstrating no aortic regurgitation. **(G)** Cine fluoroscopy after the device has been released with the platinum marker (arrow) pointing toward the patient's feet. This indicates correct orientation of the device with the flat part toward the aortic valve. **(H)** LV angiogram a few minutes after the device has been released, demonstrating good device position and minimal foaming through the device.

PROCEDURE: PROTOCOL AND TECHNIQUE

General Technique

PREPARATION

The techniques described have been reported in great detail by Hijazi and colleagues as well as Thanopoulos and colleagues *(31,42,58)*, and are illustrated in Fig. 2 and a video on the CD.

All procedures should routinely be performed under general anaesthesia for patient comfort during TEE monitoring and to avoid patient movements during crucial parts of the device delivery process. An initial complete assessment is performed to re-evaluate and reconfirm the anatomic details previously obtained by TTE. Multiple views should be applied to exactly evaluate the VSD size, such as transgastric, frontal four-chamber, and basal short-axis view. Meticulous attention should be spent evaluating valvar regurgitation and stenosis. Patients should receive appropriate antibiotic prophylaxis for the procedure (20 mg/kg Cefazolin up to 1 g).

VASCULAR ACCESS AND HEMODYNAMIC EVALUATION

The femoral artery and vein are accessed routinely for all VSDs. In addition, the right internal jugular vein is accessed if the VSD is located in mid, posterior, or apical septum.

Heparin is administered at 100 IU/kg and the activated clotting time (ACT) is maintained above 200 s throughout the procedure. A routine right and left heart catheterization is then performed to specifically evaluate the degree of left-to-right shunt as well as pulmonary vascular resistance. Evidence of a fixed pulmonary vascular resistance above 7 Wood units should be considered a contraindication for VSD closure.

ANGIOGRAPHY AND DEVICE SIZE

Initial angiography is usually performed within the left ventricle in single-plane or biplane projection. The frontal camera is positioned 60° left anterior oblique (LAO) and 20°–30° cranial angulation for VSDs in the perimembranous or anterior muscular region *(42)* and slightly less LAO (35°–45°) for other muscular VSDs. The device is chosen to be 1–2 mm larger than the largest size of VSD, as determined by TEE and angiography *(33,42)*. Some operators might want to utilize balloon sizing to determine the appropriate device size. In our opinion, this is usually not necessary because of the stiffness of the muscular ventricular septum.

For postinfarct VSDs, we recommend the use of a device 50% larger than the measured diameter of the VSD because of ongoing necrosis of the tissue surrounding the VSD. This should reduce the incidence of residual shunts or device embolization.

CROSSING THE VSD AND ARTERIOVENOUS LOOP: MUSCULAR VSD

The most common approach is to cross the VSD from the left ventricle. In our experience, the Judkins right coronary catheter is most suitable to cross the VSD. We usually use a soft-tipped angled glide wire to cross the VSD and position the wire and Judkins right coronary catheter into a branch pulmonary artery. The wire is then exchanged to a soft J-tipped exchange length 0.035"-in. wire positioned into either branch pulmonary artery. This wire is then snared using an Amplatz gooseneck snare (Microvena Corporation) and exteriorized via the right internal jugular vein (for VSDs in mid, posterior, or apical septum) or femoral vein (for all other VSD locations). The created arteriovenous loop functions as a stable rail to advance the delivery sheath. Formation of a veno-venous loop using a transseptal puncture is less suitable for device delivery because of sheath angulation and potential damage of the mitral valve apparatus.

Some larger mid-muscular or apical VSDs can be successfully crossed from the right ventricular approach, thereby placing an exchange length guide wire into the left ventricular apex. However, care should be taken to enter the appropriate communication, which can be difficult to locate within the right ventricular trabeculations.

POSITIONING OF THE DELIVERY SHEATH

A crucial part of the procedure is the placement of the delivery sheath. The sheath is usually advanced over the guide wire from the jugular or femoral venous approach, which avoids placing a larger size sheath in the femoral artery. A retrograde approach via the femoral artery is reserved for cases where placement of the delivery sheath from a right-sided approach proves difficult.

Difficulties can be encountered in the right ventricular apex because of steep angulation of the delivery sheath (muscular VSDs) and when crossing the VSD itself. Care has to be taken to overcome resistance by using only gentle forward-and-backward movements. It is at this part of the procedure that the tension of the arteriovenous loop (maintained on both ends) as well as the impingement of the delivery sheath on the ventricular septum can cause rhythm disturbances, bradycardia, and temporary drop in blood pressure. The delivery sheath should be advanced until it reaches a safe position within the ascending aorta. The dilator is then slowly withdrawn, and in cases where kinking of the delivery sheath during device advancement appear more likely, an additional 0.018-in. glide wire can be kept inside the delivery sheath.

The approach at this stage then varies according to VSD location. For VSDs approached from the internal jugular vein, the sheath is left positioned in the ascending aorta, whereas for VSDs approached from the femoral vein, the sheath is positioned within the LV apex or kept in the ascending aorta (for anterior muscular VSDs).

ADVANCEMENT OF THE DEVICE

The next stage of the procedure is the advancement of the device. The 0.035-in. J-tipped wire is being removed and the tip of the delivery system is kept in the ascending aorta or left ventricle. The device is attached to the delivery cable and pulled into the loader either under saline or blood seal. We prefer blood, as this accelerates the clotting of the device itself. If a glide wire is being used for additional stability and to prevent kinking of the delivery sheath, it has to be introduced next to the device through the loader and the Tuohy–Borst connector at the end of the loader. The loader is then flushed with blood or saline and placed inside the delivery sheath and the device slowly advanced. Advancing might require a significant force and care should be taken not to bend the delivery cable. Once the device has been advanced to the tip of the delivery sheath, the glide wire, if being used, should be removed.

DEVICE DEPLOYMENT

If the delivery sheath has been placed in the ascending aorta, it is slowly pulled back until it reaches LV mid-cavity. The left ventricular disk is then slowly deployed, taking care not to impinge on the mitral valve apparatus. TEE guidance is of paramount importance during this stage of the procedure.

In cases of high muscular VSDs where the delivery sheath is positioned in the ascending aorta, a portion of the left ventricular disk can be deployed distal to the aortic valve. This should reduce the risk of the delivery system "falling back" into the right ventricle when pulling back across the aortic valve.

Once the aortic valve has been crossed, the LV disk is deployed completely by retracting the sheath in mid-cavity position. The whole assembly consisting of delivery sheath, cable, and device is then pulled back against the ventricular septum under TEE guidance until an adequate position has been achieved, and then the waist is deployed under mild tension and continuous TEE guidance. Once adequate positioning is confirmed via angiography (via a pigtail catheter advanced from the arterial side) and TEE, the right ventricular disk is deployed. Once a good position has been confirmed by TEE and angiography, without impingement on neighboring structures and valves, the device can be released using counterclockwise rotation with the pin vise. Further confirmation of device position by TEE should be obtained after the device has been released.

CROSSING THE VSD, ARTERIOVENOUS LOOP, DEVICE DELIVERY: MEMBRANOUS VSD

Deployment of a membranous VSD device requires some considerations. Figure 2 demonstrates the various steps of closure in a patient with a large-size perimembranous

VSD (also illustrated in the video on the accompanying CD). The most important steps in the protocol are as follows:

1. Cross the VSD from the left ventricle. We use a 4F or 5F Judkins right coronary catheter of appropriate curve to cross or to point toward the VSD. We often use a 0.035-in. Terumo glide wire to cross the VSD and to advance it to the pulmonary artery. Then, we advance the catheter over this wire to either branch pulmonary artery. Once the catheter is in the pulmonary artery, the glide wire is removed and the "noodle" wire (AGA Medical Corporation, Golden Valley, MN) is advanced to the tip of the catheter.
2. Snare the noodle wire using a gooseneck snare (Microvena Corporation, MN) and exteriorize the wire out the femoral vein.
3. Delivery sheath: Over the noodle wire from the femoral vein, the appropriate size delivery sheath is advanced all the way until the tip of the sheath is in the ascending aorta. Slowly draw back the dilator to the inferior vena cava–right atrial junction. Use the Judkins catheter with the wire inside it and inside the sheath to push the tip of the sheath to the apex of the left ventricle. This might take some maneuvring to achieve this position. Once the tip of the sheath is in the left ventricle apex, the device can be loaded and advanced to the tip of the sheath. We do not remove the dilator and wire until we are ready to advance the device inside the sheath. The proper sized device is screwed into the cable. With the help of an assistant, the flat part of the microscrew is aligned with the flat part of the capsule that is located at the end of the pusher catheter. Once the device is loaded, the pin vise is securely tightened to the cable at the end of the hub of the pusher catheter. This will prevent premature disengagement of the two flat parts.
4. Deploy the left ventricle disk between the anterior mitral valve leaflet and the left ventricle outflow tract. TEE is essential to make sure that the mitral valve apparatus is not entangled with the left ventricle disk. The entire assembly is withdrawn back to the septum. This can be seen by TEE and confirmed by angiography in the left ventricle. The waist of the device is then deployed. Aligning the left ventricle disk so that the aortic end of the disk is toward the aortic valve is important. We believe that if the device is screwed properly (flat parts are aligned) and the sheath is advanced to the apex of the left ventricle, almost always the flat part of the left ventricle disk is deployed toward the aorta. The platinum marker located in the left ventricle disk should be orientated toward the patient's feet (Fig. 2). If so, this indicates proper device position. The right ventricle disk can be deployed after an angiogram to ensure good device position. TEE and repeat angiogram can confirm proper device position prior to disengagement of the two flat parts. To disengage the two flat parts, the pin vise is loosened and the pusher catheter is withdrawn over the cable. The final step is to release the device by counterclockwise rotation of the pin vise. Once the device is released, the cable and pusher should be brought inside the sheath immediately to prevent any injury from the sharp end of the cable. Repeat TEE and angiogram are performed to assess the final result in terms of closure and residual shunt and to assess the function of the tricuspid and aortic valves.

Technical and Anatomical Considerations

VSD SIZE AND LOCATION

In a recent study by Holzer and colleagues, a larger VSD size has not been found to be associated with an increased risk of complications (37). Thirty-eight percent of muscular VSDs have been found to occur in overlapping regions of the ventricular septum, whereas isolated VSDs located anterior have been described in 13%, apical in 14%, mid-muscular in 33% and posterior in only 2% of patients who underwent VSD device closure (37).

From our own experience, we encountered greater difficulties in closing posterior and some anterior muscular VSDs when compared to VSDs located in apical and mid-muscular position. These defects are frequently difficult to cross. The advancement of a wire into the main pulmonary artery in posterior defects is often hindered by the overlying tricuspid valve and positioning of the delivery sheath is more often complicated by kinking than in mid-muscular position.

Some larger mid-muscular VSDs can be successfully crossed from a right ventricular approach, thereby allowing positioning an exchange length guide wire within the LV and avoiding the need of an arteriovenous wire loop formation.

SWISS-CHEESE/MULTIPLE VSDs

Multiple muscular VSDs are associated with increased surgical morbidity and mortality (10). Although a larger number of VSDs has not been found to be associated with an increased risk for the occurrence of procedure- or device-related complications, they have been found to be associated with significantly increased fluoroscopy and procedure times (36,37). The main limitation in closing Swiss-cheese-type VSDs is the length of the procedure and the amount of contrast used. Not infrequently however, the patient can be treated successfully in multiple sessions.

CROSSING PROSTHETIC VALVES

Retrograde catheterization of the left ventricle through a prosthetic aortic valve has to be carefully considered and performed avoiding any "brute force." Some reports have described catheter entrapment with fatal outcome because of severe acute aortic regurgitation (59,60). Recently, we reported the successful closure of iatrogenic ventricular septal defects in two patients with prosthetic St. Jude and Medtronic aortic valves (53). Using a careful approach avoided significant complications in both patients and documented that device closure in patients with a prosthetic aortic valve is feasible.

Follow-up

Following the procedure, patients should usually be observed for 24 h as an inpatient. During this time, investigations should include a CXR for device position, echocardiography to assess for residual VSDs, right ventricular pressures, and left ventricular dimensions, and EKG to document any arrhythmias or conduction anomalies. Patients should receive two further doses of antibiotics and a 24-h Holter recording should be commenced directly following the procedure. All patients should receive low-dose aspirin or an equivalent antiplatelet drug for 6 mo following the procedure. Prophylaxis for bacterial endocarditis should be continued for at least 6 mo following the procedure and can subsequently be discontinued once complete closure has been documented. Follow-up visits should be scheduled at 6 mo and subsequently in 1–2 yearly intervals. Each follow-up visit should include clinical and echocardiographic assessment as well as an EKG. A chest X-ray should be repeated every 1–2 yr.

The degree of a residual shunt should be assessed by echocardiography by measuring the width of the color jet as it exits through the ventricular septum. The shunt should be classified as trivial for a width <1 mm, small for a width between 1 and 2 mm, moderate for a width between 2 and 4 mm, and large for a width ≥4 mm, as suggested by Boutin and colleagues for assessment of residual shunting after ASD device closure (61).

Complications

For muscular VSDs, procedure-related complications occurred as frequently as 37%, however, only 6.7% of patients encountered unresolved complications, such as RBBB or stroke. two patients (2.7%) died as a direct result of the procedure *(37)*. For perimembranous VSDs, device-related complications, including trivial aortic insufficiency, progression of trivial tricuspid regurgitation, and temporary ventricular arrhythmias during sheath manipulation without hemodynamic compromise, occurred with much less frequency *(40,42)*.

Postinfarct VSDs continue to carry a grave prognosis, even with percutaneous VSD device closure *(39)*. Although Holzer and colleagues recently reported the procedure to be successful in 16 of 18 patients, the 30-d mortality was as high as 28%. These results compare favorably with other reports of surgical as well as transcatheter closure of postinfarction VSDs *(17,62)*.

Cardiac arrhythmias are common and require the presence of an experienced cardiac anesthetist during these procedures. Most cases of air and clot embolization can be avoided using meticulous techniques of catheter and wire exchange, as well as keeping the ACT above 200 s. Device embolization should be a rare event in experienced centers. However, the potential for device embolization does require surgical "in-house" back-up for these procedures as well as equipment and technical skills of the interventionalist to attempt percutaneous retrieval of the device. Another potential complication not listed includes hemolysis, which is related to the presence of a residual shunt. The incidence can be reduced by presoaking the device with the patients own blood prior to heparinization. Echocardiography is extremely important for identifying device- or procedure-related valvar regurgitation as well as pericardial effusion, and a final assessment should be completed prior to discharge from the hospital.

Residual Shunts

The reported closure rates using the Amplatzer muscular and membranous VSD devices have been excellent. Arora and colleagues reported a 0% frequency of residual shunts in 90 patients after device closure of VSDs using the Amplatzer muscular VSD device (follow-up: 1–48 mo). In the largest US trial, Holzer and colleagues documented closure rates of 34/72 (47.2%) at 24 h postprocedure, increasing to 32/46 (69.6%) at 6 mo and 24/26 (92.3%) at 12 mo.

Bass et al. reported excellent closure rates when using the membranous VSD device to close perimembranous VSDs in 25 patients *(40)*. In 92%, complete occlusion was documented within 15 min of device deployment by TEE as well as angiography. Two patients had a very small residual shunt at 15 min and 24 h following the procedure.

Unfortunately, results of transcatheter device closure of postinfarct VSDs are less favorable. Immediate results demonstrated no residual shunt in 2/15 patients, a trivial residual shunt in 4/15 patients, and a small residual shunt in 9/15 patients. At subsequent outpatient follow-up, the VSD was reported as closed in 2/10 patients, 6/10 patients had a trivial or small residual shunt, and 2/10 patients had a moderate residual shunt *(39)*. These residual shunts are predominantly related to enlargement of the VSD because of ongoing necrosis after myocardial infarction.

SUMMARY

In conclusion, the most recent studies suggest that the family of Amplatzer VSD devices can be safely used to close muscular as well as perimembranous VSDs. The mortality as well as the incidence of permanent morbidity is low and closure rates are excellent.

Appropriate patient and device selection is of paramount importance to the success of the procedure and should include anatomical and morphological details of the VSDs. However, operator experience forms the basis for a successful procedure.

Device closure of VSDs should, therefore, be considered as an important alternative to the standard surgical approach to close VSDs in the pediatric and adult populations.

REFERENCES

1. McDaniel NL, Gutgesell HP. Ventricular septal defects. In: Allen HD, Gutgesell HP, Clark EB, Driscoll DJ, eds. Heart disease in infants, children and adolescents. Philadelphia: Lippincott Williams & Wilkins, 2001:636–651.
2. Crenshaw BS, Granger CB, Birnbaum Y, et al. Risk factors, angiographic patterns, and outcomes in patients with ventricular septal defect complicating acute myocardial infarction. GUSTO-I (Global Utilization of Streptokinase and TPA for Occluded Coronary Arteries) Trial Investigators. Circulation 2000;101:27–32.
3. Menon V, Webb JG, Hillis LD, et al. Outcome and profile of ventricular septal rupture with cardiogenic shock after myocardial infarction: a report from the SHOCK Trial Registry. SHould we emergently revascularize Occluded Coronaries in cardiogenic shocK? J Am Coll Cardiol 2000;36:1110–1116.
4. Pesenti-Rossi D, Godart F, Dubar A, Rey C. Transcatheter closure of traumatic ventricular septal defect: an alternative to surgery. Chest 2003;123:2144–2145.
5. Bauriedel G, Redel DA, Schmitz C, et al. Transcatheterer closure of a posttraumatic ventricular septal defect with an Amplatzer occluder device. Catheter Cardiovasc Intervent 2001;53:508–512.
6. Turner SW, Hornung T, Hunter S. Closure of ventricular septal defects: a study of factors influencing spontaneous and surgical closure. Cardiol Young 2002;12:357–363.
7. Gabriel HM, Heger M, Innerhofer P, et al. Long-term outcome of patients with ventricular septal defect considered not to require surgical closure during childhood. J Am Coll Cardiol 2002;39:1066–1071.
8. Fukuda T, Suzuki T, Kashima I, et al. Shallow stitching close to the rim of the ventricular septal defect eliminates injury to the right bundle branch. Ann Thorac Surg 2002;74:550–555.
9. Maile S, Kadner A, Turina MI, Pretre R. Detachment of the anterior leaflet of the tricuspid valve to expose perimembranous ventricular septal defects. Ann Thorac Surg 2003;75:944–946.
10. Serraf A, Lacour-Gayet F, Bruniaux J, et al. Surgical management of isolated multiple ventricular septal defects. Logical approach in 130 cases. J Thorac Cardiovasc Surg 1992;103:437–442.
11. Seddio F, Reddy VM, McElhinney DB, et al. Multiple ventricular septal defects: how and when should they be repaired? J Thorac Cardiovasc Surg 1999;117:134–139.
12. Lock JE, Block PC, McKay RG, et al. Transcatheter closure of ventricular septal defects. Circulation 1988;78:361–368.
13. Rigby ML, Redington AN. Primary transcatheter umbrella closure of perimembranous ventricular septal defect [comment]. Br Heart J 1994;72:368–371.
14. Lavoie J, Javorski JJ, Castaneda AR, et al. Intraoperative migration of a clamshell device. J Cardiothorac Vasc Anesth 1995;9:562–564.
15. Luciani GB, Starnes VA. Clamshell for pulmonary atresia, ventricular septal defect, and aortopulmonary collaterals [comment]. Ann Thorac Surg 1996;62:1247–1248.
16. Laussen PC, Hansen DD, Perry SB, et al. Transcatheter closure of ventricular septal defects: hemodynamic instability and anesthetic management. Anesth Analg 1995;80:1076–1082.
17. Landzberg MJ, Lock JE. Transcatheter management of ventricular septal rupture after myocardial infarction. Semin Thorac Cardiovasc Surg 1998;10:128–132.
18. Pienvichit P, Piemonte TC. Percutaneous closure of postmyocardial infarction ventricular septal defect with the CardioSEAL septal occluder implant [comment]. Catheter Cardiovasc Intervent 2001;54:490–494.
19. Sideris EB, Walsh KP, Haddad JL, et al. Occlusion of congenital ventricular septal defects by the buttoned device. "Buttoned device" Clinical Trials International Register. Heart 1997;77:276–279.
20. Kalra GS, Verma PK, Singh S, Arora R. Transcatheter closure of ventricular septal defect using detachable steel coil. Heart 1999;82:395–396.
21. Latiff HA, Alwi M, Kandhavel G, et al. Transcatheter closure of multiple muscular ventricular septal defects using Gianturco coils. Ann Thorac Surg 1999;68:1400–1401.
22. Chaudhari M, Chessa M, Stumper O, De Giovanni JV. Transcatheter coil closure of muscular ventricular septal defects. J Intervent Cardiol 2001;14:165–168.
23. Arora R, Trehan V, Kumar A, et al. Transcatheter closure of congenital ventricular septal defects: experience with various devices. J Intervent Cardiol 2003;16:83–91.

24. Lee EM, Roberts DH, Walsh KP. Transcatheter closure of a residual postmyocardial infarction ventricular septal defect with the Amplatzer septal occluder. Heart 1998;80:522–524.
25. Pesonen E, Thilen U, Sandstrom S, et al. Transcatheter closure of post-infarction ventricular septal defect with the Amplatzer Septal Occluder device. Scand Cardiovasc J 2000;34:446–448.
26. Mullasari AS, Umesan CV, Krishnan U, et al. Transcatheter closure of post-myocardial infarction ventricular septal defect with Amplatzer septal occluder [comment]. Catheter Cardiovasc Intervent 2001;54:484–487.
27. Rodes J, Piechaud JF, Ouaknine R, et al. Transcatheter closure of apical ventricular muscular septal defect combined with arterial switch operation in a newborn infant. Catheter Cardiovasc Intervent 2000;49:173–176.
28. Szkutnik M, Bialkowski J, Kusa J, et al. Postinfarction ventricular septal defect closure with Amplatzer occluders. Eur J Cardiothorac Surg 2003;23:323–327.
29. Chessa M, Carminati M, Cao QL, et al. Transcatheter closure of congenital and acquired muscular ventricular septal defects using the Amplatzer device. J Invasive Cardiol 2002;14:322–327.
30. Amin Z, Gu X, Berry JM, et al. New device for closure of muscular ventricular septal defects in a canine model. Circulation 1999;100:320–328.
31. Thanopoulos BD, Tsaousis GS, Konstadopoulou GN, Zarayelyan AG. Transcatheter closure of muscular ventricular septal defects with the amplatzer ventricular septal defect occluder: initial clinical applications in children. J Am Coll Cardiol 1999;33:1395–1399.
32. Tofeig M, Patel RG, Walsh KP. Transcatheter closure of a mid-muscular ventricular septal defect with an amplatzer VSD occluder device. Heart 1999;81:438–440.
33. Hijazi ZM, Hakim F, Al Fadley F, et al. Transcatheter closure of single muscular ventricular septal defects using the amplatzer muscular VSD occluder: initial results and technical considerations. Cathet Cardiovasc Intervent 2000;49:167–172.
34. Butera G, Carminati M, De Luca F, et al. Transcatheter treatment of muscular ventricular septal defect and pulmonary valvar stenosis in an infant. Cathet Cardiovasc Intervent 2002;55:212–216.
35. Fabrega SJ, Rodes-Cabau J, Piechaud JF, et al. Percutaneous closure of a mid-muscular residual ventricular septal defect using the Amplatzer(TM) device. An Esp Pediatr 2002;57:66–69 (in Spanish).
36. Waight DJ, Bacha EA, Kahana M, et al. Catheter therapy of Swiss cheese ventricular septal defects using the Amplatzer muscular VSD occluder. Cathet Cardiovasc Intervent 2002;55:355–361.
37. Holzer RJ, Balzer D, Cao QL, et al. Device closure of muscular ventricular septal defects using the Amplatzer Muscular VSD Occluder: immediate and mid term results of a US registry. J Am Coll Cardiol 2004;43:1257–1263.
38. Gupta M, Juneja R, Saxena A. Simultaneous device closure of muscular ventricular septal defect and pulmonary valve balloon dilatation. Cathet Cardiovasc Intervent 2003;58:545–547.
39. Holzer RJ, Balzer D, Amin Z, et al. Transcatheter closure of post infarction ventricular septal defects using the new Amplatzer Muscular VSD Occluder: results of a US registry. Cathet Cardiovasc Intervent 2004;61:196–201.
40. Bass JL, Kalra GS, Arora R, et al. Initial human experience with the Amplatzer perimembranous ventricular septal occluder device. Cathet Cardiovasc Intervent 2003;58:238–245.
41. Gu X, Han YM, Titus JL, et al. Transcatheter closure of membranous ventricular septal defects with a new nitinol prosthesis in a natural swine model. Cathet Cardiovasc Intervent 2000;50:502–509.
42. Hijazi ZM, Hakim F, Haweleh AA, et al. Catheter closure of perimembranous ventricular septal defects using the new Amplatzer membranous VSD occluder: initial clinical experience. Cathet Cardiovasc Intervent 2002;56:508–515.
43. Thanopoulos BD, Tsaousis GS, Karanasios E, et al. Transcatheterer closure of perimembranous ventricular septal defects with the Amplatzer asymmetric ventricular septal defect occluder: preliminary experience in children. Heart 2003;89:918–922.
44. Janorkar S, Goh T, Wilkinson J. Transcatheterer closure of ventricular septal defects using the Rashkind device: initial experience [comment]. Cathet Cardiovasc Intervent 1999;46:43–48.
45. Kalra GS, Verma PK, Dhall A, et al. Transcatheterer device closure of ventricular septal defects: immediate results and intermediate-term follow-up. Am Heart J 1999;138:339–344.
46. Bridges ND, Perry SB, Keane JF, et al. Preoperative transcatheter closure of congenital muscular ventricular septal defects. N Engl J Med 1991;324:1312–1317.
47. Bacha EA, Cao QL, Starr JP, et al. Perventricular device closure of muscular ventricular septal defects on the beating heart: technique and results. J Thorac Cardiovasc Surg 2003;126:1718–1723.
48. Fishberger SB, Bridges ND, Keane JF, et al. Intraoperative device closure of ventricular septal defects. Circulation 1993;88:II205–II209.

49. Murzi B, Bonanomi GL, Giusti S, et al. Surgical closure of muscular ventricular septal defects using double umbrella devices (intraoperative VSD device closure). Eur J Cardiothorac Surg 1997;12:450–454.
50. Coles JG, Yemets I, Najm HK, et al. Experience with repair of congenital heart defects using adjunctive endovascular devices. J Thorac Cardiovasc Surg 1995;110:1513–1519.
51. Chaturvedi RR, Shore DF, Yacoub M, Redington AN. Intraoperative apical ventricular septal defect closure using a modified Rashkind double umbrella. Heart 1996;76:367–369.
52. Okubo M, Benson LN, Nykanen D, et al. Outcomes of intraoperative device closure of muscular ventricular septal defects. Ann Thorac Surg 2001;72:416–423.
53. Holzer RJ, Latson L, Preminger T, et al. Device closure of perimembranous ventricular septal defects using the Amplatzer Membranous VSD Occluder in two patients with prosthetic aortic valve. Cathet Cardiovasc Intervent 2004, in press.
54. Benton JP, Barker KS. Transcatheter closure of ventricular septal defect: a nonsurgical approach to the care of the patient with acute ventricular septal rupture. Heart Lung 1992;21:356–364.
55. Kidd L, Driscoll DJ, Gersony WM, et al. Second natural history study of congenital heart defects. Results of treatment of patients with ventricular septal defects. Circulation 1993;87:I38–I51.
56. Wollenek G, Wyse R, Sullivan I, et al. Closure of muscular ventricular septal defects through a left ventriculotomy. Eur J Cardiothorac Surg 1996;10:595–598.
57. Snider AR, Serwer GA, Ritter SB. Defects in cardiac septation–ventricular septation. In: Snider AR, Serwer GA, Ritter SB, eds. Echocardiography in pediatric heart disease. St. Louis, MO: Mosby, 1997:246–277.
58. Hijazi ZM. Device closure of ventricular septal defects. Cathet Cardiovasc Intervent 2003;60:107–114.
59. Kober G, Hilgermann R. Catheter entrapment in a Bjork–Shiley prosthesis in aortic position. Cathet Cardiovasc Diagn 1987;13:262–265.
60. Horstkotte D, Jehle J, Loogen F. Death due to transprosthetic catheterization of a Bjork–Shiley prosthesis in the aortic position. Am J Cardiol 1986;58:566–567.
61. Boutin C, Musewe NN, Smallhorn JF, et al. Echocardiographic follow-up of atrial septal defect after catheter closure by double-umbrella device. Circulation 1993;88:621–627.
62. Deja MA, Szostek J, Widenka K, et al. Post infarction ventricular septal defect—can we do better? Eur J Cardiothorac Surg 2000;18:194–201.

12

Left Atrial Appendage Occlusion

Mark Reisman, MD

INTRODUCTION

Atrial fibrillation (AF) is the most common arrhythmia encountered in clinical practice. It has a prevalence of 0.4% in the general population, which increases with age *(1)*. Two-thirds of those with AF are considered at high risk of stroke defined as a $CHADS_2$ score of 2–6 with an adjusted stroke rate of 4.0–18% *(2)*. This score assigns one point each for the presence of congestive heart failure, hypertension, age 75 yr or older, and diabetes mellitus and assigns two points for history of stroke or transient ischemic attack. In this regard, AF accounts for approx 15% of all strokes *(3)*. Anticoagulation with warfarin has consistently demonstrated a significant reduction in stroke of approx 60% when compared to placebo *(4)*. Unfortunately, approx 23% of patients with AF are considered suboptimal candidates for warfarin therapy because of bleeding complications, increased risk of bleeding, allergies to coumarin derivatives, or fear of complications, and thus the benefits of this therapy can be unrealized *(5)*. Stafford and Singer found that anticoagulation was utilized in only about a third of outpatients with AF *(6)*.

The major source of cardiac emboli in AF has been consistently identified as the left atrial (LA) appendage as opposed to the body of the left atrium (Table 1) *(7)*. This has led to the concept of closing or obliterating the LA appendage to reduce the risk of stroke in patients with AF.

ANATOMY OF THE LEFT ATRIAL APPENDAGE

The left atrial appendage (LAA) is an elongated cul de sac lined with endothelium—a remnant of the embryonic atrium, trabeculated by pectinate muscles. The main

From: *Contemporary Cardiology: Interventional Cardiology:*
Percutaneous Noncoronary Intervention
Edited by: H. C. Herrmann © Humana Press Inc., Totowa, NJ

Table 1
Location of Left Atrial Clot in Nonrheumatic Atrial Fibrillation

Setting	N	Appendage (N [%])	LA body (N [%])	Ref.
TEE	317	66 (21%)	1 (0.3%)	Stoddard; JACC 1995
TEE	233	34 (15%)	1 (0.4%)	Manning; Circulation 1994
Autopsy	506	35 (7%)	12 (2.4%)	Aberg; Acta Med Scand 1969
TEE	52	2 (4%)	2 (3.8%)	Tsai; JFMA 1990
TEE	48	12 (25%)	1 (2.1%)	Klein; Int J Card-Imag 1993
TEE and operation	171	8 (5%)	3 (1.8%)	Manning; Circulation 1994
SPAFF III TEE	359	19 (5%)	1 (0.3%)	Klein; Circulation 1994
TEE	272	19 (7%)	0 (0%)	Leung; JACC 1994
TEE	60	6 (10%)	0 (0%)	Hart; Stroke 1994
Total	**2018**	**201 (10%)**	**21 (1.0%)**	

smooth-walled LA cavity develops later and is formed from the outgrowth of the pulmonary veins. The LAA orifice has a diameter of 10–40 mm as it enters the LA cavity and is located between the left upper pulmonary vein and the left ventricle (8). The circumflex artery runs close to the LAA basal orifice and can make surgical ligation challenging. It is a complex structure often varying in multiple planes. The appendage can be multilobar, with 54% having two lobes and 23% having three lobes. Within the pectinate muscles, there is an enormous surface area for a clot to form. Transesophageal echocardiography (TEE) has demonstrated microthrombi in approx 10% of patients with nonvalvular AF and in 20–40% of patients with recent thromboemboli. The minute size of clinically significant important thrombi (2–3 mm) makes exclusion difficult.

The LAA is best visualized by TEE, which can estimate the size of the LAA and also can be used to obtain emptying velocities. Decreased contractility of the LAA myocardium and low flow velocities (<20–25 cm/s) are assumed to result from a myopathic process and are regarded as indicators for embolic risk. TEE findings that are associated with LAA dysfunction are LAA enlargement and spontaneous echocardiographic contrast, a phenomenon indicating blood stasis.

In patients with AF at autopsy, macroscopically the LAA volumes are larger, and there are fewer pectinate muscles compared to those with sinus rhythm. Histologically, the LAA in patients with AF show endocardial thickening with fibrosis and vacuolar degeneration, myocyte hypertrophy, myocyte dystrophy with myolysis, apoptosis gap junction disorganization, and downregulation of the L-type calcium channel and sarcoplasmic reticular calcium adenosine triphosphatase gene (9). These abnormalities are also the probable substrate for "electrical remodeling," a process in chronic AF in which the atrial effective refractory period shortens and impairs its rate adaptive response (10).

PERCUTANEOUS LEFT ATRIAL APPENDAGE TRANSCATHETER OCCLUSION DEVICE

The ligation of the LAA can be performed during mitral valve or CABG surgery or by thoracoscopy to remove it as a potential source of cardiac emboli. Although complete obliteration of the LAA is the optimal goal, residual communication between the LA cavity and the LAA has been reported in as many as 36% of patients after mitral

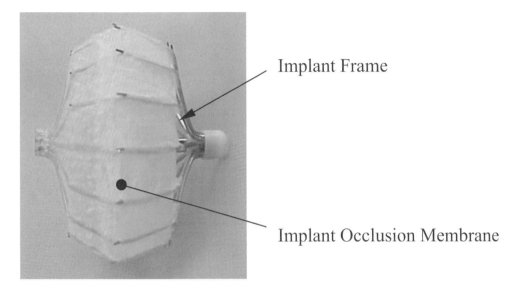

Implant Frame

Implant Occlusion Membrane

Fig. 1. The PLAATO implant.

valve surgery *(11)*. Thrombi within an incompletely ligated LAA might subsequently embolize *(12)*. The appeal of a percutaneous methodology for closure of the left atrial appendage in patients at high risk for stroke and suboptimal candidates for anticoagulation is obvious and led to the development of the percutaneous left atrial appendage transcatheter occlusion (PLAATO) device.

The PLAATO system consists of a delivery catheter and implant (Figs. 1 and 2). The PLAATO implant consists of a self-expanding nitinol frame covered with a membrane of expanded polytetreafluoroethylene (ePTFE) and a polymer. The purpose of the membrane is both to occlude the orifice of the LAA and to allow tissue incorporation into the device. Small anchors along the struts and passing through the occlusive membrane assist with the device anchoring. There are three rows of anchors proximally, mid (widest diameter), and distal. The implant is available in a variety of sizes ranging form 15 to 32 mm, with the size selected on the measured diameter of the LAA orifice.

PLAATO Implant Procedure

Premedication prior to the procedure consists of aspirin and clopidogrel, with antibiotics given 1 h prior to implantation of the device. All procedures are performed with TEE, with the majority of patients under general anesthesia. After transseptal access to the left atrium, angiograms are taken in two views to assess the size and shape of the appendage, and measurements of the orfice opening or *landing zone* for the device are determined using both angiography as well as TEE guidance (see Video 1 on accompanying CD-ROM).

An initial device is chosen that has a diameter 20–50% larger than the diameter of the LAA ostium. Once in place, the device is anticipated to not reach full dimensions, but to demonstrate at least a 15–30% compression. Thus, in the setting of increased volume or compliance of the LAA, the device has ample opportunity to further expand and remain anchored (see Video 2 on accompanying CD-ROM). Prior to release, dye injections proximal are used to demonstrate no inflow of contrast dye into the LAA and via the distal port into the LAA to demonstrate stasis of dye within the appendage (see Videos 3 and 4 on accompanying CD-ROM). This verifies adequate sealing of the appendage. If sealing is not

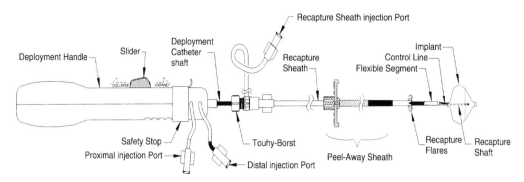

Fig. 2. The PLAATO delivery system.

adequate, as demonstrated by contrast flowing around the device or significant color flow on TEE in or exiting the appendage, the device can be collapsed, repositioned, and re-expanded, or completely removed and replaced with a more appropriately sized device.

DESIGN OF THE PLAATO FEASIBILITY STUDY

The PLAATO feasibility trial was designed to evaluate the the safety of PLAATO in patients with chronic continuous or paroxysmal AF who are at high risk for developing thromboembolic events and who are not candidates for long-term anticoagulation with warfarin. High risk was determined by the CHAD score developed by Gage et al. *(2)*, with the North American (NA) cohort requiring greater than two risk factors and the European (EU) cohort requiring one. Both the NA and EU feasibility study protocols employed a prospective, nonrandomized, single group, multicenter design.

Study Population

Patients with chronic continuous or paroxysmal AF of at least 3 mo duration, at high risk for thromboembolism, and who were not candidates for chronic anticoagulation therapy with warfarin were recruited for both studies. Patients were considered not to be candidates for warfarin therapy if they had a contraindication to warfarin based on the warfarin product label, including history of severe bleeding on warfarin therapy, excessive risk of fall or hemorrhage, or the inability to maintain a stable International Normalized Ratio (INR) as defined by an INR > 3.5 and/or <1.5 on two or more measurements in the prior year. Patients were judged to be at high risk for stroke if they met the specific clinical or echocardiographic criteria listed in Table 2. In addition, patients had to be able to undergo multiplane TEE and be candidates for emergent cardiac surgery.

Key exclusion criteria were uncontrolled hypertension, mitral or aortic stenosis, moderate to severe mitral regurgitation, left atrial diameter >6.5 cm, presence of mobile clot in the left atrium or LAA or complex aortic plaque on TEE, abnormality of the intra-atrial septum, presence of a prosthetic heart valve or inferior vena cava filter, active endocarditis or infection, acute myocardial infarction or unstable angina, recent stroke (<2 mo), history of left ventricular thrombus, symptomatic atherosclerotic carotid disease, pregnant or lactating females, and inability to complete any protocol required testing. Each participating hospital's institutional review board or ethics committee approved the study protocol and all patients gave prior written informed consent.

Table 2
High-Risk Inclusion Criteria for the European (EU) and North American (NA) Feasibility Trials

EU High-Risk Inclusion Criteria
   Patients must meet at least one of the following clinical or echocardiographic criteria.

NA High-Risk Inclusion Criteria
   Patients must meet at least two of the following clinical criteria or one of the
      echocardiographic criteria.

Clinical Criteria
   A prior history of transient ischemic attack or stroke more than 2 mo prior to the index procedure.
   Patient has been diagnosed with congestive heart failure.
   Left ventricular ejection fraction (LVEF) less than 40%.
   Patient has a history of systolic hypertension >160 mm Hg.
   Patient has Type I or Type II diabetes mellitus.
   Patient is ≥65 yr of age.
   Patient has a history of coronary artery disease, defined as previous myocardial infarction
      or known coronary stenosis ≥50%.

High-Risk Echocardiographic Inclusion Criteria
   Left atrial appendage emptying velocity ≤20 cm/s.
   Moderate or dense spontaneous echocardiographic contrast in the left atrial appendage.

Methods

Forty-eight hours prior to the PLAATO procedure, all patients received aspirin (325 mg BID.) and clopidogrel (75 mg BID.) or ticlopidine (250 mg BID). One hour prior to the PLAATO procedure, all patients received antibiotic therapy. The details of the procedure are described earlier.

Follow-up

All patients were prescribed enteric-coated aspirin indefinitely after the PLAATO procedure (300–325 mg/d). It also was recommended that patients take 75 mg clopidogrel once a day (or, if unable to take clopidogrel, 250 mg ticlopidine BID) for a period of 4–6 wk after the procedure. In the NA protocol, follow-up visits were required at 1, 3, 6, and 12 mo, and yearly thereafter for 5 yr following implantation. In the EU protocol, patients had follow-up visits at 48 h, 1 wk, and 1, 6, and 12 mo after the procedure.

A transthoracic echocardiogram (TTE) was obtained at 1 mo for all patients, and at 6 mo for patients enrolled in NA. TEE were obtained at 1 and 6 mo postprocedure for at least the first 20 patients by protocol in NA. TEE also was performed at other times at the discretion of the investigators, if clinically indicated.

Study End Points and Outcome Events

There were two primary safety end points: (1) the occurrence of a major adverse event (MAE) defined as stroke, cardiac death, or neurological death, myocardial infarction, or requirement for cardiovascular surgery related to the PLAATO procedure within 30 d of the index procedure and (2) the absence/presence of mobile left atrial thrombus or the occurrence of a MAE within 6 mo of the index procedure.

There were several primary device performance end points, including the following: (1) treatment success—defined as successful delivery and deployment of the PLAATO implant into the LAA, and LAA occlusion, as visualized by the investigator with angiography, immediately flowing placement of the implant; (2) device success—defined as successful delivery and deployment of the PLAATO implant into the LAA, or recapture and retrieval (if necessary); (3) procedural success—defined as device success and no MAEs during the index hospitalization; and (4) implantation success—defined as device success and no MAEs within 1 mo of the index procedure.

An independent echocardiographic core laboratory also evaluated echocardiographic treatment success. The percent of procedures resulting in occlusion of the LAA immediately following placement of the PLAATO implant and at 1 mo was measured.

The incidence of stroke and transient ischemic attack (TIA) throughout the follow-up period was also documented. The observed incidence of stroke was compared to the expected risk of stroke for the population based upon their $CHADS_2$ risk score at enrollment.

Statistical Analysis

Analyses were conducted on an intent-to-treat basis. Continuous variables are summarized by mean, standard deviation, and minimum and maximum values. Estimates for frequency of occurrence of events are expressed as percentages or rates with 95% confidence intervals. Comparisons between NA and EU patient characteristics were made using two-sided independent t-tests or chi-square tests, with the probability of a type 1 error set at $p = 0.05$. Time to first stroke was analyzed using standard Kaplan–Meier methodology.

RESULTS OF THE PLAATO FEASIBILITY STUDY

Patient Characteristics

Between August 2001 and November 2003, a combined total of 111 patients were enrolled. Sixty-four patients were enrolled in 8 centers in the United States and 1 center in Canada, and 47 patients were enrolled in 5 centers in Europe. Patient characteristics at baseline are summarized in Table 3. The characteristics of patients in the NA and EU trials were similar. However, patients enrolled in North America were slightly older (mean age = 73 vs 69 yr), had their diagnosis of AF for a shorter period of time (25% had AF diagnosed for less than 1 yr versus 11%), and had a higher prevalence of coronary artery disease (48% vs 30%) than patients enrolled in Europe.

Duration of Follow-up

The average follow-up was 9.5 mo. A total of 46 of 47 patients in EU and 31 of 64 patients in NA completed the 1-yr follow-up. All of the 47 patients in EU and 52 of 64 patients in NA completed the 6-mo follow-up.

Procedural Results

A total of 113 procedures were performed in 111 patients, and 108 patients received a PLAATO implant. Two patients had two procedures. One patient had a pericardial effusion during the first procedure but received the PLAATO implant during a second procedure. The other patient with two procedures was never implanted because of thrombus detected in the atrium during the first procedure and cardiac tamponade complicating the second procedure. Two additional patients were never implanted because of (1) a groin

Table 3
Patient Characteristics at Baseline

	North America (n = 64)	Europe (n = 47)	Total (n = 111)	p-Value
Mean age (yr)	73	69	71	0.03
Standard deviation	10	7	9	
Minimum	42	54	42	
Maximum	90	82	90	
% Male	61	57	60	0.71
Duration of AF				0.06
<1 yr	25%	11%	19%	
1–3 yr	23%	40%	31%	
>3 yr	52%	49%	50%	
Baseline Clinical Risk Factors				
Age ≥ 65 yr	86%	81%	84%	0.47
Age ≥ 75 yr	45%	21%	35%	0.01
CHF or LVEF <40%	44%	32%	39%	0.20
Hypertension	75%	68%	72%	0.42
Diabetes mellitus	23%	30%	26%	0.45
Prior stroke or TIA	34%	46%	38%	0.38
CAD	48%	30%	41%	0.05
High-Risk TEE	50%	43%	47%	0.44
Mean LAA Orifice Diameter (mm)	21.5	22.0	21.7	0.45
Standard deviation	3.5	3.6	3.5	
Minimum	15.0	11.4	11.4	
Maximum	30.3	27.2	30.3	

complication during venous access and (2) the detection of thrombus in the atrium. Fig. 3 displays the enrollment and procedure experience. The average total procedure time from LAA access to the end of the procedure was 68 min. In the 108 patients who were implanted, 2 patients received a 18-mm device, 1 received a 20-mm device, 7 received a 23-mm device, 15 received a 26-mm device 33 received a 29-mm device, and 50 received a 32-mm device.

Primary Safety End Points

The 30-day MAE rate was 1.8% (95% confidence interval [CI] = 0–3.2) (2 events/ 111 patients). At 30 d postprocedure, none of the European patients had a MAE. One patient from NA had two MAEs during the index hospitalization, need for emergent cardiovascular surgery 7 h postprocedure because of cardiac tamponade, and neurological death in-hospital 27 d postprocedure. This patient never received the PLAATO implant.

By 6 mo postprocedure, the rate of occurrence of MAE events and/or mobile left atrial thrombus was 3.0% (95% CI = 0–6.4) based on 3 events in 99 patients with 6-mo follow-up. No instances of mobile left atrial thrombus were observed. One patient had two MAEs during the index hospitalization as described earlier and one patient had a stroke 173 d after the implant procedure.

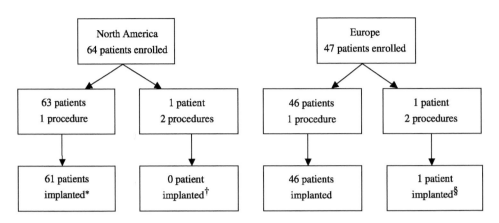

Fig. 3. Flowchart of Patient Enrollment in PLAATO Feasibility Trial. *Two patients were not implanted because of (1) a groin access complication and (2) detection of thrombus in the atrium. †One patient had two procedures but neither resulted in a successful implant. The patient experienced two MAEs during the hospitalization: emergent cardiovascular surgery because of cardiac tamponade and death because of a probable cerebral hemorrhage. §One patient had a pericardial effusion during the first procedure and was implanted successfully during a second procedure.

Primary Device Performance End Points

The PLAATO implant was successfully delivered and deployed into the LAA, with adequate LAA occlusion, as visualized by the investigator with angiography immediately following placement of the implant in 108 of 113 total procedures (95.6%) performed in 111 patients. LAA occlusion was tested using a contrast dye injection both proximal and distal to the PLAATO implant, with the degree of leak visually rated by the investigator on a four-point scale: 1 = severe leak, 2 = moderate leak, 3 = mild leak, 4 = trace to no leak. Successful occlusion of the LAA was a leak rating greater than or equal to 3. Ninety-four of 108 implanted devices were rated as a 4 (87%) and 14 devices (13%) had a rating of 3.

Device success was achieved in 108 of 113 procedures (95.6%) performed in 111 patients. Device success requires both treatment success *and* the ability to successfully recapture and retrieve the implant if required. In two procedures, an implant was never released during the procedure. Complete recapture and retrieval was performed successfully in the three procedures in which an implant was delivered but never released. Twenty procedures required multiple attempts to place the PLAATO implant before meeting implant criteria. There were no cases of unsuccessful retrieval and recapture of the PLAATO implant.

The number of procedures that resulted in device success *and* no MAEs during the hospitalization for the index procedure (procedure success) was 108 of 113 (95.6%) procedures performed in 111 patients.

The number of procedures that resulted in device success *and* no MAEs within 1 mo of the index procedure (implantation success) also was 108 of 113 (95.6%) procedures performed in 111 patients.

Treatment Success Evaluated by the Echocardiographic Core Lab

Transesophageal electrocardiography images were evaluated by the echocardiographic core laboratory to grade the degree of occlusion of the LAA immediately

Table 4
CHADS$_2$ Score Distribution at Baseline

Score	North America (n = 64) number	Europe (n = 47) number	Total (n = 111) number	CHADS$_2$ annual stroke risk[a]	Adjusted annual stroke risk[b]
0	0	2	2	1.9%	1.5%
1	16	11	27	2.8%	2.2%
2	19	14	33	4.0%	3.1%
3	12	11	23	5.9%	4.6%
4	11	7	18	8.5%	6.6%
5	6	1	7	12.5%	9.8%
6	0	1	1	18.2%	14.2%
Mean score[c]	2.6	2.4	2.5		
Standard deviation	1.3	1.3	1.3		
Minimum					
Maximum					

[a]Annual stroke risk associated based on patients' CHADS$_2$ score at baseline.

[b]Adjusted by reducing the patients' CHADS$_2$ scores by 22% to reflect the expected reduction in stroke risk for patients receiving aspirin.

[c]p-Value for the difference between NA and EU is 0.48.

postprocedure, at 1 mo, and at 6 mo. TEE testing was required for the first 20 patients in the NA protocol and also was performed at the discretion of the investigators when clinically indicated. TEE images were available for 88 patients immediately after implant, for 60 patients at 1 mo and 50 patients at 6 mo of follow-up. The degree of occlusion/persistent leak was graded on a five–point scale: 1 = severe, 2 = moderate, 3 = mild, 4 = trace, 5 = absent. Successful occlusion of the LAA was defined as a grade of 3 or higher. Immediately postprocedure, 86 of 88 (97.7%) met this criteria. At 1 mo, 60 of 60 (100%) patients and at 6 mo 50 of 50 (100%) patients met this criteria.

Incidence of Stroke and Transient Ischemic Attack

Two of 111 patients (1.8%, 95% CI = 0–4.3) enrolled experienced a stroke, and 1 patient experienced two TIAs throughout an average follow-up period of 9.5 mo. A Kaplan–Meier curve depicting time to first stroke is shown in Fig. 4. The observed stroke rate at 365 d was 2%, based on an adjusted CHAD score; the expected rate is 4.0%.

Adverse Events

All adverse events reported by the investigators were reviewed and adjudicated by an independent Clinical Events Committee. The committee determined whether an event met the definition for a serious adverse event or the end-point definition of a MAE. Serious adverse event (SAE) was defined as any event that is fatal or life threatening, results in persistent or significant disability, requires surgical intervention or ICU care to prevent permanent impairment or damage readmission, or prolongation of hospitalization. The committee also determined whether an event was device related, procedure related, or both device and procedure related. A total of six MAEs occurred in four patients (Table 5). Nine SAEs in seven patients were judged to be procedure related. None of the SAEs were judged to be device related. Procedure-related SAEs included

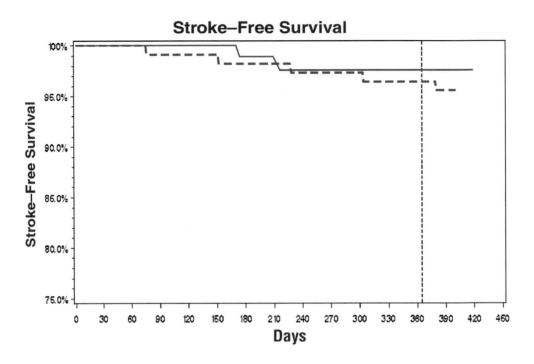

Fig. 4. Stroke-free survival. Solid line, observed; dashed line, modeled.

Table 5
Occurrence of MAEs (Cardiac/Neurological Death, Major or Minor Stroke, Myocardial Infarction, Or emergent Cardiovascular Surgery Related to the PLAATO Procedure)

MAE events	North America (n = 64)	Europe (n = 47)	Total (n = 111)
Major or minor stroke	1	1	2
Myocardial infarction,	0	0	0
Requirement for surgery, because			
of PLAATO procedure	1	0	1
Cardiac or neurological death	2	1	3
Any MAE	4	2	6
	(in 3 patients)	(in 1 patient)	(in 4 patients)

pericardial effusion (2), cardiac tamponade (2), dyspnea requiring reintubation (1), pleural effusion (1), right leg deep-vein thromboli (1), left hemothorax (1), and brachial plexus palsy (1).

Deaths

There were 6 deaths in 111 patients (5.4%) with 5 reviewed by the CEC committee and 1 pending adjudication. None were adjudicated as device or procedure related. Causes of death were cerebral hemorrhage (1), cardiac death (2), coronary artery disease (1), multisystem organ failure (2), and cause pending adjudication (1).

SUMMARY

Left atrial appendage closure via a percutaneous approach appears to be technically feasible and early data suggest potential for the reduction of stroke in patients who are at high risk for anticoagulation therapy with warfarin. The evolution of this device as well as the introduction of new devices for this application will make this an area of increasing growth and innovation.

REFERENCES

1. Anon. ACC/AHA/ESC guidelines for the management of atrial fibrillation. J Am Coll Cardiol 2001;38:1231–1266.
2. Gage BF, Waterman AD, Shannon W, et al. Validation of clinical classification schemes for predicting stroke. JAMA 2001;285:2864–2870.
3. Go AS, Hylek EM, Phillips KA, et al. Prevalence of diagnosed atrial fibrillation in adults: national implications for rhythm management and stroke prevention: the Anticoagulation and Risk Factors in Atrial Fibrillation (ATRIA) study. JAMA 2001;285:2370–2375.
4. Hart, et al. Ann Intern Med 1999;131:492–501.
5. Sudlow M, Thomson R, Thwaites B, et.al. Prevalence of atrial fibrillation and eligibility for anticoagulants in the community. Lancet 1998;352:1167–1171.
6. Stafford R, Singer D. National patterns of warfarin ue in atrial fibrillation. Arch Intern Med 1996;61:565–569.
7. Blackshear JL, Odell JA. Appendage obliteration to reduce stroke in cardiac surgical patients with atrial fibrillation. Ann Thorac Surg 1996;61(2):754–759.
8. Stollberger C, Schneider B, Finsterer J. Elimination of the left atrial appendage to prevent stroke or embolism. Chest 2003;124(6):2356–2362.
9. Shirani J, Alaeddini J. Sturctural remodeling of the left atrial appendage in patients with chronic non valvular atrial fibrillation: implications for thrombus formation, systemic embolism, and assessment by transesophageal echocardiography. Cardovasc Pathol 2000;9:95–101 (abstract).
10. Yu WC, Lee SH, Tai CT, et al. Reversal of atrial electrical remodeling following cardioversion of long standing atrial fibrillation in man. Cardiovasc Res 1999;42:470–476 (abstract).
11. Katz ES, Tsiamtsiouris T, Applebaum RM, et al. Surgical left atrial appendage ligation is frequently incomplete: a transesophgeal echocardiographic study. J Am Coll Cardiol 2000;36:468–471.
12. Rosenzweig BP, Katz E, Kort S, et al. Thromboembolus from a ligated left atrial appendage. J Am Soc Echocardiogr 2001;14:396–398.

III   ADJUNCTIVE CORONARY INTERVENTIONS

13

Devices for Myocardial Preservation

Simon R. Dixon, BHB, MBChB
and William W. O'Neill, MD

CONTENTS

INTRODUCTION

The primary goal of therapy in acute myocardial infarction is to salvage jeopardized myocardium and preserve left ventricular function *(1)*. Despite the success of contemporary reperfusion strategies, many patients with evolving myocardial infarction sustain extensive myocyte necrosis, resulting in heart failure, arrhythmia, and death. Although early restoration of blood flow to ischemic myocardium reduces infarct size, many patients with acute myocardial infarction present more than 3 h from symptom onset, beyond the timeframe when significant salvage can occur *(2–6)*. Moreover, many patients have suboptimal tissue-level perfusion despite restoration of TIMI-3 grade epicardial flow, as a result of ischemia-induced microvascular injury, distal embolization, and reperfusion injury *(7–13)*. Given that left ventricular function is the most important determinant of long-term survival *(14–16)*, there is a clear need for novel therapies that might protect the myocardium and enhance myocardial salvage. Among newer therapeutic approaches, hyperoxemic reperfusion and hypothermia appear very promising as cardioprotective strategies. This chapter will review several innovative devices used to apply these therapies, experimental data that form the scientific basis for their use, as well as recent developments in clinical investigation.

HYPEROXEMIC REPERFUSION

Hyperbaric oxygen has been shown to reduce injury and improve healing in a wide range of tissues during ischemia–reperfusion. Numerous data support the hypothesis that hyperbaric oxygen also has a protective effect in the heart.

From: *Contemporary Cardiology: Interventional Cardiology:*
Percutaneous Noncoronary Intervention
Edited by: H. C. Herrmann © Humana Press Inc., Totowa, NJ

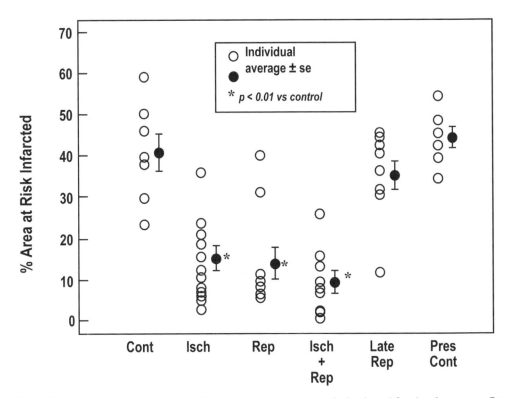

Fig. 1. Percentage of the ischemic (risk) zone that became necrotic is plotted for the six groups. Open circles represent individual experiments; closed circles represent group mean ± SEM. Cont = the ambient pressure control group; Isch = hyperbaric oxygen during ischemia only; REP = hyperbaric oxygen during reperfusion only; Isch + Rep = hyperbaric oxygen throughout the study; Late Rep = hyperbaric oxygen starting 30 min after reperfusion; Pres Cont = 2.5 atm of 40% oxygen/60% nitrogen throughout the study. (From ref. *25.*)

Hyperbaric Oxygen in Myocardial Infarction

Hyperbaric oxygen was first evaluated as a therapy for acute myocardial infarction over 40 yr ago. Investigators attempted to limit myocardial necrosis by increasing oxygen delivery to ischemic myocardium with hyperbaric oxygen. In these models of permanent coronary artery occlusion, administration of hyperbaric oxygen was shown to limit myocardial injury for up to 4 h of occlusion, reduce arrhythmia, and have a beneficial effect on hemodynamics *(17–23)*. However, the results of these experimental studies were mixed and, consequently, hyperbaric oxygen did not gain widespread acceptance as a therapeutic modality.

Studies in ischemia–reperfusion models of myocardial infarction have confirmed that administration of hyperbaric oxygen reduces infarct size *(24,25)*. In an elegant study, Sterling et al. *(25)* found that hyperbaric oxygen therapy was protective during both ischemia *and* reperfusion (Fig. 1). However, there was little effect if hyperbaric oxygen was started 30 min after reperfusion, thus suggesting there is a critical time period in which hyperbaric oxygen must be administered to be beneficial.

The precise biochemical and cellular effects of hyperbaric oxygen during ischemia–reperfusion are not well defined. However, studies in skeletal muscle and skin have shown that hyperbaric oxygen increases capillary density in postischemic muscle and

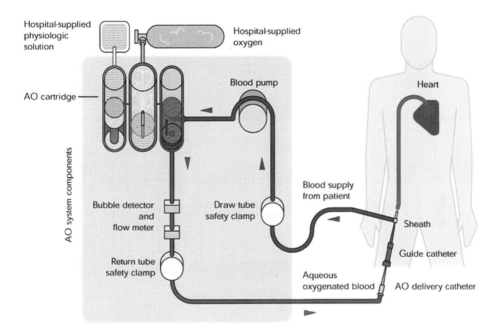

Fig. 2. Schematic diagram of the TherOx Aqueous Oxygen (AO) system.

reduces leukocyte adherence in postcapillary venules by downregulation of β_2-integrin receptors *(26–29)*. It has also been hypothesized that hyperbaric oxygen might reduce endothelial cell edema by an osmotic pump mechanism *(30)*.

One of the common questions regarding hyperbaric oxygen is the effect on free-radical production and the potential to actually increase cell necrosis. Several lines of evidence suggest that hyperoxemia does not have a detrimental effect during reperfusion. In the study by Sterling et al., administration of hyperbaric oxygen immediately before reperfusion led to a significant reduction in infarct size, similar to that achieved when hyperbaric oxygen was given during ischemia *(25)*. Moreover, tissue hypoxia *per se* is a potent stimulus for free-radical production, so augmentation of oxygen delivery might paradoxically diminish levels of reactive oxygen species *(31,32)*. In a rat model of hypoxic brain injury, hyperbaric oxygen has been shown to enhance a biochemical pathway that reduced production of lipid peroxide radicals *(33)*. Thus, it appears that the effects of hyperbaric oxygen are quite complex, but, overall, these data suggest that elevated oxygen levels are not toxic during reperfusion.

Hyperbaric oxygen was studied recently in a small, randomized clinical trial of patients treated with thrombolytic therapy *(34)*. Compared with control patients, those receiving adjunctive hyperbaric oxygen had lower creatine kinase levels at 12 and 24 h, more rapid ST-segment resolution, and higher predischarge left ventricular ejection fraction.

The TherOx® AO System

This innovative system uses Aqueous Oxygen to deliver hyperbaric levels of oxygen to ischemic tissue on a regional basis utilizing a small extracorporeal circuit (TherOx, Inc., Irvine, CA) (Fig. 2. and Video 1 on the CD). Using patented technology, the TherOx AO System produces sterile Aqueous Oxygen (AO) on demand from hospital-supplied medical-grade oxygen and sterile saline *(35)*. This physiologic solution has an oxygen concentration

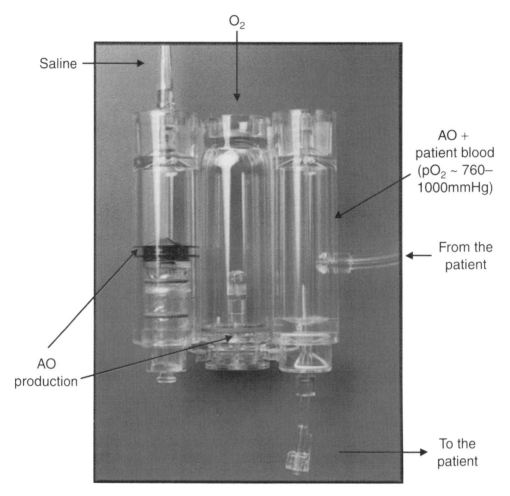

Fig. 3. The AO cartridge. Aqueous oxygen is produced in the central chamber from medical grade oxygen and physiologic saline. The AO solution is infused at 3.5 ± 1.5 mL/min into the "blood-mixing chamber" on the right to create hyperoxemic blood.

of $1–3$ mL O_2/mL saline, which is an order of magnitude greater than the O_2-carrying capacity of blood. The system uses small silica capillary tubes to infuse the AO solution into blood at ambient pressure without microbubble formation. Although hemoglobin becomes fully saturated at a pO_2 of 100 mm Hg, the oxygen content of blood increases significantly with AO solution because of the dissolution of oxygen in plasma. Thus, the AO solution can be mixed with blood to produce hyperoxemia with relatively small amounts of carrier solution.

The patient's blood is drawn from an arterial sheath and mixed with the AO solution in a sterile, single-use AO cartridge to achieve a pO_2 of $600–800$ mm Hg (Fig. 3). Hyperoxemic blood is then returned to the patient at 75 mL/min via standard PVC tubing and a subselective proprietary 4.6F AO delivery catheter. The system has a number of safety features that continuously monitor parameters such as the rate of blood flow, pressures in the fluid path, and the presence of bubbles in the AO-treated blood. The priming volume of the circuit is approx 50 mL. Compared with alternative methods of producing hyperoxemia, such as membrane oxygenators, the TherOx System has a number of advantages, including small priming volume, rapid setup, and avoidance of systemic inflammatory reactions. The TherOx AO System is approved for use in Europe, but is presently limited to investigational use in the United States.

Experimental Studies of Hyperoxemic Reperfusion with Aqueous Oxygen

Initial animal studies demonstrated that intra-arterial infusion of AO was effective for correction of hypoxemia and production of hyperoxemia, without adverse effects on blood elements or plasma chemistries (36). In a low-flow model of coronary ischemia, hyperoxemic reperfusion was associated with preservation of ventricular function compared with low-flow normoxemic perfusion. There was no significant change in coronary sinus pO_2 with the different levels of oxygen in the perfusate, suggesting that oxygen extraction might have increased with the higher arterial oxygen levels. Spears et al. then studied the effect of hyperoxemic reperfusion with AO on left ventricular function and infarct size in a porcine model of myocardial infarction (37). Following a 60-min balloon occlusion of the left anterior descending coronary artery, hyperoxemic perfusion was performed for 90 min after a 15-min period of normoxemic autoreperfusion. Hyperoxemic reperfusion with either AO or a hollow-fiber oxygenator (HFO) was associated with a significant improvement in left ventricular function at 90 min compared with normoxemic perfusion (Fig. 4). This improvement persisted after termination of hyperoxemic therapy. Infarct size and other measures of myocardial injury, including the mean hemorrhage score and myeloperoxidase levels, were significantly lower in the AO-treated animals, but not in the HFO group or normoxemic controls (Fig. 5). Electron microscopy revealed that control animals had more prominent endothelial edema, myocyte hypercontracture, and capillary luminal narrowing compared with AO-treated animals. Further studies have shown that AO hyperoxemic reperfusion is beneficial in a late reperfusion porcine model. Animals treated with a 90-min AO infusion, 24 h after coronary occlusion, had a significant improvement in left ventricular ejection fraction, compared with normoxemic controls.

Initial Human Experience with AO Hyperoxemic Reperfusion

Accordingly, we conducted a pilot study to evaluate the safety and feasibility of hyperoxemic reperfusion after primary angioplasty for acute myocardial infarction (38). Twenty-nine patients were enrolled at three centers in the United States and Europe. We included patients presenting up to 24 h from symptom onset. Hyperoxemic reperfusion was initiated immediately after angioplasty and was continued for 60–90 min. AO was successfully infused in all patients. The mean flow rate of AO solution into the patient's blood was 2.9 ± 0.5 mL/min, whereas the mean flow of blood to the infarct vessel was 82 ± 13 mL/min. Despite a high pO_2 in the coronary perfusate (728 ± 187 mm Hg), there was only a modest increase in systemic pO_2. Hyperoxemic reperfusion was safe and well tolerated. No hemodynamic instability or arrhythmia was observed; in fact, during the infusion there was a decrease in pulmonary capillary wedge pressure from 21 ± 9 mm Hg to 16 ± 7 mm Hg ($p = 0.04$). At 30 d, there were no adverse events related to the hyperoxemic therapy. An important observation from this nonrandomized study was early recovery of ventricular function after hyperoxemic reperfusion. At 24 h, there was a significant improvement in the wall motion score index of the infarct zone compared to immediately after PTCA (2.18 ± 0.32 vs 1.84 ± 0.41, $p < 0.001$), with a trend toward an

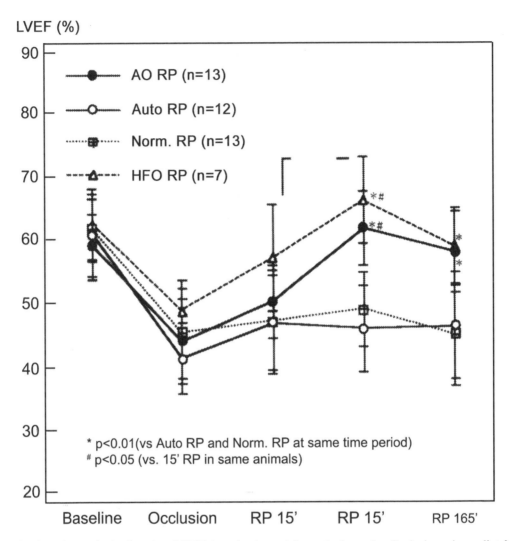

Fig. 4. Left ventricular function (LVEF) in swine by serial ventriculography. Occlusion = immediately prior to deflation of a 60-min balloon occlusion of the left anterior descending coronary artery (LAD). AO RP = AO hyperoxemic reperfusion of the LAD; Auto RP = passive reperfusion; Norm RP = active normoxemic reperfusion; HFO = hyperoxemic reperfusion with a hollow-fiber oxygenator. Error bars indicate the standard deviation. (From ref. *37*.)

increase of the left ventricular (LV) ejection fraction (Fig. 6). Progressive improvement in infarct zone function was seen at 1 and 3 mo, which was greater than was expected from historical controls, thus suggesting that the AO infusion might have promoted myocardial healing.

Similar results have been obtained in an observational study at Centro Cardiologico Monzino (Milan, Italy) *(39)*. Consecutive patients with anterior wall infarction were treated with a 90-min infusion of AO after LAD stenting. Compared with historical controls, patients treated with AO were found to have an earlier peak creatine kinase, more complete ST-segment resolution, and greater improvement of LVEF (left ventricular function) at 6 mo. Of particular interest, recovery of LVEF in this patient cohort was independent of the time to treatment. These data suggest that hyperoxemic reperfusion might enhance microvascular perfusion and thus augment myocardial salvage.

% AN/AR

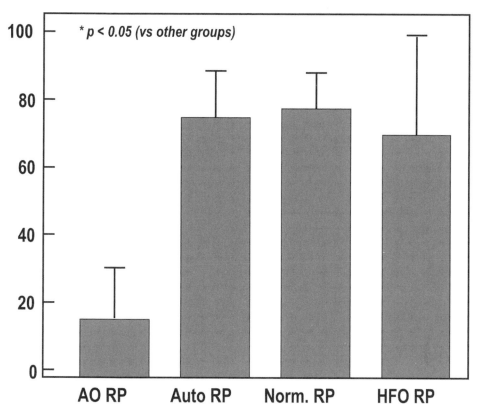

Fig. 5. Infarct size at 3 h of reperfusion in swine. % AN/AR = percent (area of necrosis)/(area at risk). (From ref. *37*.)

The AMIHOT Randomized Trial

This randomized, multicenter trial was designed to evaluate whether hyperoxemic reperfusion with Aqueous Oxygen would improve ventricular function or limit infarct size after primary percutaneous coronary intervention for acute myocardial infarction (*40*). From January 2002 to December 2003, 269 patients with anterior or large inferior myocardial infarction undergoing primary PCI were randomly assigned *after* successful PCI to receive hyperoxemic reperfusion (treatment group) or normoxemic blood autoreperfusion (control group) (Fig. 7). In contrast to most other trials evaluating adjuncts to reperfusion therapy, patients were eligible for enrollment up to 24-h from symptom-onset.The major clinical and angiographic exclusion criteria were cardiogenic shock and TIMI-3 flow in the infarct vessel at initial angiography. Hyperoxemic reperfusion was performed for 90 min utilizing intracoronary Aqueous Oxygen. The primary study endpoints were: Δ regional wall motion score index (RWM) of the infarct zone at 3 mo (using serial contrast echocardiography), ST-segment resolution (continuous ST-segment monitoring), and final infarct size at 14 d (^{99m}Tc- sestamibi SPECT imaging). At 30 d the incidence of major adverse cardiac events was similar between the control and AO groups (4.5% vs 6.0%, p=NS). There was no significant difference in the primary study endpoints with AO therapy; however, there was a trend to improved regional wall motion with AO (0.55 in the control group vs 0.65 in the AO group, p=0.16). In secondary

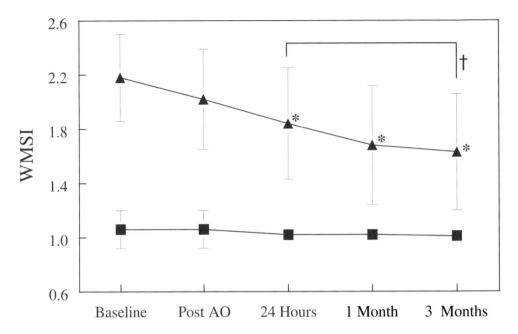

Fig. 6. Wall motion score index (WMSI) of infarct and non-infarct zones at baseline and after hyper-oxemic reperfusion with Aqueous Oxygen. Solid triangle = infarct zone; solid square = noninfarct zone. $^*p < 0.01$ vs baseline; $^\dagger p = 0.01$ vs 24 h. (From ref. *38*.)

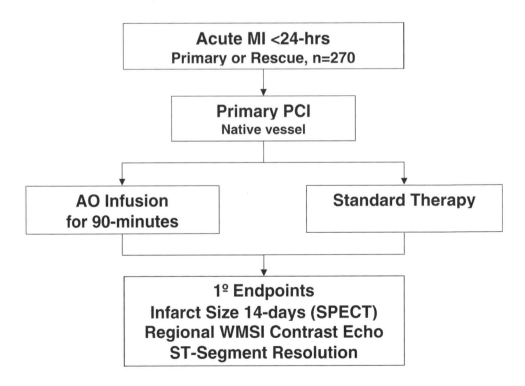

Fig. 7. Overview of the AMIHOT study design

analysis, a significant treatment benefit was observed in patients presenting within 6 h symptom-onset (infarct size: 14.3% in AO vs 18.1% in control, p=0.04; ΔRWM Score: 0.7 in AO vs 0.55 in control, p=0.05). These data suggest that hyperoxemic reperfusion improves microcirculatory flow and convalescent function in patients undergoing PCI within 6 h of symptom onset. A further study of hyperoxemic reperfusion is being planned to confirm these observations.

HYPOTHERMIA IN MYOCARDIAL INFARCTION

Cooling has been used for many years during cardiopulmonary bypass surgery, organ transplantation, and some neurosurgical procedures to limit ischemic tissue injury. Recent studies have also demonstrated that hypothermia is beneficial in survivors of cardiac arrest (41,42). Although the focus of research on therapeutic hypothermia has been as a neuroprotective strategy, there appears to be an equally sound rationale for using cooling to protect ischemic myocardium.

Relationship Between Myocardial Temperature and Necrosis

Interest in the use of therapeutic hypothermia for acute myocardial infarction was rejuvenated in the mid-1990s. At that time, several investigators demonstrated that there is an important relationship between myocardial temperature and the extent of tissue necrosis after coronary artery occlusion (43–45). Chien et al. found that small changes of temperature within the normothermic range significantly influenced myocardial infarct size, independent of changes in heart rate (43). In fact, infarct size changed by about 10% for each 1°C change in myocardial temperature (Fig. 8). These data not only highlighted the importance of controlling for myocardial temperature in experimental models of myocardial infarction but also led to further investigation into the potential therapeutic effects of mild hypothermia.

Experimental Studies of Hypothermia in Myocardial Infarction

Several animal studies have demonstrated that reducing the temperature of the heart by even a few degrees is beneficial during regional myocardial ischemia (Table 1) (46–53). However, the cardioprotective effect of mild hypothermia appears to be dependent on several factors, including the timing of cooling, depth of hypothermia, and duration of ischemia.

Hypothermia provides greatest protection when cooling is initiated *before* the onset of myocardial ischemia. In a rabbit model, Hale and Kloner induced mild hypothermia 20 min before coronary artery occlusion, using topical cooling (46). After 5 min of occlusion, the myocardial temperature in the risk region was reduced by 3.6°C. Cooling was associated with a profound reduction in mean infarct size (16 ± 3% vs 46 ± 4% of the risk zone, $p < 0.0001$) and appeared to alter the relationship between the size of the risk region and extent of necrosis. Similar results were found in another study using a pericardial catheter to cool the heart before ischemia (48).

Subsequent studies confirmed that mild hypothermia is also beneficial when applied after coronary occlusion, although the protective effect diminishes when cooling is started late after the onset of ischemia (49,50). In a 30-min rabbit occlusion model, Hale et al. started cooling either 10 min or 25 min after occlusion (49). Early cooling reduced myocardial temperature from 38.5 ± 0.1°C to 32.2 ± 0.4°C, whereas late cooling lowered the myocardial temperature to 32.5 ± 0.8°C. Compared with the control group, early cooling resulted in a significant reduction in infarct size (23 ± 4% vs 44 ± 4% of the risk

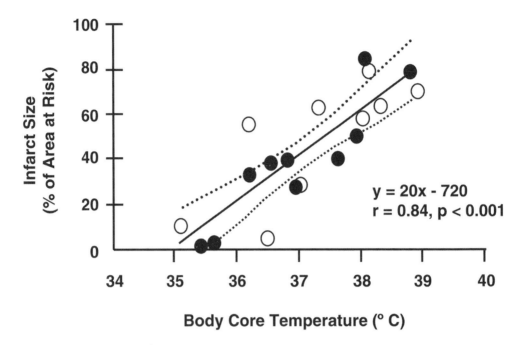

$$y = 20x - 720$$
$$r = 0.84, p < 0.001$$

Fig. 8. Relationship between body core temperature and infarct size produced by 45 min of coronary artery occlusion in 10 control swine (closed circles) and 9 swine pretreated with adenosine-receptor blocker 8-phenyltheophylline (8-PT, 5 mg/kg intravenously) and adenosine deaminase (ADA, 50 U/kg intracoronary, open circles). Relationship between temperature and infarct size was not different between the two treatment groups. The solid line represents regression line for all 19 animals. Dashed lines represent 95% confidence intervals. (From ref. *44*.)

region, $p = 0.01$); however, there was no change in infarct size in the late cooling group ($43 \pm 4\%$ vs $44 \pm 4\%$). Miki et al. also found that the protective effect of hypothermia was time dependent *(50)*. These investigators employed a novel heat exchanger between the carotid artery and jugular vein to induce hypothermia. Rabbit hearts were cooled either before coronary occlusion or 10 or 20 min after occlusion. Studies were performed at a target temperature of both 32°C and 35°C. In contrast to the study by Hale et al., late-onset cooling was associated with a significant reduction in infarct size when the temperature was lowered to 32°C, however, protection was not observed at 35°C (Fig. 9). These data suggest that cooling needs to be initiated as soon as possible after the onset of ischemia to optimally protect the myocardium from ischemic injury.

In a more recent study, Dae et al. evaluated the effect of mild hypothermia on infarct size in human-sized pigs using an endovascular heat-exchange catheter *(52)*. Cooling was started 20 min after occlusion of the left anterior descending coronary artery and was continued for 15 min after reperfusion. The catheter was used to lower the core body temperature to 34°C or to maintain normothermia (38°C). Although the size of the area at risk was similar in both hypothermic animals and normothermic controls, infarct size was significantly reduced in the hypothermic group ($9 \pm 6\%$ vs $45 \pm 8\%$, $p < 0.0001$) (Fig. 10). Moreover, additional studies with sestamibi autoradiography demonstrated that salvaged myocardium showed normal radiotracer uptake, thus suggesting that cooling exerts a protective effect for both myocytes and the microcirculation.

Table 1
Experimental Studies of Mild Hypothermia in Acute Myocardial Infarction

Author	Model	Target temp.[a]	Technique[b]	Onset of cooling	Duration of cooling	Results
Before Coronary Occlusion						
Hale and Kloner (1997) (46)	Rabbit	35°C (3.6°C)	TRH	20 min before occlusion	65 min	↓Infarct size with cooling (16% vs 46% of area at risk)
van den Doel et al. (1998) (47)	Rat	30–31°C	Surface	Before	15–120 min	Hypothermia enhanced protective effect of ischemic preconditioning, but no benefit with prolonged occlusion
Dave et al. (1998) (48)	Rabbit	34°C (5°C)	CCP	30 min before occlusion	55 min	↓Infarct size with cooling (16% vs 46% of area at risk)
After Coronary Occlusion						
Boyer (1977)	Dog	32°C	Surface	Not reported	Not reported	↓Myocardial O$_2$ consumption and LVEDP with hypothermia
Hale et al. (1997) (49)	Rabbit	32°C (6.3°C)	TRH	10 or 25 min after occlusion	5 or 25 min	Early cooling ↓infarct size (23% vs 44%); however, no benefit with late cooling
Miki et al. (1998) (50)	Rabbit	32°C or 35°C	Heat exchanger	5 min before, and 10 or 20 min after	35–40 min	Better cardioprotection at 32°C, then 35°C and with early cooling
Hale and Kloner (1998) (51)	Rabbit	30°C (10°C)	TRH	30 min after occlusion	90 min[c]	At 120 min, ↓infarct size with cooling (59% vs 72% of area at risk)
Dae et al. (2001) (52)	Pig	34°C (4°C)	Endovascular	20 min after occlusion	55 min + gradual rewarming	↓Infarct size with hypothermia (9% vs 45% of area at risk)
Hale et al. (2003) (53)	Rabbit	32°C	Surface	10 min before and 2 h after reperfusion	2 h	↓anatomic no-reflow and infarct size, and ↑regional myocardial flow in risk region with hypothermia

[a]Mean temperature reduction from baseline shown in parentheses.
[b]TRH=topical regional hypothermia; CCP=closed circuit pericardioperfusion.
[c]Model of prolonged coronary ischemia.

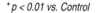

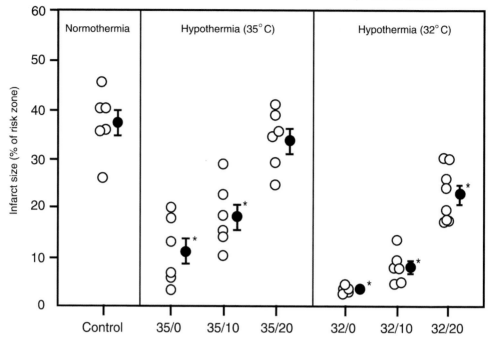

Fig. 9. Effect of mild hypothermia (32°C or 35°C) on infarct size in rabbits after a 30-min coronary artery occlusion. Hypothermia was commenced either before ischemia (0) or 10 or 20 min after occlusion. Infarct size is normalized as a percent of the risk zone and is plotted for each group. Open and closed circles indicate individual experiments and group means, respectively. Note that the protection observed depends both on the temperature and the duration of cooling. (From ref. *50.*)

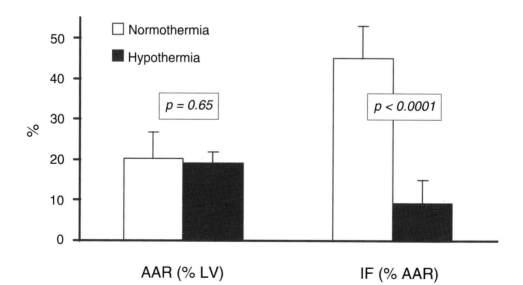

Fig. 10. Infarct size in hypothermic pigs and normothermic controls after coronary occlusion and reperfusion. The size of the area at risk (AAR) was comparable in both groups; however, infarct size (IF) was significantly reduced in the hypothermia group. (From ref. *52.*)

The optimal duration of cooling *after* reperfusion remains unclear, as no studies have directly compared the effect of short versus prolonged hypothermia in the reperfusion period. Most of the aforementioned studies have started rewarming soon after reperfusion. Nonetheless, prolonged cooling after reperfusion is likely to be beneficial, given that progressive impairment of myocardial flow associated with reperfusion injury might occur over several hours *(54)*. Prolonged hypothermia might be especially important when cooling is initiated late after the onset of myocardial ischemia. Recent data from Hale et al. suggest that maintenance of hypothermia for several hours after reperfusion attenuates reperfusion injury and protects the microvasculature *(53)*. In this model, mild hypothermia (32°C) was induced 10 min before reperfusion and continued for 2 h after reperfusion. Hypothermic treated animals had significantly higher myocardial flow in the risk region (1.21 ± 0.15 vs 0.65 ± 0.11 mL/min/g, $p = 0.0048$), less anatomic no-reflow ($11 \pm 4\%$ vs $37 \pm 5\%$, $p = 0.0001$), and smaller infarcts than normothermic controls.

Potential Mechanisms for Cardioprotection

Although it is generally believed that the beneficial effect of hypothermia is the result of lowering of metabolic demand in the risk region, the mechanisms by which cooling provides protection during myocardial ischemia–reperfusion are not well elucidated. In isolated perfused rabbit hearts, hypothermia has been shown to preserve myocardial ATP stores during ischemia, thus facilitating the maintenance of cell membrane integrity *(55)*. More recent data suggest that cooling also reduces myocyte apoptosis in response to ischemia by altering expression of antiapoptotic or proapoptotic genes *(56)*. Furthermore, hypothermia enhances production of heat shock proteins, which are believed to have a protective role in ischemia–reperfusion *(55)*. However, it is likely that the cardioprotective effects of hypothermia are far more complex, and further studies are required to determine whether myocardial cooling influences other biochemical and cellular processes such as free-radical production or the inflammatory response following reperfusion. The protective effect of myocardial cooling appears to be independent of hypothermia-induced bradycardia, as the effect persists when the heart rate is maintained with pacing *(46)*.

Devices to Induce Hypothermia During Myocardial Infarction

ENDOVASCULAR COOLING SYSTEMS

The introduction of catheter-based systems to induce hypothermia has been a major advance in this field. Three endovascular cooling systems are currently under investigation in the United States for the treatment of myocardial infarction (Table 2). These systems utilize a heat-exchange catheter that is placed in the inferior vena cava, via the femoral vein, and a central controller that circulates cool or warm saline to alter core temperature. The catheter can be placed in the emergency room or cardiac catheterization laboratory. One of the key advantages of endovascular cooling is that hypothermia can be induced rapidly and core body temperature can be maintained precisely at a desired target temperature.

SURFACE COOLING

A novel surface cooling system has also been developed to induce mild hypothermia (Artic Sun® Temperature Management System; Medivance Inc., Louisville, CO). This consists of water-based adhesive (hydrogel) pads that are applied to the patient's back, abdomen, and legs. The pads are designed to transfer heat energy by mimicking the effects of water immersion. One advantage of this system is that the nursing staff can place the hydrogel pads so that cooling can be initiated early after admission to hospital.

Table 2
Devices to Induce Hypothermia in Acute Myocardial Infarction

Cooling system	Company	Heat-exchange system	Temperature monitoring	Sheath size
Endovascular Cooling				
Reprieve™ Endovascular Temperature Therapy System	Radiant Medical Inc.	Reprieve™ catheter	Naso-esophageal probe or intravenous probe (SetProbe)	10F
CoolGard® Temperature Management System	Alsius Corporation	Fortius™ catheter	Bladder catheter	12F
Celsius Control™ System	Innercool Therapies Inc.	Celsius Control™ catheter	Catheter-based thermistor	10.7F or 14F
Surface Cooling				
Artic Sun® Temperature Management System	Medivance Inc.	Hydrogel pads	Tympanic	Not available

Clinical Experience with Cooling in Myocardial Infarction

ENDOVASCULAR COOLING

In February 2001, we initiated a pilot study (COOL-MI pilot) to evaluate the safety and feasibility of endovascular cooling in patients with acute myocardial infarction (MI) undergoing mechanical reperfusion (56). Hypothermia was induced using the Reprieve™ Endovascular Temperature Therapy System (Radiant Medical Inc., Redwood City, CA) (Fig. 11 and Video 2 on the CD). The target core body temperature was 33°C (monitored with a nasoesophageal probe). Cooling was maintained for 3 h after reperfusion, followed by controlled rewarming to 36.5°C (Fig. 12). Shivering was suppressed using skin warming with a forced-air blanket (Bair Hugger; Augustine Medical, Eden Prairie, MN), oral buspirone (30–60 mg), and intravenous meperidine (75–100 mg loading dose over 15 min, followed by an intravenous meperidine infusion at 25–35 mg/h) (Fig. 13) (57). Endovascular cooling was well tolerated, and no hemodynamic instability or increase in ventricular arrhythmia was observed in the cooling group. Mild episodic shivering was not uncommon, but was well controlled with additional meperidine.

A 20-patient feasibility study (LOWTEMP Pilot) was recently completed using the CoolGard® Temperature Management System (Alsius Corporation, Irvine, CA) (58). This consists of a collapsible, spiral-shaped balloon catheter (Fortius™) and an external temperature-control system (CoolGard®). Hypothermia was induced prior to primary percutaneous coronary intrvention (PCI) to achieve a target temperature of 32–34°C for a total of 4 h (1 h induction, 3 h maintenance) followed by active and passive rewarming to normothermia. Core body temperature was monitored using a thermistor mounted on a urinary bladder catheter. The CoolGard® System successfully reduced core body temperature (mean $33.7 \pm 0.9°C$) and there were no safety concerns, thus supporting further evaluation with this system in acute MI.

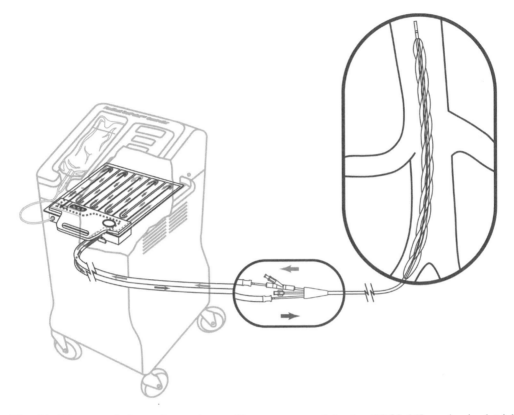

Fig. 11. Diagram of the endovascular cooling system used in the COOL-MI randomized trial (Reprieve™ Endovascular Temperature Management System.) (Courtesy of Radiant Medical Inc., Redwood City, CA.)

SURFACE COOLING

In a pilot study conducted at the Montreal Heart Institute, the Artic Sun® Temperature Management System was used to induce mild hypothermia in 11 patients undergoing primary angioplasty (Bonan, personal communication, 2003). Cooling was initiated in the emergency room and intravenous meperidine was used to suppress shivering. Results indicate that surface cooling is safe and feasible in these patients and that the core body temperature can be lowered to <35°C within 60 min.

Randomized Trials of Hypothermia

Two randomized multicenter trials of hypothermia for acute MI have been conducted: COOL-MI and ICE-IT (Table 3). Both trials were designed to evaluate the efficacy of adjunctive hypothermia during primary angioplasty, using final infarct size as the primary study end point.

COOL-MI TRIAL

In the COOL-MI trial, 392 patients with acute MI were randomly assigned to undergo primary PCI with or without adjunctive hypothermia. Cooling was performed with the Reprieve Endovascular Temperature Therapy System (Radiant Medical Inc. Redwood City, CA) using the same protocol as in the COOL-MI pilot study. Inclusion and exclusion criteria are shown in Table 4. The trial was powered to detect a 30% difference in final infarct size between the study groups.

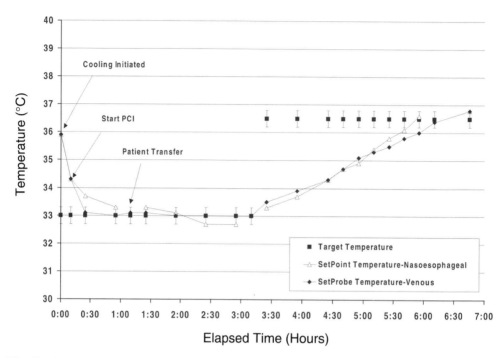

Fig. 12. Core body temperature in a patient with acute MI undergoing primary angioplasty with endovascular cooling.

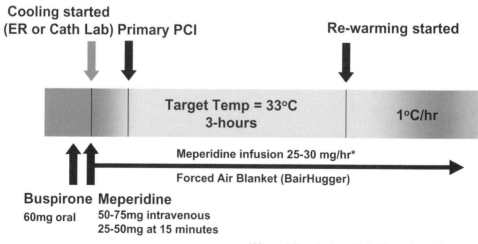

Fig. 13. Diagram of the endovascular cooling and shivering suppression protocol in the COOL-MI randomized clinical trial. Cooling was initiated in the emergency room (ER) or cardiac catheterization laboratory before primary angioplasty. Surface warming, oral buspirone, and intravenous meperidine were administered to prevent shivering (see text for details). PCI = percutaneous coronary intervention.

Table 3
Clinical Trials of Hypothermia for Acute Myocardial Infarction

Acronym	Design	Inclusion criteria	Cooling system	No. of patients	Target temp.	Duration of cooling	Primary end point
Nonrandomized Studies							
LOW TEMP	Registry	MI < 6 h	CoolGard Temperature Management System	20	32–34°C	4 h	Infarct size
NICAMI	Registry	MI < 6 h	Artic Sun Temperature Management System	11	34°C	3 h	MACE
Randomized Studies							
COOL-MI Pilot	Randomized pilot study	MI < 6 h	Reprieve Temperature Therapy System	42	33°C	3 h[a]	MACE
COOL-MI	Randomized, multicenter	MI < 6 h	Reprieve Temperature Therapy System	412	33°C	3 h[a]	Infarct size
ICE-IT	Randomized, multicenter	MI < 6 h	Celsius Control System	228	33°C	6 h	Infarct size

[a]From first balloon inflation.

Table 4
Inclusion/Exclusion Criteria for the COOL-MI Randomized Clinical Trial

Inclusion criteria	*Exclusion criteria*
Age >18 yr.	Previous MI within 1 mo.
	Cardiogenic shock
Acute MI < 6 h from symptom onset.	Hypersensitivity to hypothermia, including a history of Raynaud's disease
ST-segment elevation of ≥1 mm in two or more contiguous leads (patients with anterior or inferior infarct *only*; inferior infarcts must have ≥1 mm ST-segment depression in two or more contiguous precordial leads, V1 to V4).	Known hypersensitivity or contraindication to aspirin, heparin, contrast media, buspirone, meperidine
	Known history of severe hepatic or renal impairment
	Treatment with a monoamine oxidase inhibitor in the past 14 d
	Patient known or expected to be pregnant
	Patient has inferior vena cava filter in place
	Patient height <1.5 m (4 ft 11 in.)

Of the 392 patients, 357 underwent primary PCI. Most were treated with stent implantation and a platelet glycoprotein receptor inhibitor. In the hypothermia group, the median duration of cooling prior to reperfusion was 17 min (IQR = 10–27 min). The mean temperature at the time of the first balloon inflation was 35.1 ± 0.8°C. Eighty-seven percent of patients in the hypothermia group achieved a core temperature <34°C; however, only 72% reached the intended target temperature of 33°C. At 30 d, the primary safety end point—a composite of death, MI, and target vessel revascularization—had occurred in 3.9% of the control group and 6.2% of the hypothermia group ($p = 0.45$). The final infarct size at 30 d was 10% of the left ventricle in the control group and 10% of the left ventricle in the hypothermia group ($p = 0.47$). However, patients with anterior infarction, who had a temperature <35°C at reperfusion, has a smaller infarct size than those with a temperature >35°C at reperfusion (Fig. 14).

This study provided a number of important insights regarding the use of hypothermia in acute MI. Hypothermia was safe and well tolerated, and endovascular cooling was easily integrated into existing clinical pathways. Perhaps, the most important observation from the study relates to the duration and extent of cooling *before* reperfusion. Data from the post hoc analysis in patients with anterior infarction suggest that the heart should be cooled optimally before reperfusion to provide optimal myocyte and microvascular protection. In the trial, the median time from the onset of cooling to the first balloon inflation was only 17 min, so there was a relatively modest 1°C mean reduction of core temperature at reperfusion. At the time the COOL-MI trial was designed, we did not believe that it was ethical to delay reperfusion therapy while cooling the patient, and for this reason, we encouraged investigators to proceed with intervention as soon as possible after initiation of cooling. Based on these findings, we believe that further investigation is required to refine the cooling technique in myocardial infarction.

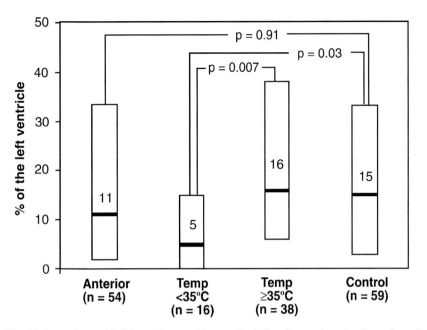

Fig. 14. Final infarct size at 30 d for patients with anterior infarction assigned to hypothermia according to the core body temperature at reperfusion. The boxes represent the 25th and 75th interquartile ranges; the median value is shown above the horizontal line.

ICE-IT TRIAL

The ICE-IT randomized trial enrolled 228 patients presenting within 6 h of symptom-onset. Patients assigned to receive hypothermia were cooled using the Celsius Control™ System. This endovascular catheter (Celsius Control™ catheter) has a gold-plated flexible heat-transfer element at the distal end and is available in two sizes depending on patient body size. One of the advantages of this system is that the Celsius Control™ catheter has a thermistor integrated into the shaft for temperature measurement and feedback, thus eliminating the need for bladder, esophageal or vascular temperature probes. Compared with the COOL-MI trial, the major difference with ICE-IT was the longer duration of cooling after reperfusion (6 vs 3 h) (Table 3). Overall, there was no difference in mean infarct size with hypothermia. However, as in the COOL-MI trial, the ICE-IT investigators noted a trend toward a treatment effect in patients who received sufficient cooling before reperfusion.

Future Directions

Based on the results of the COOL-MI trial, we believe that future studies should focus on optimizing the "dose" of cooling before reperfusion. To achieve this goal, one approach is to initiate cooling earlier after presentation, but it is likely that more powerful cooling systems will also be required. Other unresolved issues include the optimal duration of cooling after reperfusion and best methods to monitor core temperature. Additionally, there might be a role for hypothermia in cardiogenic shock to protect not only the heart but also other vital organs rendered ischemic by the low-output state.

CONCLUSION

Although extraordinary advances have been made in treatment of acute ST-segment elevation myocardial infarction, new cardioprotective strategies are required to enhance myocardial salvage and preserve ventricular function. Hyperoxemic reperfusion and hypothermia have emerged as two promising approaches that might expand the benefit of catheter-based reperfusion. Several innovative devices and systems have been developed to apply these novel therapies in clinical practice and are the subject of ongoing clinical investigation.

REFERENCES

1. Braunwald E. Myocardial reperfusion, limitation of infarct size, reduction of left ventricular dysfunction, and improved survival: should the paradigm be expanded? Circulation 1989;79:441–444.
2. Maroko PR, Libby P, Bloor CM, et al. Factors influencing infarct size following experimental coronary occlusion. Circulation 1971;43:67–82.
3. Reimer KA, Lowe JE, Rasmussen MM, Jennings RB. The wavefront phenomenon of ischemic cell death. 1. Myocardial infarct size vs duration of coronary occlusion in dogs. Circulation 1977;56: 786–794.
4. Gersh BJ, Anderson JL. Thrombolysis and myocardial salvage. Results of clinical trials and the animal paradigm—paradoxic or predictable? Circulation 1993;88:296–306.
5. Brodie BR, Stuckey TD, Hansen CJ, et al. Effect of treatment delay on outcomes in patients with acute myocardial infarction transferred from community hospitals for primary percutaneous coronary intervention. Am J Cardiol 2002;89:1243–1247.
6. Newby LK, Rutsch WR, Califf RM, et al. Time from symptom onset to treatment and outcomes after thrombolytic therapy. GUSTO-1 Investigators. J Am Coll Cardiol 1996;27:1646–1655.
7. Roe MT, Ohman EM, Maas AC, et al. Shifting the open-artery hypothesis downstream: the quest for optimal reperfusion. J Am Coll Cardiol 2001;37:9–18.
8. Kloner RA, Ganote CE, Jennings RB. The "no-reflow' phenomenon after temporary coronary occlusion in the dog. J Clin Invest 1974;54:1496–1508.
9. Forman MB, Virmani R, Puett DW. Mechanisms and therapy of myocardial reperfusion injury. Circulation 1990;81(Suppl IV):IV-69–IV-78.
10. Kloner RA. Does reperfusion injury exist in humans? J Am Coll Cardiol 1993;21:637–645.
11. Ambrosio G, Tritto I. Reperfusion injury: experimental evidence and clinical implications. Am Heart J 1999;138:S69–S75.
12. Davies MJ. A macro and micro view of coronary vascular insult in ischemic heart disease. Circulation. 1990;82(Suppl II):II-38–II-46.
13. Erbel R, Heusch G. Coronary microembolization. J Am Coll Cardiol 2000;36:22–24.
14. White HD, Norris RM, Brown MA, et al. Effect of intravenous streptokinase on left ventricular function and early survival after acute myocardial infarction. N Engl J Med 1987;317:850–855.
15. The GUSTO Angiographic Investigators. The effects of tissue plasminogen activator, streptokinase, or both on coronary artery patency, ventricular function, and survival after acute myocardial infarction. N Engl J Med 1993;329:1615–1622.
16. Burns RJ, Gibbons RJ, Yi Q, et al., CORE Study Investigators. The relationships of left ventricular ejection fraction, end-systolic volume index and infarct size to six-month mortality after hospital discharge following myocardial infarction treated by thrombolysis. J Am Coll Cardiol 2002;39:30–36.
17. Smith G, Lawson DA. Experimental coronary arterial occlusion: effects of the administration of oxygen under pressure. Scot Med J 1958;3:346–350.
18. Meijne NG, Bulterijs A, Eloff SJP, Boerema I. An experimental investigation into the influence of oxygen under increased atmospheric pressure upon coronary infarction. J Cardiovasc Surg 1963;4:521–535.
19. Trapp W, Creighton R. Experimental studies of increased atmospheric pressure on myocardial ischemia after coronary ligation. J Thorac Cardiovasc Surg 1964;47:687–692.
20. Peter RH, Rau RW, Whalen RE, et al. Effects of hyperbaric oxygenation on coronary artery occlusion in pigs. Circ Res 1966;18:89–96.
21. Cameron AJ, Hutton I, Kenmure AC, Murdoch WR. Haemodynamic and metabolic effects of hyperbaric oxygen in myocardial infarction. Lancet 1966;2:833–837.

22. Whalen RE, Saltzman HA. Hyperbaric oxygenation in the treatment of acute myocardial infarction. Prog Cardiovasc Dis 1968;10:575–583.

23. Mogelson S, Davidson J, Sobel B, Roberts R. The effect of hyperbaric oxygen on infarct size in the conscious animal. Eur J Cardiol 1980;12:135–146.

24. Thomas MP, Brown LA, Sponseller DR, et al. Myocardial infarct size reduction by the synergistic effect of hyperbaric oxygen and recombinant tissue plasminogen activator. Am Heart J 1990;120;791–800.

25. Sterling DL, Thornton JD, Swafford A, et al. Hyperbaric oxygen limits infarct size in ischemic rabbit myocardium in vivo. Circulation 1993;88(Pt 1):1931–1936.

26. Sirsjo A, Lehr HA, Nolte D, et al. Hyperbaric oxygen treatment enhances the recovery of blood flow and functional capillary density in postischemic striated muscle. Circulation Shock 1993;40:9–13.

27. Zamboni WA, Roth AC, Russell RC, et al. Morphological analysis of the microcirculation during reperfusion of ischemic skeletal muscle and the effect of hyperbaric oxygen. Plast Reconstr Surg 1993;91:1110–1123.

28. Zamboni WA, Roth AC, Russell RC, et al. The effect of hyperbaric oxygen on reperfusion of ischemic axial skin flaps: a laser Doppler analysis. Ann Plast Surg 1992;28:339–341.

29. Chen G, Banick PD, Thom SR, et al. Functional inhibition of rat polymorphonuclear leukocyte β_2 integrins by hyperbaric oxygen is associated with impaired cGMP synthesis. J Pharmacol Exp Ther 1996;276:929–933.

30. Hills BA. A role for oxygen-induced osmosis in hyperbaric oxygen therapy. Med Hypotheses 1999;52:259–263.

31. De Groot H, Noll T. The role of physiological oxygen partial pressures in lipid peroxidation. Theoretical considerations and experimental evidence. Chem Phys Lipids 1987;44:209–226.

32. Minyailenko TD, Pozharov VP, Seredenko MM. Severe hypoxia activates lipid peroxidation in the rat brain. Chem Phys Lipids 1990;55:25–28.

33. Thom SR, Elbuken ME. Oxygen-dependent antagonism of lipid peroxidation. Free Radical Biol Med 1991;10:413–426.

34. Shandling AH, Ellestad MH, Hart GB. Hyperbaric oxygen and thrombolysis in myocardial infarction: the "HOT MI" pilot study. Am Heart J 1997; 134: 544-550.

35. Spears JR. Method and apparatus for delivering oxygen into blood. US patent 5,407,426 (1995)

36. Spears JR, Wang B, Wu X, et al. Aqueous oxygen. A highly O_2-supersaturated infusate for regional correction of hypoxemia and production of hyperoxemia. Circulation 1997;96:4385–4391.

37. Spears JR, Henney C, Prcevski P, et al. Aqueous oxygen hyperbaric reperfusion in a porcine model of myocardial infarction. J Invasion Cardiol 2002;14:160–166.

38. Dixon SR, Bartorelli AL, Marcovitz PA, et al. Initial experience with hyperoxemic reperfusion after primary angioplasty for acute myocardial infarction. Results of a pilot study utilizing intracoronary Aqueous Oxygen therapy. J Am Coll Cardiol 2002;39:387–392.

39. Trabattoni D, Montorsi P, Fabbiocchi F, et al. Left ventricular function recovery after LAD hyperoxemic blood infusion in ST-elevation anterior AMI treated with primary PCI. Am J Cardiol 2002; 24:TCT-44.

40. O'Neill WW, on behalf of the AMIHOT Investigators, Acute myocardial infarction with hyperoxemic therapy (AMIHOT): a prospective, randomized, multicenter trial. Presented at the Annual Scientific Session of the American College of Cardiology, New Orleans, LA, March 2004.

41. The Hypothermia After Cardiac Arrest Study Group. Mild therapeutic hypothermia to improve the neurologic outcome after cardiac arrest. N Engl J Med 2002;346:549–556.

42. Bernard SA, Gray TW, Buist MD, et al. Treatment of comatose survivors of out-of-hospital cardiac arrest with induced hypothermia. N Engl J Med 2002;346:557–563.

43. Chien GL, Wolff RA, Davis RF, van Winkle DM. "Normothermic range" temperature affects myocardial infarct size. Cardiovasc Res 1994;28:1014–1017.

44. Duncker DJ, Klassen CL, Ishibashi Y, et al. Effect of temperature on myocardial infarction in swine. Am J Physiol 1996;270:H1189–H1199.

45. Schwartz LM, Verbinski SG, van der Heide RS, Reimer KA. Epicardial temperature is a major predictor of infarct size in dogs. J Mol Cell Cardiol 1997;29:1577–1583.

46. Hale SL, Kloner RA. Myocardial temperature in acute myocardial infarction: protection with mild regional hypothermia. Am J Physiol 1997;273:H220–H227.

47. van den Doel MA, Gho BCG, Duval SY, et al. Hypothermia extends the cardioprotection by ischaemic preconditioning to coronary artery occlusions of longer duration. Cardiovasc Res 1998;37:76–81.

48. Dave RH, Hale SL, Kloner RA. Hypothermic, closed circuit pericardioperfusion: a potential cardioprotective technique in acute regional ischemia. J Am Coll Cardiol 1998;31:1667–1671.

49. Hale SL, Dave RH, Kloner RA. Regional hypothermia reduces myocardial necrosis even when instituted after the onset of ischemia. Basic Res Cardiol 1997;92:351–357.
50. Miki T, Liu GS, Cohen MV, Downey JM. Mild hypothermia reduces infarct size in the beating rabbit heart: a practical intervention for acute myocardial infarction. Basic Res Cardiol 1998;93:372–383.
51. Hale SL, Kloner RA. Myocardial temperature reduction attenuates necrosis after prolonged ischemia in rabbits. Cardiovasc Res 1998;40:502–507.
52. Dae MW, Gao DW, Sessler DI, et al. Effect of endovascular cooling on myocardial temperature, infarct size, and cardiac output in human-sized pigs. Am J Physiol Heart Circ Physiol 2002;282:H1584–H1591.
53. Hale SL, Dae MW, Kloner RA, Hypothermia during reperfusion limits 'no-reflow' injury in a rabbit model of acute myocardial infarction. Cardiovasc Res 2003; 59:715-722.
54. Jeremy RW, Links JM, Becker LC. Progressive failure of coronary flow during reperfusion of myocardial infarction: documentation of the no reflow phenomenon with positron emission tomography. J Am Coll Cardiol 1990;16:695–704.
55. Ning XH, Xu CS, Song YC, et al. Hypothermia preserves function and signaling for mitochondrial biogenesis during subsequent ischemia. Am J Physiol 1998;274:H786–H793.
56. Ning XH, Chen SH, Xu CS, et al. Hypothermic protection of the ischemic heart via alterations in apoptotic pathways as assessed by gene array analysis. J Appl Physiol 2002;9:2200–2207.
57. Dixon SR, Whitbourn RJ, Dae MW, et al. Induction of mild systemic hypothermia with endovascular cooling during primary percutaneous coronary intervention for acute myocardial infarction. J Am Coll Cardiol 2002;40:1928–1934.
58. Mokhtarani M, Mahgoub A, Morioka N, et al. Buspirone and meperidine synergistically reduce the shivering threshold. Anesth Analg 2001;93:1233–1239.
59. Kandzari DE, Chu A, Brodie BR, et al. Feasibility of endovascular cooling as an adjunct to primary percutaneous coronary intervention (results of the LOWTEMP pilot study). Am J Cardiol 2004; 93: 636-639.
60. Grines CL, on behalf of the ICE-IT Investigators, Intravascular cooling adjunctive to percutaneous coronary intervention for acute myocardial infarction. Presented at Trancatheter Cardiovascular Therapeutics 2004, Washington DC, USA, September 2004,

14

Percutaneous Mechanical Assist Devices

Suresh R. Mulukutla, MD
and Howard A. Cohen, MD

INTRODUCTION

In 1968, the first clinical application of the intra-aortic balloon pump (IABP) was reported for treating patients with cardiogenic shock after acute myocardial infarction *(1)*. Now, just over three decades later, the IABP is routinely used by cardiologists in the cardiac care unit and in the cardiac catheterization lab as well as by cardiac surgeons in the perioperative setting. Its role in the management of congestive heart failure as a result of ischemia, infarction, or valvular heart disease has become so established that the IABP is currently the most widely used mechanical cardiac assist device. Its use is only likely to increase, given that studies have shown that aggressive IABP use is cost-effective in selected patients because of both shorter hospital stay and complication reduction *(2)*.

Other percutaneous mechanical assist devices that will be discussed in this chapter include cardiopulmonary support (CPS), the Hemopump™, and the TandemHeart™. They all function in different ways, but they all aim to achieve specific general goals,

From: *Contemporary Cardiology: Interventional Cardiology:*
Percutaneous Noncoronary Intervention
Edited by: H. C. Herrmann © Humana Press Inc., Totowa, NJ

which include reducing cardiac afterload, increasing coronary perfusion, and, over time, improving cardiac output. In this chapter, we will first review intra-aortic balloon counterpulsation given that this was the original method of mechanical cardiac assistance.

Historical Perspective

Although the first clinical use of the IABP was reported in 1968, the origins of the IABP date back to 1953. Kantrowitz and Kantrowitz *(3)* demonstrated the concept of "diastolic augmentation" by using a rubber tube connected between the femoral artery and the coronary artery that delayed the systolic pulse wave into diastole, thus increasing coronary perfusion.

Meanwhile, Harken and Claus and colleagues from Harvard University studied the concept of "counterpulsation" and demonstrated that if blood from the aorta was aspirated just prior to the opening of the aortic valve (end diastole) and returned during early diastole of the next cardiac cycle, this would result in afterload reduction and thereby decrease myocardial oxygen consumption *(4,5)*. In 1962, two groups independently published results of an intra-aortic balloon counterpulsation device. Moulopoulos et al. *(6)* and Claus et al. *(7)* described a Latex balloon that could be placed within the aorta that could be inflated during early diastole, resulting in diastolic augmentation and actively deflated during late diastole for afterload reduction.

The birth of the present-day IABP occurred in 1967. Researchers in Kantrowitz's lab designed a nondistensible polyurethane balloon driven by helium, which could be rapidly infused for balloon inflation and rapidly removed for deflation. Results of its use in dogs were published in 1967 *(8)*. In 1968, Kantrowitz and his group published results of the first clinical IABP application in patients with cardiogenic shock after acute myocardial infarction *(9)*. Although clinical outcomes were poor, hemodynamic benefits were appreciated.

In 1972, Buckley and colleagues reported the successful use of the IABP in patients who were unable to be weaned off of cardiopulmonary bypass *(10)*, and in 1973, they published their results on 87 patients with shock after myocardial infarction and reported hemodynamic benefit and relatively low complication rates *(11)*. Over the next 10 yr, the use of IABP increased; however, it was primarily limited to use by surgeons because it required surgical insertion. By 1979, Datascope Corporation introduced the percutaneous IABP, and its use was thus extended to invasive cardiologists as well. From its initial use in patients with cardiogenic shock after acute myocardial infarction, the indications for IABP have expanded to unstable angina, high-risk angioplasty, perioperative low-cardiac output syndromes, refractory heart failure, and, finally, as a bridge to cardiac transplantation.

HEMODYNAMIC AND METABOLIC BENEFITS OF MECHANICAL CARDIAC ASSIST DEVICES

Intra-aortic balloon pump counterpulsation affects several hemodynamic parameters during IABP inflation and deflation as illustrated in Fig. 1. Deflation of the IABP during end diastole is a process that involves actively drawing blood away from the central aorta and thus reducing central aortic pressure, resulting in decreased afterload, increased stroke volume, decreased end-diastolic volume, and decreased myocardial consumption. Inflation of the IABP during diastole also has several beneficial effects, including increase of diastolic pressure, which results in increased coronary flow and oxygen supply,

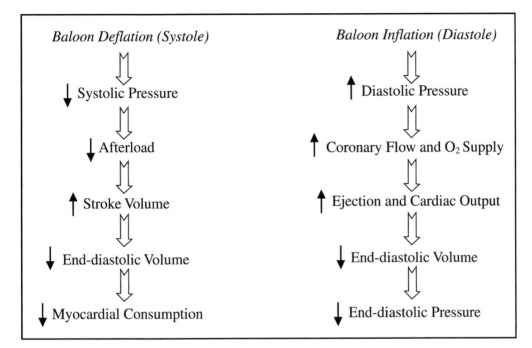

Fig. 1. Hemodynamic consequences of counterpulsation.

Table 1
Hemodynamic Parameters Affected by IABP

Aortic pressure
Left ventricular end-diastolic pressure
Left ventricular work
Tension time index
Diastolic pressure time index
Ejection fraction
Cardiac output

improved cardiac output, decreased end-diastolic volume, and decreased end-diastolic pressure, which, again, results in decreased myocardial consumption.

Table 1 illustrates some of the major hemodynamic parameters that are enhanced by balloon counterpulsation. IABP reduces aortic systolic pressure by 8.9–26.6% *(12)*. Left ventricular end-diastolic pressure decreases by 25–40% *(13)* and left ventricular work decreases by a similar 18–50% with IABP counterpulsation *(14)*. Another accurate measure of left ventricular workload is the myocardial tension time index that is reduced by 20–40% in studies of patients who require IABP therapy for hemodynamic cardiac support *(15)*. Given all of these beneficial hemodynamic effects, one would expect ejection fraction to increase as well; however, there is no experimental data to support this at this time. There are data to suggest that the IABP improves cardiac output by as much as 50%, although this is controversial *(13,16)*.

Along with the improvement in hemodynamic parameters, it is important to recognize that this is accompanied by an improvement in a number of physiologic parameters (Table 2). Coronary blood flow is augmented by 5–15% in some studies, although this

Table 2
Metabolic Parameters Affected by IABP

Coronary blood flow
Cerebral blood flow
Renal blood flow
Myocardial oxygen supply
Myocardial oxygen consumption
Lactate production

level of improvement has not been demonstrated in other studies and probably depends on the etiology of the underlying disease *(17–19)*. Cerebral blood flow does increase with IABP therapy, but renal blood flow might not be significantly altered *(20)*. The diastolic pressure time index (DPTI) is the sum of diastolic aortic pressures minus the left atrial pressures generated in 1 min, and it is proportional to the myocardial blood flow and to the amount of oxygen available to the myocardium *(21)*. IABP support results in an increase in diastolic aortic pressure (from diastolic augmentation) and a decrease in left ventricular end-diastolic pressure (and left atrial pressure). As the DPTI increases, therefore, there is a proportional increase in myocardial blood flow and myocardial oxygen supply.

INDICATIONS FOR IABP THERAPY

The indications of IABP therapy have expanded since this technique was introduced. Table 3 lists the current major indications for IABP therapy, and we will discuss only a few of these in detail.

Cardiogenic Shock

The most frequent indication for use of IABP therapy today is cardiogenic shock. Unfortunately, in spite of the improved metabolic and hemodynamic profile that results with IABP counterpulsation, the use of the device alone has failed to translate into a direct survival benefit. Studies of patients with cardiogenic shock who are treated with IABP alone have been discouraging, with overall survival rates ranging from 5% to 48% in a variety of patient populations *(22–26)*.

Because of the poor survival rates in this sick and often unstable patient population when treated with IABP alone, IABP therapy has evolved into an adjunctive strategy. Currently, in patients with cardiogenic shock, the IABP is used as a mode of ventricular support for patients with large myocardial infarctions to allow the heart to recover from the insult. It is also utilized as a bridge to next therapy in patients with shock who require percutaneous or surgical revascularization.

The most common cause of cardiogenic shock is acute myocardial infarction (MI), and considerable data have emerged with regard to the use of adjunctive IABP therapy in patients who receive thrombolytic therapy for acute MI. In community hospitals, patients with acute MI and cardiogenic shock are often managed with thrombolysis alone. In one study on patients with acute MI and cardiogenic shock, those treated with IABP and thrombolysis had a significantly higher rate of hospital survival compared with patients treated with thrombolysis alone *(27)*. Results of a larger, prospective study published in 2000 from the SHOCK registry also revealed the benefits of IABP therapy as an adjunct to thrombolysis/revascularization *(28)*. In this study, patients who received

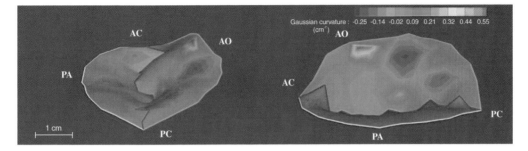

Color Plate 1, Fig. 2. (*see* discussion in Ch. 3, and full caption on p. 51). Image of a human mitral valve annulus and leaflets created with real-time three-dimensional echocardiography.

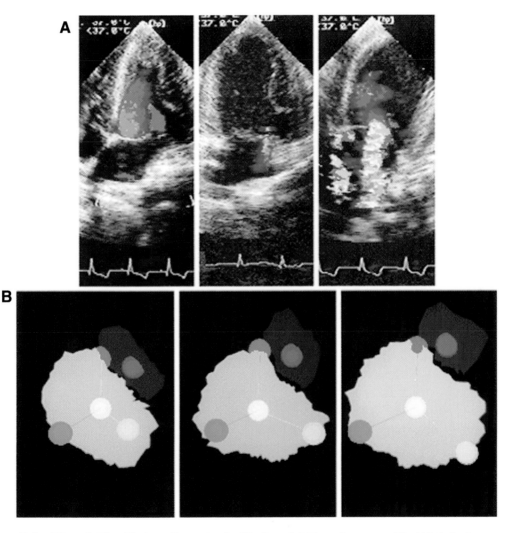

Color Plate 2, Fig. 10. (*see* discussion in Ch. 3, and full caption on p. 60). **(A)** Apical two-chamber echocardiographic images with color-flow mapping showing development. **(B)** Annular dilatation and relatio papillary muscles.

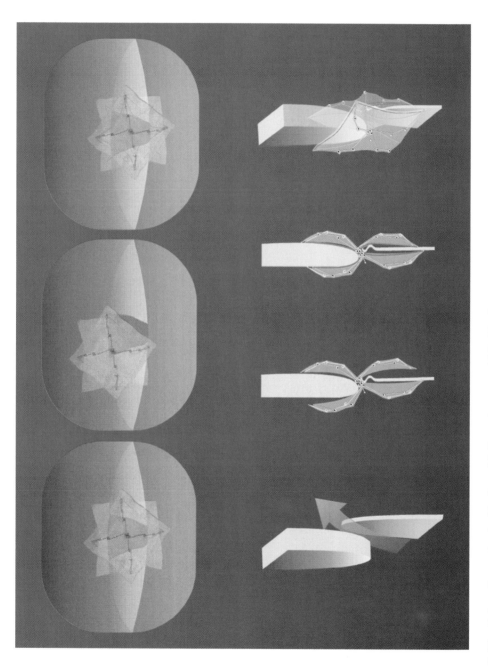

Color Plate 3, Fig. 5. (*see* discussion in Ch. 8, and full caption on p. 136). The internal autoadjusting spring mechanism unique to the CardioSEAL-STARFlex system forces the device to find, and seat within, the central portion of the FO.

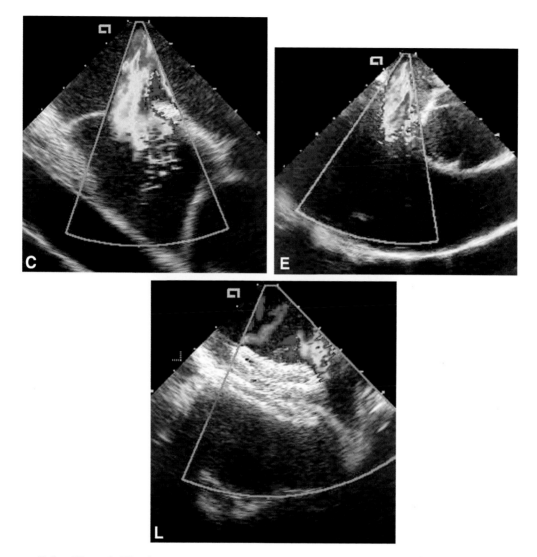

Color Plate 4, Fig. 2. (*see* discussion in Ch. 10, and full caption on p. 170). Intracardiac echocardiographic images in a patient with large secundum ASD.

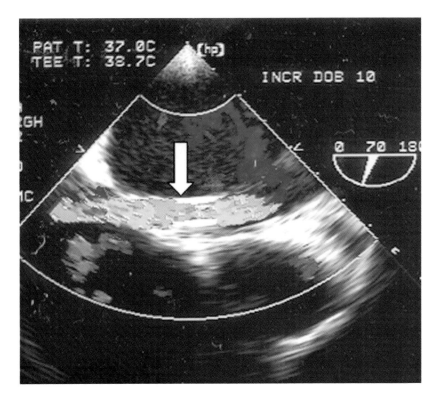

Color Plate 5, Fig. 7. (*see* discussion in Ch. 14 and caption on p. 246). Transesophageal imaging of flow across the transseptal cannula in the TandemHeart.

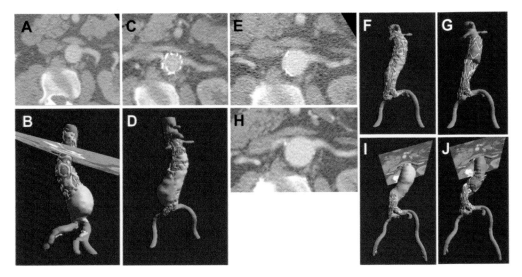

Color Plate 6, Fig. 4. (*see* discussion in Ch. 19, and full caption on p. 352). Significant migration of a Talent endograft at 4 yr of follow-up, without evidence of endoleak and with full regression of the aneurysm sac.

Table 3
Indications for IABP

Cardiogenic shock resulting from acute myocardial infarction
Acute mitral regurgitation or ventricular septal rupture
Perioperative low-cardiac-output syndrome
Unstable angina refractory to medical therapy
Bridge to cardiac surgery in patients with unstable angina
Refractory arrhythmias secondary to ischemia and/or heart failure
Bridge to cardiac transplantation
High-risk angioplasty as prophylactic support
Other
  Septic shock
  High-risk patients undergoing noncardiac surgery

IABP support had a significantly lower mortality compared to those who received no IABP therapy. Further, in the community hospital setting where percutaneous coronary intervention was not available, patients treated with both IABP support and thrombolytic therapy had the highest survival rates. Thus, given these results, it would appear that treatment of patients with cardiogenic shock with thrombolytic therapy and IABP support offers the best chance for survival when primary angioplasty is unavailable or not feasible. Although, intra-aortic counterpulsation, theoretically, would seem to benefit even patients with uncomplicated myocardial infarction by reducing left ventriculor (LV) work and improving coronary perfusion, studies have not shown such a benefit (29).

The relative ease of placement of the IABP has enhanced its utility, and it has become essential adjunctive therapy in patients who develop cardiogenic shock from mechanical complications of acute MI, including acute mitral regurgitation and rupture of the ventricular septum (30,31). The use of an IABP in acute mitral regurgitation and cardiogenic shock can result in a 30% improvement in cardiac output and blood flow to the brain while decreasing systemic vascular resistance, thereby lessening the mitral regurgitation (30). Today, IABP therapy for cardiogenic shock is often utilized as a bridge to some other mode of ventricular support, including other percutaneous ventricular assist devices, surgical means of mechanical assistance (i.e., implantable VAD), or cardiac transplantation.

Refractory Heart Failure

Intra-aortic balloon pump therapy has a role in patients with congestive heart failure who might not meet the strict criteria for cardiogenic shock. Several investigators have studied the role of IABP therapy in patients with medically refractory heart failure but without cardiogenic shock. Hagemeijer et al. studied Class III–IV heart failure patients after a recent MI and reported significant hemodynamic improvement in 80% of patients and a remarkable 56% hospital survival rate (32). Although these results were promising, more recent studies of similar patient populations have reported poorer survival rates of 25–30% (33). One explanation for these differences might be the duration of the IABP use, with patients in the Hagemeijer et al. study receiving IABP support for prolonged periods, some up to 24 d. Nonetheless, because of the relatively poor survival rates in this very sick patient population, the IABP is not sufficient as an independent mode of therapy for patients with cardiogenic shock; rather, it has been utilized effectively as an adjunct in the treatment of this condition.

Preoperative Cardiac Surgery

Patients who are scheduled to undergo cardiac surgery often benefit from preoperative insertion of an IABP. Patients with poor LV function, severe coronary artery disease, or patients who are hemodynamically compromised might benefit the greatest with preoperative IABP insertion. The indications for placement of preoperative IABPs are not standardized, but a retrospective study by Christenson et al. suggests that factors associated with increased mortality and need for placement of IABP include preoperative unstable angina, redo-CABG, LVEF <40%, diffuse coronary artery disease, and left main coronary stenosis *(34)*. Based on these results, these investigators conducted another study in which they enrolled 60 high-risk patients who had coronary artery bypass grafting with 2 or more of the following risk factors: LVEF <30%, unstable angina, left main stenosis, or prior history of bypass grafting *(35)*. Thirty patients did not receive preoperative IABP and 30 received the device. Preoperative IABP therapy was associated with higher postoperative cardiac index, lower incidence of postoperative low-cardiac-output syndrome, and shorter ICU and hospital stays. Others have come to similar conclusions, and many have suggested that preoperative IABP treatment is a cost-effective therapy *(36)*. There appears to be no consensus on how long to treat patients with intra-aortic counterpulsation. Some studies have suggested that treatment for 12 or 24 h preoperatively offers no greater advantage over treatment for 2 h prior to bypass surgery *(35)*. How long to treat patients preoperatively, however, depends a great deal on an individual patient's risk profile. Although many surgeons choose to place IABPs preoperatively, it is not entirely clear whether this offers any advantage to intraoperative or postoperative IABP insertion. Induction of anesthesia is associated with the greatest risk to the myocardium based on serial CK determinations, suggesting that preoperative IABP insertion might be beneficial in minimizing the stress on the heart caused by induction of anesthesia *(37)*. In patients with unstable angina, severe left main coronary artery stenosis, or low-cardiac-output states, prophylactic IABP use appears to be appropriate.

Postoperative Low-Cardiac-Output Syndrome

Intra-aortic ballon pump support for postcardiotomy low-cardiac-output syndromes was initially suggested by Kantrowitz's group in their seminal article from 1968 *(1)*. Buckley et al. were among the first groups to report on the successful use of IABP counterpulsation for this clinical scenario *(10)*. The definition of postcardiotomy low-cardiac-output syndrome is not standardized; however, for the purposes of this discussion, we will use the parameters used by Rao and colleagues *(38)*. They defined low-cardiac-output syndrome as a postoperative condition for which IABP or inotropic support is required to maintain a systolic blood pressure higher than 90 mm Hg or a cardiac index greater than 2.2 L/min/m^2. By these criteria, Rao et al. diagnosed postcardiotomy low cardiac output syndrome in 9.1% of post-CABG patients. This corresponds to the prevalence found in other studies *(39–41)*.

Postcardiotomy low-cardiac-output syndrome is multifactorial process resulting from inadequate myocardial protection during the perioperative period. There might be multiple reasons for lack of myocardial preservation, including recent MI, stunned myocardium, technical difficulty with bypass grafting, intraoperative infarction, coronary spasm, and prolonged periods on cardiopulmonary bypass *(42,43)*. Factors that predispose to the development of low-cardiac-output syndrome include age greater than 70, preoperative LV failure, three-vessel and/or left main coronary artery disease, and redo or emergent surgery *(42,44)*. Several other studies have found that female gender, diabetes, and length of cardiopulmonary bypass are also risk factors for the development of low-cardiac-output syndrome in the postoperative period *(45,46)*.

Studies suggest that these patients benefit greatly from IABP support. Mortality rates over 90% are reported in patients who do not receive IABP support *(47)*. However, with IABP assistance, survival rates of 40–70% are reported *(40,41,48)*. Importantly, time to IABP support is critical. Once the need for IABP assistance is recognized, it is imperative that it be initiated quickly because mortality rises if mechanical cardiac support is withheld or delayed *(49,50)*. Not surprisingly, long-term survival rates are poorer given the sick nature of this patient population. Lund et al. and Kuchar et al. reported 5-yr survival rates of 22% and 25%, respectively, in patients requiring IABP support for postcardiotomy low-cardiac-output syndrome *(45,51)*. Approximately 1% of cardiac surgical patients cannot be weaned from bypass in spite of inotropic and IABP support *(43)*, and in these patients, other ventricular assist devices might be required to provide greater hemodynamic support or to support patients as a bridge to cardiac transplantation.

Bridge to Cardiac Transplantation

In the last 20 yr, cardiac transplantation has evolved into an accepted therapy for patients with end-stage heart disease. Although potentially 40,000 patients per year die of heart disease that could have been treated with cardiac transplantation *(52)*, only about 2500 donor hearts become available annually *(53)*. Of these carefully selected patients, 1-yr survival rates are 85–90% in several analyses from different institutions *(54–56)*. The IABP has been used as a bridge to cardiac transplantation. However, as the number of patients eligible for transplantation has increased, so has the waiting period for a donor. For this reason, the IABP might be somewhat limited in its use as a bridge to transplantation; rather, devices such as the artificial heart and the ventricular assist device are often preferred at certain institutions. Nonetheless, IABPs still play a crucial role in patients awaiting cardiac transplant.

Several investigators have reported success with the IABP as a bridge to cardiac transplantation *(57–59)*. Furthermore, intra-aortic counterpulsation is an effective "bridge" for patients with ischemic cardiomyopathy as well as nonischemic cardiomyopathy *(60)*. Survival in transplant candidates who require IABP support remains quite high. Marks and colleagues from the Utah Transplant Program found no difference in 1-yr survival rates between patients who required mechanical support prior to cardiac transplantation and those who did not require such intervention *(55)*. Similarly, Birovljev et al. from Texas Heart Institute detected no significant difference in 1-yr or 2-yr survival rates between the two groups *(61)*. Although these studies revealed that survival rates were not worse if a patient required preoperative mechanical support, at least one study found that patients requiring mechanical support prior to transplantation had significantly poorer outcomes than patients who were not in need of mechanical assistance *(62)*. The higher mortality in this study was related to a higher rate of sepsis and a higher operative mortality in the group requiring mechanical support. Most of the evidence suggests that IABP support is both safe and effective. Some type of mechanical circulatory assistance is required in about 9–10% of patients awaiting cardiac transplantation *(61–64)*, and in carefully selected patients, IABP support can provide an essential bridge as they wait for a donor organ.

Table 4
Complications Associated with IABP Use

Vascular complications
    Bleeding
    Limb ischemia
    Compartment syndrome
    Arterial dissection
    Groin hematoma
Embolic events
    Cerebrovascular accident
    Bowel infarction
    Renal infarction
    Emboli to extremities
Infection
Ballon rupture or failure
Aortic rupture
Death

IABP-RELATED COMPLICATIONS

The complication rates in various studies since the introduction of the IABP vary between 11% and 45% (65–70). The more recent studies suggest that the complication rate is about 15% (65,66). Major complications occur with an incidence of between 4% and 14%, whereas minor complications occur in 17–41% of cases (65,66,68,71). Table 4 lists the some of the most common complications associated with IABP therapy. Death is also a potential complication of IABP support, but, fortunately, it occurs relatively rarely with an incidence of less than 1% (65,68).

The vast majority of IABP-related complications are vascular ones. The potential complications range from lost of distal pulse to acute arterial thrombosis to emboli with and without resultant limb loss. The potential therapies for these vascular complications also range widely from observation to possible amputation. IABP-related complications appear to be more frequent in those with peripheral vascular disease, female sex, and diabetes (65,69,71,72). In a prospective study of over 1100 patients on IABPs, Cohen et al. found that a history of peripheral vascular disease increases the risk of vascular complications by four times (65), and Gottlieb's group found that a history of peripheral vascular disease was predictive of serious vascular complications requiring surgical therapy (69). Female sex carries a relative risk of 2.3 for vascular complications, and although not clear, this might be related to the relatively smaller-caliber arteries among women (65). Diabetes is an independent risk factor for vascular complications, with complications occurring in 34% of insulin-dependent diabetics, 18% of non-insulin-dependent diabetics, and only in 14% of nondiabetic patients (65,73).

Catheter size and method of insertion are also factors that might increase the risk of complications. The early data suggested that percutaneous insertion of IABPs is associated with higher vascular complication rates than surgical insertion, and this was probably attributable to the difficulty in placing the IABP in patients with peripheral vascular disease (67,74–77). In patients with known peripheral vascular disease, the risk of vascular complications was 17.9% with a surgical cut-down technique versus 38.9% with the percutaneous method *(74)*. Not surprisingly, larger catheter sizes are also predictive for higher complication rates. 12 French catheters inserted percutaneously were associated with a 20.7% complication rate compared to 9.9% when 10.5 French catheters were used *(67)*. Over the last several years, the significant decrease in vascular complications can largely be explained by the use of catheters with smaller diameters and better patient selection in avoiding IABP placement in those with severe peripheral vascular disease. Other factors that contribute to an increased incidence of complications with IABP therapy are longer duration of IABP support, advanced age, hemodynamic instability, and emergent IABP insertion *(67)*.

Vascular complications associated with IABP therapy carry a high morbidity and mortality. Busch and Sirbu's group report a mortality rate in patients with ischemic vascular complications of 59% *(78)*. Complications in these studies included acute limb arterial occlusion, compartment syndrome, arterial dissection, and groin hematoma. Of the 524 patients evaluated in this study, 26.7% experienced vascular complications requiring surgical therapy. Surgical interventions included thromboembolectomy, profundaplasties, infrainguinal bypasses, fasciotomies, and, rarely, amputations.

Bleeding is another potentially serious complication associated with IABP use. McEnany et al. reported major bleeding in 4% of the patients studied *(79)*, and this correlated with the 4.6% reported by Cohen et al. *(65)*.

Infectious complications are also common in patients with IABPs. These include local infections, bacteremia, and sepsis. Overall, the rate of infectious complications range between 0% and 22% *(68–70,80)*. Kantrowitz's group found that the rate of infectious complications was related to the location of insertion: 26% in coronary care unit, 23% in surgical intensive care unit, 17% in cardiac catheterization laboratory, and 12% in operating room *(68)*. These findings stress the importance of aseptic technique during insertion of the IABP. Duration of IABP is also a risk factor for infection, and infection rate directly relates to the length of time that the device is left in place *(67)*. Other less common complications include paraplegia *(81)*, small-bowel infarction *(82)*, air embolism *(83,84)*, and acute ischemic hepatitis *(85)*.

Intra-aortic balloon pump-related complications should always be taken seriously and managed carefully given the wide variety of serious potential complications. Although the overall complication rate appears to be declining because of increased experience and improved technology, a high degree of awareness and a careful approach to IABP use is required to help avoid some of the potentially devastating complications associated with this and other mechanical assist devices.

CONTRAINDICATIONS TO IABP USE

The major contraindications to IABP are aortic insufficiency and aortic dissection. Peripheral vascular disease is a relative contraindication to IABP placement because of the risk of limb ischemia. However, in patients with severe diffuse peripheral vascular disease, placement of an IABP can be technically very challenging. As discussed later, other percutaneous assist devices might help to provide mechanical cardiac support even in patients with severe vascular disease. In patients with documented severe, focal stenosis in the iliac arteries or in the distal aorta, IABP insertion is possible without increase in morbidity after percutaneous angioplasty of the stenosis *(86,87)*. Limb ischemia can also be avoided by femoral–femoral bypass in patients in whom an IABP might be a life-saving maneuver.

MECHANICAL ASSISTANCE BEYOND THE IABP

Given the prevalence of coronary artery disease around the world, the concept of ventricular assistance and unloading is particularly attractive in the setting of acute MI with or without cardiogenic shock because this has the potential of helping an enormous number of patients. The treatment of acute MI (AMI) has evolved remarkably over the past 25 yr with a significant reduction in mortality, attributed largely to the institution of coronary care units, advanced pharmacology and reperfusion therapy with thrombolytic agents, and primary angioplasty *(88)*. Still, reperfusion alone does not dramatically improve global or segmental LV function *(89,90)*. Whereas in the past, successful reperfusion post-AMI was equated with restoration of epicardial vessel patency, there is a growing body of evidence that microvascular dysfunction and inadequate tissue perfusion persists despite successful opening of the epicardial vessel—the so-called "illusion of reperfusion" *(91,92)*. Optimal reperfusion has, therefore, been redefined to include restoration of microvascular flow as well as epicardial vessel patency *(93)*.

Several interventions have been evaluated for improving microvascular flow *(94,95)*. Animal models have demonstrated that the IABP restores epicardial blood flow but has little effect on microvascular flow in the setting of acute myocardial infarction (AMI) *(96)*. By contrast, the use of an LV assist device (left atrial to femoral artery bypass) in the animal model with AMI and cardiogenic shock results in complete restoration of endocardial (microvascular) as well as epicardial flow to baseline values. Further, the use of a LV assist device (LVAD) in the setting of experimental AMI results in a marked reduction in the extent of myocardial necrosis compared to controls *(97–99)*.

With this experimental evidence, implantable LVADs have been used for cardiogenic shock with AMIs; however, their use is limited by cost and the need for surgery for implantation and removal. The Jarvik 2000, the Heartmate II, and the Debakey assist device are examples of second-generation LVADs that utilize rotary pump technology to power blood flow. Although they are smaller and easier to insert than previous devices, they still require a thoracotomy for insertion and removal *(100–103)*.

The concept of left atrial to femoral artery bypass centers around the idea of reducing LV work and improving myocardial energy consumption by unloading the left ventricle. Myocardial energy consumption is maximal with the beating heart that is full and is significantly lessened with the beating heart that is empty, and oxygen consumption is minimal during cardioplegia. The importance of this is that active unloading of the left ventricle might lessen oxygen demand and oxygen consumption, thereby improving the patient's hemodynamic status.

Investigators have developed percutaneous methods of achieving the goal of ventricular unloading. Left heart bypass with left atrial cannulation was reported in 1960 by Salisbury *(104)*. Dennis in 1962 also described a method of cannulating the left atrium for left heart bypass (LHB) *(105)*. Glassman and colleagues employed a method of closed-chest transseptal cannulation of the left atrium (LA) for LHB in dogs and in three patients *(106)*. Pavie et al. studied three patients who underwent finger-guided transseptal left atrial cannulation for LV support *(107)*. They used a transseptal cannula placed in the LA and femoral artery (FA) cannulation to support three patients' post-cardiotomy and attained flows of nearly 2 L/min. The TandemHeart™ was then developed after considerable research and has the potential to offer hemodynamic support well beyond that of the IABP alone.

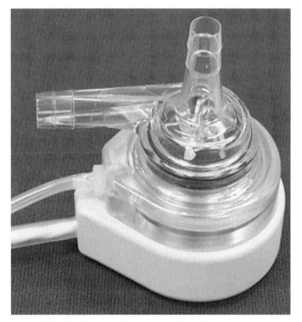

Fig. 2. TandemHeart centrifugal pump.

PERCUTANEOUS LEFT VENTRICULAR ASSIST WITH THE TANDEMHEART

The TandemHeart percutaneous LVAD, manufactured by CardiacAssist Inc., was recently approved by the Food and Drug Administration (FDA) in June 2003 as a short-term circulatory support system. It is a relatively inexpensive left atrial to femoral artery bypass system that can be inserted percutaneously. The device consists of a small centrifugal pump (Fig. 2) with a specially designed transseptal inflow cannula (Fig. 3) and outflow conduit for percutaneous femoral artery placement. The device is powered by a DC-brushless motor and typically operates at 3000–7500 rpm. It functions as a hydrodynamic bearing, with its moving surfaces suspended in a heparinized sterile water lubricant. Figure 4 is a cutaway section of the TandemHeart pump. The device is connected to a controller that operates based on a back-EMF (electromagnetic force) algorithm and has several built-in safety features (Fig. 5). Figure 6 is a diagram of the transseptal cannula after placement in the left atrium. Standard transseptal technique is used to enter the left atrium. An Inoue guide wire is used to maintain access safely in the left atrium while the interatrial septum is dilated with a graduated progressive dilator. The transseptal cannula, a 21 French polyurethane cannula with a large endhole and 14 side holes is then passed into the left atrium. Care must be taken to be certain that all side holes are situated in the left atrium in order to avoid right-to-left shunting. Less than 20 cm^3 is used to prime the pump and 60 cm^3 for the entire system. Once all air has been removed from the system and the lines are secured, the cannulae are connected to the TandemHeart using standard Tygon tubing. The power line for the device is then connected to the controller, and ventricular assist can begin. Experienced operators can insert the device and institute LV assistance in less than 30 min.

Patients must be maintained on systemic anticoagulation with heparin with ACT maintained at 200–250 s. When it is decided to terminate use of the device, heparin is

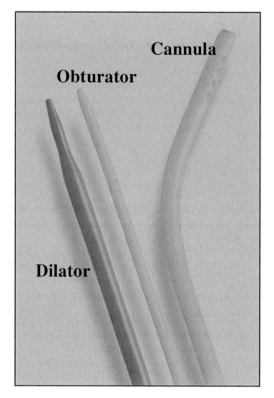

Fig. 3. TandemHeart cannula that crosses the atrial septum. The septum is predilated with a dilator.

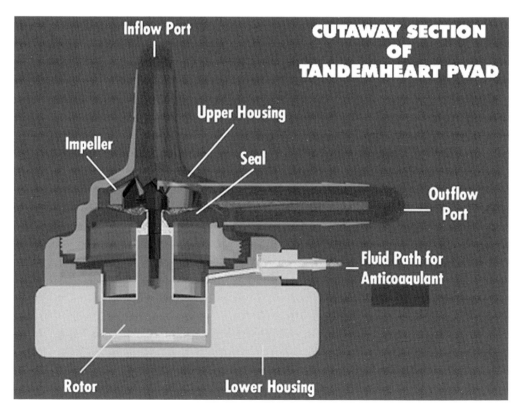

Fig. 4. Cutaway section of the TandemHeart.

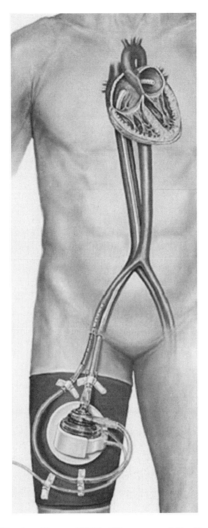

Fig. 5. The TandemHeart pVAD. (Courtesy of CardiacAssist, Inc.)

discontinued, and the cannulae removed, with hemostasis achieved with direct manual pressure over the puncture sites. Figure 7 shows transesophageal images of the transseptal cannula in the left atrium during support with the TandemHeart with color-flow Doppler demonstrating the flow in the cannula. Because the TandemHeart removes oxygenated blood from the left atrium and replaces it in the femoral artery, an important issue is to verify that adequate flow is maintained in the carotid artery for cerebral perfusion and that flow in the aorta is well preserved. Figures 8 shows Doppler flow within the carotid artery during varying flow rates from the TandemHeart. The figure illustrates that continuous flow within the carotid artery improves with increasing flow rates from the TandemHeart. Figure 9 shows Doppler flow in the descending thoracic aorta at varying flow rates. With increasing support, there is more retrograde (continuous) flow and less anterograde (native) flow as the device takes over the pumping function of the heart.

A Phase I study of the TandemHeart device was performed at five different institutions around the United States *(108)*. Thirteen patients were enrolled with a mean age of 66.3 yr, and eight patients had post-MI cardiogenic shock. All patients were on maximal pharma-

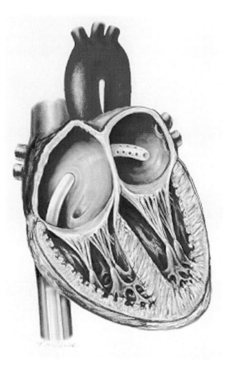

Fig. 6. Close-up of TandemHeart transseptal catheter in the left atrium.

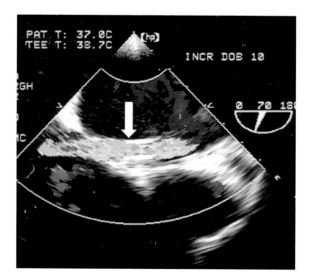

Fig. 7. Transesophageal imaging of flow across the transseptal cannula in the TandemHeart. (Color illustration is printed in insert following page 236.)

cologic therapy and nine of them were refractory to IABP therapy. The device resulted in significant improvement in cardiac index and significant reduction in pulmonary capillary wedge pressure. It caused no significant hemolysis or thrombocytopenia. This feasibility study demonstrated that the TandemHeart can be implanted quickly and safely and that it was potentially effective in reversing cardiogenic shock and stabilizing patients as a bridge to definitive therapy.

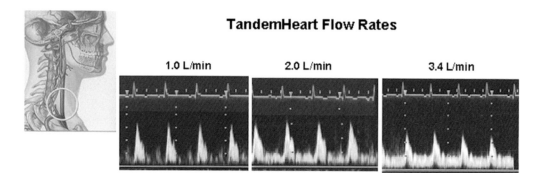

Fig. 8. Carotid Doppler flow during TandemHeart support.

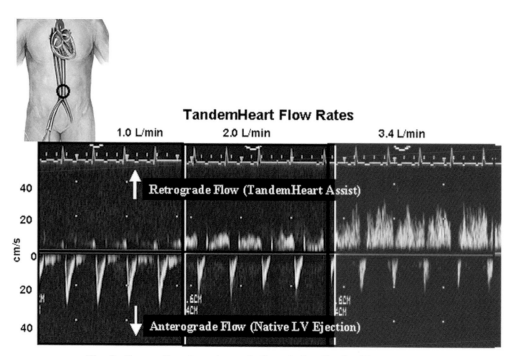

Fig. 9. Descending thoracic aortic flow during TandemHeart support.

Following these promising Phase I results, Thiele et al. reported on the reversal of cardiogenic shock with the TandemHeart device *(109)*. Eighteen consecutive patients were enrolled with cardiogenic shock and AMI. Five of 18 patients had ventricular septal rupture. The mean duration of support was 4 ± 3 d. Survival in this study was 56% at 30 d. Eliminating the 5 patients with ventricular septal rupture, 10 of 13 patients with AMI and cardiogenic shock survived. Flow of up to 4 L/min can be provided with the device. The major result of this study was the demonstration of significant increases in cardiac output (3.5–4.8 L/min) and blood pressure (63.1–80.2 mm Hg). They also showed significant reductions in heart rate (108–103 bpm), pulmonary capillary wedge pressure (20.8–14.2 mm Hg), and lactate (4.7–3.0). Thus, the TandemHeart was successful in improving several hemodynamic and metabolic parameters of cardiogenic shock.

As opposed to the cardiopulmonary support system (discussed later), the TandemHeart could be used to support patients in cardiogenic shock for prolonged periods of time. Currently, Phase II studies in the United States are ongoing. This is a multicenter trial of the treatment of cardiogenic shock despite therapy with or without IABP randomized to TandemHeart versus conventional therapy. The results of this trial might potentially alter our treatment of patients with cardiogenic shock.

Another exciting potential application of the TandemHeart is its use for supported percutaneous coronary intervention (PCI) Preliminary studies have shown promise in this regard. Serruys' group studied seven patients, two with acute myocardial infarction and cardiogenic shock and five with stable angina but undergoing high-risk coronary intervention (110). Device use was associated with a tendency toward decreasing LV filling pressures and increasing systemic arterial pressures. Overall, the study demonstrated that the TandemHeart might constitute a promising option to reduce PCI-related complications.

HEMOPUMP™

In 1988, Wampler and colleagues first described a retrograde, catheter-mounted LVAD intended for surgical placement via the femoral artery (111). The device is based on the ancient concept of a screw pump first described by the Egyptians and later by Archimedes. The pump system is intracorporeal with a disposable catheter with a turbine at its tip driven by an external motor that is connected to an electrical console (Fig. 10). The disposable pumping system consists of an inlet cannula, an axial flow blood pump, and a drive cable in a polymeric sheath and a rotor motor. The sheath also serves as a conduit for purge fluid that lubricates the drive cable and hydrodynamic bearings. Purge fluid flows outward through the pump seal to prevent any blood entry into the pumping mechanism. Axial blood flow is achieved by a rapidly turning the Archimedes screw turbine within the catheter. At speeds of up to 45,000 rpm, blood is withdrawn from the left ventricle and pumped into the descending aorta. The miniature cable-driven axial flow pump is passed across the aortic valve to provide transvalvular left ventricular assistance. The catheter, available initially in the 21F size, was subsequently miniaturized to 14F. Nonpulsatile flow rates of up 3.5–4.5 L/min can be achieved. Figure 11 is a diagram of the Hemopump catheter assembly. Figure 12 demonstrates the Hemopump catheter positioned in the left ventricle and the ascending aorta, the aortic arch, and descending aorta.

Smalling and colleagues investigated the use of the Hemopump in the canine infarct model and reported significant infarct salvage compared with reperfusion alone (112). In addition, the Hemopump appeared to provide superior systolic and diastolic unloading compared with intra-aortic counterpulsation. In another study, Smalling et al. reported on the use of the Hemopump in the clinical setting of cardiogenic shock associated with AMI (113). Hemodynamics, including pulmonary capillary wedge pressure, cardiac index, and dopamine requirements, improved significantly during the first 24 h of LV assistance. Four of 11 patients (36%) survived. This study demonstrated the feasibility of use of the Hemopump in patients with cardiogenic shock complicating AMI. The results supported the conclusion that LV unloading might decrease infarct expansion and improve LV function over the long term.

With promising pilot data, the device was further studied in clinical trials. Scholz et al., in a multicenter registry, reported on the clinical experience of the Hemopump utilized

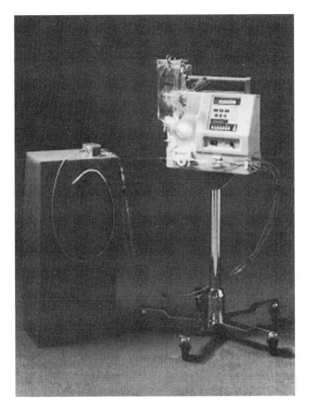

Fig. 10. Hemopump controller. (Reprinted with permission from Kluwer Academic Publishers: Supported complex and high risk coronary angioplasty. Shawl F, ed. 1991.)

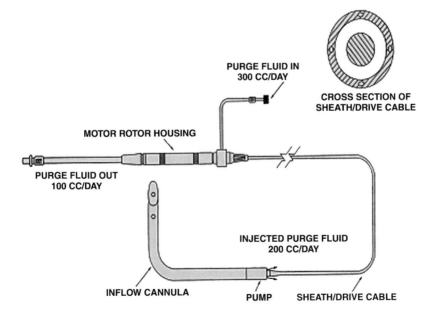

Fig. 11. Schematic of the Hemopump system. (Reprinted with permission from Kluwer Academic Publishers: Supported complex and high risk coronary angioplasty. Shawl F, ed. 1991.)

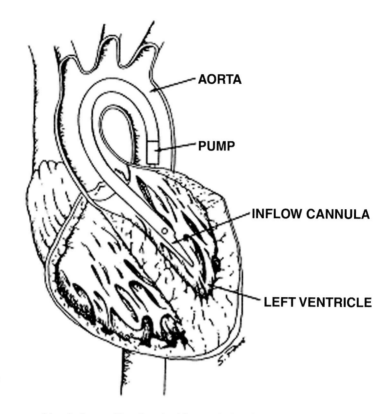

Fig. 12. Hemopump position in heart. (Reprinted with permission from Kluwer Academic Publishers: supported complex and high risk coronary angioplasty. Shawl F, ed. 1991.)

during high-risk PTCA *(114)*. The device on maximum pump speed resulted in a decrease in pulmonary artery wedge pressure from 15 ± 6 to 13 ± 6 mm Hg ($p < 0.001$). Cardiac index, mean aortic pressure, and systolic pressure did not change significantly during support. Plasma-free hemoglobin rose significantly from 4.9 ± 2.8 to 30.0 ± 21.7 mg/DL (normal range-0–10; $p < 0.001$). Serum haptoglobin did not change significantly immediately postassistance, but LDH rose significantly from 163 ± 35 to 301 ± 103 U/L ($p < 0.001$). The overall procedural mortality was 12.5% (4 of 32 patients). Two patients died of cardiogenic shock following reocclusion of the angioplasty vessel after removal of the Hemopump. One patient died after surgery for vascular repair of femoral artery occlusion and another patient died 3 d after PTCA complicated by periprocedural cardiovascular accident (CVA), which was attributed to pre-existing severe stenosis of the middle cerebral artery and prolonged cerebral hypoperfusion during the PTCA. There was no histologic evidence of atheromatous debris or thromboembolism secondary to the device. In a study from Belgium, 61 patients with postcardiotomy LV failure who failed IABP therapy were treated with the Hempump system *(115)*. In this study, one-third of patients improved, suggesting that this device might be beneficial in patients who require additional support beyond that of the IABP. Although this device does appear to provide hemodynamic support for many patients, significant procedure-related vascular access problems in reports may limit its use. Furthermore, hemolysis was a potential problem, particularly for long-term use. The Hemopump has not received FDA approval and further investigation is ongoing.

CARDIOPULMONARY SUPPORT (PERCUTANEOUS)

Counterpulsation with an IABP can help to achieve hemodynamic stability in patients with cardiogenic shock, but it is incapable of supporting a patient with complete hemodynamic collapse resulting from severe ventricular dysfunction. More complete cardiopulmonary support systems have been developed for patients with hemodynamic or potential hemodynamic collapse *(116)*. Figures 13 and 14 show the Bard percutaneous cardiopulmonary support (CPS) system. It utilizes an 18 French arterial cannula in the descending aorta and an 18 French venous cannula in the right atrium with these cannula connected to an external pump and membrane oxygenator to achieve full cardiopulmonary bypass *(117)*. Vogel et al. first reported on the use of CPS using this system in patients undergoing high-risk coronary angioplasty *(118)*. In this initial report, the cannulae were inserted via surgical cutdown on the femoral artery and femoral vein. Shawl et al. reported on the percutaneous insertion of these cannulae for patients undergoing high-risk and emergency percutaneous intervention *(119)*. In 1990, Vogel and colleagues published a report from 14 centers, all part of a national registry of elective CPS during coronary angioplasty *(120)*. Indications for this group of patients included an ejection fraction <25%, a target vessel supplying more than half of the myocardium, or both. During the period of the registry, technological improvements in the CPS system gradually allowed for percutaneous insertion and removal of the circulatory support cannulae, obviating the need for surgical cutdown for insertion of equipment. Although the angioplasty success rate was high (95%) in this group of very high-risk patients, morbidity was frequent (39%), and in most cases the result of cannulae insertion or removal. Hospital mortality was 7.6%, with half of these deaths occurring in patients with both age >75 yr and left main coronary artery stenosis. In patients without these two factors, the mortality rate was only 2.6%. Teirstein et al. reported on the use of "standby" versus "prophylactic" use of CPS in high-risk patients and found that in, most cases, high-risk angioplasty could be performed safely as long as emergency initiation of CPS was immediately available *(121)*.

Rapid institution of CPS allows for stabilization of patients who have cardiovascular collapse in the cardiac catheterization laboratory. Patients who have abrupt closure of a vessel can be supported until the situation is remedied either in the cardiac catheterization laboratory or in the operating room. CPS obviously does not provide myocardial blood flow beyond acutely obstructed arteries, but it allows for circulatory support until the situation can be remedied with successful percutaneous intervention. If the cause of cardiovascular collapse cannot be rapidly corrected in the catheterization laboratory, the patient can be transferred in a stable condition to the operating room for emergency surgery. Revascularization needs to be performed emergently, however, to enhance myocardial salvage, because CPS provides hemodynamic support but not distal perfusion. The duration of hemodynamic support is limited, as percutaneous CPS of more than 6 h duration leads to severe hematological and pulmonary complications *(122)*.

Initiation of CPS results in a predictable hemodynamic response *(122)*. After the pump is primed with approx 1.3 L of normosol, blood is withdrawn from the right atrium and pumped through a heat exchanger and then a membrane oxygenator and ultimately infused into the femoral artery. There is a fall in the right atrial, pulmonary arterial, pulmonary capillary wedge, and systemic arterial pressures. The pump provides continuous flow with maintenance of a pulsatile arterial pressure unless the circulation is being completely supported by the CPS system. Systemic anticoagulation with heparin is crucial and must be meticulously monitored to avoid thromboembolic and bleeding complications.

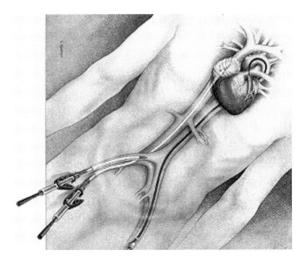

Fig. 13. Schematic representation of the appropriate position of the arterial and venous cannulae. Note placement of the tip of the venous cannula just above the junction of the inferior vena cava and right atrium. The arterial cannula is advanced until the hub is flush with the skin. Also note that the right femoral approach is shown in the diagram, whereas the left femoral approach is more commonly used in elective cases with PTCA performed from the contralateral side. (Reprinted with permission from Kluwer Academic Publishers: Supported complex and high risk coronary angioplasty. Shawl F, ed. 1991.)

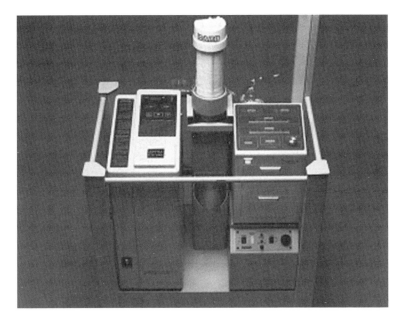

Fig. 14. Portable cardiopulmonary bypass support system. (Reprinted with permission from Kluwer Academic Publishers: Supported complex and high risk coronary angioplasty. Shawl F, ed. 1991.)

Although percutaneous CPS has been suggested for potential use in the setting of high-risk valvuloplasty, cardiogenic shock as a result of AMI, electrophysiologic testing producing hemodynamically compromising ventricular arrhythmias, hypothermia, prior to high-risk CABG, near drowning, drug overdose, and as a bridge to other mechanical assist devices or cardiac transplant, its primary use has been in the setting of abrupt vessel closure with hemodynamic collapse and refractory cardiac arrest in the

Table 5
Contraindications to the Institution of Percutaneous Cardiopulmonary Support

Severe peripheral atherosclerotic disease
History of recent cerebral vascular accident
Pre-existing coagulopathy
Active bleeding
Untreatable or terminal disease
Suspected traumatic closed head injury
Unwitnessed normothermic cardiac arrest
Refractory cardiac arrest of long duration
Severe aortic regurgitation

cardiac catheterization laboratory *(123,124)*. Contraindications to the use of CPS are listed in Table 5.

The percutaneous CPS system has been life-saving for a small percentage of patients treated in the cardiac catheterization laboratory who have experienced hemodynamic collapse, but it has not been extensively studied in other patient populations. Ultimately, its use has been limited by a relatively high morbidity rate associated with vascular access as well as by the limited duration of time that the device can be employed.

OTHER PERCUTANEOUS MECHANICAL ASSIST DEVICES

Research on other mechanical assist devices is progressing quickly. A-Med Systems, Inc. has introduced a percutaneous ventricular assist device, that is a newer iteration of the Hemopump. The FDA has not reviewed this device, but it is designed for rapid and easy placement of an intravascular micropump to provide temporary left ventricular and circulatory support. Trials are underway testing this device in patients with MI and cardiogenic shock. Percutaneous extracorporeal life support (ECLS) is another cardiac support technology that is being investigated. Veno-venous access and perfusion has been utilized for cardiopulmonary failure, especially in neonates and has had promising results *(125,126)*. Veno-arterial ECLS is being studied in adult patients with cardiac failure. Another device on the horizon is the Kantrowitz CardioVAD™, which requires surgical implantation currently but has recently shown some promise in Phase I trials *(127)*.

CONCLUSIONS

Mechanical cardiac assist devices have evolved rapidly over the last 40 yr. For patients with cardiogenic shock, the IABP remains the "standard" device and is likely to remain so because of its ease of placement, the rapidity with which therapy can be instituted, and the relatively low morbidity rates associated with it. However, although the IABP is excellent in providing hemodynamic and metabolic support, for many patients IABP support is not sufficient and other mechanical assist devices need to be considered. Furthermore, clinical outcomes remain somewhat poor with IABP therapy alone. In the past, patients who required more support than an IABP could provide were referred for surgical implantation of ventricular assist devices. However, today, exciting new devices such as the TandemHeart and the Hemopump are being investigated for their potential role in a variety of clinical scenarios. Although the initial data for these new devices are promising, it still remains to be proven whether they will improve long-term outcomes in patients. Cardiogenic shock remains an enormous health problem, and with improved technology and further research, mechanical cardiac assist devices will better allow us to treat patients effectively to lessen the devastating consequences associated with this condition.

REFERENCES

1. Kantrowitz A, Tjønneland S, Freed PS, et al. Initial clinical experience with intraaortic balloon pumping in cardiogenic shock. JAMA 1968;203:35–140.
2. Mehlhorn U, Kroner A, de Vivie ER. 30 Years clinical intra-aortic balloon pumping: facts and figures. Thorac Cardiovasc Surg. 1999;4:298–330.
3. Kantrowitz A, Kantrowitz A. Experimental augmentation of coronary flow by retardation of the arterial pressure pulse. Surgery 1953;34:678–687.
4. Harken DE. Counterpulsation: foundation and future, with tribute to William Clifford Birtwell (1916–1978). In Unger F, ed. Assisted circulation. New York: Springer-Verlag, 1979:20–23.
5. Claus RH, Birtwell WC, Albertal G, et al. Assisted circulation I: The arterial counterpulsator. J Thorac Cardiovasc Surg 1961;41:447–458.
6. Moulopoulos SD, Topaz SR, Kolff WJ. Extracorporeal assistance to the circulation and intraaortic balloon pumping. Trans Am Soc Artif Intern Organs 1962;8:85–89.
7. Claus RH, Missier P, Reed GE, Tice D. Assisted circulation by counter-pulsation with an intra-aortic balloon. Methods and effects. In: Digest, 15th annual conference on engineering in medicine and biology. Vol. 4. Chicago; IL: Northwestern University;1962:44.
8. Schilt W, Freed PS Khalil G, Kantrowitz A. Temporary non-surgical intraarterial cardiac assistance. Trans Am Soc Artif Intern Organs 1967;13:322–327.
9. Kantrowitz A, Tjønneland S, Freed PS, Phillips SJ, Butner AN, Sherman JL Jr. Initial clinical experience with intraaortic balloon pumping in cardiogenic shock. JAMA 1968;203:135–140.
10. Buckley MJ, Craven JM, Gold HK. IABP assist for cardiogenic shock after cardiopulmonary bypass. Circulation 1972;46 (Suppl):II76
11. Scheidt S, Wilner G, Mueller H, et al. Intraaortic balloon pumping in cardiogenic shock. Report of a cooperative clinical trial. N Engl J Med 1973;288:979–984.
12. Talpins NL, Kripke DC, Goetz RH. Counterpulsation and intraaortic balloon pumping in cardiogenic shock. Circ Dyna Arch Surg 1968;97:991–999.
13. Kantrowitz A, Krakauer J, Zorzi G, et al. Current status of intraaortic balloon pump and initial clinical experience with aortic patch mechanical auxiliary ventricle. Transplant Proc 1971;3:1459–1471.
14. Chatterjee S, Rosensweig J. Evaluation of intraaortic balloon counterpulsation. J Thorac Cardiovasc Surg 1971;61:405–410.
15. McDonald RH Jr, Taylor RR, Cingolani HE. Measurement of myocardial developed tension and its relation to oxygen consumption. Am J Physiol 1966;211:667–673.
16. Hedayat N, Sherwood JT, Schomisch SJ, Carino JL, Cmolik BL. Circulatory benefits of diastolic counterpulsation in an ischemic heart failure model after aortomyoplasty. J Thorac Cardiovasc Surg 2002;123(6):1067–1073.
17. Powell WJ Jr, Daggett WM, Margo AE, et al. Effects of intraaortic balloon counterpulsation on cardiac performance, oxygen consumption, and coronary blood flow in dogs. Circ Res 1970;26:753–764.
18. Shaw J, Taylor DR, Pitt B. Effects of intraaortic balloon counterpulsation on regional coronary blood flow in experimental myocardial infarction. Am J Cardiol 1974;34:552–556.
19. Kimura A, Toyota E, Songfang L, et al. Effects of intraaortic balloon pumping on the septal arterial blood flow velocity waveform during severe left main coronary artery stenosis. J Am Coll Cardiol 1996;27:810–816.
20. Bhayana JN, Scott SM, Sethi GK, Takaro T. Effects of intraaortic balloon pumping on organ perfusion in cardiogenic shock. J Surg Res 1979;26:108–113.
21. Mueller H, Ayres SM, Conklin EF, et al. The effects of intraaortic counterpulsation on cardiac performance and metabolism in shock associated with acute myocardial infarction. J Clin Invest 1971;50:1885–1900.
22. Wajszczuk WJ, Krakauer J, Rubenfire M, et al. Current indications for mechanical circulatory assistance on the basis of experience with 104 patients. Am J Cardiol 1974;33:176 (abstract).
23. Kantrowitz A. The physiologic basis of in-series cardiac assistance and the clinical application of intra-aortic devices. In: Davila JC, ed. 2nd Henry Ford Hospital international symposium on cardiac surgery. New York: Appleton-Century-Croft, 1977:640–643.

24. Willerson JT, Curry GC, Watson JT, et al. Intra-aortic balloon counterpulsation in patients with cardiogenic shock, medically refractory heart failure and/or recurrent ventricular tachycardia. Am J Med 1975;58:183–191.
25. DeWood MA, Notske RN, Hensley GR, et al. Intra-aortic balloon counterpulsation with and without reperfusion for myocardial infarction shock. Circulation 1980;61:1105–1112.
26. Torchiana DF, Hirsch G, Buckley MJ, et al. Intraaortic balloon pumping for cardiac support: trends in practice outcome, 1968–1995. J Thorac Cardiovasc Surg 1997;113:758–769.
27. Kovack PJ, Rasak MA, Bates ER, et al. Thrombolysis plus aortic counterpulsation: improved survival in patients who present to community hospitals with cardiogenic shock. J Am Coll Cardiol 1997;29(7): 1454–1458.
28. Sanborn TA, Sleeper LA, Bates ER, et al. Impact of thrombolysis, intraaortic balloon pump counterpulsation, and their combination in cardiogenic shock complicating acute myocardial infarction: a report from the SHOCK Trial Registry. J Am Coll Cardiol 2000;36(3 Suppl A):1123–1129.
29. Flaherty JT, Becker LC, Weiss JL, et al. Results of a randomized prospective trial of intra-aortic balloon counterpulsation and intravenous nitroglycerin in patients with acute myocardial infarction. J Am Coll Cardiol 1985;6:434–436.
30. Dekker AL, Reesink KD, van der Veen FH, et al. Intra-aortic balloon pumping in acute mitral regurgitation reduces aortic impedance and regurgitant fraction. Shock 2003;19(4):334–338.
31. Bouchart F, Bessou JP, Tabley A, et al. Urgent surgical repair of postinfarction ventricular septal rupture: early and late outcomes. J Cardiac Surg 1998;13(2):104–112.
32. Hagemeijer F, Larid JD, Haalebos MMP, Hugenholtz PG. Effectiveness of intra-aortic balloon pumping without cardiac surgery for patients with severe heart failure secondary to a recent myocardial infarction. Am J Cardiol 1977;40:951–956.
33. Moulopoulos S, Stametelopoulos S, Petrou P. Intraaortic balloon assistance in intractable cardiogenic shock. Eur Heart J 1986;7:396–403.
34. Christenson JT, Simonet F, and Schmuziger M. The effect of preoperative intra-aortic balloon pump support in high risk patients requiring myocardial revascularization. J Cardiovasc Surg 1997;38: 397–402.
35. Christenson JT, Simonet F, Badel P, Schmuziger M. Optimal timing of preoperative intraaortic balloon pump support in high-risk coronary patients. Ann Thorac Surg 1999;68:934–939.
36. Gutfinger DE, Ott RA, Miller M, et al. Aggressive preoperative use of intraaortic balloon pump in elderly patients undergoing coronary artery bypass grafting. Ann Thorac Surg 1999;67:610–613.
37. Oldham, HN Jr, Roe CR, Young WG, et al. Intraoperative detection of myocardial damage during coronary artery surgery by plasma creatine phosphokinase isoenzyme analysis. Surgery 1973;74:917–925.
38. Rao V, Ivanov J, Weisel R, et al. Predictors of low cardiac output syndrome after coronary artery bypass. J Thorac Cardiovasc Surg 1996;112:38–51.
39. The Warm Heart Investigators. Normothermic versus hypothermic cardiac surgery: a randomized trial of 1732 coronary bypass patients. Lancet 1994;343:559–563.
40. McGee NG, Zillgitt SL, Trono R, et al. Retrospective analyses of the need for mechanical circulatory support (intraaortic balloon pump/abdominal left ventricular assist device or partial artificial heart) after cardiopulmonary bypass. A 44 month study of 14,168 patients. Am J Cardiol 1980;46:135–142.
41. Norman JC, Cooley DA, Igo SR, et al. Prognostic indices for survival during postcardiotomy intra-aortic balloon pumping. Methods of scoring and classification, with implications for left ventricular assist device utilization. J Thorac Cardiovasc Surg 1977;74:709–720.
42. Lund O, Johansen G, Allermand H, et al. Intraaortic balloon pumping in the treatment of low cardiac output following open heart surgery—immediate results and long-term prognosis. Thorac Cardiovasc Surg 1988;36:332–337.
43. Campbell CD, Tolitano DJ, Weber KT, et al. Mechanical support for postcardiotomy heart failure. J Cardiac Surg 1988;3:181–191.
44. Kurki TS, Kataja M. Preoperative prediction of postoperative morbidity in coronary artery bypass grafting. Ann Thorac Surg 1996;61:1740–1745.
45. Royster RL. Myocardial dysfunction following cardiopulmonary bypass: recovery patterns, predictors of inotropic need, theoretical concepts of inotropic administration. J Cardiothorac Vasc Anesth 1993;7:19–25.
46. Charlson M, Krieger KH, Peterson JC, Hayes J, Isom OW. Predictors and outcomes of cardiac complications following elective coronary bypass grafting. Proc Assoc Am Physicians 1999:111(6):622–632.
47. Najafi H, Henson D, Dye WS, et al. Left ventricular hemorrhagic necrosis. Ann Thorac Surg 1969;7: 550–561.

48. Hedenmark J, Ahn H, Henze A, et al. Intra-aortic balloon counterpulsation with special reference to determinants of survival. Scand J Thorac Cardiovasc Surg 1989;23;57–62.
49. Bolooki H, William W, Thurer RJ, et al. Clinical and hemodynamic criteria for use of intraaortic balloon pump in patients requiring cardiac surgery. J. Thorac Cardiovasc Surg 1976;72:756–758.
50. Hausmann H, Potapov EV, Koster, et al. Prognosis after the implantation of an intra-aortic balloon pump in cardiac surgery calculated with a new score. Circulation 2002:106(12 Suppl 1):I203–I206.
51. Kuchar DL, Campbell TJ, O'Rourke MF. Long-term survival after counterpulsation for medically refractory heart failure complicating myocardial infarction and cardiac surgery. Eur Heart J 1987;8: 490–502.
52. Kottke TE, Pesch DG, Frye RL. The potential contribution of cardiac replacement to the control of cardiovascular disease: a population based estimate. Arch Surg 1990;125:1148–1151.
53. Hosenpud JD, Bennett LE, Keck BM, et al. The Registry of the International Society for Heart and Lung Transplantation: Fourteenth official report—1997. J Heart Lung Transplant 1997;16:691–712.
54. Carrier M, White M, Pelletier G, et al. Ten-year follow-up of critically ill patients undergoing heart transplantation. J Heart Lung Transplant 2000;19:439–443.
55. Marks JD, Karwande SV, Richenbacher WE, et al. Perioperative mechanical circulatory support for transplantation. J Heart Lung Transplant 1992;11:117–128.
56. Kaye MP. The registry of the International Society for Heart Transplantation: fourth official report—1987. J Heart Transplant 1987;6:64–67.
57. Hardesty RL, Griffith BP, Trento A, et al. Mortally ill patients and excellent survival following cardiac transplantation. Ann Thorac Surg 1986;41:126–129.
58. O'Connell JB, Renlunnd DG, Robinson JA, et al. Effect of preoperative hemodynamic support on survival after cardiac transplantation. Circulation 1988;78(Suppl III):78–82.
59. Kavarana MN, Sinha P, Naka Y, Oz MC, Edwards NM. Mechanical support for the failing cardiac allograft: a single-center experience. J Heart Lung Transplant 2003:22(5):542–547.
60. Rosenbaum AM, Murali S, Uretsky BF. Intra-aortic balloon counterpulsation as a "bridge" to cardiac transplantation. Effects in nonischemic and ischemic cardiomyopathy. Chest 1994;106:1683–1688.
61. Birovljev S, Radovancevic B, Burnett CM, et al. Heart transplantation after mechanical circulatory support: Four years' experience. J Heart Lung Transplant 1992;11:240–245.
62. Carrier M, White M, Pelletier G, et al. Ten-year follow-up of critically ill patients undergoing heart transplantation. J Heart Lung Transplant 2000;19:439–443.
63. Minich LL, Tani LY, Hawkins JA, Orsmond GS, Di Russo GB, Shaddy RE. Intra-aortic balloon pumping in children with dilated cardiomyopathy as a bridge to transplantation. J Heart Lung Transplant 2001:20(7):750–754.
64. Schmid C, Welp H, Klotz S, et al. Left ventricular assist stand-by for high-risk cardiac surgery. Thorac Cardiovasc Surg 2002:50(6):342–346.
65. Cohen M, Dawson MS, Kopistansky C, McBride R. Sex and other predictors of intra-aortic balloon counterpulsation-related complications: prospective study of 1119 consecutive patients. Am Heart J 2000;139:282–287.
66. Cook L, Pillar B, McCord G, Josephson R. Intra-aortic balloon pump complications: a five-year retrospective study of 283 patients. Heart Lung 1999;28:195–202.
67. Scholz KH, Ragab S, von zur Muhlen F, et al. Complication of intra-aortic balloon counterpulsation. The role of catheter size and duration of support in a multivariate analysis of risk. Eur Heart J 1998;19:458–465.
68. Kantrowitz A, Wasfie T, Freed PS, et al. Intraaortic balloon pumping 1967 through 1982: analysis of complications in 733 patients. Am J Cardiol 1986;57:976–983.
69. Gottlieb SO, Brinker JA, Borkon AM, et al. Identification of patients at high risk for complications of intraaortic balloon counterpulsation: a multivariate risk factor analysis. Am J Cardiol 1984;53:1135–1139.
70. Lefemine AA, Kosowsky B, Madoff I, et al. Results and complications of intraaortic balloon pumping in surgical and medical patients. Am J Cardiol 1977;40:416–420.
71. Arafa OE, Pedersen TH, Svennevig JL, et al. Vascular complications of the intraaortic balloon pump in patients undergoing open heart operations: 15-year experience. Ann Thorac Surg 1999;67:645–651.
72. Arafa OE, Pedersen TH, Svennevig JL, et al. Vascular complications of the intraaortic balloon pump in patients undergoing open heart operations: 15-year experience. Ann Thorac Surg 1999;67:645–651.
73. Wasfie T, Freed PS, Rubenfire M, et al. Risk associated with intraaortic balloon pumping in patients with and without diabetes mellitus. Am J Cardiol 1988;61:558–562.
74. Miller JS, Dodson TF, Salam AA, Smith RB 3rd. Vascular complications following intra-aortic balloon pump insertion. Am Surg 1992;58:232–238.
75. Curtis JJ, Bolan M, Bliss D, et al. Intra-aortic balloon cardiac assist: complication rates for the surgical and percutaneous insertion techniques. Am Surg 1988;54:142–147.

76. Goldberg MG, Rubenfire M, Kantrowitz A, et al. Intraaortic balloon pump insertion: A randomized study comparing percutaneous and surgical techniques. J Am Coll Cardiol 1987;9:515–523.

77. Pelletier LC, Pomar JL, Bosch X, et al. Complications of circulatory assistance with intra-aortic balloon pumping: A comparison of surgical and percutaneous techniques. J Heart Transplant 1986;5:138–142.

78. Sirbu H, Busch T, Aleksic I, et al. Ischaemic complications with intraaortic balloon counter-pulsation: Incidence and management. Cardiovasc Surg 2000;8:66–71.

79. McEnany MT, KayHR, Buckley MJ, et al. Clinical experience with intraaortic balloon pump support in 728 patients. Circulation 1978;58(Suppl I):124–132.

80. Beckman CB, Geha AS, Hammond GL, Baue AE. Results and complications of intraaortic balloon counterpulsation. Ann Thorac Surg 1977;24:550–559.

81. Seifert PE, Silverman NA. Late paraplegia resulting from intra-aortic balloon pump. [letter]. Ann Thorac Surg 1986;41:700.

82. Jamolowski CR, Poirier RL. Small bowel infarction complicating intra-aortic balloon counterpulsation via the ascending aorta. J Thorac Cardiovasc Surg 1980;79:735–737.

83. Tomatis L, Nemiroff M, Riahi M, et al. Massive air embolism due to rupture of pulsatile assist device: successful treatment in the hyperbaric chamber. Ann Thorac Surg 1981;32:604–608.

84. Haykal HA, Wang AM. CT diagnosis of delayed cerebral air embolism following intraaortic balloon pump catheter insertion. Comput Radiol 1986;10:307–309.

85. Shin H, Yozu R, Sumida T, Kawada S. Acute ischemic hepatic failure resulting from intraaortic balloon pump malposition. Eur J Cardiothorac Surg 2000;17:492–494.

86. Lewis BE, Sumida C, Hwang MH, Loeb HS. New approach to management of intraaortic balloon pumps in patients with peripheral vascular disease: case reports of four patients requiring urgent IABP insertion. Cathet Cardiovasc Diagn 1992;26:295–299.

87. Coyler WR Jr, Moore JA, Buket MW, Cooper CJ. Intraaortic balloon pump insertion after percutaneous revascularization in patients with severe peripheral vascular disease. Cathet Cardiovasc Diagn 1997;42:1–6.

88. Grines CL, Browne KF, Marco J, et al. A comparison of immediate angioplasty with thrombolytic therapy for acute myocardial infarction. N Engl J Med 1993;328:673–679.

89. Christian TF, Schwartz RS, Gibbons RJ. Determinants of infarct size in reperfusion therapy for acute myocardial infarction. Circulation 1992;86:81–90.

90. Miller TD, Christian TF, Hopfenspirger MR, et al. Infarct size after acute myocardial infarction measured by quantitative tomographic ^{99m}Tc sestamibi imaging predicts subsequent mortality. Circulation 1995;92:334–341.

91. Kloner RA, Ganote CE, Jennings RB. The "no-reflow" phenomenon after temporary occlusion in the dog. J Clin Invest 1974;54:1496–1508.

92. Lincoff AM, Topol EJ. "Illusion of reperfusion": does anyone achieve optimal reperfusion during acute myocardial infarction? Circulation 1993;88:1361–1374.

93. Roe MT, Ohman EM, Maas AC, et al. Shifting the open-artery hypothesis downstream: the quest for optimal reperfusion. J Am Coll Cardiol 2001;37:9–18.

94. Lincoff AM, Popma JJ, Ellis SG, et al. Percutaneous support devices for high risk or complicated coronary angioplasty. J Am Coll Cardiol 1991;17:770–780.

95. Vogel JH, Ruiz CE, Jahnke EJ, et al. Percutaneous (nonsurgical) supported angioplasty in unprotected left main disease and severe left ventricular dysfunction. Clin Cardiol 1989;12:297–300.

96. Stone GW, Marsalese D, Brodie BR, et al. A prospective, randomized evaluation of prophylactic intraaortic balloon counterpulsation in high risk patients with acute myocardial infarction treated with primary angioplasty. Second Primary Angioplasty in Myocardial Infarction (PAMI-II) Trial Investigators. J Am Coll Cardiol 1997;29:1459–1467.

97. Catinella FP, Cunningham JN, Glassman E, et al. Left atrium-to-femoral artery bypass: effectiveness in reduction of acute experimental myocardial infarction. J Thorac Cardiovasc Surg 1983;86: 887–896.

98. Grossi EA, Krieger KH, Cunningham JN, et al. Time course of effective interventional left heart assist for limitation of evolving myocardial infarction. J Thorac Cardiovasc Surg 1986;91:624–629.

99. Laschinger JC, Grossi EA, Cunningham JN, et al. Adjunctive left ventricular unloading during myocardial reperfusion plays a major role in minimizing myocardial infarct size. J Thorac Cardiovasc Surg 1985;90:80–85.

100. Frazier OH, Rose EA, Macmanus Q, et al. Multicenter clinical evaluation of the HeartMate 1000 IP left ventricular assist device. Ann Thorac Surg 1992;53:1080–1090.

101. Vetter HO, Kaulbach HG, Schmitz C, et al. Experience with the Novacor left ventricular assist system as a bridge to cardiac transplantation, including the new wearable system. J Thorac Cardiovasc Surg 1995;109:74–80.

102. Farrar DJ, Hill JD. Univentricular and biventricular Thoratec VAD support as a bridge to transplantation. Ann Thorac Surg 1993;55:276–282.

103. Marelli D, Laks H, Amsel B, et al. Temporary mechanical support with the BVS 5000 assist device during treatment of acute myocarditis. J Cardiac Surg 1997;12:55–59.

104. Salisbury PF. Comparison of two types of mechanical assistance in experimental heart failure. Circ Res 1960;8:431.

105. Dennis C. Left atrial cannulation without thoractomy for total left heart bypass. Acta Chir Scand 1962;123:267–279.

106. Glassman E, Engelman RM, Boyd AD, et al. A method of closed-chest cannulation of the left atrium for left atrial-femoral artery bypass. J Thorac Cardiovasc Surg 1975;69:283–290.

107. Pavie A, Leger P, Nzomvuama A, et al. Left centrifugal pump cardiac assist with transseptal percutaneous left atrial cannula. Artif Organs 1998;22:502–507.

108. CardiacAssist, Inc. Phase I study—internal industry data. Pittsburgh, PA: CardiacAssist, Inc.

109. Thiele H, Lauer B, Hambrecht R, Boudriot E, Cohen HA, Schuler G. Reversal of cardiogenic shock by percutaneous left atrial-to-femoral arterial bypass assistance. Circulation 2001:104:2917–2922.

110. Lemos PA, Cummins P, Lee C, et al. Usefulness of percutaneous left ventricular assistance to support high-risk percutaneous coronary interventions. Am J Cardiol 2003;91:479–491.

111. Wampler RJ, Moise JC, Frazier OH, et al. In vivo evaluation of a peripheral vascular access axial flow blood pump. Trans ASAIO 1988;34:450–455.

112. Smalling RW, Cassidy DB, Barrett R, et al. Improved regional myocardial blood flow, left ventricular unloading, and infarct salvage using an axial-flow, transvalvular left ventricular assist device. A comparison with intraaortic balloon counterpulsation and reperfusion alone in a canine infarction model. Circulation 1992;85:1152–1159.

113. Smalling RW, Sweeney M, Lachterman B, et al. Transvalvular left ventricular assistance in cardiogenic shock secondary to acute myocardial infarction—evidence for recovery from near fatal myocardial stunning. J Am Coll Cardiol 1994;23:637–644.

114. Scholz KH, Figulla HR, Schweda F, et al. Mechanical left ventricular unloading during high risk coronary angioplasty—first use of a new percutaneous left ventricular assist device. Cathet Cardiovasc Diagn 1994;31:61–65.

115. Meyns B, Sergeant P, Wouters P, et al. Mechanical support with microaxial blood pumps for postcardiotomy left ventricular failure: can outcome be predicted. J Thorac Cardiovasc Surg 2000;120(2):393–400.

116. Figulla HR. Circulatory support devices in clinical cardiology. Cardiology 1994;84:149–155.

117. Shawl F. Percutaneous cardiopulmonary bypass support: technique, indications and complications. In: Shawl FA, ed. Supported complex and high risk coronary angioplasty. Boston: Kluwer Academic, 1991:65–100.

118. Vogel RA, Tommaso CL, Gundry SR. Initial experience with coronary angioplasty and aortic valvuloplasty using elective semi-percutaneous cardiopulmonary support. Am J Cardiol 1988;62:811–813.

119. Shawl FA, Domanski MJ, Punja S. Percutaneous cardiopulmonary bypass support in high risk patients undergoing percutaneous transluminal coronary angioplasty. Am J Cardiol 1989;64:1258–1263.

120. Vogel RA, Shawl FA, Tommaso CL, et al. Initial report of the National Registry of Elective Cardiopulmonary Bypass Supported Coronary Angioplasty. J Am Coll Cardiol 1990;15:23–29.

121. Teirstein PS, Vogel RA, Dorros G, et al. Prophylactic versus standby cardiopulmonary support for high risk percutaneous transluminal coronary angioplasty. J Am Coll Cardiol 1993;21:590–596.

122. Ronan JA, Shawl FA. Echocardiographic and hemodynamic changes during percutaneous cardiopulmonary bypass. In: Shawl FA, ed. Supported complex and high risk coronary angioplasty. Boston: Kluwer Academic, 1991:57–63.

123. Shawl FA, Domanski MJ, Hernandez TJ, et al. Emergency percutaneous cardiopulmonary bypass with cardiogenic shock from acute myocardial infarction. Am J Cardiol 1989;64:967–970.

124. Shawl FA, Domanski MJ, Wish MH, et al. Emergency cardiopulmonary bypass support in patients with cardiac arrest in the catheterization laboratory. Cathet Cardiovasc Diagn 1990;19:8–12.

125. Reickert CA, Schreiner RJ, Bartlett RH, Hirschl RB. Percutaneous access for venovenous extracorporeal life support in neonates. J Pediatr Surg 1998:33(2):365–369.

126. Pranikoff T, Hirschl RB, Remenapp R, Swaniker F, Bartlett RH. Venovenous extracorporeal life support via percutaneous cannulation in 94 patients. Ches 1999;115(3):818–822.

127. Jeevanandam V, Jayakar D, Anderson AS, et al. Circulatory assistance with a permanent implantable IABP: initial human experience. Circulation 2002:106(12 Suppl 1):I183–I188.

15

Alcohol Septal Ablation for Hypertrophic Obstructive Cardiomyopathy

Haran Burri, MD and Ulrich Sigwart, MD

CONTENTS

INTRODUCTION

About 25% of patients with hypertrophic cardiomyopathy (HCM) have left ventricular outflow obstruction under resting conditions *(1,2)*. Medical therapy with negative inotropic drugs might alleviate symptoms in many of these patients; however, a certain number might remain refractory to drug therapy. This subset of patients could represent 5–10% of the total population with this disease *(3)*. Surgical myectomy has been shown to reduce outflow gradients and has been practiced since the 1960s. However, some patients might not be regarded as favorable candidates for this major intervention because of advanced age, concomitant medical conditions, or previous cardiac surgery *(4)*. In 1994, a catheter treatment (known as a variety of terms listed in Table 1) using absolute alcohol to induce a myocardial infarction localized to the interventricular septum has been introduced as an alternative to surgery. An alcohol-induced septal branch ablation procedure was first described as therapy for ventricular tachycardia *(5)*. This technique was applied to HCM after noting clinical improvement in a patient with septal hypertrophy who suffered an anterior myocardial infarction, as well as the transient reduction in left ventricular outflow pressure gradients observed with temporary septal artery balloon occlusion. Since the first series of three patients reported in 1995 *(6)*, there has been growing enthusiasm in this technique. During the first 5 yr, over 800 cases had been performed *(7)*; the number is probably several thousand now. Although initially confined to Europe and North America, this technique is now being practiced worldwide.

From: *Contemporary Cardiology: Interventional Cardiology:
Percutaneous Noncoronary Intervention*
Edited by: H. C. Herrmann © Humana Press Inc., Totowa, NJ

259

Table 1
Acronyms for Percutaneous Transluminal Septal Myocardial Ablation

Percutaneous transluminal septal myocardial ablation (PTSMA)
Transcoronary ablation of septal hypertrophy (TASH)
Transcoronary alcohol ablation (TAA)
Alcohol septal reduction (ASR)
Nonsurgical septal reduction therapy (NSRT)
Nonsurgical myocardial reduction (NSMR)

PATIENT SELECTION

In addition to stable patients, those at high risk of surgical morbidity and mortality (including patients of advanced age or with comorbidities such as pulmonary or renal disease) can be evaluated for alcohol ablation. The following criteria can be used to select candidates:

- Patients in NYHA or CCS Class III or IV despite drug therapy with a resting gradient of >30 mm Hg or >60 mm Hg under stress (8)
- Patients in NYHA or CCS Class II with a resting gradient of >50 mm Hg or >30 mm Hg at rest and ≥100 mm Hg under stress (9)
- Patients who are symptomatic after having to discontinue medication because of side effects
- Previous but hemodynamically unsuccessful surgical myectomy or pacemaker therapy

Septal wall thickness should be ≥18 mm, and the anatomy of the septal perforator branches should be adequate.

It has been a subject of debate whether patients with gradients that are present only by provocation benefit from alcohol ablation. A report compared patients in NYHA Class III and IV with gradients of >30 mm Hg at rest to those who whose gradient was only present after an extrasystolic beat; it found that the hemodynamic and functional benefit was similar in both groups (10).

Little experience with alcohol ablation has been reported so far in patients with midventricular obstruction, although this is technically feasible.

Surgical myectomy is preferable to ablation in patients with concomitant cardiac conditions requiring surgery such as extensive coronary artery disease or valvular disease and morphological changes of the mitral valve and papillary muscles responsible for gradient formation or mitral regurgitation.

MECHANISMS OF TREATMENT EFFICACY

Alcohol ablation induces a well-demarcated subaortic necrosis, corresponding to approximatively 10% of the left ventricle by PET and SPECT imaging (11–13). Despite the creation of a septal infarct, new Q-waves in the septal leads are rarely seen (14).

The left ventricular outflow tract (LVOT) gradient usually falls immediately after alcohol ablation, with a further fall in the gradient over the following months (Fig. 1). The mechanisms of acute reductions in gradients have been studied by echocardiography. First, alcohol ablation induces a decrease in septal contraction, thus reducing subaortic narrowing in systole (15–17). Second, there appear to be global changes in left ventricular ejection, with a slower acceleration and a later peak ejection velocity (15). This may be

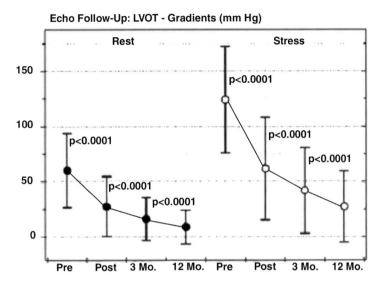

Fig. 1. Acute effect of alcohol septal ablation with evolution of outflow gradient over time. (Reproduced, with permission, from ref. *9*.)

due to a reduced septal contribution to left ventricular ejection. Alternatively, changes in electromechanical activation secondary to right bundle-branch block or left anterior hemiblock might induce inhomogeneous left ventricular contraction.

The long-term relief in outflow obstruction is probably linked to LVOT remodeling with widening resulting from infarction necrosis and myocardial scar formation *(15,16)*. Furthermore, there appear to be geometrical changes in the left ventricle, resulting in a more parallel angle between ejection flow and the mitral valve, with less drag forces that lead to systolic anterior motion *(15)*.

In addition to relief of LVOT obstruction, changes in diastolic function also seem to improve long-term hemodynamics resulting from alcohol ablation. This may be due to more favorable relaxation *(18–20)* as well as a reduction in left ventricular stiffness secondary to regression of hypertrophy *(21–23)* and a decrease in interstitial collagen *(22)*.

Outflow obstruction relief results in higher aortic diastolic pressure along with a lower left ventricular end-diastolic pressure. This serves to increase coronary flow, thus decreasing ischemia, which might participate in the patients' symptoms *(18)*. Finally, reductions in the severity of mitral regurgitation might contribute to clinical improvement *(24)*.

TECHNIQUE

Measurement of Outflow Gradient

A 5F pigtail catheter with side holes situated close to the tip introduced retrogradely in the left ventricle (placed so as to avoid entrapment) can be used to measure the prestenotic pressure. Many operators prefer this approach to the technique described initially whereby a Brockenbrough catheter is placed in the left ventricular inflow tract after a transseptal puncture *(6)*. The poststenotic pressure is measured via a 7F guiding catheter (e.g., Judkins L4, Cordis) placed in the ascending aorta. After having excluded a valvular gradient, the peak-to-peak intraventricular gradient should be measured at rest, during isoproterenol infusion, and after extrasystoles (Fig. 2). A temporary pacing wire should be placed in the

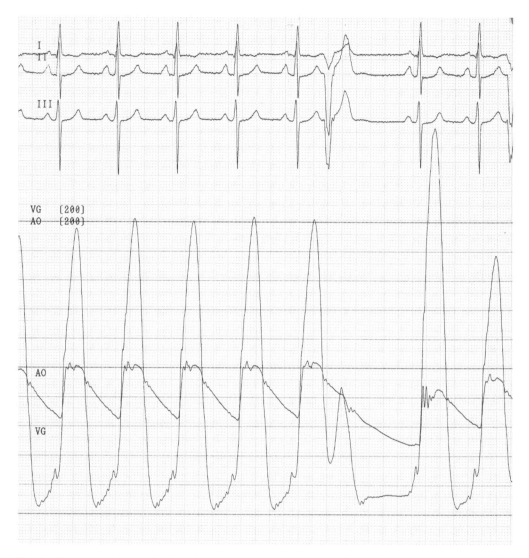

Fig. 2. Hemodynamic monitoring showing a resting peak-to-peak gradient of 100 mm Hg, with a postextrasystolic gradient of about 170 mm Hg.

right ventricle to ensure backup pacing in the advent of AV block. The pacing wire can also serve to measure the postextrasystolic gradient by programmed stimulation (with coupling intervals of about 370 ms) if extrasystoles are not observed spontaneously.

Positioning and Testing of the Balloon Catheter

A left coronary angiogram is performed (Fig. 3A and Video 1 on accompanying CD). Milking of the septal perforators supplying the hypertrophied segments is often observed. Positioning the guide wire in the septal branch can sometimes be difficult because of a steep take-off angle (see Video 2 on accompanying CD). Preshaping the guide wire through a needle with two angles as shown in Fig. 3 (rather than a curve) might be of help. The septal branch should be of ≥1.5 mm in diameter. The balloon catheter is then placed in the proximal segment of the first septal perforator over a 0.014-in. guide wire after

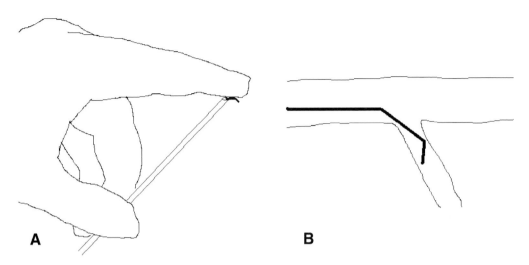

Fig. 3. (A) Preshaping the 0.014-in. guide wire with two angles through a blunt needle. **(B)** Positioning of the guide wire in a septal branch.

intravenous administration of heparin (see Video 3 on accompanying CD). The balloon should be slightly oversized (usually 1.5–3 mm), and adapted to the dimension of the vessel (a 10 × 2-mm balloon is suitable for most cases). In case of proximal branching of the septal perforator, a short balloon (e.g., 5 mm) can be used. The balloon should be inflated with a pressure of 4–6 atm and correct positioning verified by injecting contrast agent into the left coronary artery (Fig. 4B), and then distally via the lumen of the balloon catheter using about 1 cm^3 of contrast dye (Fig. 4C and Video 4 on accompanying CD). Absence of retrograde leakage and stability of balloon position (especially with shorter balloons) should be verified attentively. Furthermore, the extent of myocardium supplied by the septal branch and shunting of flow to nontargeted regions can also be analyzed, ideally using two different projections. The injection of a contrast agent also serves to accentuate ischemia to the territory of the septal branch. The outflow gradient should be monitored continuously to check for a drop in the resting gradient by >30 mm Hg or the postextrasystolic gradient by >50 mm Hg within 5 min of balloon occlusion. If these criteria are not met [as is the case in about 20% of patients *(21)*], the balloon catheter can be positioned in another septal branch. Occasionally, the culprit vessel might originate from an intermediate or diagonal branch *(25)*.

Myocardial Contrast Echocardiography

Myocardial contrast echocardiography has proved to be extremely useful for targeting the culprit septal branch, increasing success rates despite a reduced infarct size, which, in turn, avoids complications *(13,25,26)*. Before injecting alcohol, 1–2 mL of echo contrast (e.g., Sonovue®, Levovist®, Optison®, Albunex®, etc.) is injected via the inflated balloon catheter under transthoracic echography in the apical four- and five-chamber views. This serves to verify whether the opacified myocardium is adjacent to the region of maximal flow acceleration and to withhold alcohol injection in case of a mismatch, such as when the right side of the interventricular septum is opacified *(27)*. Furthermore, this technique also helps in delineating the infarct zone and to rule out retrograde leakage or involvement of myocardium distant from the expected target region *(28)* such as the

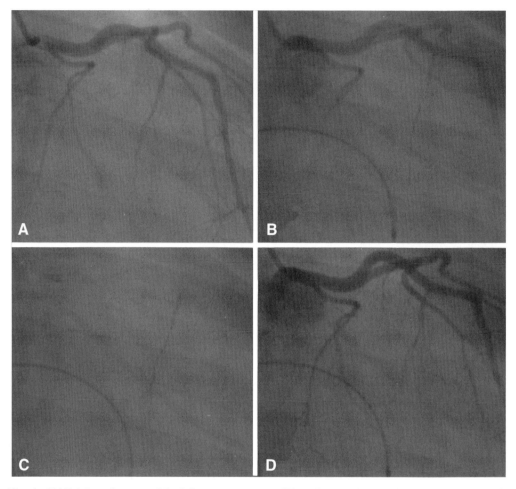

Fig. 4. **(A)** RAO angiogram of the left coronary artery. **(B)** Balloon catheter inflated and positioned in the first septal branch over a 0.014-in. guide wire. **(C)** Contrast dye is injected via the balloon catheter to confirm the absence of retrograde leakage. **(D)** Angiogram after alcohol injection. Note that the first septal branch is patent.

ventricular free wall *(13,26)* or papillary muscles *(26,29)*. Transcapillary passage of echo contrast into the ventricles is usually observed during the injection. If echo contrast is not available, echocardiography may also be performed during regular contrast dye injection in the septal perforator via the occluded balloon catheter.

Alcohol Injection

Once the septal perforator is considered suitable, 0.7–3 mL of 96% alcohol may be slowly injected through the inflated balloon catheter. The electrocardiogram should be monitored closely and the injection aborted upon the development of atrioventricular block. There has been a tendency over the last years to reduce the amount of alcohol injected to a maximum of 2 cm^3 *(11,21)*, which might help reduce complications. The balloon should be left inflated for 5 min. Chest pain may be relieved by administering analgesics. Left coronary angiography should be repeated after balloon deflation in order to confirm patency of the left anterior descending artery (Fig. 4D). The target septal vessel

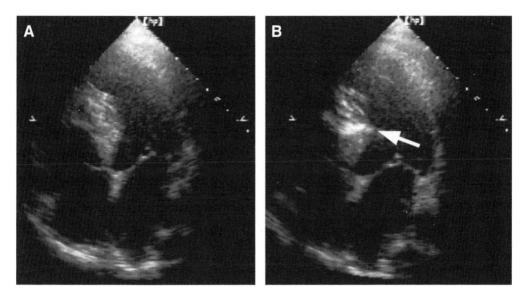

Fig. 5. (A) Apical four-chamber echocardiogram showing the hypertrophied septum. **(B)** After alcohol injection, the area of necrosis becomes echodense (arrow).

might not necessarily be occluded, although flow is usually slowed down. Injection of alcohol results in a significant contrast effect that is easily visible by echocardiography (Fig. 5 and Video 5 on accompanying CD).

If the residual gradient after alcohol injection is >30 mm Hg at rest, the balloon can be positioned more proximally, or a shorter balloon used if branches of the septal perforator were occluded by the balloon during the first injection. Alternatively, a second septal perforator might be targeted using the same procedure as for the first branch. Most patients will only require one target perforator branch, especially since the advent of myocardial contrast echocardiography. A residual gradient of <30 mm Hg is acceptable, as it has been shown that a further decrease in outflow gradient might be observed over the following months because of ventricular remodeling *(26,30)* (Fig. 1) in about 50% of patients *(31)*.

Postprocedural Management

Vascular sheaths may be removed after normalization of coagulation parameters and then heparin resumed to prevent intracavitary thrombus formation at the site of ablation. Creatinine kinase (CK) levels should be dosed every 4 h. Peak rises are usually observed in the range of 750–1500 U/L. Patients should be observed in the coronary care unit for 48 h, with removal of the temporary pacing wire at the end of this period in the absence of atrioventricular block. The patient can then be transferred to a telemetry unit for the remainder of the hospital stay.

TREATMENT EFFICACY

There is growing evidence to indicate that alcohol ablation is comparable to surgical myectomy with respect to hemodynamic and functional improvement *(20,32–34)*, although no randomized comparative studies exist to date. Gradient reduction can be achieved acutely in about 90% of patients *(24,25,35,36)*. In a series of 241 patients, acute reductions in mean rest gradients from 72 to 20 mm Hg and mean postextrasystolic gradients from 148 to 62 mm Hg were achieved *(37)*.

Although very long-term follow-up data are still lacking, reports indicate maintenance of clinical and hemodynamic benefits for at least a year *(21,24,35,38,39)*. In a series of 178 patients observed for 2–5 yr *(39)*, gradients at baseline compared to last follow-up were 60 ± 35 mm Hg versus 7 ± 14 mm Hg ($p < 0.001$) at rest and 127 ± 50 mm Hg versus 20 ± 28 mm Hg ($p < 0.001$) with Valsalva. The outflow gradient might even decrease over time *(25,26,30,31)*, indicating a remodeling process (Fig. 1). Functional class, exercise capacity, and quality of life are also significantly improved over follow-up *(24,30,35,39–41)*.

Redo procedures may sometimes be required due to recurring gradient and symptoms despite initial success, as was necessary in a series in 7 of 50 patients *(24)*.

RISKS OF THE PROCEDURE

Mortality associated with the procedure is low, ranging from 0% to 4%, which is comparable to that with surgical myectomy. In the registry from the German Society of Cardiology *(36)*, of 242 patients, there were 3 (1.2%) in-hospital deaths. There are also reports of death as a result of stroke *(35,38)*, complete heart block *(35,38)*, dissection of the left anterior descending artery *(24)*, and right coronary artery thrombosis *(24)*. A dreaded complication is retrograde leakage of alcohol into the left anterior descending artery, which could result in a massive infarct *(42,43)*. However, this complication is extremely rare, and the importance of the different precautions mentioned previously to check for leakage before alcohol injection cannot be overemphasized.

Spontaneous ventricular fibrillation and tachycardia has been reported to occur within 48 h of the procedure *(35,40,42)*. The most frequent complication of alcohol ablation, however, is transient or permanent complete atrioventricular block, which has been reported to occur in up to 70% of patients *(25)*. The block is usually observed shortly after alcohol injection [but might even appear at 72 h *(44)*] and is most often transient. Complete heart block might resolve within the first 12 h of alcohol ablation, and then recur within the following week, requiring pacemaker implantation *(21)*. We and others *(10,45)* implant a pacemaker if the block persists for >48–72 h, although with longer observation, atrioventricular conduction might recover in many patients. About 10–20% of patients ultimately require a pacemaker. In a recent series of 224 patients, the incidence of pacemaker implantation was 14% *(45)*. Baseline conduction abnormalities (especially left bundle-branch block) might increase the risk for complete heart block after ablation *(12,14,45)*. Other factors found to be independently predictive of pacemaker implantation are female gender, bolus injection of ethanol, and injection into more than one septal artery *(45)*. Use of myocardial contrast echography helps limit infarct size, and in one series, it reduced the need for permanent pacemaker implantation from 17% to 7% *(25)* which is still higher than the 2% incidence with surgical myectomy *(33,46)*.

Right bundle-branch block might be observed in over half of the patients *(14,21,47)*. This is not surprising, as the right bundle is a discrete structure that is vascularized by septal branches from the left anterior coronary artery in 90% of patients, whereas the left bundle is fanlike and receives a dual blood supply from perforator branches of both the left anterior descending and posterior descending arteries. The left conduction system might nevertheless be involved, and left anterior fascicular block is reported to appear in 11% of patients *(14)*.

Alcohol ablation could result in the loss of capture in patients implanted with a pacemaker if the ventricular lead is placed near the septum *(48)*. It might be prudent to increase pacing to maximal output during the first days following the procedure in these patients.

There was no evidence for the creation of an arrhythmogenic substrate by alcohol ablation as assessed by serial electrophysiological studies before and after the procedure in a total of 78 patients in 2 different series *(21,35)* and none of the published reports indicate an increase in incidence of ventricular arrhythmias or sudden death over follow-up.

CONCLUSION

Alcohol ablation is progressively replacing surgical myectomy as the first treatment of choice for drug-resistant obstructive HCM. Data indicate that procedural success is high and comparable to that of surgery, with the advantage that it can be performed in patients in whom major surgery might be considered unsuitable. Benefits in comparison to myectomy also include shorter hospitalization, minimal pain, and avoidance of complications associated with surgery and cardiopulmonary bypass. Alcohol ablation has an important learning curve, with potentially serious complications, the most frequent of which is atrioventricular block requiring a pacemaker in 10–20% of patients. Although these rates are declining with continuing experience and with the advent of imaging techniques such as myocardial contrast echocardiography, the procedure should only be practiced by experienced operators and on carefully selected patients.

REFERENCES

1. Maron BJ, Olivotto I, Spirito P, et al. Epidemiology of hypertrophic cardiomyopathy-related death: revisited in a large non-referral-based patient population. Circulation 2000;102:858–864.
2. Maron MS, Olivotto I, Betocchi S, et al. Effect of left ventricular outflow tract obstruction on clinical outcome in hypertrophic cardiomyopathy. N Engl J Med 2003;348:295–303.
3. Maron BJ, Bonow RO, Cannon RO 3rd, et al. Hypertrophic cardiomyopathy. Interrelations of clinical manifestations, pathophysiology, and therapy (1). N Engl J Med 1987;316:780–789.
4. Maron BJ. Hypertrophic cardiomyopathy: a systematic review. JAMA 2002;287:1308–1320.
5. Brugada P, de Swart H, Smeets JL, et al. Transcoronary chemical ablation of ventricular tachycardia. Circulation 1989;79:475–482.
6. Sigwart U. Non-surgical myocardial reduction for hypertrophic obstructive cardiomyopathy. Lancet 1995;346:211–214.
7. Spencer WH, III, Roberts R. Alcohol septal ablation in hypertrophic obstructive cardiomyopathy: the need for a registry. Circulation 2000;102:600–601.
8. Braunwald E, Seidman CE, Sigwart U. Contemporary evaluation and management of hypertrophic cardiomyopathy. Circulation 2002;106:1312–1316.
9. Seggewiss H. Medical therapy versus interventional therapy in hypertropic obstructive cardiomyopathy. Curr Control Trials Cardiovasc Med 2000;1:115–119.
10. Gietzen FH, Leuner CJ, Obergassel L, et al. Role of transcoronary ablation of septal hypertrophy in patients with hypertrophic cardiomyopathy, New York Heart Association functional class III or IV, and outflow obstruction only under provocable conditions. Circulation 2002;106:454–459.
11. Kuhn H, Gietzen FH, Schafers M, et al. Changes in the left ventricular outflow tract after transcoronary ablation of septal hypertrophy (TASH) for hypertrophic obstructive cardiomyopathy as assessed by transoesophageal echocardiography and by measuring myocardial glucose utilization and perfusion. Eur Heart J 1999;20:1808–1817.
12. Lakkis NM, Nagueh SF, Kleiman NS, et al. Echocardiography-guided ethanol septal reduction for hypertrophic obstructive cardiomyopathy. Circulation 1998;98:1750–1755.
13. Nagueh SF, Lakkis NM, He ZX, et al. Role of myocardial contrast echocardiography during nonsurgical septal reduction therapy for hypertrophic obstructive cardiomyopathy. J Am Coll Cardiol 1998;32:225–229.
14. Runquist LH, Nielsen CD, Killip D, et al. Electrocardiographic findings after alcohol septal ablation therapy for obstructive hypertrophic cardiomyopathy. Am J Cardiol 2002;90:1020–1022.

15. Flores-Ramirez R, Lakkis NM, Middleton KJ, et al. Echocardiographic insights into the mechanisms of relief of left ventricular outflow tract obstruction after nonsurgical septal reduction therapy in patients with hypertrophic obstructive cardiomyopathy. J Am Coll Cardiol 2001;37:208–214.

16. Henein MY, O'Sullivan CA, Ramzy IS, et al. Electromechanical left ventricular behavior after nonsurgical septal reduction in patients with hypertrophic obstructive cardiomyopathy. J Am Coll Cardiol 1999;34:1117–1122.

17. Park T-H, Lakkis NM, Middleton KJ, et al. Acute effect of nonsurgical septal reduction therapy on regional left ventricular asynchrony in patients with hypertrophic obstructive cardiomyopathy. Circulation 2002;106:412–415.

18. Nagueh SF, Lakkis NM, Middleton KJ, et al. Changes in left ventricular diastolic function 6 months after nonsurgical septal reduction therapy for hypertrophic obstructive cardiomyopathy. Circulation 1999;99:344–347.

19. Nagueh SF, Lakkis NM, Middleton KJ, et al. Changes in left ventricular filling and left atrial function six months after nonsurgical septal reduction therapy for hypertrophic obstructive cardiomyopathy. J Am Coll Cardiol 1999;34:1123–1128.

20. Sitges M, Shiota T, Lever HM, et al. Comparison of left ventricular diastolic function in obstructive hypertrophic cardiomyopathy in patients undergoing percutaneous septal alcohol ablation versus surgical myotomy/myectomy. Am J Cardiol 2003;91:817–821.

21. Boeksteegers P, Steinbigler P, Molnar A, et al. Pressure-guided nonsurgical myocardial reduction induced by small septal infarctions in hypertrophic obstructive cardiomyopathy. J Am Coll Cardiol 2001;38:846–853.

22. Nagueh SF, Stetson SJ, Lakkis NM, et al. Decreased expression of tumor necrosis factor-alpha and regression of hypertrophy after nonsurgical septal reduction therapy for patients with hypertrophic obstructive cardiomyopathy. Circulation 2001;103:1844–1850.

23. Mazur W, Nagueh SF, Lakkis NM, et al. Regression of left ventricular hypertrophy after nonsurgical septal reduction therapy for hypertrophic obstructive cardiomyopathy. Circulation 2001;103:1492–1496.

24. Lakkis NM, Nagueh SF, Dunn JK, et al. Nonsurgical septal reduction therapy for hypertrophic obstructive cardiomyopathy: one-year follow-up. J Am Coll Cardiol 2000;36:852–855.

25. Faber L, Seggewiss H, Gleichmann U. Percutaneous transluminal septal myocardial ablation in hypertrophic obstructive cardiomyopathy: results with respect to intraprocedural myocardial contrast echocardiography. Circulation 1998;98:2415–2421.

26. Faber L, Seggewiss H, Ziemssen P, et al. Intraprocedural myocardial contrast echocardiography as a routine procedure in percutaneous transluminal septal myocardial ablation: detection of threatening myocardial necrosis distant from the septal target area. Cathet Cardiovasc Intervent 1999;47:462–466.

27. Okayama H, Sumimoto T, Morioka N, et al. Usefulness of selective myocardial contrast echocardiography in percutaneous transluminal septal myocardial ablation: a case report. Jpn Circ J 2001;65:842–844.

28. Faber L, Ziemssen P, Seggewiss H. Targeting percutaneous transluminal septal ablation for hypertrophic obstructive cardiomyopathy by intraprocedural echocardiographic monitoring. J Am Soc Echocardiogr 2000;13:1074–1079.

29. Harada T, Ohtaki E, Sumiyoshi T. Papillary muscles identified by myocardial contrast echocardiography in preparation for percutaneous transluminal septal myocardial ablation. Acta Cardiol 2002;57:25–27.

30. Faber L, Meissner A, Ziemssen P, et al. Percutaneous transluminal septal myocardial ablation for hypertrophic obstructive cardiomyopathy: long term follow up of the first series of 25 patients. Heart 2000;83:326–331.

31. Seggewiss H, Faber L, Meissner A, et al. Improvement of acute results after percutaneous transluminal septal myocardial ablation in hypertrophic obstructive cardiomyopathy during mid-term follow-up. J Am Coll Cardiol 2000;35:188A (abstract).

32. Firoozi S, Elliott PM, Sharma S, et al. Septal myotomy–myectomy and transcoronary septal alcohol ablation in hypertrophic obstructive cardiomyopathy. A comparison of clinical, haemodynamic and exercise outcomes. Eur Heart J 2002;23:1617–1624.

33. Nagueh SF, Ommen SR, Lakkis NM, et al. Comparison of ethanol septal reduction therapy with surgical myectomy for the treatment of hypertrophic obstructive cardiomyopathy. J Am Coll Cardiol 2001;38:1701–1706.

34. Qin JX, Shiota T, Lever HM, et al. Outcome of patients with hypertrophic obstructive cardiomyopathy after percutaneous transluminal septal myocardial ablation and septal myectomy surgery. J Am Coll Cardiol 2001;38:1994–2000.

35. Gietzen FH, Leuner CJ, Raute-Kreinsen U, et al. Acute and long-term results after transcoronary ablation of septal hypertrophy (TASH). Catheter interventional treatment for hypertrophic obstructive cardiomyopathy. Eur Heart J 1999;20:1342–1354.

36. Faber L, Seggewiss H, Kuhn H, et al. Catheter interventional septal ablation for hypertrophic obstructive cardiomyopathy: an analyisis of the follow-up data from the registry of the German Society of Cardiology. J Am Coll Cardiol 2002;39:3A (abstract).

37. Seggewiss H, Faber L, Ziemssen P, et al. Age related acute results of percutaneous septal ablation in hypertrophic obstructive cardiomyopathy. J Am Coll Cardiol 2000;35:188A (abstract).

38. Oomman A, Ramachandran P, Subramanyan K, et al. Percutaneous transluminal septal myocardial ablation in drug-resistant hypertrophic obstructive cardiomyopathy: 18-month follow-up results. J Invasive Cardiol 2001;13:526–530.

39. Welge D, Faber L, Werlemann B, et al. Long-term outcome after percutaneous septal ablation for hypertrophic obstructive cardiomyopathy. J Am Coll Cardiol 2002;39:173A (abstract).

40. Kim JJ, Lee CW, Park SW, et al. Improvement in exercise capacity and exercise blood pressure response after transcoronary alcohol ablation therapy of septal hypertrophy in hypertrophic cardiomyopathy. Am J Cardiol 1999;83:1220–1223.

41. Knight C, Kurbaan AS, Seggewiss H, et al. Nonsurgical septal reduction for hypertrophic obstructive cardiomyopathy: outcome in the first series of patients. Circulation 1997;95:2075–2081.

42. Knight C, Kurbaan AS, Seggewiss H, et al. Nonsurgical septal reduction for hypertrophic obstructive cardiomyopathy: outcome in the first series of patients. Circulation 1997;95:2075–2081.

43. Dimitrow PP, Dudek D, Dubeil JS. The risk of alcohol leakage into the left anterior descending coronary artery during non-surgical myocardial reduction in patients with obstructive hypertrophic cardiomyopathy. Eur Heart J 2001;22:437–438.

44. Kern MJ, Holmes DG, Simpson C, et al. Delayed occurrence of complete heart block without warning after alcohol septal ablation for hypertrophic obstructive cardiomyopathy. Cathet Cardiovasc Intervent 2002;56:503–507.

45. Chang SM, Nagueh SF, Spencer I, et al. Complete heart block: determinants and clinical impact in patients with hypertrophic obstructive cardiomyopathy undergoing nonsurgical septal reduction therapy. J Am Coll Cardiol 2003;42:296–300.

46. ten Berg JM, Suttorp MJ, Knaepen PJ, et al. Hypertrophic obstructive cardiomyopathy. Initial results and long-term follow-up after Morrow septal myectomy. Circulation 1994;90:1781–1785.

47. Kazmierczak J, Kornacewicz-Jach Z, Kisly M, et al. Electrocardiographic changes after alcohol septal ablation in hypertrophic obstructive cardiomyopathy. Heart 1998;80:257–262.

48. Valettas N, Rho R, Beshai J, et al. Alcohol septal ablation complicated by complete heart block and permanent pacemaker failure. Cathet Cardiovasc Intervent 2003;58:189–193.

49. Seggewiss H, Faber L, Gleichmann U. Percutaneous transluminal septal ablation in hypertrophic obstructive cardiomyopathy. Thorac Cardiovasc Surg 1999;47:94–100.

16

Therapeutic Angiogenesis and Myocardial Regeneration

G. Chad Hughes, MD
and Brian H. Annex, MD

CONTENTS

SCOPE OF CLINICAL PROBLEM

Ischemic heart disease is the leading cause of morbidity and mortality in the Western world. The term "ischemic heart disease" covers a broad spectrum of manifestations ranging from effort-induced angina without myocardial damage, through stages of chronic myocardial ischemia with associated reversible impairment in ventricular function, to states of irreversible myocardial injury and necrosis resulting in congestive heart failure (CHF). Ischemic heart disease, therefore, is the leading cause of CHF, a disease process that affects approx 1% of adults in the United States, with 550,00 new cases diagnosed annually and an incidence of 10 cases per 1000 population after age 65 *(1)*. With the aging of the population, the incidence of this problem is increasing, as evidenced by the number of discharges for CHF, which rose from 377,00 in 1979 to 999,000 in 2000 (165% increase) *(1)*. In addition, >50,000 deaths per year in the United States are directly attributable to CHF *(1)*. Likewise, the costs of caring for these patients is enormous, with $3.6 billion ($5471 per discharge) paid to Medicare beneficiaries for CHF-related treatment based on the most recently available data from 1998 *(1)*. Currently, median survival after diagnosis of CHF is 1.7 yr for men and 3.2 yr for women *(1)*, indicating a general inadequacy of presently available treatment options for the majority of these patients. Consequently, novel therapies are needed to improve the outlook for this patient population.

From: *Contemporary Cardiology: Interventional Cardiology:*
Percutaneous Noncoronary Intervention
Edited by: H. C. Herrmann © Humana Press Inc., Totowa, NJ

Another patient population with ischemic heart disease presently underserved by percutaneous and surgical therapy are those individuals with so-called "end-stage" coronary artery disease (CAD) (2). These patients typically have diffuse coronary disease, small distal vessels, or other comorbidities, making them poor candidates for traditional methods of treatment. By definition, end-stage CAD refers to patients with the persistence of severe anginal symptoms (Canadian Cardiovascular Society Class III and IV) despite maximal conventional antianginal combination therapy and coronary atherosclerosis not amenable to revascularization by percutaneous means or surgical bypass (2). These patients generally have a relatively large amount of viable myocardium and only moderately impaired left ventricular function and are not candidates for cardiac transplantation (3). Patients with end-stage CAD could represent as many as 12% of all patients with symptomatic coronary disease (4) and, similar to those patients with CHF, an increase in this cohort can be expected with the continued aging of the general population.

As can be seen from the above-mentioned statistics, there is an ever-increasing need for novel effective therapies for both CHF and CAD. The term "angiogenesis" refers to the growth and proliferation of blood vessels (2). Therapeutic angiogenesis seeks to improve perfusion via new blood vessel growth in order to treat disease states such as ischemic heart disease. Therapeutic angiogenesis might be achieved through mechanical and pharmacological approaches, as well as via cell-based therapies. In addition, cellular approaches might be particularly valuable in the treatment of end-stage CHF, where viable myocardium able to respond to improved blood flow is lacking. This chapter will review several of the more promising options, including transmyocardial laser revascularization (TMR), percutaneous myocardial revascularization (PMR), angiogenic growth factor-based therapy, and various stem cell transplant approaches to the treatment of both end-stage CAD and CHF.

TRANSMYOCARDIAL LASER REVASCULARIZATION AND PERCUTANEOUS MYOCARDIAL LASER REVASCULARIZATION

Transmyocardial laser revascularization was initially described as an alternative therapy for coronary artery disease in patients who were not candidates for traditional modes of revascularization, including bypass surgery or angioplasty (5). The technique was based directly on the work of Sen and colleagues, who, in 1965, described "direct ventricular revascularization" using a "transmyocardial acupuncture" procedure in dogs (6). The rationale behind the procedure was an attempt to surgically mimic the pattern of myocardial circulation of reptiles, in which blood flows directly into the myocardial tissue from the ventricular cavity (5).

Numerous experimental and clinical studies have now disproven this concept of patent channels perfusing the left ventricular myocardium by demonstrating that the laser channels become occluded in the early postoperative period (5). Although still somewhat controversial, the mechanism of action of TMR appears to involve some combination of improved blood flow via laser injury-induced neovascularization and/or regional myocardial denervation. Numerous groups (7–17) have investigated changes in regional myocardial perfusion and function in long-term follow-up after experimental TMR. Chronic myocardial ischemia models in rats (17), dogs (7), sheep (8), and pigs (9–16) have all demonstrated improved myocardial perfusion weeks to months after TMR using various techniques, including radioactive (11) and colored (7,8) microspheres, ^{99m}Tc-sestamibi perfusion scanning (12), magnetic resonance imaging (MRI) (13,17), and positron emission tomography (PET) *(14–16)* to directly measure regional myocardial blood flow. These studies have generally demonstrated some degree of improvement in either rest or stress function concomitant with the increased perfusion. In addition, the changes in regional perfusion and function have been associated with histologic evidence for neovascularization in regions of the myocardium treated with laser therapy (Fig. 1).

Denervation also appears to be a plausible mechanism for the marked anginal reductions reported in the very early postoperative period in some patients, at a time when significant angiogenesis would not yet have occurred. Experimental studies investigating whether denervation occurs post-TMR have produced evidence both for *(18,19)* and against *(20–22)* this hypothesis. A clinical study using PET to assess regional sympathetic innervation found evidence for denervation in a group of patients 2 months after holmium : YAG TMR *(23)*. Likewise, there appears to be a significant incidence of silent ischemia in the early postoperative period after TMR *(24)*, which might represent further clinical evidence of myocardial denervation. However, analysis of electrocardiograms obtained during symptom-limited exercise in a group of patients 12 mo after either TMR or PMR found that neither procedure was associated with silent ischemia at long-term follow-up *(25)*. Recent work from our laboratory *(26)* using a porcine model to evaluate regional myocardial sympathetic innervation both early (3 d) and late (6 mo) after TMR found evidence for short-term denervation after TMR, as there was a significant reduction in tyrosine hydroxylase protein concentration in the lased regions 3 d after TMR. Tyrosine hydroxylase is a neural-specific enzyme found in sympathetic efferent nerves and a commonly used anatomic marker of regional innervation that has been used in prior studies investigating denervation after TMR *(18,19)*. However, this same study also supports other work suggesting that denervation is not the long-term mechanism of action of TMR *(20–22)*, as both immunohistochemical staining and Western blot analysis confirmed the presence of tyrosine hydroxylase in the regions of myocardium 6 mo following laser therapy (Fig. 2). Thus, one hypothesis for the symptom relief after TMR would include denervation as an explanation for the early relief of symptoms seen in some patients, with angiogenesis becoming the dominant mechanism in the months that follow as mature collateral vessels develop in the treated regions.

At the present time, three different types of laser (defined by their photon-emitting active mediums) are being used for surgical TMR. These include carbon dioxide (CO_2), holmium : YAG, and xenon : chloride excimer. The CO_2 and holmium : YAG lasers are classified as infrared lasers and rely on thermal ablation to create transmyocardial channels. Excimer lasers, on the other hand, are "cold" lasers that operate in the deep ultraviolet spectrum and produce tissue ablation via dissociation of molecular bonds *(5)*. From the clinician's perspective, excimer lasers might be considered as more purely ablative and producing less collateral damage of surrounding myocardium than either of the two infrared lasers. Of the two infrared lasers, holmium : YAG produces greater lateral thermal damage than CO_2 *(5)*. At the present time, there are no studies comparing the various lasers in terms of clinical efficacy, and experimental studies have demonstrated evidence for neovascularization in myocardium lased with each of the three lasers *(27–29)*. However, only the CO_2 and holmium: YAG lasers are currently approved by the US Food and Drug Administration (FDA) for clinical use for surgical TMR.

Both TMR and PMR are currently being used as treatment for patients with end-stage coronary disease. These patients have severe, medically refractory angina pectoris usually

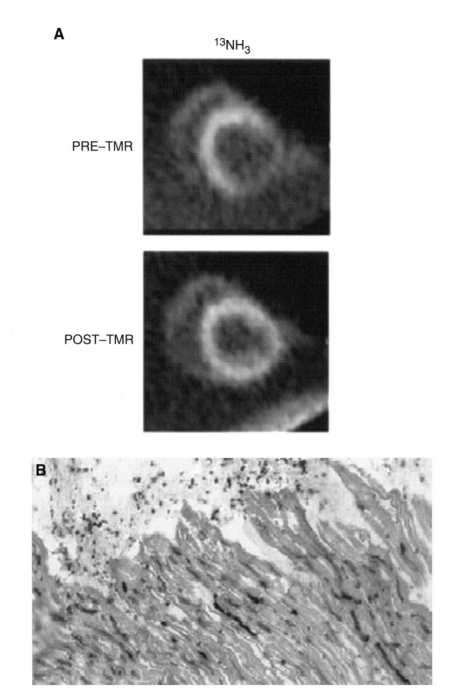

Fig. 1. (A) Positron emission tomographic scan pre-TMR and 6 mo post-TMR in a mini-swine with an experimentally produced high-grade stenosis of the left circumflex coronary artery. Note significant improvement in regional perfusion 6 mo post-TMR. **(B)** Histology of lased left circumflex distribution demonstrating neovascularization in and around TMR channel remnant at 6 mo postoperatively. (Reproduced from refs. *14* and *16* with permission.)

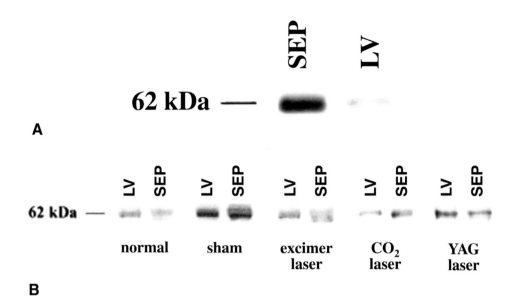

Fig. 2. Western blot analysis for tyrosine hydroxylase protein (TYR-OH), a neural-specific enzyme found in sympathetic efferent nerves and a commonly used anatomic marker of regional innervation **(A)** 3 d and **(B)** 6 mo after TMR in swine. Note marked reduction in TYR-OH levels at 3 d with return to normal by 6 mo following TMR with any of the three clinically available lasers. SEP, non-laser septum; LV, laser lateral wall of left ventricle; normal, non-operated control; sham, sham thoracornary control. (Reproduced from ref. *26* with permission.)

secondary to diffuse three-vessel coronary atherosclerosis *(5,30)*. The majority have had at least one prior myocardial infarction and undergone multiple prior revascularization procedures with either percutaneous angioplasty (PTCA) and/or coronary artery bypass grafting (CABG). To be considered a candidate for TMR/PMR, patients must demonstrate the following: Canadian Cardiovascular Society (CCS) Class III–IV angina pectoris on maximally tolerated medical therapy, recent coronary angiography demonstrating anatomy unfavorable for PTCA or CABG, and ischemic, viable (hibernating) myocardium in regions to be treated *(5,30)*. Because of higher complication rates among patients with unstable angina and CHF, patients requiring intravenous nitrates to remain pain-free and patients with an ejection fraction <30% should generally be excluded *(5)*. An additional requirement for PMR patients is a myocardial wall thickness ≥8 mm in the area to be treated to minimize the chance of left ventricular perforation with the laser. A recent study on the use of surgical TMR in "real-world" community practice analyzing data from the Society of Thoracic Surgeons National Cardiac Database found a 30-d mortality rate of 3.7% for patients meeting the above criteria *(31)*. No such data are currently available for PMR owing to lack of FDA approval.

Surgical TMR involves using a laser to create transmural channels extending from the epicardial to endocardial surface of the left ventricular free wall of the beating heart. The technique is most commonly performed via a small left anterior thoracotomy. To date, there have been six prospective, randomized, controlled trials of surgical TMR versus best medical therapy *(32–37)* (Table 1). These studies have randomized patients with CCS Class III or IV angina to either TMR or continued medical management. The studies have consistently demonstrated significant improvements in anginal class and exercise time in

Table 1

Published Prospective, Randomized, Controlled, Clinical Trials of TMR versus Medical Therapy with 12 mo Follow-up. Modified from Ref. 30 with Permission

Author (ref.)	No. of patients	Crossover allowed?	Laser used (mean number of channels produced)	% of patients with a decrease of ≥2 CCS angina classes: TMR vs control (p-value)	Improvement in exercise time (s): TMR vs control (p-value)	Survival: TMR vs control (p-value)	Perfusion Modality Change
Allen et al. (33)	275	Yes	Ho : YAG (39)	76 vs 32 ($p < 0.001$)	+5.0 vs +3.9 MET[a] ($p = 0.05$)	84% vs 89% (p = NS)	^{201}T1 : SPECT: no change
Frazier et al. (32)	192	Yes	CO_2 (30)	72 vs 13 ($p < 0.001$)	NA	85% vs 79% (p = NS)	^{201}T1 : SPECT: improved
Schofield et al. (34)	188	No	CO_2 (30)	25 vs 4 ($p < 0.001$)	NA[b]	89% vs 96% (p = NS)	^{99m}Tc : SPECT: no change
Burkhoff et al. (35)	182	No	Ho : YAG (18)	48 vs 14 ($p < 0.001$)	+65 vs –46 ($p < 0.0001$)	95% vs 90% (p = NS)	^{201}T1 : SPECT: no change
Aaberge et al. (37)	100	No	CO_2 (48)	39 vs 0 ($p < 0.01$)	+8 vs –10[c] (p = NS)	88% vs 92% (p = NS)	NA
Jones et al. (36)	86	No	Ho : YAG (NA)	NA[d]	+119 vs –85 ($p = 0.0001$)	NA	^{201}T1 : SPECT: no change

[a]Exercise treadmill testing was not part of the original study design, and no treadmill tests were performed at baseline; analysis of total exercise time included only 81 patients who underwent Naughton testing.

[b]Exact data not available; however, the difference in exercise times between the two groups was 40s (in favor of TMR) at 12 mo (p = NS).

[c]Time to chest pain during exercise increased by 66s in the TMR group and decreased by 3s in the control group ($p < 0.01$).

[d]Mean CCS class at the conclusion of the 12-mo follow-up period was 1.7 among patients treated with TMR and 3.8 among the medically treated group ($p < 0.0001$).

CCS = Canadian Cardiovascular Society; CO_2 = carbon dioxide; Ho : YAG = holmium : yttrium–aluminum–garnet; MET = metabolic equivalent; NA = data not available; NS = statistically not significant; SPECT = single-photon emission computed tomography, TMR = transmyocardial laser revascularization.

276

TMR versus medically treated patients at 12-month follow-up. However, improvements in myocardial perfusion as measured using single-photon emission computed tomography (SPECT) have not been consistently observed. Of the five studies *(32–36)* measuring myocardial perfusion with SPECT, only one *(32)* reported a significant improvement in the TMR-treated patients as compared to medically managed controls. In none of the trials was TMR associated with a survival benefit at 1-yr follow-up.

Percutaneous myocardial revascularization creates channels via advancement of a fiber-optic catheter against the endocardial surface from the left ventricular cavity. Unlike surgical TMR, complete transmural penetration of the left ventricular myocardium is avoided. Catheter position is determined using one of two techniques: (1) a combination of coronary angiography and biplane left ventriculography or (2) the Biosense electromechanical mapping system. The latter creates a real-time three-dimensional image of the left ventricle, which allows catheter movements to be tracked and the location on the endocardial surface visualized throughout the procedure *(30)*. Only the holmium : YAG and excimer lasers allow the laser beam to be transmitted via an optical fiber and can, thus, be used in PMR, although all of the catheter-based PMR systems developed to date are based on the holmium : YAG laser. As noted earlier, no PMR devices have as yet obtained FDA approval. There are currently three published prospective, randomized, controlled trials of PMR versus medical therapy *(38–40)*. Two of the three trials *(38,40)* found a significant benefit at 12 mo follow-up with regard to both exercise tolerance time and anginal scores in patients randomized to PMR as compared to medically treated controls. The third trial *(39)*, however, found no significant differences in either anginal scores or exercise tolerance at 6 mo follow-up. In addition, the as-yet unpublished but widely publicized Direct myocardial revascularization In Regeneration of Endomyocardial Channels Trial (DIRECT) failed to show any benefit in the laser-treated group *(41)*. No assessment of myocardial perfusion was performed as part of any of the published PMR trials *(42,43)*.

GROWTH FACTOR-BASED TREATMENT STRATEGIES

Until recently, neovascularization in the chronically ischemic adult heart had been thought to be the result of the processes of angiogenesis and arteriogenesis. Angiogenesis refers to the sprouting of new capillaries from pre-existing ones and, in the adult, is mainly caused by hypoxia and mediated via activation of hypoxia-inducible factor-1α (HIF-1α), which serves to increase transcription of vascular endothelial growth factor (VEGF) and its receptors and stabilize VEGF mRNA *(44)*. Arteriogenesis, on the other hand, is the type of vascular growth responsible for maturation of collateral conduits and produces vessels capable of carrying significant blood flow as well as being visualized with angiography *(44,45)*. Primary arteriogenic stimuli include shear stress and inflammation where an invasion of monocytes and other white blood cells leads to the production of growth factors such as the fibroblast growth factors (FGFs) with subsequent vascular growth *(46,47)*. Recent work *(48,49)*, however, has demonstrated that neovascularization in adults is not restricted to angiogenesis and arteriogenesis, but, rather, involves vasculogenesis as well. Vasculogenesis refers to the process of *in situ* formation of blood vessels from endothelial progenitor cells (EPCs) termed "angioblasts" *(45,50)*. Angioblasts are stem cells recruited from the bone marrow that migrate and fuse with other EPCs and capillaries to form a primitive network of vessels known as the primary capillary plexus. After this primary capillary plexus is formed, it is remodeled by sprouting and branching via the process

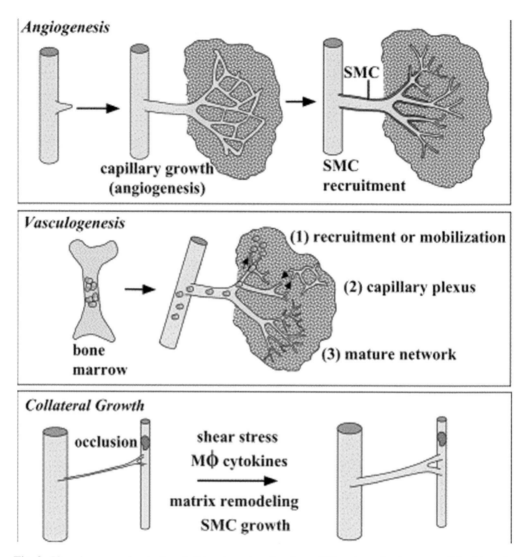

Fig. 3. Vascular expansion in the adult heart can involve three different mechanisms, possibly driven by distinct signals: (1) angiogenesis (top), which is the growth of new blood vessels from pre-existing ones; (2) arteriogenesis (bottom), which is the growth of arteries from pre-existing arterioles; and (3) vasculogenesis (middle), which refers to the formation of new blood vessels by fusion and differentiation of EPCs originating in the bone marrow. (Reproduced from ref. *51* with permission.)

of angiogenesis. Thus, angiogenesis, vasculogenesis, and arteriogenesis all potentially contribute to neovascularization in the adult heart *(45,51)* (Fig. 3), although some authors *(47)* have suggested that arteriogenesis is necessary for significant improvements in myocardial blood flow.

The adult myocardial endothelium normally exists in a quiescent state. Only when provoked by stress or pathologic conditions does the coronary vascular bed expand via the processes of angiogenesis, vasculogenesis, and arteriogenesis as outlined earlier *(51)*. This neovascularization represents a highly ordered physiological mechanism under tight regulation, with many factors active at the molecular level to influence the process including numerous soluble polypeptides such as the VEGFs, the angiopoietins, FGFs,

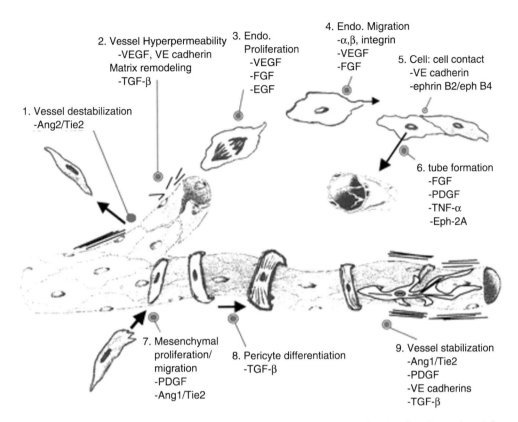

Fig. 4. Physiologic processes involved in neovascularization. See text for details. (Reproduced from ref. *50* with permission.)

platelet derived growth factors (PDGFs), transforming growth factor-β (TGF-β), tumor necrosis factor-α (TNF-α), the colony-stimulating factors, as well as many others (Fig. 4) *(50)*. In addition, several membrane-bound proteins play prominent roles in angiogenesis, including various members of the integrin, cadherin, and ephrin families. Finally, mechanical forces acting on the endothelium also contribute to the regulation of neovascularization via shear-stress-induced upregulation of angiogenic and inflammatory mediators, primarily serving to stimulate adaptive arteriogenesis *(50,51)*. However, even though the myocardial vascular bed can expand via the neovascularization process, this expansion is limited and myocardial ischemia results. This could then lead to the process of myocardial hibernation whereby regional cardiac contractility is downregulated to restore the balance between myocardial oxygen supply and demand *(52,53)*. Hibernating myocardium is viable, but in the absence of revascularization, progressive myocyte apoptosis, ventricular remodeling, and structural alterations, including the loss of contractile material within cardiomyocytes as well as increases in the amount of interstitial connective tissue, occur, eventually resulting in irreversible myocardial fibrosis *(53)*. Experimental studies in genetically engineered mice lacking normal VEGF production have demonstrated progressive cardiac failure over time as a result of insufficient angiogenic growth factor availability *(54)* and provide a rationale for the administration of angiogenic growth factors or their genes to rescue hibernating myocardium *(51)*.

As can be seen from the list of molecular mediators of the neovascularization process outlined earlier, there are a wide variety of therapeutic options available when one considers growth factor-based treatment strategies for the induction of new blood vessel growth in the heart. The growth of the therapeutic angiogenesis field has exploded in the past decade as a result of the development of recombinant growth factors, the best characterized of which are the ligands of the FGF and VEGF families. A large body of preclinical evidence exists supporting the efficacy of both VEGF and FGF as angiogenic agents and these latter two cytokines will be the focus of this discussion.

The VEGFs are a family of glyocproteins of which VEGF-1 (or VEGF-A) has been studied most extensively with regard to use as a pro-angiogenic agent. The other VEGFs, which are structurally similar to VEGF-1, include VEGF-2 (VEGF-C), VEGF-3 (VEGF-B), VEGF-D, VEGF-E, and placental growth factor *(45)*. At least four isoforms of VEGF-1 are produced as a result of alternative splicing containing 121 ($VEGF_{121}$), 165 ($VEGF_{165}$), 189 ($VEGF_{189}$), and 206 ($VEGF_{206}$) amino acids. The isoforms, which differ in their heparin-binding capacity, appear to have similar angiogenic potency *(45,50)*. $VEGF_{121}$ and $VEGF_{165}$ are secreted into the extracellular environment, whereas $VEGF_{189}$ and $VEGF_{206}$ remain cell or matrix associated via their affinity for heparan sulfates *(45,50)*. VEGF binds to at least three known tyrosine kinase receptors: Flt-1 (VEGFR-1), KDR/Flk-1 (VEGFR-2), and Flt-4 (VEGFR-3) *(50)*. VEGFR-2 is thought to transduce angiogenic signals, whereas the role of VEGFR-1 is less well defined and VEGFR-3 is involved in lymphangiogenesis *(45,50)*. The primary cellular target of VEGF is the endothelial cell, although functional VEGF receptors are also present on vascular smooth muscle cells and monocytes/macrophages. Consequently, VEGF could utilize endothelial as well as other cell types as effectors *(45,50)*.

Vascular endothelial growth factor exerts several effects on endothelial cells, including enhanced migration, increased permeability, and increased production of plasminogen activators, plasminogen activator inhibitor-1, and interstitial collagenase, all of which contribute to angiogenesis *(50)*. VEGF can also stimulate endothelial cell proliferation, an effect specific to vascular endothelial cells, as VEGF does not induce proliferation of other cells types such as smooth muscle cells or fibroblasts *(50)*. VEGF production is regulated by local oxygen concentration with hypoxia stimulating VEGF production via the binding of HIF-1α to the VEGF promoter with subsequent increased VEGF gene transcription and mRNA stability, as mentioned earlier *(45,50)*. Thus, low oxygen tension acts to stimulate angiogenesis via VEGF.

Acidic FGF (FGF-1) and basic FGF (FGF-2) are members of a large family of structurally related polypeptide growth factors (FGF-1 to FGF-23) *(55)*. Both FGF-1 and FGF-2 are potent endothelial cell mitogens and, similar to VEGF, induce processes in endothelial cells critical to angiogenesis *(45,50)*. The biologic functions of FGFs are mediated primarily by specific cell surface receptors of the tyrosine kinase family *(55)*. Like VEGF, FGF is involved in endothelial cell proliferation, migration, and production of plasminogen activator and collagenase *(50,55)*. Unlike VEGF, which is mitogenic primarily for endothelial cells, FGF stimulates proliferation of most cells derived from embryonic mesoderm and neuroectoderm, including pericytes, fibroblasts, myoblasts, chrondrocytes, and osteoblasts *(50)*. Also, unlike VEGF, FGFs lack a signal sequence and are not secreted proteins *(45,50)*. Thus, FGF does not appear to play a general role in all angiogenic processes, but, rather, is normally involved in blood vessel remodeling associated with tissue repair *(50)*.

Table 2
Differences Between Gene- and Protein-Based Angiogenic Therapies.
Reproduced from Ref. *56* with Permission

	Gene therapy	Protein therapy
Temporal exposure	Sustained presence	Finite
Dose response	Unpredictable	Defined
Administration	Single	Repeated?
Targeting	Possible	Possible
Slow release	Yes	Possible through fossculation
Inflammatory response	Yes	No, unless effect of protein
Foreign material	Yes	No
Serum half-life	Long	Short
Tissue half-life	Unpredictable	Short, subject to engineering
Induence patient serology	Yes	No

Angiogenic cytokines utilized for therapeutic angiogenesis may be administered either as recombinant human protein or the gene encoding the protein may be transferred into target myocardium, with subsequent protein production by transfected cells. Each approach has its own advantages and disadvantages (Table 2). With protein therapy, a known quantity of protein is administered and, thus, a more precise dose–response relationship can be attained *(45)*. Unlike gene therapy, protein therapy avoids the need for transfection, transcription, and translation necessary with gene therapy approaches and assumes that the presence of the protein in a therapeutic concentration is sufficient to induce the desired angiogenic response. The major disadvantage of protein therapy is the short tissue half-life of angiogenic proteins, which might be insufficient for the sustained stimulation and multiple cell cycling required for the growth and remodeling of new collateral vessels *(56)*. Conversely, the advantage of gene therapy techniques is that sustained local production may lead to prolonged elevation of tissue protein levels beyond that which may be obtained using protein-based approaches. Gene therapy techniques utilized to date generally involve either plasmid DNA or replication-defective adenovirus containing the gene of interest. These vectors have a limited duration of expression on the order of 1–2 wk *(56)*. This limited duration of expression may be ideal for therapeutic angiogenesis where prolonged exposure to elevated levels of angiogenic protein raises concern over promotion of malignancy and pathologic neovascularization, as well as acceleration of atherosclerosis. The main disadvantages of the gene therapy techniques include the inflammatory response to adenoviral proteins and inconsistent level of gene expression in different patients with a given dose of vector *(56)*.

Finally, consideration of the route of administration is important with angiogenic therapies. Angiogenic proteins may be administered systemically (i.e., intravenously through a peripheral vein), intracoronary, or via direct intramyocardial injection. Intramyocardial injection is required in the case of naked plasmid DNA, as the plasmid undergoes prompt degradation if delivered into circulating blood. In addition, plasmid DNA gene transfer is less efficient than with adenoviral vectors, although the clinical differences are uncertain. Viral vectors are not subject to similar intravascular degradation and can be delivered either via an intracoronary route or intramyocardial injection.

To date there have been five Phase II prospective, randomized, double-blind, placebo-controlled trials of angiogenic growth factor therapy for the induction of therapeutic

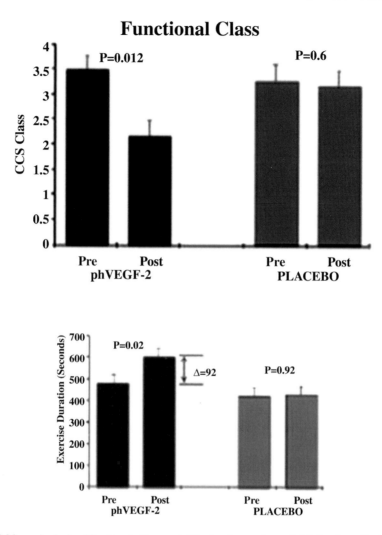

Fig. 5. (A) CCS anginal classification before and 12 wk after endocardial injection of naked plasmid DNA encoding for VEGF2. See text for details. **(B)** Exercise tolerance data. See text for details. (Reproduced from ref. 59 with permission.)

angiogenesis in the myocardium *(57–61)* including two VEGF *(59,60)* and three FGF *(57,58,61)* trials. Losordo et al. *(59)* investigated the use of percutaneous catheter-based gene transfer via direct endocardial injection of naked plasmid DNA encoding for VEGF2 in no-option patients (*n* = 19) with CCS Class III or IV angina. A twelve-week follow-up demonstrated a statistically significant improvement in CCS angina class (Fig. 5A) in VEGF2-treated versus placebo-treated patients. VEGF2-treated patients also had a statistically significant increase in their mean duration of exercise tolerance (Fig. 5B) over the 12-wk period, whereas no change occurred in the placebo group. Left ventricular electromechanical mapping using the NOGA system demonstrated a significant reduction in the area of myocardial ischemia at 90 d posttreatment in the VEGF2 patients, whereas no change was seen in controls. Similarly, a trend toward improved perfusion was observed in a subset of VEGF2 patients undergoing SPECT myocardial perfusion imaging at 90 d. The Vascular endothelial growth factor in Ischemia for Vascular Angiogenesis trial (VIVA trial) *(60)* randomized 178 no-option patients to placebo, low-dose $VEGF_{165}$, or high-dose $VEGF_{165}$ protein with follow-up out to 120 d. Patients in the VEGF group received an intracoronary infusion on d 0, followed by intravenous infusions on d 3, 6, and 9. There was no significant improvement in exercise treadmill time (ETT), the primary end point of the study, from baseline to 60 d in VEGF-treated patients. By 120 d, there was a trend toward improved ETT in the high-dose VEGF group versus placebo. Similarly, 60 d posttreatment, there was no difference in angina class improvement from baseline in VEGF versus control patients, whereas at 120 d, a statistically significant improvement in angina class for high-dose VEGF treated patients compared with placebo was present. Myocardial perfusion studies performed at d 60 demonstrated no significant improvement in VEGF-treated patients versus placebo-treated patients.

The FGF Initiating RevaScularization Trial (FIRST) randomized 337 patients considered to be suboptimal candidates for standard surgical or catheter-based revascularization to a single intracoronary infusion of placebo or one of three escalating doses of recombinant FGF2 with a 180-d follow-up *(57)*. There was no significant improvement in ETT in FGF-2- versus placebo-treated patients at 90 d follow-up, the primary study end point. Likewise, there was no evidence for a treatment effect on ETT at 180 d. Angina frequency and CCS angina scores were significantly improved in FGF-2- versus placebo-treated patients at 90 d follow-up, although this difference was lost at the 180-d follow-up. The improvements in anginal scores were more pronounced in highly symptomatic (CCS Class III–IV) patients. Nuclear perfusion imaging demonstrated no significant changes in rest or stress perfusion at 90 or 180 d. The Angiogenic GENe Therapy (AGENT) trial *(58)* examined the effects of single intracoronary administration of placebo or five escalating doses of replication-defective adenovirus containing the human FGF-4 gene in 79 patients with CCS Class II–III angina with a 12-wk follow-up. Unlike the other four randomized, placebo-controlled angiogenesis trials *(57,59–61)*, the AGENT trial did not enroll no-option patients, but, rather, patients with one-, two-, or three-vessel CAD, the majority of whom had anatomy suitable for CABG or PTCA. There was a trend toward improved ETT in FGF- versus placebo-treated patients at both 4 and 12 wk follow-up, although the differences did not reach statistical significance. Post hoc analysis revealed that when patients with a baseline ETT time >10 min were excluded, ETT improvement was significantly greater for FGF patients at both 4 and 12 wk. There was no difference in time to angina during ETT for FGF versus placebo. However, as with the ETT time data, when patients with ETT > 10 min were excluded, there was an overall significant improvement in time to angina in FGF patients. A follow-up study from this same group (AGENT-2 trial) *(61)* randomized 52 patients to intracoronary infusion of 10^{10} adenoviral particles containing the human FGF-4 gene or placebo. The dose of adenovirus used was based on the dose-escalation results from the preceding AGENT trial *(58)*. Unlike the AGENT trial, patients enrolled were not optimal candidates for revascularization by surgical or percutaneous means. The primary end point was change in myocardial perfusion as assessed using stress adenosine SPECT 8 wk posttreatment. There was a strong trend toward greater reduction in the size of reversible perfusion defect by SPECT in the FGF-4-treated patients versus controls (Fig. 6). Likewise, there was a trend toward greater angina reductions and less nitroglycerin use in the FGF-4 group.

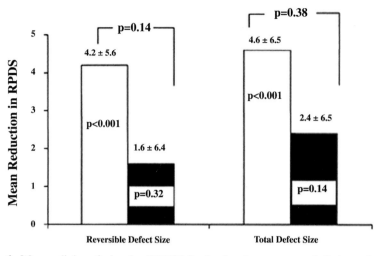

Fig. 6. Myocardial perfusion by SPECT 8 wk after intracoronary infusion of placebo or adenovirus containing the human FGF-4 gene. See text for details. RPDS, reversible perfusion defect size; white bars, Ad5FGF-4; black bars, placebo. (Reproduced from ref. *61* with permission.)

CELLULAR-BASED TREATMENT STRATEGIES FOR THERAPEUTIC ANGIOGENESIS AND MYOCARDIAL REGENERATION

Theoretically, angiogenesis in the myocardium could be achieved via a process whereby all of the elements necessary for the angiogenic response could be derived from the myocardium itself. In their seminal work, Asahara et al. *(48,49)* demonstrated that cells derived from the peripheral circulation and bone marrow were present in the angiogenic response occurring after experimentally induced hind-limb ischemia. This work established that postnatal neovascularization involves circulating EPCs that hone to sites of neovascularization and contribute to vasculogenesis. These circulating EPCs derive from hematopoietic stem cells and contribute to reparative processes such as neovascularization after ischemia.

Studies subsequent to those of Asahara and colleagues have demonstrated that the exogenous administration of angiogenic growth factors leads to increases in EPCs and that these cells could contribute to the effects of therapeutic angiogenesis *(62)*. Interestingly, patient risk factors such as diabetes, aging, and hypercholesterolemia that are associated with an impaired "endogenous" response to ischemia are also associated with reduced numbers of circulating EPCs *(51)*. Thus, lack of sufficient availability of angiogenic growth factors might not be the only reason for these patients to develop myocardial ischemia, as underlying conditions might prevent the adult endothelium from responding normally to angiogenic stimuli *(51)*. Furthermore, therapies designed to modify these risk factors (e.g., statin medications) lead to increases in circulating EPC numbers *(63)*. If stem cells contribute or are even essential for therapeutic angiogenesis, it follows that stem-cell-based therapies for angiogenesis might be sufficient to produce the desired angiogenic response and reduce or even reverse the sequelae of ischemic heart disease.

The heart has a limited capacity for regeneration because of the inability of adult cardiac myocytes to routinely re-enter the cell cycle and proliferate and, as a result, ventricular remodeling and ultimately heart failure are the inexorable consequences of substantial myocardial infarction *(64)*. Because stem cells have also been demonstrated to differentiate into cardiac muscle, there is intense interest in their use for promoting myogenesis.

Table 3
Adult Human Stem Cells and Their Primary Direction of Differentiation

Cell type	Tissue-specific location	Cells or tissues produced
Hematopoietic stem cells	Bone marrow, peripheral blood	Bone marrow and blood lymphohematopoietic cells
Mesenchymal stem cells	Bone marrow, peripheral blood	Bone, cartilage, tendon, adipose tissue, muscle, marrow stroma, neural cells
Neural stem cells	Ependymal cells, astrocytes (subventricular zone) of the central nervous system	Neurons, astrocytes, oligodendrocytes
Hepatic stem cells	In or near the terminal bile ductules (canals of Hering)	Oval cells that subsequently generate hepatocytes and ductular cells
Pancreatic stem cells	Intraislet, nestin-positive cells, oval cells, duct cells	Beta cells
Skeletal-muscle stem cells or satellite cells	Muscle fibers	Skeletal muscle fibers
Stem cells of the skin (keratinocytes)	Basal layer of the epidermis, bulge zone of the hair follicles	Epidermis, hair follicles
Epithelial stem cells of the lung	Tracheal basal and mucus-secreting cells, bronchiolar Clara cells, alveolar type II pneumocyte	Mucous and ciliated cells, type I and II pneumocytes
Stem cells of the intestinal epithelium	Epithelial cells located around the base of each crypt	Paneth's cells, brush-border enterocytes, mucus-secreting goblet cells, enteroendocrine cells of the villi

Source: Reproduced from ref. *66* with permission.

Therefore, patients with established infarcts or end-stage myocardial hibernation with fibrosis represent another population where stem-cell-based treatment strategies hold particular promise.

Stem cells are defined as undifferentiated cells with the capacity for proliferation and self-renewal as well as an ability to regenerate multiple cell types and tissues *(64–66)*. Embryonic stem cells are derived from mammalian embryos in the blastocyst stage and have the ability to generate any terminally differentiated cell in the body. Adult stem cells are part of the tissue-specific cells of the postnatal organism into which they are committed to differentiate (Table 3) *(64–66)*. Stem cells are capable of maintaining, generating, and replacing terminally differentiated cells lost as a result of physiologic cell turnover or tissue injury. Stem cells have clonogenic and self-renewing capabilities and can differentiate into multiple cell lineages, a phenomenon known as stem cell plasticity. The means by which circulating stem cells are recruited into various solid-organ tissues and differentiate into the tissue-specific cells subsequently generated are not fully understood

(64,66). Tissue injury results in changes in the microenvironment that could play an important role in stem cell recruitment. After tissue injury in organs such as the liver, skin, or intestine, which have their own supply of intrinsic stem cells, resident stem cells at the site of tissue damage contribute to tissue repair. If the pool of endogenous stem cells is exhausted, exogenous circulating stem cells are then signaled to replenish the pool and participate in tissue repair, thus serving as a backup rescue system *(66)*. However, in organs such as the heart, which appear to lack resident stem cells, the release of chemokines such as VEGF following ischemic injury stimulate mobilization of bone-marrow-derived stem cells. These mobilized stem cells are then attracted to ischemic areas by locally elevated VEGF or stromal-cell-derived factor-1 levels *(62,66)*. Thus, the processes of neovascularization and myocardial regeneration in ischemic tissue are dependent on the mobilization and integration of stem cells.

Embryonic stem cells have been demonstrated in vitro to differentiate into cardiomyocytes that express cardiac-specific genes, beat spontaneously, respond to chronotropic drugs, and form a functional syncytium capable of electrical conduction *(64)*. However, the clinical use of embryonic stem cells is currently limited by practical issues such as immunological rejection following embryonic stem-cell-derived cell transplantation as well as possible teratoma formation *(67)*. Ethical issues surrounding the use of human embryos might also limit their use and, consequently, widespread utilization of embryonic stem cells for cardiovascular therapy in the near future is unlikely *(64–66)*.

Adult stem cells, on the other hand, are present within the adult organism and are an attractive option for clinical use. These cells retain the ability to differentiate beyond their own tissue boundaries and are present within multiple organs, including the bone marrow, peripheral blood, brain, liver, and skeletal muscles, among others, where they normally participate in tissue repair (Table 3) *(64–66)*. Multipotent adult progenitor cells are similar to embryonic stem cells in that they can be extensively expanded in vivo and form cells of all three germ cell layers. In contrast to embryonic stem cells, autologous adult stem cells avoid the rejection resulting from the expression of major histocompatability complex (MHC) proteins in human embryonic stem cells *(66)*. Also, unlike embryonic stem cells, tumorigenicity has not been observed with adult stem cells. With regard to cardiovascular therapeutics, the adult stem cells most likely to be useful for myocardial regeneration and neovascularization are skeletal myoblasts and bone-marrow-derived and peripheral-blood-derived stem cells (Fig. 7). Experimental transplantation of stem cells has been carried out via percutaneous means using an intracoronary or coronary sinus route, direct endocardial injection, epicardially via a surgical approach, or systemically, and the preferable route for delivery at the present time remains unclear and awaits further study *(64)*.

Skeletal myoblasts are stem cells residing in skeletal muscle. They can be obtained from muscle biopsy and cultured for expansion and have been used in human subjects *(68)*. Preclinical studies have demonstrated engraftment of myoblasts within the heart, with formation of new striated muscle, myotube formation, long-term graft survival, and augmentation of ventricular function (Fig. 8) *(64,68,69)*. However, expression of cardiac-specific markers did not occur and no gap junctions were detected, which has raised concerns over potential arrhythmogenicity *(70)*. Indeed, myoblasts and bone-marrow-derived stem cells differ in their electrophysiologic properties and ability to couple electromechanically among themselves and with host cardiomyocytes. These findings suggest that arrhythmias might be more likely to occur after myoblast than other types of stem cell transplantation and some have suggested restricting their use to patients with an implanted cardiac defibrillator *(70)*. One advantage of using

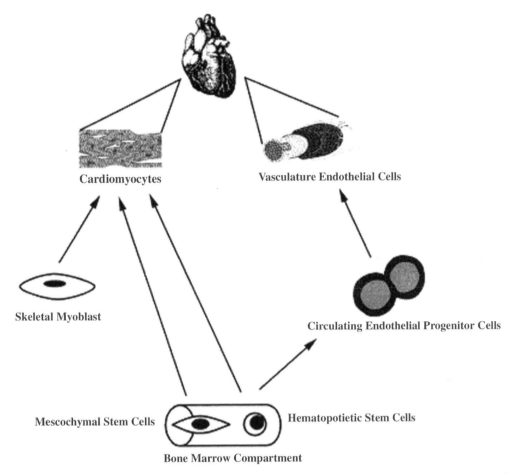

Fig. 7. Bone-marrow-derived hematopoietic and mesenchymal stem cells and autologous skeletal myoblasts represent the adult stem cells most likely to be useful for cardiovascular therapeutics, including angiogenesis and myogenesis. (Reproduced from ref. *64* with permission.)

skeletal myoblasts is that they are relatively more resistant to ischemia than cardiomyocytes, which favors their engraftment in ischemic or infarcted myocardium *(68)*.

Adult bone marrow cells represent the other major stem cell option for cardiovascular therapeutics at the present time. Bone marrow contains both hematopoietic and mesenchymal stem cells (Table 3), both of which have the capacity for multilineage differentiation *(64,66)*. Mesenchymal stem cells, also known as marrow stromal cells, are pluripotent progenitor cells, which can form cardiomyocytes. Hematopoietic stem cells can be found in both the bone marrow and peripheral blood and have the capacity to differentiate into both cardiomyocytes and endothelial cells *(64)*. Hematopoietic stem cells are the source of circulating EPCs or angioblasts, which, as previously described, are now felt to contribute to angiogenesis and vasculogenesis in the adult organism.

The published clinical experience to date with stand-alone stem-cell-based therapies consists mainly of small, mostly uncontrolled, Phase I clinical series *(68,71–74)*. Assmus and colleagues *(74)* treated a total of 20 patients with intracoronary infusion of either autologous bone-marrow- or peripheral-blood-derived progenitor cells into the infarct-related artery several days after reperfused acute myocardial infarction (MI) and found

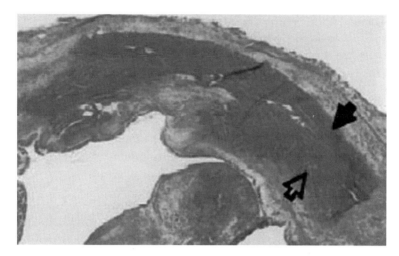

Fig. 8. Engraftment of autologous skeletal myoblasts within infarcted rabbit myocardium. Engraftment resulted in an island of cells which improved regional systolic and diastolic function in this animal model. (Reproduced from ref. *69* with permission.)

evidence for improved regional and global function 4 mo posttreatment. There did not appear to be any difference between patients treated with bone-marrow- versus peripheral-blood-derived cells. Tse et al. *(71)* injected autologous bone marrow cells into regions of chronic myocardial ischemia using a catheter-based technique with NOGA guidance in eight patients with medically refractory angina pectoris and found a reduction in angina along with small improvements in regional function and myocardial perfusion by magnetic resonance imaging (MRI) in an uncontrolled study with a 3-mo follow-up. Similar results were reported by Fuchs et al. *(73)* in 10 no-option patients receiving transendocardial injections of autologous bone marrow. Using the same NOGA-guided transendocardial injection technique, Smits et al. *(68)* investigated the use of autologous skeletal myoblasts injected into a region of old MI in five patients with chronic CHF and found evidence for improved regional function 6 mo posttreatment. In the only study to date with a control group (although not concurrently enrolled), Perin and colleagues enrolled 21 no-option patients with ischemic cardiomyopathy (mean ejection fraction = 20%) in a prospective, nonrandomized study of NOGA-guided transendocardial injection of autologous bone marrow cells. They found a significant reduction in myocardial ischemia and improved function by SPECT in treated versus control patients at 2 month follow-up *(72)*.

CURRENT TRIAL STATUS AND FUTURE DIRECTIONS

Results of clinical trials of pro-angiogenic therapies (TMR, PMR, angiogenic growth factors) have generally been positive with regard to anginal scores, whereas the majority of these same trials have failed to consistently demonstrate concomitant improvements in perfusion in treated patients. One potential explanation holds that the conventional nuclear imaging techniques (i.e., thallium, sestamibi) used in these clinical trials have lower spatial resolution and assess perfusion only semiquantitatively, thus limiting their ability to detect small changes in myocardial perfusion in patients with end-stage CAD *(13,17,42)*. In addition, there appears to be a large variability in the measured percent myocardial ischemia (up to 50% variability) over time, which might limit the utility of scintigraphic techniques to detect improved myocardial perfusion in response to therapy *(42)*. Consequently, improvements in perfusion in human subjects might be too small to be detected with radionuclide scanning yet still be able to decrease the pain of angina pectoris. MRI, with its high spatial resolution and potential for quantification of myocardial perfusion, might be better suited to the detection of perfusion changes within regions of the heart treated with pro-angiogenic therapies. MRI has been useful in experimental studies to detect improved myocardial blood flow after TMR *(13,17)*, and preliminary clinical data suggest that MRI might be superior to nuclear perfusion scans as well. Laham et al. *(43)* utilized MRI to examine 15 patients undergoing PMR and found a significant improvement in regional perfusion in the region of the myocardium treated with laser therapy at 30 d and 6 mo posttreatment, despite no change in nuclear perfusion scans in these same patients. Thus, in future studies evaluating the utility of the various novel therapies outlined in this chapter, consideration should be given to the use of more sensitive techniques such as MRI when assessing myocardial blood flow pretreatment and posttreatment.

Trials of angiogenic growth factor therapy have established the safety of this approach. The ideal growth factor(s), their optimal dose, as well as route of administration remain undefined. Work is still needed to more clearly define the time-course of angiogenesis, especially given the significant improvements seen from d 60 to 120 posttreatment in the high-dose VEGF group in the VIVA study *(60)*.

Similar to the situation with angiogenic growth factors, the best possible stem cell for cardiovascular use has yet to be defined. The ideal route of administration and dose are unclear. Given the well-described reduction in EPC number and function with age, techniques aimed at stimulating the EPC pool in vivo or expanding it ex vivo will likely be necessary for meaningful responses to angiogenic growth factor therapies. Much additional clinical work is needed as well with randomized, controlled trials similar to those performed previously with TMR, PMR, and the angiogenic growth factors, as definitive data on human clinical efficacy are lacking at the present time. Finally, efficacy of stem cell therapy at the present time is indirect, as there is currently no available method to determine engraftment in the living patient.

Given the complex and highly ordered physiological regulation involved in the processes of angiogenesis and myogenesis, it is difficult to envision that any single growth factor, stem cell, or mechanical therapy will be the "magic bullet" to cure end-stage coronary disease or ischemic heart failure. Rather, combination therapy with multiple growth factors, mechanical means such as transmyocardial laser revascularization, or stem cell transplantation might be necessary to achieve consistent clinical benefits for patients with CAD and CHF.

REFERENCES

1. American Heart Association. Heart disease and stroke statistics—2003 update. Dallas, TX: American Heart Association, 2002.
2. Hughes GC, Post MJ, Simons M, Annex BH. Porcine models of human coronary artery disease: implications for pre-clinical trials of therapeutic angiogenesis. J Appl Physiol 2003;94:1689–1701.
3. Schoebel FC, Frazier OH, Jessurun GAJ, et al. Refractory angina pectoris in end-stage coronary artery disease: evolving therapeutic concepts. Am Heart J 1997;134:587–602.
4. Mukherjee D, Bhatt DL, Roe MT, et al. Direct myocardial revascularization and angiogenesis-how many patients might be eligible? Am J Cardiol 1999;84:598–600.
5. Hughes GC, Abdel-aleem S, Biswas SS, et al. Transmyocardial laser revascularization: experimental and clinical results. Can J Cardiol 1999;15:797–806.

6. Sen PK, Udwadia TE, Kinare SG, Parulkar GB. Transmyocardial acupuncture. A new approach to myocardial revascularization. J Thorac Cardiovasc Surg 1965;50:181–189.

7. Yamamoto N, Kohmoto T, Gu A, et al. Angiogenesis is enhanced in ischemic canine myocardium by transmyocardial laser revascularization. J Am Coll Cardiol 1998;31:1426–1433.

8. Ozaki S, Meyns B, Racz R, et al. Effect of transmyocardial laser revascularization on chronic ischemic hearts in sheep. Eur J Cardio-thorac Surg 2000;18:404–410.

9. Horvath KA, Greene R, Belkind N, et al. Left ventricular functional improvement after transmyocardial laser revascularization. Ann Thorac Surg 1998;66:721–725.

10. Horvath KA, Belkind N, Wu I, et al. Functional comparison of transmyocardial revascularization by mechanical and laser means. Ann Thorac Surg 2001;72:1997–2002.

11. Martin JS, Sayeed-Shah U, Byrne JG, et al. Excimer versus carbon dioxide transmyocardial laser revascularization: effects on regional left ventricular function and perfusion. Ann Thorac Surg 2000;69:1811–1816.

12. Hamawy AH, Lee LY, Samy SA, et al. Transmyocardial laser revascularization dose response: enhanced perfusion in a porcine ischemia model as a function of channel density. Ann Thorac Surg 2001;72:817–822.

13. Mühling OM,Wang Y, Panse P, et al. Transmyocardial laser revascularization preserves regional myocardial perfusion: an MRI first pass perfusion study. Cardiovasc Res 2003;57:63–70.

14. Hughes GC, Kypson AP, St Louis JD, et al. Improved perfusion and contractile reserve after transmyocardial laser revascularization in a model of hibernating myocardium. Ann Thorac Surg 1999;67:1714–1720.

15. Hughes GC, Kypson AP, Annex BH, et al. Induction of angiogenesis after TMR: a comparison of holmium: YAG, CO_2, and excimer lasers. Ann Thorac Surg 2000;70:504–509.

16. Hughes GC, Biswas SS, Yin B, et al. A comparison of mechanical and laser transmyocardial revascularization for induction of angiogenesis and arteriogenesis in chronically ischemic myocardium. J Am Coll Cardiol 2002;39:1220–1228.

17. Nahrendorf M, Hiller K-H, Theisen D, et al. Effect of transmyocardial laser revascularization on myocardial perfusion and left ventricular remodeling after myocardial infarction in rats. Radiology 2002;225:487–493.

18. Kwong KF, Kanellopoulos GK, Nickols JC, et al. Transmyocardial laser treatment denervates canine myocardium. J Thorac Cardiovasc Surg 1997;114:883–890.

19. Kwong KF, Schuessler RB, Kanellopoulos GK, et al. Nontransmural laser treatment incompletely denervates canine myocardium. Circulation 1998;98(19 Suppl)II-67–II-71.

20. Hirsch GM, Thompson GW, Arora RC, et al. Transmyocardial laser revascularization does not denervate the canine heart. Ann Thorac Surg 1999;68:460–468.

21. Minisi AJ, Topaz O, Quinn MS, Mohanty LB. Cardiac nociceptive reflexes after transmyocardial laser revascularization: implications for the neural hypothesis of angina relief. J Thorac Cardiovasc Surg 2001;122:712–719.

22. Arora RC, Hirsch GM, Hirsch K, Armour JA. Transmyocardial laser revascularization remodels the intrinsic cardiac nervous system in a chronic setting. Circulation 2001;104:I-115–I-120.

23. Al-Sheikh T, Allen KB, Straka SP, et al. Cardiac sympathetic denervation after transmyocardial laser revascularization. Circulation 1999;100:135–140.

24. Hughes GC, Landolfo KP, Lowe JE, et al. Diagnosis, incidence, and clinical significance of early postoperative ischemia after transmyocardial laser revascularization. Am Heart J 1999;137: 1163–1168.

25. Myers J, Oesterle SN, Jones J, Burkhoff D. Do transmyocardial and percutaneous laser revascularization induce silent ischemia? An assessment by exercise testing. Am Heart J 2002;143:1052–1057.

26. Hughes GC, Baklanov DV, Biswas SS, et al. Regional cardiac sympathetic innervation early and late after transmyocardial laser revascularization. J Cardiac Surg 2004;19:1–7.

27. Mack CA, Magovern CJ, Hahn RT, et al. Channel patency and neovascularization after transmyocardial revascularization using an excimer laser. Results and comparisons to nonlased channels. Circulation 1997;96(Suppl II):II-65–II-69.

28. Fisher PE, Kohmoto T, DeRosa CM, et al. Histologic analysis of transmyocardial channels: comparison of CO_2 and homium : YAG lasers. Ann Thorac Surg 1997;64:466–472.

29. Hughes GC, Lowe JE, Kypson AP, et al. Neovascularization after transmyocardial laser revascularization in a model of chronic ischemia. Ann Thorac Surg 1998;66:2029–2036.

30. Saririan M, Eisenberg MJ. Myocardial laser revascularization for the treatment of end-stage coronary artery disease. J Am Coll Cardiol 2003;41:173–183.

31. Peterson ED, Kaul P, Kaczmarek RG, et al. From controlled trials to clinical practice: monitoring transmyocardial revascularization use and outcomes. J Am Coll Cardiol 2003;42:1611–1616.

32. Frazier OH, March RJ, Horvath KA. Transmyocardial revascularization with carbon dioxide laser in patients with end-stage coronary artery disease. N Engl J Med 1999;341:1021–1028.
33. Allen KB, Dowling RD, Fudge TL, et al. Comparison of transmyocardial revascularization with medical therapy in patients with refractory angina. N Engl J Med 1999;341:1029–1036.
34. Schofield PM, Sharples LD, Caine N, et al. Transmyocardial laser revascularization in patients with refractory angina: a randomized controlled trial. Lancet 1999;353:519–524.
35. Burkhoff D, Schmidt S, Schulman SP, et al. Transmyocardial laser revascularization compared with continued medical therapy for treatment of refractory angina pectoris: a prospective randomized trial. ATLANTIC investigators: angina treatments—lasers and normal therapies in comparison. Lancet 1999;354:885–890.
36. Jones JW, Schmidt SE, Richman BW, et al. Holmium:YAG laser transmyocardial revascularization relieves angina and improves functional status. Ann Thorac Surg 1999;67:1596–1602.
37. Aaberge L, Nordstrand K, Dragsund M, et al. Transmyocardial revascularization with CO_2 laser in patients with refractory angina pectoris: clinical results from the Norwegian randomized trial. J Am Coll Cardiol 2000;35:1170–1177.
38. Oesterle SN, Sanborn TA, Ali N, et al. Percutaneous transmyocardial laser revascularization for severe angina: the PACIFIC randomised trial. Lancet 2000;356:1705–1710.
39. Stone GW, Teirstein PS, Rubenstein R, et al. A prospective, multicenter, randomized trial of percutaneous transmyocardial laser revascularization in patients with nonrecanalizable chronic total occlusions. J Am Coll Cardiol 2002;39:1581–1587.
40. Gray TJ, Burns SM, Clarke SC, et al. Percutaneous myocardial laser revascularization in patients with refractory angina pectoris. Am J Cardiol 2003;91:661–666.
41. Leon MB. DIRECT (DMR In Regeneration of Endomyocardial Channels Trial). Presented at Late-Breaking Trials, Transcatheter Cardiovascular Therapeutics, 2000.
42. Burkhoff D, Jones JW, Becker LC. Variability of myocardial perfusion defects assessed by thallium 201 scintigraphy in patients with coronary artery disease not amenable to angioplasty or bypass surgery. J Am Coll Cardiol 2001;38:1033–1039.
43. Laham RJ, Simons M, Pearlman J, et al. Magnetic resonance imaging demonstrates improved regional systolic wall motion and thickening and myocardial perfusion of myocardial territories treated by laser myocardial revascularization. J Am Coll Cardiol 2002;39:1–8.
44. Schaper W, Buschmann I. Arteriogenesis, the good and bad of it. Cardiovasc Res 1999;43:835–837.
45. Freedman SB, Isner JM. Therapeutic angiogenesis for coronary artery disease. Ann Intern Med 2002;136:54–71.
46. Schaper W, Ito WD. Molecular mechanisms of coronary collateral vessel growth. Circ Res 1996;79:911–919.
47. Schaper W. Quo vadis collateral blood flow? A commentary on a highly cited paper. Cardiovasc Res 2000;45:220–223.
48. Asahara T, Murohara T, Sullivan A, et al. Isolation of putative progenitor endothelial cells for angiogenesis. Science 1997;275:964–967.
49. Asahara T, Masuda H, Takahashi T, et al. Bone marrow origin of endothelial progenitor cells responsible for postnatal vasculogenesis in physiological and pathological neovascularization. Circ Res 1999;85:221–228.
50. Papetti M, Herman IM. Mechanisms of normal and tumor-derived angiogenesis. Am J Physiol Cell Physiol 2002;282:C947–C970.
51. Luttun A, Carmeliet P. De novo vasculogenesis in the heart. Cardiovasc Res 2003;58:378–389.
52. St.Louis JD, Hughes GC, Kypson AP, et al. An experimental model of chronic myocardial hibernation. Ann Thorac Surg 2000;69:1351–1357.
53. Hughes GC. Cellular models of hibernating myocardium: implications for future research. Cardiovasc Res 2001;51:191–193.
54. Carmelit P, Ng YS, Nuyens D, et al. Impaired myocardial angiogenesis and ischemic cardiomyopathy in mice lacking the vascular endothelial growth factor isoforms VEGF164 and VEGF188. Nature Med 1999;5:495–502.
55. Detillieux KA, Sheikh F, Kardami E, Cattini PA. Biological activities of fibroblast growth factor-2 in the adult myocardium. Cardiovasc Res 2003;57:8–19.
56. Post MJ, Laham R, Sellke FW, Simons M. Therapeutic angiogenesis in cardiology using protein formulations. Cardiovasc Res 2001;49:522–531.
57. Simons M, Annex BH, Laham RJ, et al. Pharmacological treatment of coronary artery disease with recombinant fibroblast growth factor-2. Double-blind, randomized, controlled clinical trial. Circulation 2002;105:788–793.

58. Grines CL, Watkins MW, Helmer G, et al. Angiogenic gene therapy (AGENT) trial in patients with stable angina pectoris. Circulation 2002;105:1291–1297.

59. Losordo DW, Vale PR, Hendel RC, et al. Phase 1/2 placebo-controlled, double-blind, dose-escalating trial of myocardial vascular endothelial growth factor 2 gene transfer by catheter delivery in patients with chronic myocardial ischemia. Circulation 2002;105:2012–2018.

60. Henry TD, Annex BH, McKendall GR, et al. The VIVA trial. Vascular endothelial growth factor in ischemia for vascular angiogenesis. Circulation 2003;107:1359–1365.

61. Grines CL, Watkins MW, Mahmarian JJ, et al. A randomized, double-blind, placebo-controlled trials of Ad5FGF-4 gene therapy and its effect on myocardial perfusion in patients with stable angina. J Am Coll Cardiol 2003;42:1339–1347.

62. Dimmeler S, Vasa-Nicotera M. Aging of progenitor cells: limitation for regenerative capacity? J Am Coll Cardiol 2003;42:2081–2082.

63. Rupp S, Badorff C, Koyanagi M, et al. Statin therapy in patients with coronary artery disease improves the impaired endothelial progenitor cell differentiation into cardiomyogenic cells. Basic Res Cardiol 2004;99:61–68.

64. Abbott JD, Giordano FJ. Stem cells and cardiovascular disease. J Nucl Cardiol 2003;10:403–412.

65. Perin EC, Geng Y-J, Willerson JT. Adult stem cell therapy in perspective. Circulation 2003;107:935–938.

66. Körbling M, Estrov Z. Adult stem cells for tissue repair-a new therapeutic concept? N Engl J Med 2003;349:570–582.

67. van der Heyden MAG, Hescheler J, Mummery CL. Spotlight on stem cells-makes old hearts fresh. Cardiovasc Res 2003;58:241–245.

68. Smits PC, van Geuns R-JM, Poldermans D, et al. Catheter-based intramyocardial injection of autologous skeletal myoblasts as a primary treatment of ischemic heart failure. J Am Coll Cardiol 2003;42:2063–2069.

69. Atkins BZ, Lewis CW, Kraus WE, et al. Intracardiac transplantation of skeletal myoblasts yields two populations of striated cells in situ. Ann Thorac Surg 1999;67:124–129.

70. Makkar RR, Lill M, Chen P-S. Stem cell therapy for myocardial repair. Is it arrhythmogenic? J Am Coll Cardiol 2003;42:2070–2072.

71. Tse H-F, Kwong Y-L, Chan JKF, et al. Angiogenesis in ischaemic myocardium by intramyocardial autologous bone marrow mononuclear cell implantation. Lancet 2003;361:47–49.

72. Perin EC, Dohmann HFR, Borojevic R, et al. Transendocardial, autologous bone marrow cell transplantation for severe, chronic ischemic heart failure. Circulation 2003;107:2294–2302.

73. Fuchs S, Satler LF, Kornowski R, et al. Catheter-based autologous bone marrow myocardial injection in no-option patients with advanced coronary artery disease. J Am Coll Cardiol 2003;41:1721–1724.

74. Assmus B, Schächinger V, Teupe C, et al. Transplantation of progenitor cells and regeneration enhancement in acute myocardial infarction (TOPCARE-AMI). Circulation 2002;106:3009–3017.

IV   PERIPHERAL INTERVENTIONS

17

Renal and Iliac Intervention

Michael T. Caulfield, MD,
Dharsh Fernando, MD,
and Kenneth Rosenfield, MD

INTRODUCTION

Because atherosclerosis is a systemic disease process, it is not surprising that cardiologists find themselves treating patients with peripheral vascular problems in addition to the more traditional cardiovascular issues. Of the 64.4 million Americans with cardiovascular disease, 8–12 million are affected by peripheral arterial disease (PAD), which is estimated to encompass 12–20% of Americans over age 65. Identification of these patients is extremely important, as up to 70% of patients with PAD have significant coronary artery disease (CAD)*(2)*, and the primary cause of mortality in PAD patients is myocardial infarction, stroke, and complications from diabetes *(3)*. Evidence of PAD, therefore, should be a "red flag" signaling the need for further cardiovascular evaluation.

RENAL ARTERY DISEASE

Background

Unlike angina in patients with CAD and claudication in patients with lower extremity PAD, there is no "signature" symptom associated with renal artery stenosis (RAS). Thus, RAS is largely underrecognized and underdiagnosed. Furthermore, as there is no established population screening test for the disease, the true prevalence is unknown. Nonetheless, the impact of this disease is profound. In a study by Conlon et al. 3987 patients undergoing cardiac catheterization had abdominal aortography performed to assess for RAS *(5)*. "Significant" RAS (defined as greater than 75% stenosis) was detected in 4.8% and severe bilateral disease was found in 0.8%. Importantly, RAS was shown to be an independent predictor of mortality. Four-year survival in

From: *Contemporary Cardiology: Interventional Cardiology:*
Percutaneous Noncoronary Intervention
Edited by: H. C. Herrmann © Humana Press Inc., Totowa, NJ

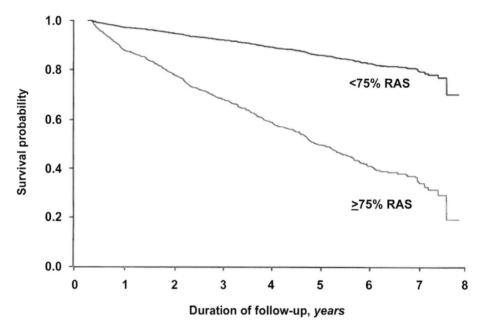

Fig. 1. Kaplan–Meier survival curve showing survival according to presence or absence of signficant RAS. (From ref. *5.*)

patients with RAS was only 57% compared to 89% in patients without RAS (*p*<0.001). Prognosis worsened with increasing degree of stenosis and in the presence of bilateral stenosis (Fig. 1).

Atherosclerotic RAS (ARAS) is also believed to account for 12–18% of patients reaching end-stage renal disease in Western countries *(6).* Ischemic nephropathy from ARAS leads to renal atrophy and dysfunction as measured by elevation in serum creatinine *(7).* The clinical significance of this problem is underscored by the fact that end-stage renal disease (ESRD) patients treated with dialysis or transplantation have a 10–30 times higher risk of cardiovascular mortality than the general population *(8,9).*

The goal of revascularization of the renal arteries has been to preserve or restore renal function, facilitate the control of hypertension, and treat cardiac perturbations associated with RAS, such as congestive heart failure, angina, and recurrent pulmonary edema. Since Gruntzig first reported percutaneous transluminal angioplasty (PTA) therapy for RAS in 1978 *(10),* this has progressively become the treatment of choice over surgery. However, the treatment modality must be tailored to each patient, based on lesion etiology, morphology, and location, as well as patient comorbidities. The two main etiologies, fibromuscular dysplasia (FMD) and atherosclerotic disease, will be addressed separately, as their presentations, treatments, and prognoses differ.

FIBROMUSCULAR DYSPLASIA

FMD occurs primarily in women between the ages of 15 and 50 yr. Several pathologic subtypes exist, the most common being medial or perimedial fibroplasia of the renal artery *(11).* The angiographic morphology of this subtype is the appearance of a "string of beads" in the body of the renal artery *(12)* (Fig. 2).

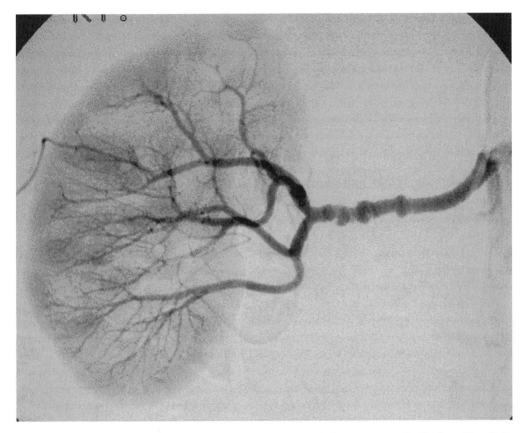

Fig. 2. Fibromuscular dysplasia of a renal artery, with typical appearance of a "string of beads."

Although FMD can be treated by surgical revascularization, the success of angioplasty in these patients has made endovascular therapy the method of choice for disease involving the main renal artery or its primary branches. In a representative series, Kling and colleagues *(13)* described their experience of treating FMD with balloon angioplasty. Of the 52 patients in their series undergoing PTA for FMD, initial technical success exceeded 90%, and initial clinical success (elimination or significant reduction in hypertension at 6-mo follow-up) occurred in 87%. During 5 yr of follow-up, only three patients (6%) of the initially successful cohort experienced a recurrence. When the FMD involves the more peripheral renal artery branches or there is associated aneurysmal disease, the preferred method of revascularization is not as clear. Traditionally, these lesions were treated surgically, sometimes requiring the "bench" technique (e.g., extracorporeal reconstruction of the branch vessels). This, however, is highly technical work and is only performed in select centers. Angioplasty of these smaller branches has also been investigated, as Cluzel et al. reported successful technical and clinical outcomes in 21 of 25 (84%) renal branch arteries dilated for treatment of hypertension *(14)*. This might offer an effective alternative treatment for selected patients, although the decision to attempt PTA on smaller branch vessels must be weighed against the potential to cause dissection, thrombosis, and loss of the kidney. For main artery lesions, acute technical success in excess of 95% and long-term clinical benefit can be expected in 80–90% of patients with FMD. Based on these favorable results, the threshold for PTA in patients with FMD is relatively low; patients with persistent, even modest, hypertension on medications should be treated, especially if they are young, so as to avoid the long-term consequences of hypertension.

The use of endovascular stents has not generally been advocated in FMD patients for two main reasons: First, the results with balloon angioplasty alone for FMD have been excellent. Occasionally, PTA must be repeated, but the recurrence rate is far less than that for PTA of atherosclerotic lesions. Second, the biologic effects and long-term consequences of placing endovascular stents in these lesions are unknown. There have, nonetheless, been anecdotal reports of the use of stents for FMD lesions that are either refractory to PTA or recurrent.

ATHEROSCLEROTIC RENAL ARTERY STENOSIS

Since its conception over 25 yr ago, PTA for ARAS has become the preferred method of revascularization. In a meta-analysis of multiple early studies, acute improvement in renal function occurred in 43%, stabilization occurred in 35%, and continued worsening (e.g., no beneficial effect of PTA) occurred in 22% (15). The mortality rate in most series was less than 1%, and contrast-related and recognized atheroembolic complications were infrequent. Although the short-term results of PTA were acceptable, it became clear that the major shortcoming of renal angioplasty for ARAS was the high restenosis rate, which approached 70% in the short or intermediate term (6–12 mo) in some series. The high restenosis rate is felt to be secondary to the high prevalence (approx 80–90%) of aorto-ostial plaque, which is thick, calcified, and resistant to balloon expansion. Thus, during balloon inflation, the plaque is only temporarily displaced and then demonstrates a predilection for immediate and delayed elastic recoil upon removal of the balloon. The high restenosis rate following balloon angioplasty previously served as a compelling reason to recommend primary surgical revascularization in appropriately selected patients who were good surgical candidates, in spite of reported surgical mortality rates (2–17%) considerably higher than for PTA (<1%) (15–18).

In the only prospective randomized trial comparing PTA to surgical reconstruction in ARAS, Weibell and colleagues found that in 58 nondiabetic patients with unilateral aorto-ostial ARAS under the age of 70 yr, there was no statistically significant difference in acute patency (19). At 24 mo, however, the primary patency in the angioplasty group was only 62%. Secondary patency, achieved by either repeat PTA or surgery, was 90%, comparable to that of patients who had initially been randomized to surgery (97%). The results with regard to clinical outcome, including cure or improvement of hypertension, were similar in PTA and surgical cohorts, as was the frequency of complications. The authors concluded that a strategy of initial treatment with PTA is appropriate, followed by close clinical follow-up and either additional PTA or surgical revascularization for cases of restenosis. There are several limitations of this study as it applies to current practice. First, the study utilized surgeons who were highly experienced in renal artery revascularization and thus produced the best results. Such individuals experienced in renal artery surgery are not available at most institutions. Second, in order to qualify for randomization, patients had to be considered surgical candidates. All were less than 70 yr of age and in reasonable health. In contrast, many patients currently evaluated for renal artery revascularization are older than 70, infirm, have coronary artery disease and/or congestive heart failure, or are otherwise poor surgical candidates. Such patients would not have been enrolled. Third, the Weibell study was carried out prior to the routine use of stents, which dramatically enhance the outcome of percutaneous revascularization. Any comparison between surgery and percutaneous therapy in the current era would need to include the use of stents in the PTA arm. Such a study is unlikely ever to be performed, primarily because of the excellent results now obtained using stents and the striking difference in morbidity and mortality between surgery and PTA.

The greatest limitations to PTA of ARAS are elastic recoil and significant restenosis rates. This is especially true of ostial lesions, in which the plaque is primarily aortic in origin (20–22). These limitations began to be addressed in the 1990s, with the advent of stenting for ARAS (23–28). Studies quickly revealed not only that the immediate problem of elastic recoil was resolved but also that restenosis rates were dramatically decreased. With stenting, binary restenosis was reported to be between 10% and 25% (23–29). In 1999, van de Ven and colleagues reported a prospective randomized study comparing PTA with PTA/stent for ostial ARAS (28). They described a higher primary success rate (<50% residual stenosis) with stenting versus PTA (88% vs 57%) and a lower rate of restenosis at 6 mo (14% vs 48%). Complications were similar in the two groups. A recent study from Shammas and colleagues confirmed these restenosis rates, and identified smoking, time to evaluate for restenosis, and vessel diameter of 4 mm or less as predictors of its occurrence (73).

History and Exam

Most patients with RAS are asymptomatic. They often present with new or increasingly refractory hypertension or worsening renal function. Although some present with symptoms of congestive heart failure or flash pulmonary edema, most complaints stem from associated disease states (e.g., diabetes mellitus) or atherosclerosis involving other organ systems (e.g., angina from coronary artery disease, transient ischemia attack [TIA]/stroke from carotid artery disease, claudication from PAD). Examination might reveal an abdominal bruit, best auscultated utilizing the diaphragm for detection of a higher pitched arterial bruit while depressing the head of the stethoscope deep into the abdomen.

Noninvasive Evaluation

Functional studies, such as nuclear perfusion and renin–captopril studies have been used to assess for renovascular hypertension and changes in renal perfusion suggestive of RAS. However duplex ultrasound, magnetic resonance angiography (MRA), and computed tomography angiography (CTA) have become the preferred diagnostic imaging modalities over the past several years (30–35). There are advantages and limitations to each of these studies, which should be recognized when individualizing care. MRA is often preferred, although some patients cannot lie in the magnet (e.g., obesity, claustrophobia, metallic implants). Duplex ultrasonography can be technically difficult (e.g., in obese patients or those with intestinal gas or pathology) and is heavily operator dependent. CTA uses iodinated contrast that can be nephrotoxic and should be minimized or avoided in patients with renal dysfunction.

Interventional Options

INDICATIONS

In the current era, the percutaneous approach is the initial choice of therapy for ARAS. Furthermore, the evidence is overwhelming that stents, whether used primarily or provisionally, greatly enhance the results of PTA when deployed by competent and skilled interventionalists. Surgery is reserved for patients in whom PTA is less suitable, such as those with branch vessel disease, total occlusions, and stenosis in a renal artery that arises from within an abdominal aortic aneurysm.

The degree to which a renal artery must be narrowed to induce a clinically relevant pathologic state has been greatly debated. Nonetheless, the goals for renal artery revascularization

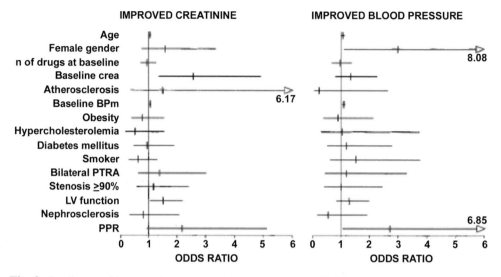

Fig. 3. Predictors of improved serum creatinine concentration **(left)** or improved mean arterial blood pressure **(right)** by multivariate logistic regression analysis. Graphs show odds ratios and their 95% confidence intervals. BPm = mean arterial blood pressure; crea = creatinine; PTRA = percutaneous transluminal renal angioplasty; LV = left ventricle function; PPR = parenchymal/pelvic ratio. (From ref. *38.*)

by PTA and stenting remain clear: (1) control of hypertension, (2) elimination of congestive heart failure/flash pulmonary edema, and (3) preservation or salvage of renal function.

Despite these clear goals, it is less clear which patients will have a favorable response to revascularization. In order to weigh the risks and benefits of a procedure, it is always desirable to identify patient characteristics that predict procedural benefit. Careful selection of patients for renal artery revascularization is even more critical, given that there is a subset of patients (10–20%) in whom renal function will worsen immediately following revascularization, presumably the result of cholesterol embolization or contrast toxicity *(6).* Based on past studies, certain factors have been considered predictors of successful outcome for PTA: (1) recent difficulty controlling of hypertension, (2) malignant hypertension (e.g., "end-organ" effects), (3) episodic flash pulmonary edema, (4) recent deteriorations in renal function, (5) azotemia in response to ACE inhibitors therapy, and (6) bilateral RAS (or unilateral RAS to a solitary kidney) *(25,36).* It has also been considered to be of lesser benefit to revascularize patients with (1) normal renal function, (2) unilateral RAS, (3) significant nephrosclerosis, or (4) diabetes mellitus *(37).*

A recent, prospective study by Zeller and colleagues specifically addressed the question of which baseline patient characteristics predict improvement of renal function after stenting of ostial ARAS *(38).* They found that among the characteristics that they examined, elevated serum creatinine and impaired left ventricular function were the only independent predictors of improved renal function. With respect to improved blood pressure control, the only independent predictors were female sex, preserved renal parenchymal thickness, and mean blood pressure at baseline (Fig. 3). Contrary to previous beliefs, PTA for bilateral ARAS was not predictive of improved renal function, and nephrosclerosis and diabetes mellitus were not associated with less favorable blood pressure and renal functional outcomes.

As a general rule, if renal failure and/or hypertension is the result of intrinsic kidney disease, a favorable clinical response to revascularization is less likely, no matter how tight the stenosis. Nonetheless, many patients, even with advanced nephrosclersosis, achieve a benefit from renal artery revascularization. One of the central challenges in managing patients with ARAS is the inability to discern how much intrinsic kidney disease is present and, more importantly, to predict what is the likelihood of a beneficial response to intervention. One index that might predict a less dramatic impact is the presence of a low parenchymal/pelvic ratio, as described by Zeller and colleagues. This ratio is often concordant with kidney atrophy to less than 7 or 8 cm in length, which is also assumed to be associated with less favorable outcome.

TECHNIQUE

Access. The approach toward renal artery cannulation can be from either femoral or brachial artery access. The choice should be made according to anatomical orientation of the arteries and the pathology of the adjacent structures, which can often be determined by preprocedure noninvasive imaging. Femoral access is most familiar to interventionalists, but could be precluded by an occluded abdominal aorta or could carry an increased procedural risk if there is a thrombus-laden abdominal aortic aneurysm or significant atheromatous disease just below the ostia of the renal arteries. Additionally, if the proximal renal artery is directed in an extreme inferior angulation, it might be difficult to achieve the coaxial catheter position needed to successfully deliver a stent. The brachial artery approach, however, has limitations as to the size of sheaths and catheters that can be accepted by the smaller artery, and manipulation of catheters is more difficult from this approach. It is also associated with more complications at the puncture site. Furthermore, brachial access is not protective against atheroembolism, which can involve the cerebral territory. Unless the aorta is occluded or unusually diseased or the renal artery origin is extremely angulated, most interventionalists prefer the femoral approach.

Diagnostic Angiography. Nonselective abdominal arteriography is recommended prior to selective canulation of the renal arteries. This is advantageous for several reasons: (1) Location of the renal artery ostia and identification of anatomical variations, such as accessory renal arteries, will guide the remainder of the procedure, and minimize catheter manipulation while searching for the ostia. (2) Orientation of the renal arteries to the aorta is important information in choosing the appropriate catheter shape and approach. (3) Defining the architecture of the abdominal aorta (e.g., atheromatous disease of the aorta or iliac arteries, abdominal aortic aneurysm, and overall appearance and size of the aorta) might be essential in formulating a strategy for successful canulation of the renal arteries and for minimizing complications. (4) Nonselective images might be sufficient to exclude significant RAS, thus eliminating the need for selective canulation.

Although a conventional pigtail catheter can be used for abdominal aortography, it can lead to retrograde flow of contrast and subsequent filling of the superior mesenteric artery (SMA) or celiac artery. This could cause overlap, thus obscuring of the origins of the renal arteries. In order to avoid filling these vessels, one can use a tennis racket /omni-flush-shaped catheter for a more lateral and less cephalad contrast flow. The appropriate positioning of these catheters is usually achieved when the top of the catheter aligns with the top of the first lumbar vertebral body. A "test puff" of dilute hand-injected contrast can be performed under fluouroscopy in order to confirm that the catheter is in the correct position.

Typically, 20–30 mL of iodinated contrast is injected at a rate between10 and 17 mL/s. In patients with significant renal insufficiency, the contrast can be diluted, such that only

10–15 mL are used for the aortogram. In severe renal failure, the aortogram can be performed using carbon dioxide (CO_2) rather than iodinated contrast. This can be accomplished by forceful hand-injection of the gas via a 60-mL syringe. Such an aortogram is not optimal for defining the architecture of the aorta, but it does locate the renal artery ostia quite sufficiently. Gadalinium can also be substituted for iodinated contrast, although it is more expensive and yields less optimal images.

Selective arteriography should be performed by careful (so as to minimze contact with the aortic wall) canulation of the renal artery with a soft-tipped diagnostic catheter that has a shape compatible with the vessel's orientation to the aorta (e.g., renal double curve [RDC], cobra, Judkins right 4, internal mammary, Sos omni, hockey stick, or multipurpose catheter). Once engaged, arteriography can be performed by hand-injections of contrast (Fig. 4A). A good renal arteriogram should also contain a baseline nephrogram, which should be compared to a postintervention image. A new defect in the nephrogram might indicate the presence of a subcapsular hematoma. It is not uncommon for the catheter to disengage during the diagnostic injection. Passing a small caliber (0.014-in.) soft-tip guide wire into the distal vessel will serve to anchor the catheter into the ostium during injection through a rotating "Y" adaptor. This will serve to improve angiogram quality and to avoid further catheter manipulation. Additionally, this could allow for the diagnostic catheter to be advanced across an ostial lesion in order to measure a baseline pressure gradient (Fig. 4B). If there is no gradient between the aorta and the renal artery beyond the lesion, then it is likely to be hemodynamically insignificant and should usually not be instrumented futher. A significant pressure gradient is, by convention, considered to be anything in excess of 10 mm Hg mean and/or 20 mm Hg peak, as measured through a 4 French catheter. If the stenosis is severe (>80%), the diagnostic catheter need not be advanced; the lesion is considered significant enough to warrant intervention.

Intervention. If there is a guide wire already across the lesion, the diagnostic catheter can be removed over the wire, and the guide catheter or shaped sheath can be positioned in its place. If there is difficulty with wire support, a "buddy" wire can be useful for the exchange. The guide can be "loaded" with a 4 French diagnostic or hydrophilic catheter by placing the smaller catheter through a rotating hemostatic Y adapter attached to the guide. This can minimize the trauma that might occur by advancing a larger French guide up the aorta alone. Once the smaller catheter engages the vessel, the guide can be transitioned into place. By using this coaxial technique, the guiding catheter itself is not manipulated within the abdominal aorta. The smaller catheter is then removed, leaving the guide wire in place and the guiding catheter situated close to the renal artery ostium. Care must be taken at this point, however, to maintain the guiding catheter in a coaxial position with respect to the guide wire and the renal artery.

Balloon angioplasty of the lesion can then be performed. In the case of ARAS and planned stenting, it is recommended to predilate the lesion with an undersized balloon. This is preferred for several reasons: (1) to facilitate stent delivery, (2) to identify a lesion that is "resistant" to dilatation (e.g., bulky, calcified lesions) and might benefit from rotational atherectomy prior to stent placement or (more rarely) consideration of a surgical alternative, (3) to aid in optimal size selection of the stent, by comparing to the diameter and length of the inflated balloon, and (4) to determine the optimal angulation of the C-arm to show the balloon most enlongated, thereby revealing the best view of the aorto-ostial junction. Because the renal arteries arise from the postero-lateral aspect of the aorta, this angle will often be slightly left anterior oblique (LAO) for the left renal artery and AP or slightly right

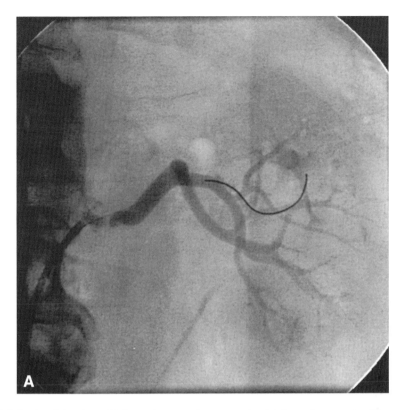

Fig. 4. (A) Selective injection of left renal artery, demonstrating high-grade stenosis; **(B)** measurement of significant pressure gradient across stenosis; **(C)** selective injection poststent; **(D)** resolution of pressure gradient poststent.

anterior oblique (RAO) for the right renal artery. The angle can vary, however, as a result of tortuosity, elongation, and/or ectasia within a diseased abdominal aorta. This technique avoids the contrast usage of optimizing the angle by multiple test injections. In the past, following predilation, the guide catheter was typically advanced atraumatically over the balloon during deflation, in order to position the guiding catheter beyond the lesion to facilitate delivery of bulky, stiff hand-mounted stents. This technique was necessary to "protect" the stent during delivery and to minimize the chance of stent dislodgment as the stent is advanced around a sharply angulated renal artery origin. With the current iteration of premounted, flexible, and low-profile stents, crossing the lesion with the guiding catheter is rarely required, although the technique is still useful at times. In the current era, the appropriately selected stent is delivered to the target site, with the guide maintained slightly retracted from the renal ostium. If the stent is advanced too distal during positioning, it could be "stripped" off of the balloon as it is pulled back to the lesion. After confirmation of appropriate stent position, taking into account the expected amount of foreshortening and the need to extend the stent 0.5–2 mm into the aorta (ostial lesions), the stent is deployed. During balloon inflation, the patient should be asked whether he or she has discomfort, such as back, flank, or abdominal pain. If so, this implies that the balloon might be oversized and further inflation to higher pressure should be avoided. If the pain persists after deflation of the balloon, immediate investigation for evidence of dissection/occlusion or rupture should ensue.

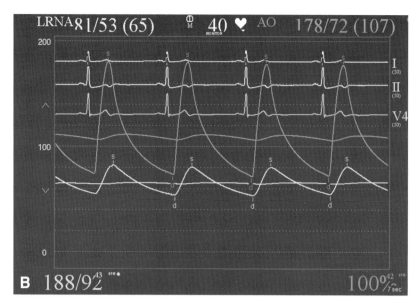

Fig. 4. *(Continued)*

The stent delivery balloon is then withdrawn into the guiding catheter. Care should be exercised not to disrupt the stent with the guiding catheter. If the guiding catheter migrates inferiorly into the aorta, withdrawing the stent delivery balloon will pull the catheter toward the ostium and potentially cause the guide catheter to crush the stent. There are two methods to keep the guide catheter coaxial to the stent and to avoid damage to the stent from occurring: (1) inflating the balloon to low pressure within the stent and gently advancing (transitioning) the guide over the balloon catheter as the balloon is withdrawn and (2) rotating the guide catheter in the axial plane approx 90° away from the ostium, then advancing it to the level of the renal while turning it back toward the ostium. A third method, that of advancing the guide while kicking it off the aortic wall by means of advancing the soft-tipped guide wire into the distal renal bed, can also be used, but carries with it a small chance of disrupting the distal renal vasculature.

Postdilation to high pressure can be performed (based on angiographic results, intravascular ultrasound [IVUS], or pressure gradient measurements), but care should be taken to avoid overdilation of the distal, nonstented vessel. Dissection beyond the stent can easily propagate into distal branches. Pressures can be measured to confirm elimination of the gradient, and final angiography is performed with careful attention to the distal vasculature and nephrogram, confirming that neither has changed from baseline (Figs. 4C and 4D). The guide catheter is then removed over a wire.

Periprocedural Care. Intravenous (IV) fluids should be given liberally before, during, and after the procedure, even if diuretics are also needed. Prior to the procedure, patients should be treated with aspirin. During the procedure, IV heparin, bivalirudin, or alternative thrombin inhibitor should be administered. If an intervention is performed, a goal activated clotting time (ACT) of 200–300 s should be achieved. Most interventionalist use a thiopyridine (e.g., clopridogrel) after stenting, although no data are available to support its use in renal artery interventions. The use of glycoprotein 2b3a inhibitors is also not established in renal artery interventions and, therefore, is not recommended at this time. Volume monitoring should be strict, as some patients have a significant postrevascularization diuresis

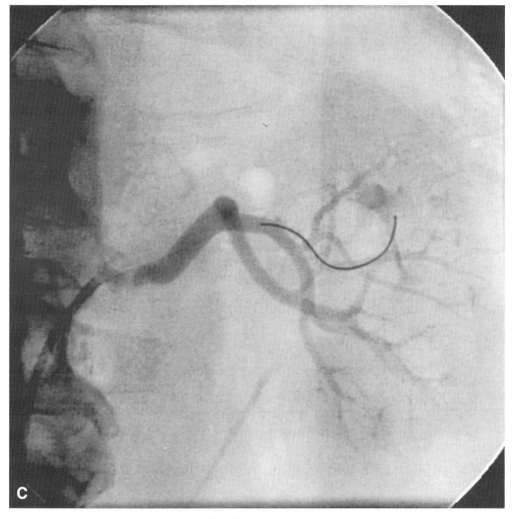

Fig. 4. *(Continued)*

and could become hypovolemic if this is not recognized. Blood pressure should also be closely monitored postprocedure. Occasionally, if antihypertensive medications are given prior to the procedure, hypotension could occur as the high-renin state recedes postrevascularization. Finally, the clinical response to renal artery revascularization could occur in a delayed fashion, over a 1–2 wk period. Therefore, blood pressure, creatinine, and medications should be reevaluated at 2–4 wk during follow-up.

Complications

Complications of percutaneous treatment of RAS have been reported to occur in 5–15% of patients and include atheroembolization, renal artery thrombosis, dissection or perforation, renal infarction, renal failure, subcapsular or retroperitoneal bleeding, and access site issues *(28,39,40)*. Additionally, there is a learning curve associated with the technical performance of PTA/stenting for RAS *(41)*. The complication of most concern is that of atheroembolism, which probably occurs more frequently than is clinically appreciated. Cholesterol embolization, into either renal vascular or peripheral vascular

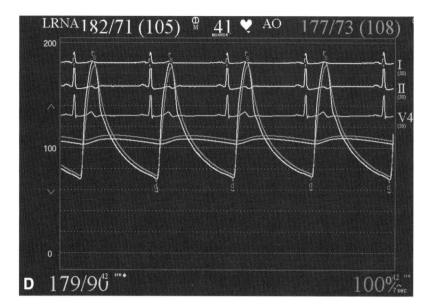

Fig. 4. *(Continued)*

beds, is more likely to occur with aggressive catheter manipulation. To minimize this, efforts should be made to study the nonselective images in order to avoid contact with the wall of the aorta when using to over-the-wire transitioning, telescoping of catheters, and "no-touch" techniques when engaging the ostia. Atheroembolization can be seen acutely or in a delayed fashion *(44)*. Clinical findings include blue toes, livedo reticularis, distal extremity pain, abdominal/flank/back pain, hematuria, accelerated hypertension, and renal failure. Extreme manifestations have included gangrene, nonhealing foot ulcers, spinal cord infarction, penile gangrene, and hematochezia. Cholesterol emboli can be associated with fever, elevated erythrocyte sedimentation rate, and peripheral eosinophilia. Other delayed findings include progressive rise in the serum creatinine and persistent hypertension despite adequate angiographic revascularization. There is no known effective treatment for the renal manifestations of cholesterol embolization. Adequate hydration is recommended, with the possible addition of sodium bicarbonate if there is severe rhabdomyolysis. Intravenous prostacyclin has been used for the treatment of lower extremity pain and ulceration resulting from cholesterol emboli *(42)*. Prevention of embolization to the renal vascular bed might be enhanced with the use of distal protection devices (balloon occlusion devices and filter wires).

Renal failure could also occur as a consequence of the toxic effects of radiographic dye. Because RAS patients are already at increased risk for dye-induced nephrotoxicity because of their underlying pathologic condition, they should be vigorously hydrated before, during, and after the procedure to avoid dye-related complications. Drugs with renal toxic effects should be avoided. The use of Mucomist to prevent toxic effects from the contrast dye has not yet been studied for renal procedures.

Renal artery dissection could lead to thrombosis or occlusion. Perforation through the distal renal artery into the renal parenchyma could be caused by the guide wire, with subsequent formation of a perinephric or subcapsular hematoma. The patient might have symptoms of flank or abdominal pain, nausea, and hypotension. Evidence of an expanding perinephric hematoma might by seen on the nephrogram initially as a local invagination that appears less "full" than preprocedure. At later stages, the distal vascular tree will appear "compressed" as a result of the space-occupying hematoma and impaired filling of the capillary bed. Heparin should be reversed with protamine, and close hemodynamic monitoring is required. Balloon occlusion of a proximal vessel can be used to curtail blood loss. Surgical consultation is recommended, as urgent surgery might be required. Rupture of the body of the renal artery is infrequent but might occur from balloon oversizing. This complication usually requires urgent surgical repair, although covered stents might be useful.

Restenosis

Restenosis after stenting of ARAS occurs in 10–25% of patients. In-stent restenosis is initially best managed by repeat balloon angioplasty. Use of a relatively long balloon or a cutting balloon might be preferred in order to avoid a "watermelon seed" effect. Caution must be exercised to avoid edge dissections, which can easily propagate into the distal renal artery. IVUS guidance for appropriate balloon sizing might be prudent in this lesion subset. Stenting within a stent can be performed in circumstances where recoil is severe; however, the long-term outcome of this approach is unknown. There is currently no data for the employment either debulking strategies (i.e., atherectomy), drug-eluting stents, or brachytherapy, although all strategies have been used successfully in anecdotal cases.

Outcomes

Although the beneficial effects of renal artery stenting have been evident for years, the use of stents for ARAS was only approved by the Food and Drug Administration (FDA) in July 2002 (43). This is, perhaps, a reflection on the paucity of prospective randomized trials comparing alternative treatments. In a comprehensive assessment of prior (mainly older) studies, only 10% of patients with renovascular hypertension were "cured," but almost 50% required less medication to control their blood pressure (44). At 1 yr, over 60% continued to have improved or "cured" hypertension. Additionally, in patients with azotemia from RAS, approx 30% experienced improvement and almost 50% achieved stabilization of their renal function after stenting. Although clinical outcomes were similar between percutaneous and surgical revascularization, major complications were about twice as frequent in the surgical group. In a cost-effectiveness analysis, they found stenting to be roughly twice as expensive as PTA, but surgery was 15 times more than PTA. Their analysis confirmed the accepted preference for the percutaneous approach.

Future Directions

Although there is a large body of data supporting stenting for ARAS, prospective, randomized clinical trials are clearly still needed. The National Institutes of Health (NIH)-funded Cardiovascular Outcomes for Renal Atherosclerotic Lesions Trial (CORAL) will examine the effect on major cardiovascular events (e.g., death, myocardial infarction [MI], stroke, renal failure) of combined stenting with best medical therapy versus best medical therapy alone for patients with hypertension and RAS. Other trials in progress or planned will examine the potential benefits of drug eluting stents (GREAT Trial) and distal embolic protection.

Summary

Advances in device technology, refinement in technique, and better understanding of the deleterious consequences of renal artery disease have all led to a large increase in the performance of renal artery stenting procedures. The technique is associated with a learning curve and must be performed with caution and in appropriately selected patients. Ongoing trials and basic research will enhance our understanding of this complex disorder and help to further delineate the role of newer devices and the indications and potential benefit in specific subsets of patients.

AORTO-ILIAC OBSTRUCTIVE DISEASE

Background

Most disease in the infrarenal abdominal aorta and iliac arteries is atherosclerotic in origin. The pathophysiology of atherosclerosis of the peripheral arteries is identical to that of coronary atherosclerosis and is associated with the same risk factors of tobacco smoking, diabetes mellitus, hypertension, and hyperlipidemia.

The prevalence of peripheral arterial obstructive disease is less than 3% in those under 60 yr but is more than 20% in those over 75 yr of age *(45)*. However, the prevalence of atherosclerotic disease of the lower extremeties is underestimated in the general population, as the process might exist in an asymptomatic form for many years. After the superficial femoral artery, the terminal aorta and iliac arteries are the most common site for atherosclerotic involvement. Diabetics tend to develop more tibioperoneal disease, a similar degree of femoropopliteal disease and possibly less aorto-iliac disease compared to the nondiabetic population. Diabetics also have a greater likelihood of developing critical limb ischemia and have a 12-fold increase risk of requiring an amputation *(46)*.

The natural history of symptomatic peripheral arterial obstructive disease is variable. Over 5–10 yr, without intervention, 70% or more patients report no interval change or an improvement in their symptoms, 20–30% have progressive symptoms requiring intervention, and less than 10% need amputation. There is, however, an up to a threefold increase in morbidity and mortality in patients with symptomatic peripheral arterial obstructive disease that is related to concomitant coronary and cerebrovascular disease *(47)*.

Leriche first recognized the effects of impaired inflow at the level of the terminal aorta and iliac arteries in his classic 1923 publication *(48)*. Surgical revascularization for aorto-iliac disease began with endarterectomy in the 1940s and bypass surgery in the 1950s. Nearly two decades later, in 1979, Gruentzig and Kumpe described their experience with balloon angioplasty of iliac lesions, which yielded an 87% patency rate at 2 yr *(49)*. Since then, the percutaneous approach has been applied not just to aorto-iliac disease, but to atherosclerotic disease at every site in the body. Nowhere, however, are the results superior to those achieved at the site originally selected by Gruentzig—the aorto-iliac vessels.

Clinical Presentation

Clinical symptoms of obstructive arterial disease do not usually develop until the arterial lumen is narrowed by at least 50%. Symptoms, such as intermittent claudication, will also depend on the presence or absence of collateral arterial supply and the severity of distal disease. Claudication is usually described as an ache, pain, tightness, or soreness involving the calf, hip, buttocks, or arch of the foot on ambulation and relieved with rest. With progressive aorto-iliac disease, pain in the buttock, hip, thigh, and even the low back, mimicking degenerative joint disease of the lumbosacral spine, could develop. With involvement of the internal iliac (hypogastric) arteries, symptoms

Table 1
Clinical Categories of Chronic Limb Ischemia

Grade	Category	Clinical description	Objective criteria
0	0	Asymptomatic	Normal treadmill/stress test
	1	Mild claudication	Completes treadmill exercise[a] ankle pressure after exercise <50 mm Hg but >25 mm Hg less than brachial
I	2	Moderate claudication	Between categories 1 and 3
	3	Severe claudication	Cannot complete treadmill exercise and ankle pressure after exercise <50 mm Hg
II	4	Ischemic rest pain	Resting ankle pressure <60 mm Hg, ankle or metatarsal pulse volume recording flat or barely pulsatile; toe pressure <40 mm Hg
	5	Minor tissue loss–nonhealing ulcer, focal gangrene with diffuse pedal ischemia	Resting ankle pressure <40 mm Hg, flat or barely pulsatile ankle or pulse volume recording; toe pressure <30 mm Hg
III	6	Major tissue loss–extending above transmetatarsal level, functional foot no longer salvageable	Same as category 5

[a]Five min at 2 mph on a 12% incline.
Source: Adapted from ref. *50.*

of impotence could also occur. With progression of disease and more advanced ischemia, rest pain develops where the metabolic demands of the skin, muscle, and other tissues at rest are not met by the existing blood supply to the affected limb. Tissue necrosis manifest as painful skin ulceration and frank gangrene could develop. Rutherford and colleagues developed a classification for chronic limb ischemia (Table1) *(50).*

Physical examination findings could include the presence of abdominal and femoral bruits and diminished femoral, popliteal, pedal pulses. The level at which there is diminution of the pulse allows some estimation on the level of the arterial obstruction. Pallor of the feet and dependent rubor as well as trophic skin changes—thin, hairless, pale, cool skin with slow capillary return—might be found. With critical limb ischemia, there may be absent capillary return and skin marbling, tenderness, edema of the affected region, ulceration, and gangrene.

Although intermittent claudication is the most common presentation of peripheral arterial obstructive disease, acute limb ischemia is another possible and often dramatic presentation. Acute limb usually occurs as a result of embolic occlusion of either a diseased or nondiseased vessel. This can result from a cardioembolic source, *in situ* thrombosis of a diseased vessel, or spontaneous thrombosis in the setting of a hypercoagulable state. Clinical features include a cold, pale, pulseless limb. The limb is painful and develops paresthesias and, finally, motor dysfunction or paralysis.

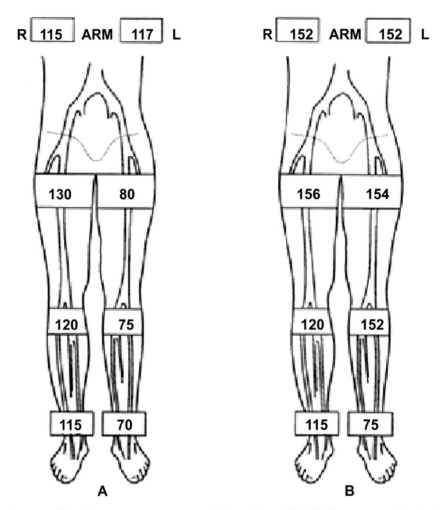

Fig. 5. Segmental blood pressure measurement. (Adapted from Wilt TJ. Current strategies in the diagnosis and management of lower extremity peripheral vascular disease. J Gen Intern Med 1992;7:91.)

Noninvasive Investigation

SEGMENTAL DOPPLER PRESSURES AND PULSE VOLUME RECORDINGS

Segmental Doppler pressure assessments at the thigh, calf, and ankle compared with the brachial pressure can be measured, initially at rest and subsequently with exercise (Fig. 5). Comparing arm pressure to thigh, calf, and ankle pressures gives a systolic pressure index that can then be used to delineate the level of obstruction in either inflow (aorto-iliac), outflow (femoro-popliteal), or runoff (tibio-peroneal) vessels. An ankle brachial index (ABI) of 0.85 or more is associated with asymptomatic PAD. An ABI of 0.5–0.8 is associated with intermittent claudication and a values below 0.5 are usually associated with rest pain, critical limb ischemia, and a threatened limb.

In conjuction with segmental Doppler pressure measurements, pulse volume recordings are a useful noninvasive method of assessing arterial flow. With arterial obstruction, the arterial wave form becomes more rounded and of a lower amplitude and there is loss of the dicrotic notch. Pulse volume recordings are particularly useful in the setting of calcified, noncompressible lower extremity vessels where segmental Doppler pressure measurements are not accurate.

IMAGING

Noninvasive imaging by gadolinium-enhanced magnetic resonance angiography (MRA) is helpful in defining disease severity and anatomical location *(51)*. It is also useful in the development of a percutaneous revascularization strategy with regard to planning whether access should be ipsilateral or contralalteral to the site of the lesion. Because MRA with gadolinium also obviates the need to give an iodinated contrast load, as would be needed for CT angiography, it is becoming an increasingly important imaging modality (Fig. 6).

Duplex ultrasound scanning is also a useful modality to noninvasively assess PAD severity and anatomic location of stenoses. With a skilled operator, the arterial tree can be imaged from the abdominal aorta to the proximal crural vessels *(45)*.

Treatment of Aorta-Iliac Disease

MEDICAL THERAPY

The management of patients with aorto-iliac and other lower extremity obstructive arterial disease is based on the appropriate modification of cardiovascular risk factors and symptom control with a combination of exercise programs, pharmacotherapy, and revascularization where appropriate. Cessation of tobacco use, control of lipids, blood sugar, and blood pressure should be undertaken with appropriate lifestyle and pharmacotherapeutic interventions. Antiplatelet therapy should be administered with aspirin or Clopidogrel *(52,53)*. Pentoxifylline, by improving red blood cell deformability as well as lowering fibrinogen levels and a mild antiplatelet effect, has shown some improvement over placebo in increasing walking distance *(54)*. The phosphodiesterase inhibitor Cilostazol has antiplatelet and vasodilatory properties, which improve walking distance and quality of life over placebo *(53)*.

Exercise programs are important and were traditionally the mainstay of therapy for those with only mild to moderate claudication (Rutherford category 1 and 2). Exercise can promote the development of collaterals, improve skeletal muscle capillary density, and cause metabolic adaptations. Finally, endovascular revascularization, with its low morbidity and mortality, can offer prompt relief of symptoms.

INDICATIONS FOR REVASCULARIZATION

The major indications for aorto-iliac revascularizations are as follows:

1. Relief of symptomatic lower extremity ischemia, including claudication, rest pain, ulceration or gangrene, or embolization
2. Restoration and/or preservation of inflow to the lower extremity in the setting of pre-existing or anticipated distal bypass
3. Procurement of access to more proximal vascular beds for anticipated invasive procedures (e.g., cardiac catheterization/PTCA, intra-aortic balloon insertion).

REVASCULARIZATION STRATEGY: ENDOVASCULAR VERSUS SURGERY

Current surgical options for aorto-iliac disease include aortobifemoral bypass surgery, aorto-iliac endarterectomy, and fem-fem bypass. The endovascular options for treatment are PTA alone or PTA and stent. Aortobifemoral bypass and variants thereof have been considered to be the "gold standard" for revascularization of the aorto-iliac vessels. The

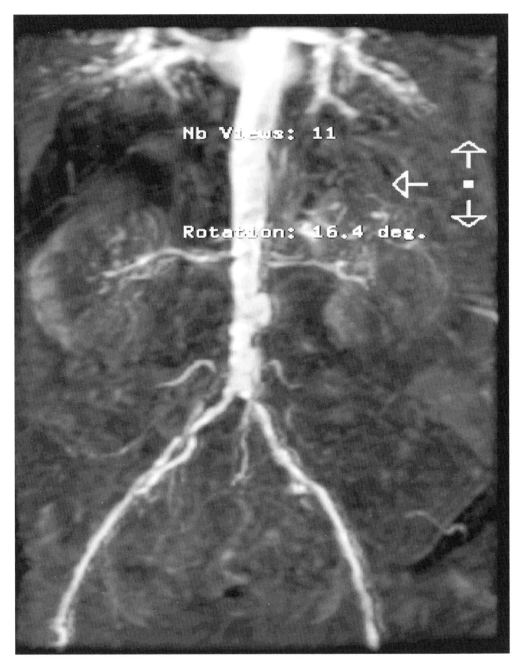

Fig. 6. Gadolinium-enhanced MRA of the abdominal aorta and iliac arteries showing severe atherosclerotic disease of the aorto-iliac bifurcation and infra-renal aorta with a deep plaque ulcer in the infrarenal aorta.

TASC group found the 1-, 3-, and 5-yr patency of aorto-iliac surgical reconstruction to be 89%, 86% and 86% respectively. This compared with data collected contemporaneously in a group of patients treated with iliac stenting that showed patency rates of 85%, 72% and 64% for 1-, 3-, and 5-yr patency, respectively *(52)*.

However, the better long-term patency rate with surgery is associated with an increased mortality and morbidity compared to an endovascular approach. These patients, with a high likelihood of coexisting coronary artery disease, have a mortality rate between 1.6% and 3.3% and a morbidity of approx 8–10% with surgical revascularization *(57–60)*. Accordingly, the threshold for surgical intervention has remained high, reserved for patients with critical limb ischemia or advanced degrees of disability (Rutherford category 3 or above).

ENDOVASCULAR INTERVENTION

Most aortic disease is nonfocal and involves the aortic bifurcation and iliac arteries. As the merits of PTA and stenting have become evident over the years, revascularization strategies for this disease have evolved and practice patterns have changed significantly. Nonetheless, considerable controversy remains in some circles concerning the "optimal" treatment *(61)*. Interventionalists generally support a primary strategy of angioplasty and stenting. Vascular surgeons generally support a more traditional approach of "definitive" revascularization with aortobifemoral bypass, especially in young patients or those with advanced or diffuse disease. The TASC group has recommended an endovascular approach for Type A lesions, with Type B and C lesions having insufficient data to recommend endovascular therapy over surgery. With complex aorto-iliac disease (Type D) lesions, surgery was recommended *(62)*.

The results of balloon angioplasty alone for iliac stenoses, particularly focal lesions, are excellent, with acute technical and clinical success in excess of 90% *(63,64)*. The 1-, 3-, and 5-yr patency rates are in the of range approx 75–95%, 60–90%, and 55–85%, respectively. The wide ranges of these results reflects variations in selection criteria, discrepancies in measurements of outcome, and the evolution of technique over time.

Several factors have been identified that affect short- and long-term patency. Factors associated with good results include short, focal lesions, large vessel size, common iliac (as opposed to external iliac), single lesion (as opposed to multiple serial lesions), male gender, lower Rutherford category (claudication as opposed to critical limb ischemia), and presence of good runoff. The results in patients with diffuse disease, smaller vessels, diabetes mellitus, female gender, critical limb ischemia, poor runoff, and total occlusions are less favorable. Nonetheless, patients in these categories might still benefit from PTA as the initial strategy.

In 1993, the FDA approved the use of Palmaz balloon expandable stents (P-308 series) for iliac arteries. Specific indications were for failed PTA, defined as a residual mean gradient of greater than or equal to 5 mm Hg, residual stenosis of more than 30%, or presence of a flow limiting dissection *(65)*. The self-expanding Wallstent prosthesis was approved for similar indications in 1996 *(66)*. There are a number of both balloon-expandable and self-expanding stents now available that are appropriate for use in the treatment of aorto-iliac obstructive disease. A recent randomized trial comparing one of the newer self-expanding nitinol stents (S.M.A.R.T. stent) with a stainless-steel self-expanding Wallstent for the treatment of aorto-iliac disease, showed that, at 12 mo, both stents were very efficacious. Vessel patency was 95% for the nitinol self-expanding stent and 91% for the Wallstent. There was a higher procedural success rate for the nitinol stent versus the Wallstent (98% vs 88%) which was largely the result of the ability to place the nitinol stent more accurately *(67)*. With regard to balloon-expandable versus self-expanding stents in the treatment of ostial common iliac stenoses and where kissing stents are needed to reconstruct the aorto-iliac bifurcation, many prefer to use balloon-expandable stents, as they offer the greatest radial strength and the most precision in placement. Other have had success with self-extracting stents.

The favorable acute results (>90%), relative ease of use, paucity of complications, and high long-term patency (75% at 3 yr) observed with aorto-iliac stenting has led to expanded use of these devices. Many interventionalists have adopted a strategy of primary stent deployment for aortoiliac vessels. However, in a randomized trial of balloon angioplasty with provisional stenting versus primary stenting for aorto-iliac disease, Tetteroo and colleagues demonstrated that a strategy of "selective" or "provisional" stenting might be appropriate (63).

The most compelling evidence in favor of primary stenting comes from Bosch and Hunink (64), who performed metanalysis on 14 recent studies (all published after 1990) involving more than 2100 patients undergoing aorto-iliac PTA. The meta-analysis showed greater immediate success rate for stents than for PTA alone (96% vs 91%). For patients with claudication, the 4-yr primary patency rate for *stenotic* lesions was 77% for stenting and 65% for PTA alone. For *occlusions*, 4-yr patency rates were 61% for stents and 54% for PTA. Thus, stenting yielded better acute results and, furthermore, reduced the risk of 4-yr failure by nearly 40% over PTA alone. For complex aorto-iliac stenoses and for occlusions, stenting is the primary therapy preferred by most interventionalists.

ENDOVASCULAR TECHNIQUE

Prior to undertaking aorto-iliac PTA, careful consideration should be given to the issue of arterial access. With unilateral disease that ends above the common femoral artery, ispilateral retrograde access provides the simplest approach with the best mechanical advantage to facilitate stent deployment to the stenotic (or occlusive) lesion. The contralateral approach using "crossover" sheaths, such as the Balkan sheath and guiding catheters, is selected in cases where the lesion is located near the common femoral artery. The contralateral approach is also employed where the ipsilateral groin is either scarred or in cases where there is particular concern about impeding the "outflow" during sheath removal, after revascularizing an iliac lesion. In addition, if more distal revascularization is to be pursued in the same sitting, then a contralateral approach is necessary. Contralateral access should be avoided in cases of acutely angulated aortic bifurcations and for stenoses at the origin of the common iliac artery. For iliac occlusions, either retrograde or contralateral access is appropriate and, frequently, both are required to successfully recanalize occluded segments (Fig. 7). The ability to advance stents over angulated bifurcations has been greatly enhanced by two factors: first, the availability of contralateral sheaths and, second, the availability of more flexible stents, both of the self-expanding and balloon-expandable variety.

For lesions involving the aortic bifurcation, a bilateral retrograde femoral approach is recommended in order to enable placement of "kissing stents" (Fig. 8). Although bifurcation stenting using a kissing stent technique is the treatment advocated for aorto-iliac bifurcation disease, this does come at the cost of a technically more challenging procedure, compromise of subsequent contralateral access and an unknown long-term outcome. Haulon and colleagues reported that of 106 patients treated with aortic bifurcation kissing stents, the primary and secondary patency rates at 3 yr were 79% and 98%, respectively. Of the 18 patients needing repeat revascularization, 17 of the 18 patients were able to be treated with repeat endovascular intervention and only 1 needed to have aortobifemoral bypass (68).

Occasionally, brachial access can be useful for patients with aortic occlusion or, for example, a target lesion that involves the distal iliac artery in one leg (near the femoral head), with the coexistent occlusion of the contralateral iliac (precluding a contralateral approach).

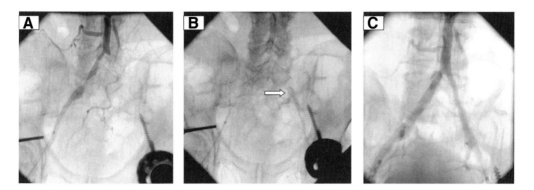

Fig. 7. (**A**) Left common iliac occlusion. A stenosis of the right common iliac is also seen. (**B**) Late filling of the left external iliac via collaterals (white arrow). A stenosis of the distal right common iliac is also seen. (**C**) After PTA and stenting of the left and right common iliac arteries.

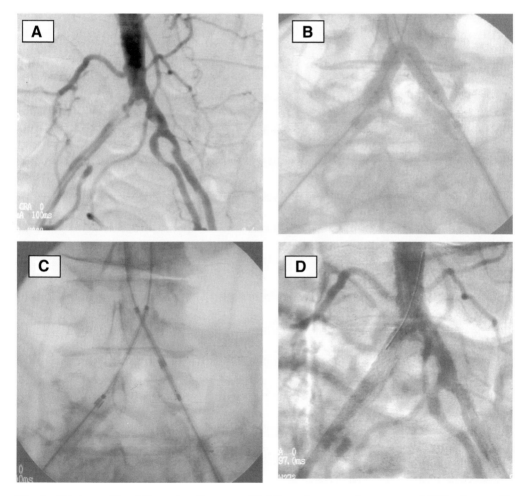

Fig. 8. (**A**) Aorto-iliac bifurcation diesease; (**B**) bilateral retrograde access and PTA of aorto-iliac bifurcation; (**C**) "kissing stent" technique using ballon-expandable stents to reconstruct the aortic bifurcation; (**D**) final result.

Pressure gradients are routinely measured across iliac and aortic lesions. In spite of their regular use, objective data regarding what constitutes a significant hemodynamic stenosis do not yet exist. By convention, most interventionalists use a threshold of 5 mm Hg mean resting pressure gradient as indicative of a significant residual stenosis. If the resting gradient is borderline, administration of a vasodilator (100–300 mg of nitroglycerin or 25 mg of papaverine) and induction of a mean pressure gradient of more than 15 mm Hg is considered significant. It is advisable to obtain pressure gradients routinely following aortoiliac intervention; it is not uncommon that a residual gradient will uncover an occult stenosis that was not well defined on the uniplanar completion angiogram (Fig. 9).

Intravascular ultrasound (IVUS) can be of great utility during aortoiliac angioplasty. Not only can IVUS detect plaque and other details that are angiographically "silent," but it also can identify with great accuracy the dimensions of the reference site, the degree of narrowing, and the characteristics of the vessel wall (e.g., calcium) *(69,70)*.

AORTOILIAC PTA IN CONJUNCTION WITH SURGERY

Many patients with aortoiliac disease also have infra-inguinal disease. In such cases, the aorto-iliac disease is treated first, based on the premise that improving inflow might secondarily improve outflow augmenting perfusion pressure to the distal segments. This might obviate the need for reconstruction more distally. Implicit in this strategy is the lesser degree of technical difficulty, high rate of procedural success, and low incidence of restenosis associated with aorto-iliac PTA, in comparison to that for more distal segments. The same strategy underlies the preparatory role of iliac angioplasty in patients undergoing surgical revascularization for treatment of distal disease. As surgeons become more proficient in endovascular techniques, they are bringing these techniques into the operating room and employing them in conjunction with more conventional bypass procedures. There are several reports now describing the technique of common femoral artery cutdown, intraoperative balloon angioplasty, and stent deployment of iliac arteries, followed by fem-pop or fem-fem bypass. Revascularization can be staged with proximal PTA first, followed by surgery some 3–4 wk later. This approach is a natural extension of the use of endovascular techniques to minimize morbidity and mortality and maximize the benefit for the patient.

Complications

Complications are relatively infrequent with aorto-iliac angioplasty (less than 6% based on multiple series). Most common are access site complications, including local or retroperitoneal bleeding, pseudoaneurysm, and AV fistula. At the site of angioplasty, thrombotic occlusion is extremely rare, as is rupture. The latter, however, can have devastating consequences. This, as well as retroperitoneal bleeding, can be fatal if not controlled. Arterial rupture must be recognized promptly and controlled by inflation of a balloon within the lesion (balloon tamponade), reversal of anticoagulation, and volume resuscitation. Surgery might be required infrequently (approx 2%). In the future, stent-grafts might be readily available to treat this complication. Other complications include distal embolization, which was said to occur with alarming frequency in early studies of recanalized total iliac occlusion. More recent studies indicate an incidence of less than 5% *(71)*. Systemic complications, such as contrast or atheroembolic-induced renal failure, myocardial infarction, cardio vascular accedent (CVA), and death all occur with very low frequency, less than 0.5%.

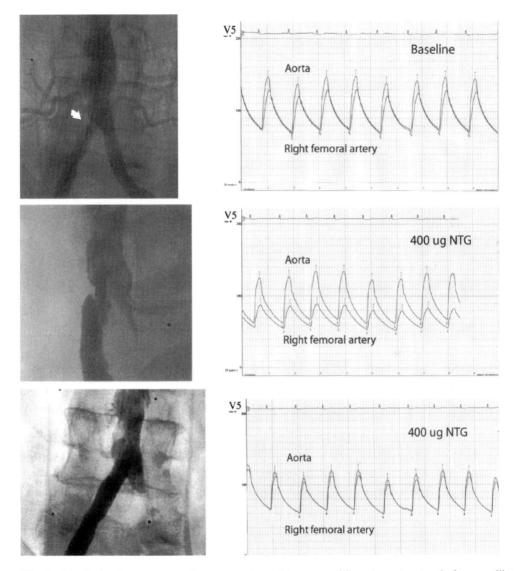

Fig. 9. Translesional pressure gradients across the right common iliac artery at rest and after vasodilator administration before and after stent placement.

Summary

In summary, endovascular revascularization represents the first line of invasive therapy for aorto-iliac obstructive disease. With the exception of patients with very extensive disease, PTA with or without stent deployment is associated with a highly successful acute and long-term outcome. Furthermore, in the event that this strategy fails, subsequent surgical intervention remains feasible. In the guidelines for peripheral PTA published by the AHA in 1994 *(72)*, four categories of iliac disease were described. Category 1 included stenoses of less than 3 cm in length, concentric and noncalcified, for which PTA is recommended. Category 2 include stenoses 3–5 cm in length or calcified or eccentric stenoses less than 3 cm in length. For these, PTA was also felt to be well suited. For category 3 lesions, stenoses 5–10 cm in length or occlusions of less than 5 cm in length, it was recommended that PTA could be performed but that the initial chance of technical success or long-term benefit might not be as good as with bypass surgery. However, PTA as a first approach might be indicated in these patients, depending on the patient risk-factor profile. Category 4 lesions included stenoses greater than 10 cm in length, occlusion greater than 5 cm in length, extensive bilateral aortoiliac atherosclerosis, or lesions in association with abdominal aortic aneurysm or other lesion requiring surgical repair. For category 4 lesions, the percutaneous approach was not recommended. In the future, it is likely that these guidelines will continue to evolve as technological improvements extend the benefits of percutaneous stenting.

REFERENCES

1. American Heart Association. Heart disease and stroke statistics—2004 update. Dallas, TX: American Heart Association, 2003.
2. Valentive RJ, et al. Coronary artery disease is highly prevalent among patients with premature peripheral vascular disease. J Vasc Surg 1994;19(4):668–674, Apr.
3. Coffman JD. Intermittent claudication-be conservative. N Engl J Med 1991;325:577–578.
4. Beller GA, Bonow RO, Fuster V, et al. ACC revised recommendations for training in adult cardiovascular medicine core cardiology training II (COCATS 2) (revision of the 1995 COCATS Training Statement). 2002.
5. Conlon PJ, Little MA, Pieper K, Mark DB. Severity of renal vascular disease predicts mortality in patients undergoing coronary angiography. Kidney Int 2001;60:1490–1497.
6. Textor SC, Wilcox CS. Ischemic nephropathy/azotemic renovascular disease. Semin Nephrol 2000;20(5):489–502.
7. Caps MT, Zierler RE, Polissar NL, et al. Risk of atrophy in kidneys with atherosclerotic renal artery stenosis. Kidney Int 1998;53:735–742.
8. Sarnak MJ, Levey AS, Schoolwerth AC, et al. Kidney disease as a risk factor for development of cardiovascular disease: a statement from the American Heart Association Councils on Kidney in Cardiovascular Disease, High Blood Pressure Research, Clinical Cardiology, and Epidemiology and Prevention. Hypertension 2003;42:1050–1065.
9. Foley RN, Parfrey PS, Sarnak MJ. Clinical epidemiology of cardiovascular disease in chronic renal disease. Am J Kidney Dis 1998;32:S112–S119.
10. Gruntzig A, Kuhlmann U, Lutolf U, et al. Treatment of renovascular hypertension with percutaneous transluminal dilation of a renal-artery stenosis. Lancet 1978;1:801–802.
11. Rudd P, Dzau VJ. Hypertension: Evaluation and Management. In: (Loscalzo, Creager, Dzau, eds.), Vascular medicine: a textbook of vascular biology and diseases, 2nd ed. Boston; Little, Brown and Company, 1996.
12. Harrison EG, McCormac LJ. Pathologic classification of renal artery disease in renovascular hypertension. Mayo Clin Proc 1971;46:161–167.
13. Klinge J, Mail Wp, Puijlaert CB, et al. Percutaneous translumenal renal angioplasty: initial and long-term results. Radiology 1989;171:501.
14. Cluzel P, Raynaud A, Beyssen B, et al. Stenoses of renal branch arteries in fibromuscluar dysplasia: results of percutaneous transluminal angioplasty. Radiology 1994;193:227–232.
15. Rimmer JM, Gennari, FJ. Atherosclerotic renovascular disease and progressive renal failure. Ann Intern Med 1993;118:712–719.
16. Libertino JA, Flam TA, Zinman, LN, et al. Changing concepts in surgical management of renovascular hypertension. Arch Intern Med 1988;148:357–359.
17. Messina LM, Zelenock GB, Yao KA, Stanley JC. Renal revascularization for recurrent pulmonary edema in patients with poorly controlled hypertension and renal insufficiency. J Vasc Surg 1992;15:73–82.
18. Libertino JA, Bosco PJ, Ying CY, et al. Renal revascularization to preserve and restore renal function. J Urol 1992;147:1485–1487.
19. Weibull H, Bergqvist D, Bergentz S, et al. Percutaneous transluminal renal angioplasty versus surgical reconstruction of atherosclerotic renal artery stenosis: a prospective randomized study. J Vasc Surg 1993;18:841–852.
20. Sos TA, Pickering TG, Phil D. Percutaneous transluminal renal angioplasty in renovascular hypertension due to atheroma or fibromuscular dysplasia. N Engl J Med 1983;309:274–279.
21. Tegtmeyer CJ, Dyer R, Teates CD, et al. Percutaneous transluminal dilatation of the renal arteries. Radiology 1980;135:589–599.

22. Sos TA Angioplasty for the treatment of azotemia and renovascular hypertension in atherosclerotic renal artery disease. Circ 1991;83(Suppl I):I-162–I-166.

23. Rees CR, Palmaz JC, Becker GJ, et al. Palmaz stent in atherosclerotic stenoses involving the ostia of the renal arteries: preliminary report of a multicenter study. Radiology 1991;181:507–514.

24. Dorros G, Jaff M, Jain A, et al. Follow-up of primary palmaz & Chatz stent placement for atherosclerotic renal artery stenosis. Am J Cardiol 1995;75:1051–1055.

25. White CJ, Ramee SR, Collins TJ, et al. Renal artery stent placement: utility in lesions difficult to treat with balloon angioplasty. J Am Coll Cardiol 1997;30:1445–1450.

26. Blum U, Krumme B, Flugel P, et al. Treatment of ostial renal-artery stenoses with vascular endoprostheses after unsuccessful balloon angioplasty. N Engl J Med 1997;336:459–465.

27. Rundback JH, Gray RJ, Rozenblit G, et al. Renal artery stent placement for the management of ischemic nephropathy. J Vasc Interv Radiol 1998;9(3):413–420.

28. van de Ven PJ, Kaatee R, Beutler JJ, et al. Arterial stenting and balloon angioplasty in ostial atherosclerotic renovascular disease: a randomised trial. Lancet 1999;353:282–286.

29. Lim ST, Rosenfield K. Renal artery stent placement: indications and results. Curr. Intervent Cardiol Rep 2000;2:130–139.

30. Oei HY, Geyskes GG, Mees EJ, Puylaert CB. The significance of captopril renography in renovascular hypertension. Contrib Nephrol 1987;56:95–103.

31. Setaro JF, Chen CC, Hoffer PB, Black HR. Captopril renography in the diagnosis of renal artery stenosis and the prediction of improvement with revascularization: the Yale Vascular Center experience. Am J Hypertens 1991;4:698S–705S.

32. Olin JW, Piedmonte MR, Young JR, et al. The utility of duplex ultrasound scanning of the renal arteries for diagnosing significant renal artery stenosis. Ann Intern Med 1995;122:833–838.

33. Gedroyc WMW, Neerhut P, Negus R, et al. Magnetic resonance angiography of renal artery stenosis. Clin Radiol 1995;50:436–439.

34. Beregi JP, Elkohen M, Deklunder G, et al. Helical CT angiography compared with arteriography in the detection of renal artery stenosis. Am J Roentgenol 1996;167:495–501.

35. Qanadli SD, Soulez G, Therasse E, et al. Detection of renal artery stenosis: prospective comparison of captopril-enhanced Doppler sonography, captopril-enhanced scintigraphy, and MR angiography. Am J Roentgenol 2001;177(5):1123–1129.

36. Harden PN, Macleod MJ, Rodgers RS, et al. Effect of renal-artery stenting on progression of renovascular renal failure. Lancet 1997;349:1133–1136.

37. Palmaz JC. The current status of vascular intervention in ischemic nephropathy. J Vasc Intervent Radiol 1998;9:539.

38. Zeller T, Frank U, Müller C, et al. Predictors of improved renal function after percutaneous stent-supported angioplasty of severe atherosclerotic ostial renal artery stenosis. Circulation 2003;108:2244–2249.

39. Isles CG, Robertson S, Hill D. Management of renovascular disease: a review of renal artery stenting in ten studies. Q J Med 1999;92:159–167.

40. Lederman RJ, Mendelsohn FO, Santos R, et al. Primary renal artery stenting: characteristics and outcomes after 363 procedures. Am Heart J 2001;142:314–323.

41. Beek FJ, Kaatee R, Beutler JJ, et al. Complications during renal artery stent placement for atherosclerotic ostial stenosis. Cardiovasc Intervent Radiol 1997;20:184–190.

42. Ramos R, Cruzado JM, Palom X, et al. Cholesterol embolism associated with macroscopic renal infarction. Nephrol Dial Transplant 1999;14:962–965.

43. Tillman DB. Letter of approval for Cordis PALMAZ Balloon Expandable Stent. Department of Health and Human Services, July 10, 2002.

44. Kandarpa K, Becker GJ, Hunink MG, et al. Transcatheter interventions for the treatment of peripheral atherosclerotic lesions: part I. J Vasc Intervent Radiol 2001;12:683–695.

45. Halperin JL, Creager MA. Arterial obstructive diseases of the extremities. In: Loscalzo J, Creager MA, Dzau, VJ. eds. Boston: Vascular medicine: a textbook of vascular biology and diseases. Little, Brown and Company, 1996:825–852.

46. Humphrey LL, Palumbo PJ, Butters MA, et al. The contributuion of non-insulin dependent diabetes to lower-extremity amputation in the community. Archi Intern Med 1994;154:885–892.

47. Weitz J, Byrne J, Clagett P, et al. AHA scientific statement: diagnosis and treatment chronic arterial insufficiency of the lower extremeties: a critical review. Circulation 1996;94:3026–3049.

48. Leriche, R. Des obliterations arterielles hautes (obliteration de la terminaison de l'aorte) come causes des insuffances circulatoires des membres inferieurs. Bull Mem Soc Chir 1923;1404.

49. Gruntzig A, Kumpke DA. Technique of percutaneous transluminal angioplasty with the Gruntzig balloon catheter. Am J Roentgenol 1979;132:547.
50. Rutherford RB, Flanigan DP, Guptka SK. Suggested standards for reports with lower extremity ischemia. J Vasc Surg 1986;4:80–94.
51. Nelemans PJ, Leiner T, et al. Peripheral arterial disease: meta-analysis of the diagnostic performance of MR angiography. Radiology 2000;217(1):105–114.
52. Antiplatelet Trialists' Coollaboration. Collaborative Overview of randomized trials of antiplatelet therapy: I. Prevention of death, myocardial infarction and stroke by prolonged antiplatelet therapy in various categories of disease. Br Med J 1994;308:81–106.
53. CAPRIE Steering Committee. A randomized, blinded trial of clopidogrel versus aspirin in patients at risk of ischemic events (CAPRIE). Lancet 1996;348:1329–1339.
54. Porter JM, Cutler BS, Lee BY, et al. Pentoxifylline efficacy in the treatment of intermittent claudication: multicenter controlled double-blind trial with objective assessment of chronic occlusive arterial disease patients. Am Heart J 1982;104(1):66–72.
55. Beebe HG, Dawson DL, Cutler BS, et al. A new pharmacological treatment for intermittent claudication: results of a randomized, multicenter trial. Arch Intern Med 1999;159(17):2041–2050.
56. Timaran CH, Prault TL, Stevens SL, et al. Iliac artery stenting versus surgical reconstruction for TASC (Transatlantic Inter-Society Consensus) type B and type C iliac lesions. J Vasc Surg 2003;38:272–278.
57. St Goar FG, Joye JD, Laird JR. Percutaneous arterial aortoiliac intervention. J Intervent Cardiol 2001;14(5):533–537.
58. Baird RJ, Johnston KW, Walker PM, et al. Aortoiliofemoral occlusive disease. In: Wilson SE, Veith FJ, Hobson RW, Williams RA, eds. Vascular surgery: principles and practice. New York: McGraw-Hill, 1987:344–352.
59. Crawford ES, Bomberger RA, Glaeser DH, et al. Aortoiliac occlusive disease: factors influencing survival and function following reconstructive operation over a 25-year period. Surgery 1981;90:1055–1066.
60. de Vries SO, Hunink MGM. Results of aortic bifurcation grafts for aortoiliac occlusive disease: a meta-analysis. J Vasc Surg 1997;26:558–569.
61. Brewster MD. Current controversies in the management of aortoiliac occlusive disease. J Vasc Surg 1997;25:365.
62. Transatlantic Inter-Society Concensus (TASC). J Vasc Surg 2001;31:S1–S296.
63. Tetteroo E, van der Graaf Y, Bosch JL, et al. Randomised comparison of primary stent placement versus primary angioplasty followed by selective stent placement in patients with iliac-artery occlusive disease. Dutch Iliac Stent Trial Study Group. Lancet 1998;351:1153–1159.
64. Bosch JL, Hunink MG. Meta-analysis of the results of percutaneous transluminal angioplasty and stent placement for aortoiliac occlusive disease. Radiology 1990;174:969.
65. Palmaz JC, Garcia OIJ, Schatz RA, et al. Placement of balloon expandable intraluminal stents in iliac arteries: first 171 procedures. Radiology 1990;174:969–975.
66. Martin EC, Katzen BT, Benenati JF, et al. Multicenter trial of the wallstent in the iliac and femoral arteries. J Vasc Intervent Radiol 1995;6(6):843–849.
67. Ponec D, et al. Cordis Randomized Iliac Stent Project (CRISP) study In: Society of Interventional Radiology 28th annual scientific meeting, 2003.
68. Haulon S, Mounier-Vehier C, Gaxotte V, et al. Percutaneous reconstruction of the aortoiliac bifurcation with the "kissing stents" technique: long-term follow-up in 106 patients. J Endovasc Ther 2002;9:363.
69. Rosenfield K, Losordo DW, Ramaswamy, K, et al. Three dimensional reconstruction of human coronary and peripheral arteries from images recorded with two-dimensional intravascular ultrasound examination. Circulation 1991;84:1938.
70. Losordo DW, Rosenfield K, Pieczek A, et al. How does angioplasty work? Serial analysis of human iliac arteries using intravascular ultrasound. Circulation 1992;86:1845.
71. Weaver F, Comerota A, Youngblood M, Froehlich J, et al. Surgical revascularization versus thrombolysis for nonembolic lower extremity native artery occlusions: results of a prospective randomized trial. J Vasc Surg 1996;24(4):513–523.
72. Pentecost MJ, Criqui MH, Dorros G, et al. Guidelines for peripheral percutaneous transluminal angioplasty of the abdominal aorta and lower extremity vessels. A statement for health professionals from a special writing group of the Councils on Cardiovascular Radiology, Arteriosclerosis, Cardio-Thoracic and Vascular Surgery, Clinical Cardiology, and Epidemiology and Prevention, the American Heart Association. Circulation 1994;89:511–531.
73. Shammas NW, Kapalis MJ, Dippel EJ, et al. Clinical an angiographic predictors of restenosis following renel artery stending. J Invasive Cardiol. 2004;16(1):10–13.

18

Percutaneous Carotid Artery Stenting

Cameron Haery, MD and Jay S. Yadav, MD

CONTENTS

INTRODUCTION
RATIONALE FOR CAROTID REVASCULARIZATION
DIAGNOSTIC EVALUATION OF CAROTID STENOSIS
CEREBROVASCULAR ANATOMY
PROCEDURAL TECHNIQUE
COMPLICATIONS OF CAROTID ARTERY STENTING
CONCLUSION
REFERENCES

INTRODUCTION

Stroke is a major cause of mortality and disability. It is the third leading cause of death in the United States. In fact, the annual incidence of new or recurrent stroke in the United States is about 700,000. Almost 25% of stroke victims will die within 1 yr of the event. About 70% of all strokes represent first attacks, making identification of those at greatest risk for stroke before the first event critical to impacting its overall incidence. Moreover, health care costs linked both directly and indirectly to stroke were estimated to exceed $51 billion in the United States in 2003, representing about 14% of the total expenditure for cardiovascular disease *(1)*.

Although carotid endarterectomy (CEA) remains the most commonly performed procedure aimed at relieving carotid stenoses predisposing to risk of hemispheric stroke, percutaneous endovascular carotid intervention is emerging as an attractive treatment modality for many patients. Carotid stenting is generally less expensive, more comfortable for patients (avoiding neck dissection), and associated with reduced hospital length of stay, and it avoids many complications of neck surgery as well as the augmented risk of general anesthesia in a patient population that has elevated risk of myocardial infarction and death. Likewise, the endovascular carotid artery stent (CAS) procedure continues to evolve, meeting the challenges to reduce procedure-related complications. CAS holds promise to emerge as a standard therapy for treatment of carotid artery stenosis.

From: *Contemporary Cardiology: Interventional Cardiology:
Percutaneous Noncoronary Intervention*
Edited by: H. C. Herrmann © Humana Press Inc., Totowa, NJ

RATIONALE FOR CAROTID REVASCULARIZATION

The mechanism of stroke can be generally categorized as being either ischemic or hemorrhagic (intracerebral or subarachnoid). Eighty-eight percent of all strokes are ischemic, with atherothrombotic brain infarction accounting for 61% of all complete strokes and cerebral embolus accounting for another 24% *(1)*.

Carotid artery stenosis increases the risk for ischemic cerebrovascular events, and an increasing degree of stenosis correlates with increased risk of future stroke and death. The annual stroke risk for asymptomatic patients with carotid stenosis greater than 60% is approx 2% *(2,3)*. The annual stroke risk for asymptomatic carotid stenosis ≥80% have been reported to be between 4% and 5.5% *(4,5)*. Patients with a history of transient ischemic attack (TIA) or stroke have a significant incremental risk of recurrent events that correlates with stenosis severity. The North American Symptomatic Carotid Endarterectomy Trial (NASCET) demonstrated a 13% annual incidence of recurrent stroke in patients with ≥70% stenoses who were treated medically. The recurrence rate of ipsilateral stroke is 22.2% at 5 yr for patients with 50–69% stenosis *(6,7)*. The adjusted relative risk of dying is 2.22 for carotid stenoses 45–74% and 3.24 for stenoses 75–99% *(8–10)*.

The rationale that mechanical revascularization to relieve carotid artery stenosis is beneficial stems from several well designed surgical trials. CEA has been shown to reduce the risk of stroke in significant symptomatic and asymptomatic lesions when compared to medical management alone. Although CEA has been performed in the United States since 1954, definitive evidence demonstrating its benefit in stroke reduction came in 1991 with the publication of the NASCET study. In NASCET, 659 patients with high-grade carotid stenosis (70–99%) and history of ipsilateral hemispheric, retinal TIA, or nondisabling stroke underwent randomization to treatment with CEA or medical therapy. At 30 d, the risk of stroke or death in the CEA arm was 5.8% versus 3.3% in the medical group. At 2 yr however, the risk of any ipsilateral stroke was 26% in the medical therapy arm and 9% with CEA ($p < 0.001$). The risk of major stroke or death was 18.1% in the medical arm and 8% in the surgical group ($p < 0.001$) *(6)*. Moreover, of patients enrolled in NASCET with moderate (50–69%) carotid narrowing and history of ipsilateral TIA or nondisabling stroke within 120 d, the 5-yr risk of ipsilateral stroke was reduced from 22.2% in the medical arm to 15.7% with CEA ($p = 0.045$). It appears that the benefit in this subset is derived from men, nondiabetics, and those suffering nondisabling stroke as the antecedent event *(7)*. The benefit derived was not significant in symptomatic patients with ipsilateral stenosis of 30–49% (18.7% medical therapy vs 14.9% CEA, $p = 0.16$).

The Veterans Affairs Cooperative Study (VACS) *(11)* and European Carotid Surgery Trialists' (ECST) Collaborative group studies provided corroborative evidence that CEA reduces the risk of stroke and death in patients with moderate to severe internal carotid artery (ICA) stenosis and ipsilateral hemispheric symptoms. In VACS, 189 men with ICA stenoses >50% and ipsilateral symptoms were randomized to receive either CEA or medical therapy within 120 d of the sentinel event. The 30-d stroke or death rate was 6.6% in the surgical group and 2.2% in the medical therapy group. At a mean of 11.9 mo of follow-up, however, the overall incidence of stroke or TIA was 7.7% in the CEA group and 19.4% in the medical group ($p = 0.011$). Similarly, the 3-yr ipsilateral ischemic stroke rate for patients with symptomatic carotid stenosis 70–99% randomized to CEA versus medical therapy was 2.8% vs 16.8%, respectively, in ECST ($p < 0.0001$) *(12)*. Pooled data from 6092 patients enrolled in the 3 major randomized trials comparing CEA and medical therapy for symptomatic carotid stenosis revealed a 16% absolute risk reduction ($p < 0.001$)

in the 5-yr risk of ipsilateral stroke for stenosis >70% without near occlusion. Modest benefit was also evident for stenoses 50–69% (ARR = 4.6%, p = 0.04). No benefit is seen when CEA is applied to carotid stenosis <50% *(13)*.

Asymptomatic patients with carotid artery stenosis are also at risk for cerebrovascular events. The ACAS trial randomized 1662 patients 40–79 yr old with carotid artery stenoses >60% without ipsilateral cerebrovascular symptoms to undergo CEA or medical therapy (325 mg aspirin daily). At 5 yr (median follow-up = 2.7 yr), there was a 5.1% risk of ipsilateral stroke for the surgical arm, compared to 11% in the medical management group (relative risk reduction = 53%, p = 0.004). In the VA Asymptomatic Carotid Artery Stenosis study, 444 men with asymptomatic carotid stenosis ≥50% were randomized to CEA versus medical therapy with aspirin alone. At 48 mo, the rate of ipsilateral stroke was 4.7% in the surgical group versus 9.4% in the medical group (p = NS).

Carotid Angioplasty and Stenting

The era of percutaneous carotid revascularization has evolved significantly since the first reported carotid angioplasty procedures in 1980 and 1981 *(14–16)*. Early reports of carotid angioplasty reserved the use of stents for complications of balloon angioplasty, namely dissection) *(17–22)*. Not until the routine use of the carotid stent did endovascular intervention become a viable approach to carotid revascularization. The earliest prospective series of carotid artery stenting in 1997 demonstrated favorable acute outcomes when CAS was performed for patients who were determined to be high risk for CEA *(23)*. Between 1997 and September 2002, the global registry of CAS procedures totaled over 12,700, and the reported technical procedural success rate was 98.9% *(24)*. In this heterogeneous population of patients and operators, the overall combined 30-d rate of stroke and procedure-related death was 3.98%. The worldwide use of cerebral embolic protection devices (EPD) appeared to limit the complication rate of 30-d stroke and procedure-related death from 5.29% to 2.23%. At 4 yr, the reported rate of ipsilateral neurological events, including TIA, minor or major stroke, and neurologic related death, was 4.5%. The worldwide registry is self-reported data and cannot be used as an independent confirmation of the superiority of any device or technique over another *(24)*.

The Carotid and Vertebral Artery Transluminal Angioplasty Study (CAVATAS) *(25)* is the only significant published randomized trial comparing carotid angioplasty to CEA. Patients were enrolled between March 1992 and July 1997, prior to the era of EPD use or routine stenting. In the study, 254 patients were randomized to undergo either percutaneous carotid intervention (251) or CEA (253). Patients met NASCET eligibility criteria for enrollment and were randomized only after determination by a surgeon, interventional radiologist, and neurologist that successful revascularization could be performed by either method. Of patients enrolled in the endovascular therapy arm, only 26% received stents. The remaining 74% underwent balloon angioplasty alone. Ninety percent of patients had symptoms within 6 mo of randomization. The 30-d outcome of disabling stroke or death did not differ between groups (6.4% endovascular vs 5.9% CEA, p = NS) nor did the rate of disabling stroke lasting more than 7 d (10% endovascular vs 9.9% CEA, p = NS). At 3 yr, the rate of death or disabling stroke was also comparable between groups (14.3% endovascular vs 14.2% CEA [hazard ratio = 1.03; 95% confidence interval {CI} 0.64–1.64; p = 0.9]). The complications of cranial neuropathy and significant neck hematoma occurred more frequently in the surgical arm. Although restenosis occurred more frequently with angioplasty, repeat interventions were comparable between the two groups.

The complication rate in the CEA arm was higher than previously seen in NASCET and ACAS; however, this is probably a more accurate reflection of complication rates seen in general community practice. It has been postulated that the low stent use rate in the endovascular therapy arm might account for the higher restenosis rates. Comparable outcomes between endovascular intervention, with limited stent use and without any use of EPDs, and CEA in this randomized controlled trial has led to enthusiastic speculation that routine stenting with concomitant use of EPD will result in improved outcomes relative to CEA in certain patient populations.

Emboli Protection Devices

Mechanical disruption of the carotid atherosclerotic plaque frequently results in the liberation of atheroembolic debris to the cerebral circulation, predisposing to periprocedural stroke *(26–32)*. Histopathologic study of debris liberated during carotid revascularization has demonstrated the presence of cholesterol vacuoles, calcium, foam cells, as well as platelet and fibrin aggregates *(33)*. EPDs have been effectively designed to prevent atheromatous debris from embolizing to the cerebral circulation *(34)*. Current devices are based on three differing designs, each with specific advantages and impediments. Categories are (1) "basket" or "umbrella" filter, (2) distal balloon occlusion and aspiration, and (3) proximal balloon occlusion with flow-reversal systems. EPDs available either commercially or in investigational trails in the United States are depicted in Fig. 1.

The "basket" or "umbrella" filter devices are mounted on the distal end of a 0.014-in. guide wire. The undeployed device is contained within a microsheath, which is retracted once the lesion has been crossed with the device. When the device is deployed distal to the stenosis, the interventional procedure can be performed without compromise of antegrade blood flow while still capturing liberated debris. At the conclusion of the intervention, the device is retrieved using a specially designed sheath, and the wire can be removed. Disadvantages of this design include the need to traverse friable stenoses with the guide wire–microsheath assembly before it can be deployed in the distal carotid artery. "Umbrella" and "basket" devices might not circumferentially oppose the vessel wall, allowing embolic debris to escape around the edges of the device. Newer-generation devices are being designed to overcome this limitation. Although microscopic, the fenestrations designed to allow antegrade blood flow while capturing embolic particles might allow microscopic emboli to pass directly through the pores. Theses devices might also become overwhelmed with atheroembolic debris during intervention, resulting in obstruction of antegrade cerebral blood flow and a static column of blood in the carotid artery between the stenosis and the device. Unless this column of stagnant blood and debris is aspirated, retrieval of the device into the capture sheath could result in cerebral embolization. The AngioGuard Guidewire™ (Cordis, Miami, FL) was the first umbrella device specifically designed for use in percutaneous carotid artery intervention. The pores in the umbrella measure 100 μm in diameter. It has undergone rigorous study, demonstrating efficacy in carotid stenting procedures. The Stenting and Angioplasty with Protection in Patients at High Risk for Endarterectomy (SAPPHIRE) trial *(35)* randomized 334 patients with comorbidity criteria classifying them as high risk for CEA to undergo stenting with the AngioGuard Guidewire XP™ or CEA. Patients were either asymptomatic with ≥80% stenosis by ultrasound or symptomatic with ≥50% stenosis. Patients met eligibility only if one or more of the following high-risk characteristics were present: congestive heart failure (class III or IV), left ventricular ejection fraction less than 30%, need for open heart surgery within 6 wk, recent myocardial infarction (MI), unstable angina, age greater than 80 yr, pre-

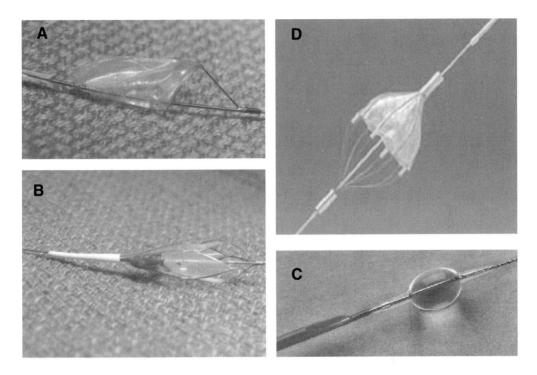

Fig. 1. Emboli protection devices currently available for use in the United States: (**A**) FilterWire, (**B**) AccuNet, (**C**) PercuSurge GuardWire, and (**D**) AngioGuard.

vious CEA with restenosis, previous radiation therapy or radical neck surgery, or lesions distal or proximal to the usual cervical location. One-third of patients were symptomatic. The technical success rate AngioGuard EPD use was 98.6%. The composite end point of death, stroke, or MI at 30 d was seen in 4.4% of CAS patients versus 9.9% of CEA patients ($p = 0.06$). At 1 yr, the primary end point of death, stroke, or MI at 30 d plus stroke or death at 360 d was 12.0% for CAS and 20.1% for CEA ($p = 0.048$). These randomized data confirm that CAS with EPD is safer than CEA in patients with significant comorbid conditions.

The nonrandomized registry arm of the SAPPHIRE study comprised patients who, after meeting clinical entry inclusion criteria, were deemed unsuitable for randomization to either CEA or CAS. Four hundred six patients were deemed unsuitable for CEA by a vascular surgeon and, therefore, underwent CAS. Seven patients were considered unsuitable for CAS and underwent CEA. Compared to those in the randomized arm of the trial, patients entered into the stent registry had a higher incidence of prior CEA, greater incidence of radiation treatment, higher occurrence of anatomically high or low lesions, as well as the presence of more than one high risk criteria for enrollment.

The Carotid Revascularization Endarterectomy versus Stent Trial (CREST) is a randomized multicenter trial designed to compare CAS using the AccuNet™ filter EPD and Acculink™ stent (Guidant Corp., Menlo Park, CA), with CEA. The CREST study patient cohort is designed to be similar to those enrolled in NASCET. The primary eligibility criteria for enrollment is a carotid artery stenosis greater than or equal to 50% in patients with transient ischemic attack or ipsilateral nondisabling stroke within 180 d of revascularization. Unlike those enrolled in SAPPHIRE, they are at relatively low risk for CEA-related complications *(36)*.

Table 1
Trials of Emboli Protection Devices in Carotid Artery Stenting

Registry study trials	EPD used	Stent used	Patient population enrolled	Status of Trial
ARCHeR	AccuNet OTW	Acculink OTW	High surgical risk	Published data unavailable
ARCHeR RX	AccuNet RX	Acculink RX	High surgical risk	Currently enrolling
BEACH	FilterWire EX or Filter Wire EZ	Carotid Wallstent	High surgical risk	Currently enrolling
CABERNET	Filter Wire EX	NexStent	High surgical risk	Currently enrolling
MAVErIC II	GuardWire	Exponent	High surgical risk	Published data unavailable
SECuRITY	MedNova EmboShield	MedNova Exact	High surgical risk	Published data unavailable
MAVErIC	Interceptor	Exponent	High surgical risk	CE mark approved
SAPPHIRE	AngioGuard XP	Precise	High surgical risk	Completed
CREST	AccuNet	Acculink OTW	Symptomatic carotid artery stenosis without high surgical risk	Enrolling

Several other trials of carotid stenting with EPD use are underway. Many are designed as prospective registry studies of consecutively treated patients, without a comparison treatment group (e.g., CEA or medical therapy alone). Other filter EPDs undergoing such trials include the FilterWire™ (Boston Scientific, Natick, MA), MedNova Neuroshield/Emboshield™ (MedNova, Inc., Galway, Ireland), MDT-Filter (Medtronic), Microvena-Trap (Microvena), SPIDER™ (ev3), and Interceptor (Medtronic) (Table 1).

The distal balloon occlusion and aspiration systems involve an occlusion balloon on the distal end of a guide wire, arresting flow during percutaneous intervention. The stagnant column of blood and atheroembolic debris is then aspirated prior to removal of the occlusive device. The major limitation of such systems include the mandatory arrest of cerebral blood flow through the target internal cartoid artery (ICA) during intervention. The PercuSurge GuardWire® (Medtronic/AVE, Santa Rosa, CA), has been successfully employed in CAS procedures but is not Food and Drug Administration (FDA) approved for use in CAS (37–39). It has proven efficacious in reducing adverse events after aorto-coronary saphenous vein graft intervention (40).

Proximal balloon occlusion and flow-reversal systems occlude flow proximal to the target lesion by inflating a balloon at the end of a sheath. By obstructing carotid inflow, cerebral circulation in the target vessel is reversed, allowing extraction of atheroembolic material through the sheath. In theory, if the retrieval limb of the sheath is connected to the femoral vein, retrieved debris can be safely diverted to the pulmonary circulation. The

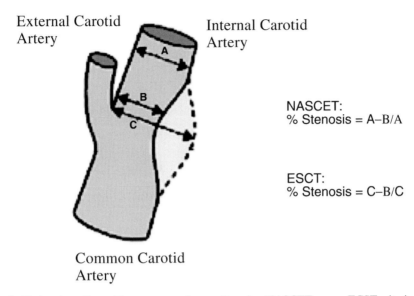

NASCET:
% Stenosis = A–B/A

ESCT:
% Stenosis = C–B/C

Fig. 2. Estimation of carotid artery stenosis severity using NASCET versus ECST criteria. (From ref. *41*.)

Parodi Anti-Emboli System (Arteria Medical Science, Inc., San Francisco, CA), has been used with success in CAS *(37)*. Although a theoretical advantage of such devices is avoiding the need to cross the target lesion with a guide wire before the device is deployed, reversal of flow in the target vessel might predispose to complications of prolonged cerebral ischemia. Further study is needed before such a device is likely to become standard of care for CAS.

DIAGNOSTIC EVALUATION OF CAROTID STENOSIS

Determination of Stenosis Severity

Considerable heterogeneity exists among diagnostic modalities used to evaluate carotid atherosclerosis. There are nonuniform standards used to calculate stenosis severity. Two accepted criteria might be used to calculate stenosis severity, depending on the diameter of the reference segment used (Fig. 2). NASCET criteria utilized the widest diameter of the ICA distal to the lesion and beyond any poststenotic dilation as the reference diameter, excluding the carotid bulb from the calculation. ECST criteria utilized the largest diameter of the carotid bulb as the reference segment. Because of the larger reference segment diameter, using ECST criteria to determine carotid stenosis severity will relatively overestimate the determination of stenosis severity.

Noninvasive Diagnostic Modalities

ULTRASOUND

Duplex ultrasound remains the standard noninvasive tool for assessment and quantification of carotid artery stenosis. Among diagnostic centers that employ strict and routine quality control measures with properly trained ultrasound technicians, sensitivity and specificity for detection of high-grade stenosis has been reported to be as high as 100%

Table 2
Ultrasound-Based Classification of Internal Carotid Artery Stenosis Severity
at the Cleveland Clinic Vascular Laboratory, 2004

Diameter reduction	Peak systolic velocity (cm/s)	End-diastolic velocity (cm/s)	Flow character
0–19%	<105	*a	Minimal or no spectral broadening
20–39%	<105	*	Increased spectral broadening
40–59%	105–149	*	Increased spectral broadening until the whole window is filled
60–79%	150–240	*	Marked spectral broadening
80–99%	>240	>135	Marked spectral broadening
Total occlusion	Not applicable	Not applicable	No flow signal in ICA

Note: Velocity values based on use of 5 MHz pulsed Doppler carrier frequency with a 1.5-mm sample volume at a 60° flow angle.
[a] The asterisk indicates that the end-diastolic velocity values are only used as stenosis classification criteria for 80–99% diameter stenosis lesions.

and >85%, respectively. Duplex scanning also imparts the ability to provide physiologic blood flow data as well as intimal pathology data that contrast angiography does not provide. Assessment of stenosis severity using duplex ultrasound data involves an incorporation of several measured parameters. These include peak systolic velocity (PSV), end-diastolic velocity (EDV), PSV_{ICA}/PSV_{CCA} ratio, as well as EDV_{ICA}/EDV_{CCA} ratio. No single parameter of duplex scanning velocity is universally sufficient to accurately assess carotid stenosis severity. Individual variations in cardiac output, blood pressure, arterial collateralization, ipsilateral common carotid stenosis, and contralateral ICA stenosis might influence PSV, reducing accuracy in diagnosis. Although PSV is regarded as the most important parameter of duplex scanning for determination of stenosis severity, EDV also provides a high degree of specificity for ICA stenosis detection. In 2004, the Cleveland Clinic Vascular Laboratory classified the degree of ICA stenosis using the criteria listed in Table 2. The PSV_{ICA}/PSV_{CCA} ratio is also reported. NASCET criteria for prediction of severe ICA stenosis (70–99%) included PSV > 250 cm/s, but it has been criticized for marginal sensitivity (68%) and specificity (67%). Although ultrasound has been used as the sole diagnostic test for patient selection for CEA, it is susceptible to significant error. Duplex scanning might interpret a subtotal occlusion as complete occlusion because of the lack of turbulence and severe limitation of flow. Such an error might result in the denial an opportunity for revascularization for a patient, when it might indeed be beneficial. Adequate imaging of patients who have undergone recent neck surgery (i.e., endarterectomy) can be limited, as well as in patients with very thick or muscular necks.

General considerations for maintaining consistent carotid duplex scanning results include strict adherence to locally determined scanning protocols. A constant-angle measurement between the ultrasound beam and the longitudinal axis of the vessel should be maintained prior to spectral waveform recording, and the sample volume should be moved through the area of stenosis to determine the highest peak systolic and end-diastolic velocities. Spectral waveforms taken at an angle greater than 60° from the longitudinal axis will cause significant errors in peak velocity calculations. Sample volume size should be minimized whenever possible to obtain the most discrete spectral information, and the sample volume placement should be in the center of the vessel or flow channel. In very tight lesions, the sample volume size might be expanded in order to locate the channel of flow.

Magenetic Resonance Angiography

Modern magnetic resonance angiography (MRA) techniques have become very effective in providing information regarding carotid artery stenoses as well as the intracranial vasculature. The two complementary techniques most commonly used are (1) contrast-enhanced (CE) MRA and (2) three-dimentional time-of-flight (TOF).

The CE MRA is effective in the evaluation of the carotid artery from the arch origin as well as the carotid bifurcation to the circle of Willis. The CE MRA acquisition time is short and less susceptible to artifact from patient movement. Despite its ability to accurately visualize the site and length of stenosis, it might also overestimate stenosis severity because turbulent flow in high-grade stenoses might not be detected, resulting in complete signal loss, erroneously overestimating true severity. Injection of contrast must be precisely timed; otherwise, early return from the jugular vein may result in obscuration of arterial vessels. Three-dimentional TOF images provide high spatial resolution in small arterial vessels and those with high flow velocity. The circle of Willis and extracranial ICA are well visualized *(42)*.

A meta-analysis comparing MRA and duplex ultrasound with digital subtraction angiography by Nederkoorn et al. *(43)* reported a pooled sensitivity of 95% (95% CI = 92–97) and pooled specificity of 90% (95% CI = 86–93) for MRA in the detection of carotid stenoses with severity 70–99%. Despite the progress in MRA, we have found it to generally overestimate stenosis severity and we use ultrasound as our primary screening test.

CEREBROVASCULAR ANATOMY

The aortic arch usually gives rise to three major vessels supplying the arterial circulation to the head and neck. The first branch of the aortic arch is the brachiocephalic artery (innominate artery), which gives rise to the right common carotid artery and the right subclavian artery. The left common carotid artery (LCCA) typically arises as the second major branch of the aorta. Many variations of the origin and course of the large vessels supplying the head and neck exist. The most common variant origin of the LCCA involves takeoff of the LCCA from the innominate artery. This is commonly referred to as the bovine aortic arch and occurs in about 27% of people. Finally, the left subclavian artery is the third branch of the aorta and gives rise to the left vertebral artery. The aortic arch can be classified according to the origin of the great vessels in relation to the arch apex. To determine arch type, the widest diameter of the LCCA is used as a reference unit. The type 1 arch is technically the least challenging arch for performing carotid stenting. Here, the origin of the innominate artery arises within one reference unit of the arch apex. In the type 2 arch, the origin of the innominate arises between one and two reference units of the apex. Type 3 arches are technically challenging, and the origin of the innominate arises beyond two reference units from the arch apex (Fig. 3). The common carotid artery most commonly (in about 50% of individuals) bifurcates at the level of the C4–C5 intervertebral space, giving rise to the ICA and

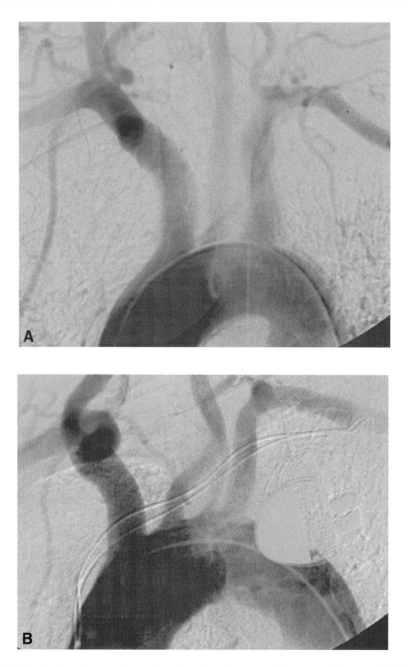

Fig. 3. Digital subtraction angiography of aortic arch types: (**A**) type 1, (**B**) type 2, (**C**) type 3.

external carotid artery (ECA). In about 38% of individuals, the carotid bifurcation will arise higher, at about C3–C4, and the remainder might arise lower. The origin of the ICA commonly has a somewhat fusiform dilation, known as the carotid bulb, comprising a rich network of neurofibers and highly sensitive baroreceptors that exert control over peripheral vascular tone and cardiac chronotropy.

The ECA supplies much of the extracranial head and facial circulation. The external carotid artery and its branches have a broadly redundant circulation and excellent arterial

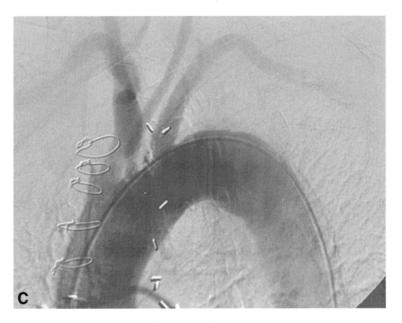

Fig. 3. *(continued).*

collaterals, so atherosclerosis or impingement during ICA revascularization is usually of little clinical consequence. Jaw or tongue claudication can occur if bilateral ECA insufficiency exists.

The ICA typically courses posteriorly and laterally to the ECA. It is divided into five segments before giving rise to the intracerebral circulation. In ascending order, they are cervical, petrous, cavernous, clinoid, and supraclinoid (Fig. 4). The cervical and petrous segments have no branches. The ICA enters the cranial vault through the foramen lacerum in the petrous bone. Then, the ICA traverses the cavernous sinus with the abducens nerve and supplies branches to the posterior pituitary artery via the meningo-hypophyseal artery. The ICA penetrates the dura mater in the supraclinoid segment. Branches of the supraclinoid ICA include the ophthalmic artery, anterior choroidal artery, and posterior communicating artery before terminating in the anterior cerebral and middle cerebral arteries.

The Circle of Willis

The circle of Willis is an anastomotic network at the base of the brain, surrounding the optic chiasm and the pituitary stalk (Fig. 5). There are significant anatomic variations of the circle of Willis, without clinical consequence in otherwise healthy patients. The posterior communicating artery (PCOM), arising from the terminal portion of the supraclinoid ICA, provides the major collateral connection between the anterior circulation (from the ICA) and posterior circulation (to the posterior cerebral artery). Although the PCA typically arises from the basilar artery of the posterior circulation, the PCA could arise directly from the ICA, without any PCOM connection of the anterior and posterior circulation. By definition, this is known as fetal PCA. If the PCOM is larger in caliber than the segment of the PCA between the basilar artery bifurcation and the PCOM (known as the P1 segment), the term "fetal PCA" can also be applied.

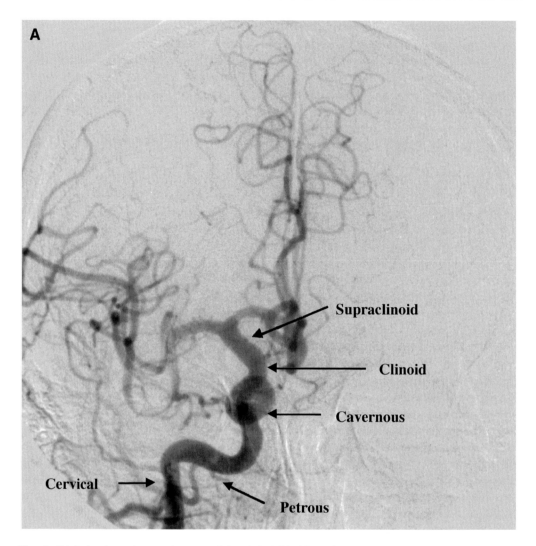

Fig. 4. Digital subtraction angiogram of the right ICA. Note the contralateral left anterior cerebral artery filling via a patent anterior communicating artery. **(A)** Cross-table 90° lateral projection; **(B)** postero-anterior cranial projection.

   The terminal ICA bifurcates into the anterior cerebral (ACA) and middle cerebral arteries (MCA). The ACA is divided into five segments: A1–A5. The anterior communicating artery (ACOM) arises from the A1 segment of the ACA and provides communication of right and left anterior hemispheres. The MCA provides circulation to territories responsible for motor and sensory function, language centers, and cognition. It is divided into four segments: M1–M4. The M1 segment is the first segment after the ICA bifurcation and courses horizontally until it turns superiorly into the insula, where it branches into M2–M4 segments. The M1 segment gives rise to the lenticulostriate arteries.

   The vertebral artery courses superiorly from the subclavian artery through the transverse foramen of the C6 vertebrae. It then courses posteriorly along the posterior arch of the atlas and enters the skull through the foramen magnum. It then begins an antero-medial

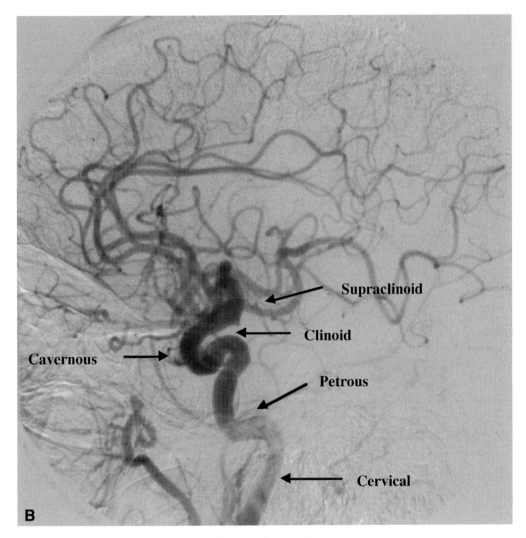

Fig. 4. *(Continued)*

course to the level of the ponto-medullary junction, where it fuses with the contralateral vertebral artery to form the basilar artery. The distal vertebral artery gives rise to the posterior inferior cerebellar artery (PICA). PICA supplies the infero-lateral cerebellum, lower portion of the medulla, inferior fourth of the ventricle, vermis, and tonsils. The anterior inferior cerebellar artery (AICA) originates from the proximal or mid-basilar artery. It supplies the pons, middle cerebellar peduncle, cranial nerves VI–III, and choroid. The superior cerebellar artery (SCA) originates in the distal basilar artery and supplies portions of the upper pons, lower midbrain, upper vermis, and part of the superior cerebellum.

When a hemisphere of the anterior circulation is supplied by only one source (i.e., from only one of the following: ICA, ACOM, PCOM) because of atherosclerotic disease or congential variation, the term "isolated hemisphere" is applied, signifying patients at increased risk for hyperperfusion syndrome after carotid revascularization and those at elevated risk for stroke, seizure, or loss of consciousness during intraprocedural vessel occlusion (see the section Complications of Carotid Artery Stenting).

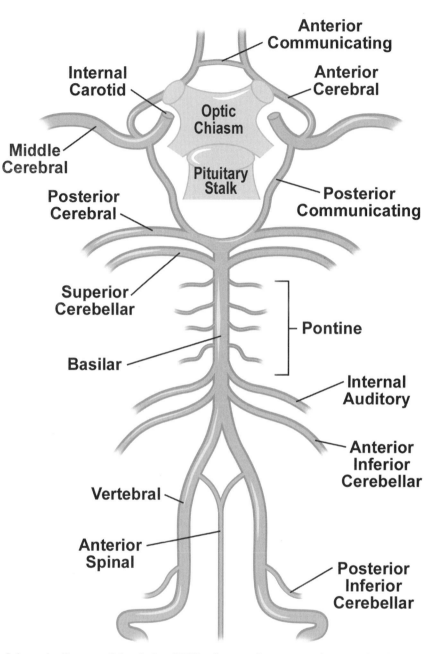

Fig. 5. Schematic diagram of the circle of Wills; Symmetric anastomotic network without anomalies shown.

PROCEDURAL TECHNIQUE

Angiography

After careful patient selection based on synthesis of information obtained from history and physical examination, diagnostic imaging studies (including baseline brain computed tomography [CT] or magnetic resonance imaging [MRI] scan), and consultation with appropriate neurological and surgical specialists, the safe and

Table 3
Commonly Used Diagnostic Catheters Used for Selective Engagement
of Aortic Arch Vessels

	Arch type	Risk of aorta and great arch vessel trauma
Judkins Right	I–II	Low
Vitek	II–III	Low
Simmons	III	High
Headhunter	III	Intermediate

effective percutaneous carotid intervention procedure begins with angiographic evaluation. Anatomic origin of great arch vessels (aortic arch type), disease of the great vessels of the aortic arch, curvature of the aorta, vertebral artery dominance, target lesion characteristics, target vessel tortuosity, and understanding of intracerebral and collateral arterial circulation should all be considered in planning the approach and anticipating complications.

Arch aortography is the most effective means for evaluating the origin of the great vessels and is usually performed in the left anterior oblique 40°–50° projection. The field-of-view should include the arch of the aorta to the base of the skull, when possible. A basic cerebrovascular study will include selective angiography of each of the common carotid arteries, the innominate artery, and one or both subclavian arteries to visualize the vertebrobasilar circulation. Diagnostic catheters used for selective engagement of the great vessels are determined by the arch type (Table 3).

When the common carotid artery is engaged, ipsilateral 30° and 90° cross-table lateral projections are typically adequate to visualize the carotid artery bifurcation. Subsequent angiography of the intracerebral circulation should include the arterial filling and venous drainage phases, as well attention to possible delayed filling of contralateral hemisphere or branches of the posterior circulation. The A1 segment of the ACA is commonly visualized in the PA (0°) cranial projection. The A2–A5 segments can be seen in the cross-table 90° lateral view. The MCA segments M1–M4 can be seen in the standard PA cranial projection. On the cross-table 90° lateral view, the superior limit of the branches of the MCA that traverse the circular sulcus forms an imaginary line that is the base of a triangle whose apex is inferior to the base, at the limen insulae. This imaginary triangle is termed the "Sylvian triangle."

Engagement of the innominate artery is usually performed in the left anterior oblique (LAO) projection. A right anterior oblique (RAO) projection might then facilitate visualization of the innominate bifurcation and selective engagement of either the right CCA or right subclavian arteries. The origin of either vertebral artery is frequently best viewed in the contralateral oblique projection. The vertebrobasilar system is visualized in the PA cranial and cross-table 90° lateral projections.

Carotid Stenting Procedure

Various techniques have been used to perform safe and effective carotid artery stenting. Procedural technique must be tailored to the individual. Strict adherence to an algorithmic approach to the procedure, without modification of technique based on sound clinical judgment and operator experience, should be avoided.

The proper guide catheter or sheath is determined by the arch type and location of the target lesion. In the event of type 1 or type 2 aortic arch, CAS can usually be performed through a flexible 6 French long guide sheath (e.g., 90 cm Cook Shuttle sheath; Cordis, Miami, FL.) positioned in the common carotid artery. The technique is usually accomplished engaging the origin of the CCA with a 5F diagnostic catheter, typically 110 cm JR4 or VTK, and using a 0.035-in. stiff guide wire (e.g., Terumo stiff angled Glidewire) to carefully engage the external carotid artery under road-mapping angiographic guidance. Meticulous care must be taken not to disrupt the target lesion, commonly at the ICA origin and frequently involving the distal CCA. The diagnostic catheter may then be advanced into the mid-ECA and the guide wire removed. An extra support 0.035-in. guide wire (e.g., 0.035-in. (260-cm)-long Super stiff Amplatz guide wire) might then be carefully advanced through the diagnostic catheter to its distal tip, and the diagnostic catheter removed over the wire. The femoral arterial sheath can then be removed and the long guide sheath back-loaded over the superstiff Amplatz guide wire, where it is positioned in the common carotid artery, proximal to the target lesion. While the guide wire and sheath-introducing dilator are being removed under fluoroscopic visualization, manual-retracting tension should be maintained on the guide sheath once it is positioned in the CCA, because elimination of the stiffness provided by the guide wire and dilator during their removal could cause the sheath to lunge forward in the CCA.

Another commonly used technique involves performing CAS through a preformed guide catheter that is positioned proximal to the target lesion using a "telescoping" method. This technique is particularly useful in the event of type 2 or 3 aortic arch, where extra support is needed to prevent prolapse of the guide wire or guide catheter into the aorta during intervention or when CCA tortuosity or target vessel angulation requires a torqueable preformed guide catheter to aid in direction of the equipment through the target vessel. The telescoping technique is usually performed through an 8F sheath in the femoral artery. A 5F long diagnostic catheter that can be used to engage the origin of the target CCA (e.g., JR4, VTK, Simmons curve, or Headhunter) is advanced through an 8F guide catheter (typically an H1 guide). The diagnostic catheter is advanced over a 0.035-in. guide wire into the descending thoracic aorta, where its shape can be reconfigured to engage the target CCA. The diagnostic catheter is then used to engage the target CCA, and a 0.035-in. guide wire (e.g., Terumo stiff angled Glidewire) can be used to engage the ECA using road-mapping angiographic guidance. The diagnostic catheter is then advanced into the CCA, and the guide catheter can then be advanced over the diagnostic catheter into the mid-CCA. This technique commonly requires slight counterclockwise rotation of the guide catheter during advancement while attention is paid to maintaining position of the diagnostic catheter and guide wire, to prevent prolapse into the aorta. The guide catheter telescoping technique can increase the risk of inadvertent disruption of arch or CCA atheroma when compared to the guide sheath technique because of the more abrupt transition between the diagnostic catheter and the guide catheter compared to the snug fit between the dilator and the sheath. The guide catheter technique, however, is faster and provides more flexibility and control during the procedure.

After adequate position of the guide catheter or sheath, the lesion may be crossed with the EPD guidewire. The EPD filter or occlusive balloon is usually positioned in a straight portion of the distal cervical ICA without atherosclerotic disease. Once proper position and apposition to the ICA wall has been confirmed by angiographic contrast injection, balloon PTA of the target lesion prior to stent placement is recommended. Balloon PTA ensures minimal resistance of stent delivery into the target lesion, as well as giving important information regarding patient response to temporary cerebral ischemia, and the hemodynamic significance of the baroreceptor reflex. After predilation PTA, the decision can be made to pretreat with intravenous atropine or vasopressors prior to stent deployment and poststent dilation. Predilation PTA is typically performed using a 4.0/20-mm or 4.0/30-mm balloon dilation catheter.

All stents used for bifurcation CAS today are self-expanding and commonly made of nitinol or elgiloy. Balloon-expandable stents provide the advantage of precise positioning but are prone to deformation and compression as a result of the superficial nature of the carotid artery. Self-expanding stents conform to the vessel wall and the appropriate size should be chosen such that the unconstrained diameter of the stent (as described by the manufacturer's label) exceeds the reference vessel diameter by 1–2 mm. Appropriate sizing might be challenging in the event of aneurysmal dilatation or extensive atherosclerotic disease beyond the stent margins.

Poststent balloon dilation is frequently performed but not obligatory. Self-expandable stents are usually postdilated using a 5.5- or 6.0/20-mm balloon dilation catheter in the ICA. The distal edge of the stent should be fully expanded, but the poststent balloon should be maintained within the stent bounds as much as possible, and nominal inflation pressure should not be greatly exceeded near the stent edges, to minimize risk of dissection.

If an umbrella/basket filter-type EPD is used, angiography should be performed immediately after stent deployment and postdilation is complete, to delineate whether slow reflow or no reflow exists, so that prompt aspiration of the target vessel could be performed if necessary. Aspiration is performed using a 4F or 5F multipurpose catheter with side holes connected to a Touhy–Borst or Copilot Y-adapter or the PercuSurge Export aspiration catheter. Once the EPD is retrieved, final target lesion and intracerebral angiographic images should be obtained.

Example angiograms of a right internal carotid artery with a bifurcation stenosis are shown in the videos on the accompanying CD-ROM before and after deployment of an 8.0/30 mm Precise stent (Cordis, Miami, FL) using Angioguard (Cordis, Miami, FL) distal emboli protection and postdilation using a 5.5-mm Aviator (Cordis, Miami, FL) balloon dilation catheter.

COMPLICATIONS OF CAROTID ARTERY STENTING

The most devastating complications of percutaneous carotid revascularization are stroke and death. The development of new techniques and equipment specially designed for use in cerebrovascular intervention as well as more experienced operators has led to a reduction in the frequency of complications. Stroke rates during endovascular stent procedures seem to be reduced when EPDs are employed. In a meta-analysis of reported CAS procedures performed between January 1990 and June 2002, Kastrup et al. *(44)* documented that the combined stroke and death rate at 30 d in both symptomatic and asymptomatic patients was 1.8% in patients treated with EPD versus 5.5% for patients not treated with EPD ($p < 0.001$). This was primarily attributable to a reduction in the rate of minor strokes (3.7% without EPD vs 0.5% with EPD, $p < 0.001$) and major strokes (1.1% without EPD vs 0.3% with EPD, $p < 0.05$). Death rates were not significantly different between the two groups (approx 0.8%, $p = 0.6$) *(44)*. Advanced age (>80 yr old) and long or multiple stenoses appear to be independent predictors of procedural stroke *(45)*.

Although the use of EPD has led to a reduction of embolic complications of CAS and is an essential component of contemporary CAS procedures, EPDs present an additional step during the procedure that could pose additional challenges and potential for complications. The crossing profile of most EPDs is larger than that of a standard 0.014-in. guide wire because of the encasing microsheath. Excessively angulated lesions or those with severe proximal tortuosity might preclude effective delivery. In complex lesions, crossing the lesion with the device is not a "protected" step in the procedure. Also, if the EPD is eccentrically positioned in the distal vessel, atheroembolism could occur around the device. Patients are frequently able to tolerate brief periods of carotid obstruction during CAS; however, in the case of percutaneous intervention of an isolated hemisphere, loss of consciousness seems to occur more frequently (23). Severe movement or dislodgement of the EPD during CAS could, itself, injure the endothelium and cause endoluminal wall dissection and embolization.

In the event of slow reflow or no reflow after CAS, intracerebral angiography should be performed. If no identifiable occlusion is identified, supportive therapy with airway management, fluid resuscitation, and hemodynamic support is recommended. If, however, embolic occlusion of the proximal MCA is identified, an attempt at interventional restoration of flow using a soft hydrophilic guide wire such as the Whisper (Guidant, Temecula, CA) and a small balloon PTA catheter or embolus snare device can be attempted. Direct intraarterial infusion of glycoprotein IIb/IIIa inhibitors could predispose to intracerebral hemorrhage and death and should be done only with careful consideration of risk-to-benefit ratio (46).

Even in angiographically successful CAS procedures, transient cerebral ischemia could occur. In a single-center prospective series of patients undergoing neuroprotected CAS, postprocedural ischemic brain lesions were detected using diffusion-weighted MRI scanning in 23% of patients. Ninety percent of these cases were clinically silent. In those patients with clinically silent ischemia, however, follow-up MRI at 4.1 mo did not identify any residual ischemia indicating that these were silent TIAs and not strokes (47).

Acute vessel closure as a result of vessel or stent thrombosis is a rare but potentially devastating complication of CAS (23) and is associated with inadequate anticoagulation and antiplatelet regimens. Angiographic features that could predispose to acute vessel closure include vessel dissection, presence of thrombus, and deployment of a stent in a vessel without TIMI 3 flow. Patients should be pretreated with aspirin and a thienopyridine (namely Clopidogrel) prior to the procedure. With once-daily dosing, plasma concentrations of Clopidogrel reach a steady state in 5–7 d (48). In vivo pharmacokinetics of Clopidogrel is variable depending on the dose administered. For example, when a Clopidogrel dose was administered to subjects with coronary artery disease undergoing stent implantation who were already taking aspirin, platelet aggregation at 4 h (measured by ADP 20 µmol/L-induced aggregation assay) was inhibited by up to 59% with a 600-mg loading dose, compared with 38–40% inhibition with 300 mg (49). Inhibition of platelet aggregation is approx 50% at 2 h with a 450-mg loading dose of Clopidogrel (50). The degree of evoked platelet inhibition in humans might be quite variable (51), and the clinical impact of intersubject heterogeneity of Clopidogrel responsiveness has not been extensively studied. For this reason, in patients undergoing CAS at The Cleveland Clinic who have not been receiving 75 mg Clopidogrel daily for at least 5 d prior to the procedure, a loading dose of 300–450 mg is administered at least 4 h prior to the procedure. Aspirin is continued indefinitely and Clopidogrel should be continued for at least 4 wk after stent implantation. Randomized trials have not been performed to determine the most effective procedural heparin dose during CAS procedures. At The Cleveland Clinic, 50–60 units/kg intravenous heparin is administered to achieve an activated clotting time of 275–300s during the procedure.

Data regarding the utility of glycoprotein IIb/IIIa (GP IIb/IIIa) use during CAS is sparse. In a prospective series of 151 consecutive patients undergoing CAS prior to the introduction of EPDs, 128 of whom received intravenous abciximab (0.25 mg/kg bolus before the lesion was crossed with the guide wire and 0.125 mg/kg/min infusion for 12 h), Kapadia et al. (52) reported an 8% rate of 30 d stroke and death in the control group, compared to 1.6% in the group receiving abciximab ($p < 0.05$). One patient in the abciximab group suffered a delayed intracranial hemorrhage by 30 d follow-up (52). Hofmann et al. subsequently reported a randomized series of 74 patients undergoing CAS, receiving either abciximab infusion or placebo (53). There was a 19% periprocedural ischemic event rate in the abciximab group versus 8% in the control group (53). There is no current standard regarding use of GP IIb/IIIa use during neuroprotected CAS and it is not routinely used at The Cleveland Clinic for patients not deemed to be at high risk for platelet-mediated atherothrombotic events.

Reflex bradycardia and hypotension are well-recognized sequelae of CAS (54). Stimulation of carotid baroreceptors of the afferent glossopharyngeal nerve results in efferent vagal nerve stimulation and a decrease in sympathetic outflow via the spinal cord. About 71% of patients have hypotension or bradycardia during balloon inflation of the carotid sinus (23). Severe cases of prolonged bradycardia and high-grade atrioventricular block are rare; however, pretreatment with intravenous atropine could be used if severe bradycardia is anticipated after predilation PTA of the carotid bulb or proximal ICA. Temporary transvenous pacemakers are rarely necessary. Efferent pathways of the spinal cord might also stimulate a reflex vasodilatory response and hypotension. Hypotension is common after CAS and often lasts several hours to days after intervention. Vasodepressor-mediated hypotension is usually self-limited, and patients can gradually resume antihypertensive medications 24 h after the procedure. If hypotension is profound, hemodynamic support with intravenous fluids, and IV vasopressors (norepinephrine, dopamine, neosynephrine) or oral pseudoephedrine could be used.

Chronic limitation of intracerebral blood flow and ischemia results in chronic loss of autoregulation and vasomotor tone. As a result, sudden restoration of intracerebral flow could predispose to symptoms of ipsilateral headache, altered mental status, stupor, epileptic seizure, focal neurologic deficits, hypertension, intracerebral hemorrhage, or death (55–60). The true incidence of cerebral hyperperfusion syndrome is unknown; however, in a Cleveland Clinic series of 450 patients undergoing CAS, the rate of postprocedural intracerebral hemorrhage was 0.67%. All affected patients had periprocedural hypertension as well as severe target lesion stenosis (95.6% + 3.7%) and concomitant contralateral ICA stenosis greater than 80% (61). Preprocedural and postprocedural hypertension, severe ipsilateral stenosis with contralateral ICA stenosis, or the target lesion supplying an isolated cerebral hemisphere appear to be predisposing features for cerebral hyperperfusion syndrome. Attentive blood pressure control (maintenance of systolic blood pressure between 90 and 140 mm Hg) in the immediate and short-term postprocedural period might reduce the frequency of this potentially catastrophic complication.

In-stent restenosis is not as frequent as it is in the coronary and lower extremity arterial beds. In the worldwide registry of CAS procedures, the restenosis rates (defined as greater than 50% restenosis) at 1, 2, 3, and 4 yr were 2.70%, 2.60%, 2.40%, and 5.60%, respectively (24). The rate of target lesion revascularization at 1 yr in the CAS arm of the SAPPHIRE trial was 0.6%. The rate was similarly low in the CAS registry arm of SAPPHIRE (0.7%). Repeat balloon angioplasty might be warranted in the case of carotid stent restenosis, and we have successfully performed gamma radiation brachytherapy in severe cases (62).

CONCLUSION

Carotid endarterectomy for patients with significantly stenotic symptomatic and asymptomatic carotid artery disease continues to be the standard revascularization strategy today. Relatively healthy patients have well-established rates of good outcomes with open surgical revascularization; however, those with comorbid medical conditions have a more significant surgical risk. With the development of self-expanding stents, embolic protection devices, and technical expertise, the carotid stenting procedure appears to be safer and more effective than CEA in those high-risk patients. The optimal revascularization strategy for patients without high-risk medical comorbidities and extracranial carotid artery disease is a subject of debate. The outcomes of randomized trials comparing the two treatment modalities in a wide array of patient populations as well as registry-type trials designed to evaluate various CAS techniques and equipment are much anticipated and likely to alter the way carotid artery revascularization is approached in the future.

REFERENCES

1. Heart disease and stroke statistics—2003 update Dallas, TX: American Heart Association, 2003.
2. O'Holleran LW, Kennelly MM, McClurken M, Johnson JM. Natural history of asymptomatic carotid plaque. Five year follow-up study. Am J Surg 1987;154:659–662.
3. Executive Committee for the Asymptomatic Carotid Atherosclerosis Study Group. Endarterectomy for asymptomatic carotid artery stenosis. Executive Committee for the Asymptomatic Carotid Atherosclerosis Study. JAMA 1995;273:1421–1428.
4. Chambers BR, Norris JW. Outcome in patients with asymptomatic neck bruits. N Engl J Med 1986;315:860–865.
5. Norris JW, Zhu CZ, Bornstein NM, Chambers BR. Vascular risks of asymptomatic carotid stenosis. Stroke 1991;22:1485–1490.
6. North American Symptomatic Carotid Endarterectomy Trial Collaborators. Beneficial effect of carotid endarterectomy in symptomatic patients with high-grade carotid stenosis. North American Symptomatic Carotid Endarterectomy Trial Collaborators. N Engl J Med 1991;325:445–453.
7. Barnett HJ, Taylor DW, Eliasziw M, et al. Benefit of carotid endarterectomy in patients with symptomatic moderate or severe stenosis. North American Symptomatic Carotid Endarterectomy Trial Collaborators. N Engl J Med 1998;339:1415–1425.
8. Joakimsen O, Bonaa KH, Mathiesen EB, et al. Prediction of mortality by ultrasound screening of a general population for carotid stenosis: the Tromso Study. Stroke. 2000;31:1871–1876.
9. Taylor LM Jr, Loboa L, Porter JM. The clinical course of carotid bifurcation stenosis as determined by duplex scanning. J Vasc Surg 1988;8:255–261.
10. Fabris F, Poli L, Zanocchi M, et al. A four year clinical and echographic follow-up of asymptomatic carotid plaque. Angiology 1992;43:590–598.
11. Mayberg MR, Wilson SE, Yatsu F, et al. Carotid endarterectomy and prevention of cerebral ischemia in symptomatic carotid stenosis. Veterans Affairs Cooperative Studies Program 309 Trialist Group. JAMA 1991;266:3289–3294.
12. Randomised trial of endarterectomy for recently symptomatic carotid stenosis: final results of the MRC European Carotid Surgery Trial (ECST). Lancet 1998;351:1379–1387.
13. Rothwell PM, Eliasziw M, Gutnikov SA, et al. Analysis of pooled data from the randomised controlled trials of endarterectomy for symptomatic carotid stenosis. Lancet 2003;361:107–116.
14. Kerber CW, Cromwell LD, Loehden OL. Catheter dilatation of proximal carotid stenosis during distal bifurcation endarterectomy. Am J Neuroradiol 1980;1:348–349.
15. Mullan S, Duda EE, Patronas NJ. Some examples of balloon technology in neurosurgery. J Neurosurg 1980;52:321–329.
16. Hasso AN, Bird CR, Zinke DE, Thompson JR. Fibromuscular dysplasia of the internal carotid artery: percutaneous transluminal angioplasty. Am J Roentgenol 1981;136:955–960.

17. Gil-Peralta A, Mayol A, Marcos JR, et al. Percutaneous transluminal angioplasty of the symptomatic atherosclerotic carotid arteries. Results, complications, and follow-up. Stroke 1996;27:2271–2273.

18. Numaguchi Y, Puyau FA, Provenza LJ, Richardson DE. Percutaneous transluminal angioplasty of the carotid artery. Its application to post surgical stenosis. Neuroradiology 1984;26:527–530.

19. Bergeon P, Rudondy P, Benichou H, et al. Transluminal angioplasty for recurrent stenosis after carotid endarterectomy. Prognostic factors and indications. Int Angiol 1993;12:256–259.

20. Brown MM, Butler P, Gibbs J, et al. Feasibility of percutaneous transluminal angioplasty for carotid artery stenosis. J Neurol Neurosurg Psychiatry 1990;53:238–243.

21. Ahuja A, Blatt GL, Guterman LR, Hopkins LN. Angioplasty for symptomatic radiation-induced extracranial carotid artery stenosis: case report. Neurosurgery 1995;36:399–403.

22. Marks MP, Dake MD, Steinberg GK, et al. Stent placement for arterial and venous cerebrovascular disease: preliminary experience. Radiology 1994;191:441–446.

23. Yadav JS, Roubin GS, Iyer S, et al. Elective stenting of the extracranial carotid arteries. Circulation 1997;95:376–381.

24. Wholey MH, Al-Mubarek N. Updated review of the global carotid artery stent registry. Catheter Cardiovasc Intervent 2003;60:259–266.

25. CAVATAS Investigators. Endovascular versus surgical treatment in patients with carotid stenosis in the Carotid and Vertebral Artery Transluminal Angioplasty Study (CAVATAS): a randomised trial. Lancet 2001;357:1729–1737.

26. Jordan WD Jr, Voellinger DC, Doblar DD, et al. Microemboli detected by transcranial Doppler monitoring in patients during carotid angioplasty versus carotid endarterectomy. Cardiovasc Surg 1999;7:33–38.

27. Rapp JH, Pan XM, Sharp FR, et al. Atheroemboli to the brain: size threshold for causing acute neuronal cell death. J Vasc Surg 2000;32:68–76.

28. McCleary AJ, Nelson M, Dearden NM, et al. Cerebral haemodynamics and embolization during carotid angioplasty in high-risk patients. Br J Surg 1998;85:771–774.

29. Markus HS, Clifton A, Buckenham T, Brown MM. Carotid angioplasty. Detection of embolic signals during and after the procedure. Stroke 1994;25:2403–2406.

30. Jansen C, Ramos LM, van Heesewijk JP, et al. Impact of microembolism and hemodynamic changes in the brain during carotid endarterectomy. Stroke 1994;25:992–997.

31. Gaunt ME, Martin PJ, Smith JL, et al. Clinical relevance of intraoperative embolization detected by transcranial Doppler ultrasonography during carotid endarterectomy: a prospective study of 100 patients. Br J Surg 1994;81:1435–1439.

32. Ackerstaff RG, Jansen C, Moll FL, et al. The significance of microemboli detection by means of transcranial Doppler ultrasonography monitoring in carotid endarterectomy. J Vasc Surg 1995;21:963–969.

33. Angelini A, Reimers B, Della Barbera M, et al. Cerebral protection during carotid artery stenting: collection and histopathologic analysis of embolized debris. Stroke 2002;33:456–461.

34. Al-Mubarak N, Roubin GS, Vitek JJ, et al. Effect of the distal-balloon protection system on microembolization during carotid stenting. Circulation 2001;104:1999–2002.

35. Yadav JS, et al. Stenting and angioplasty with protection in patients at high risk for endarterectomy. The American Heart Association Scientific Sessions, Chicago, IL, 2002.

36. Hobson RW 2nd. Carotid angioplasty-stent: clinical experience and role for clinical trials. J Vasc Surg 2001;33:S117–S123.

37. Adami CA, Scuro A, Spinamano L, et al. Use of the Parodi anti-embolism system in carotid stenting: Italian trial results. J Endovasc Ther 2002;9:147–154.

38. Henry M, Amor M, Henry I, et al. Carotid stenting with cerebral protection: first clinical experience using the PercuSurge GuardWire system. J Endovasc Surg 1999;6:321–331.

39. Henry M, Henry I, Klonaris C, et al. Benefits of cerebral protection during carotid stenting with the PercuSurge GuardWire system: midterm results. J Endovasc Ther 2002;9:1–13.

40. Baim DS, Wahr D, George B, et al. Randomized trial of a distal embolic protection device during percutaneous intervention of saphenous vein aorto-coronary bypass grafts. Circulation 2002;105:1285–1290.

41. Donnan GA, Davis SM, Chambers BR, Gates PC. Surgery for prevention of stroke. Lancet 1998;351:1372–1373.

42. Szabo K, Gass A, Hennerici MG. Diffusion and perfusion MRI for the assessment of carotid atherosclerosis. Neuroimaging Clin North Am 2002;12:381–390.

43. Nederkoorn PJ, van der Graaf Y, Hunink MG. Duplex ultrasound and magnetic resonance angiography compared with digital subtraction angiography in carotid artery stenosis: a systematic review. Stroke 2003;34:1324–1332.

44. Kastrup A, Groschel K, Krapf H, et al. Early outcome of carotid angioplasty and stenting with and without cerebral protection devices: a systematic review of the literature. Stroke 2003;34:813–819.
45. Mathur A, Roubin GS, Iyer SS, et al. Predictors of stroke complicating carotid artery stenting. Circulation 1998;97:1239–1245.
46. Qureshi AI, Saad M, Zaidat OO, et al. Intracerebral hemorrhages associated with neurointerventional procedures using a combination of antithrombotic agents including abciximab. Stroke 2002;33:1916–1919.
47. Schluter M, Tubler T, Steffens JC, et al. Focal ischemia of the brain after neuroprotected carotid artery stenting. J Am Coll Cardiol 2003;42:1007–1013.
48. Savcic M, Hauert J, Bachmann F, et al. Clopidogrel loading dose regimens: kinetic profile of pharmacodynamic response in healthy subjects. Semin Thromb Hemost 1999;25 (Suppl 2):15–19.
49. Muller I, Seyfarth M, Rudiger S, et al. Effect of a high loading dose of clopidogrel on platelet function in patients undergoing coronary stent placement. Heart 2001;85:92–93.
50. Gawaz M, Seyfarth M, Muller I, et al. Comparison of effects of clopidogrel versus ticlopidine on platelet function in patients undergoing coronary stent placement. Am J Cardiol 2001;87:332–336.
51. Gurbel PA, Bliden KP, Hiatt BL, O'Connor CM. Clopidogrel for coronary stenting: response variability, drug resistance, and the effect of pretreatment platelet reactivity. Circulation 2003;107:2908–2913.
52. Kapadia SR, Bajzer CT, Ziada KM, et al. Initial experience of platelet glycoprotein IIb/IIIa inhibition with abciximab during carotid stenting: a safe and effective adjunctive therapy. Stroke 2001;32: 2328–2332.
53. Hofmann R, Kerschner K, Steinwender C, et al. Abciximab bolus injection does not reduce cerebral ischemic complications of elective carotid artery stenting: a randomized study. Stroke 2002;33:725–727.
54. Qureshi AI, Luft AR, Sharma M, et al. Frequency and determinants of postprocedural hemodynamic instability after carotid angioplasty and stenting. Stroke 1999;30:2086–2093.
55. Schoser BG, Heesen C, Eckert B, Thie A. Cerebral hyperperfusion injury after percutaneous transluminal angioplasty of extracranial arteries. J Neurol 1997;244:101–104.
56. Phatouros CC, Meyers PM, Higashida RT, et al. Intracranial hemorrhage and cerebral hyperperfusion syndrome after extracranial carotid artery angioplasty and stent placement. Am J Neuroradiol 2002;23:503–504.
57. McCabe DJ, Brown MM, Clifton A. Fatal cerebral reperfusion hemorrhage after carotid stenting. Stroke 1999;30:2483–2486.
58. Meyers PM, Higashida RT, Phatouros CC, et al. Cerebral hyperperfusion syndrome after percutaneous transluminal stenting of the craniocervical arteries. Neurosurgery 2000;47:335–343; discussion 343–345.
59. Ho DS, Wang Y, Chui M, et al. Epileptic seizures attributed to cerebral hyperperfusion after percutaneous transluminal angioplasty and stenting of the internal carotid artery. Cerebrovasc Dis 2000;10:374–379.
60. Morrish W, Grahovac S, Douen A, et al. Intracranial hemorrhage after stenting and angioplasty of extracranial carotid stenosis. Am J Neuroradiol 2000;21:1911–1916.
61. Abou-Chebl AM, Yadav JS, Reginelli JP, et al. Intracranial hemorrhage and hyperperfusion syndrome following carotid artery stenting: risk factors, prevention, and treatment. J Am Coll Cardiol 2004;43:1596–1601.
62. Chan AW, Roffi M, Mukherjee D, et al. Carotid brachytherapy for in-stent restenosis. Cathet Cardiovasc Intervent 2003;58:86–92.

19

Aortic Stent Grafting
Percutaneous and Surgical Approaches

Omaida C. Velazquez, MD, Edward Woo, MD, and Ronald M. Fairman, MD

CONTENTS

INTRODUCTION

Parodi published the first series of abdominal aortic aneurysms repaired using endovascular techniques *(1)*. Since then, the field of aortic aneurysm treatment has been revolutionized by fast technological advancements in catheter-based covered stent-grafts. In the United States, clinical studies began only a few years after Parodi's pioneering work *(2,3)* and trials have progressed rapidly since then, fueled by industry support and cheered by both physicians and patients. To date, four devices have been approved by the Food and Drug Administration (FDA) (Ancure, Guidant/EVT, Menlo Park, CA; AneuRx, Medtronics, Santa Rosa, CA; Excluder, W.L. Gore & Associates, Flagstaff, AZ; Zenith,

From: *Contemporary Cardiology: Interventional Cardiology:
Percutaneous Noncoronary Intervention*
Edited by: H. C. Herrmann © Humana Press Inc., Totowa, NJ

Cook, Bloomington, IN). One of the four (Ancure) has been withdrawn from the market by Guidant. In addition, numerous other devices are currently undergoing clinical trials. The FDA-approved devices can be used for the abdominal aorta, but ongoing trials are exploring the use of similar endovascular technologies for aneurysms of the thoracic aorta. Currently, a length of at least 15 mm for the proximal aortic neck and a 20-mm-long landing zone in the common iliac arteries away from any major named arterial branch are a prerequisite for being able to exclude an aneurysm by endovascular approaches. However, ongoing experimental techniques continue to push the frontiers of the endovascular approach by attempting to design ways in which one can maneuver around aortic branches, move them out of the way, or reconstruct stent-graft branches as part of the repair. Similarly, although currently a femoral cut-down is routinely used for endovascular aneurysm exclusion, the frontier of completely percutaneous aneurysm repair is actively being sought by numerous investigators and industry bioengineers. Currently, despite some early setbacks and still evolving technology, commercially manufactured endovascular systems are employed to treat abdominal aortic aneurysms (AAAs) in about 50% of elective aneurysm repairs and are continuing to spread widely throughout the world *(4)*.

EVOLUTION AND SETBACKS

Technology has advanced rapidly since the advent of endovascular repair of abdominal aortic aneurysms, but rapid progress came with occasional significant setbacks. The initially unbridled excitement in Australia and Europe over the Vanguard endograft (Boston Scientific Corp., Natick, MA) was curtailed before the graft was widely used in the United states markets when a high incidence of graft-component disconnections was noted. The contralateral docking segment of this modular bifurcated graft and the length of intussusception were short, leading to a propensity for separation of the components of the contralateral limb. Subsequently, despite resolution of this design issue, fabric erosion leading to type III endoleaks became a major problem for this endograft. Yet, the Vanguard device, composed of a modular polyester graft supported with a nitinol frame, had initially yielded encouraging trial reports after analysis of the French Vanguard trial *(5)*. This multicenter trial reported 100% success rate of implantation, no perioperative deaths, and an 8% rate of early reoperation. A 30% endoleak rate was noted on immediate perioperative computed tomography (CT) scans. One patient died of AAA rupture during the mean follow-up of 18 mo. An additional 12% and 11% endovascular reinterventions were required for the treatment of graft limb occlusions or endoleaks, respectively. Significant AAA expansion was noted in patients with persistent endoleaks.

The first endograft approved in the United states (Ancure) also had some limitations related to the deployment complexity of the unibody design. Specifically, the unsupported limbs had a predisposition to kink, and the infrarenal fixation with hooks limited candidates without calcification or thrombus at the proximal aortic neck. However, as time passed and issues of ongoing infrarenal aortic neck dilatation with possible endograft migration have been recognized in other types of graft design, the Ancure hook fixation is now regarded as the most positive attribute of this endograft. Regrettably, issues of the deployment complexities among other FDA-related inquiries prompted Guidant to stopped marketing the device.

The thoracic Excluder graft (W. L. Gore & Associates, Flagstaff, AZ) was initially very well received (during clinical trials), because the great ease of the delivery and

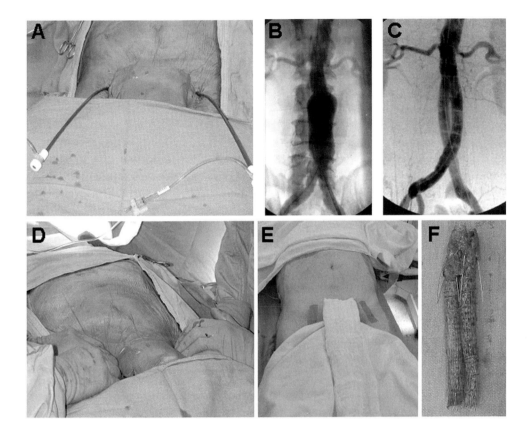

Fig. 1. Completely percutaneous endovascular repair of infrarenal AAA—"the hope for the future." **(A)** Photograph of patient from the Cordis phase I trial with delivery sheaths in place. **(B,C)** Intraoperative arteriograms **(B)** of the AAA before repair and **(C)** after endovascular exclusion with the Cordis device. **(D)** Application of femoral pressure after removal of the delivery sheaths. **(E)** Photograph at the completion of the case, with small Band-Aids over access punctures after the completely percutaneous technique. **(F)** Photograph of an explanted Cordis Endograft (explanted after placement of bilateral proximal stents failed to correct a proximal type I endoleak).

deployment systems were a true innovation. However, this endograft exhibited problems with materials fatigue. A similar story lead to the early discontinuation of the phase I clinical trial of the Cordis endograft (Johnson & Johnson). The Cordis endograft main innovation was that of very low profile 12 French (F) delivery sheath, making it the first completely percutaneous stent-graft. The design consisted of a polyurethane-covered gasket and two endolegs. The Cordis clinical trial was stopped in phase I because of endoleg occlusions and uncorrectable proximal type 1 endoleaks. However, the promise and allure of the percutaneous endograft concept for AAA repair remains very much alive, despite these potential pitfalls (Fig. 1).

SURGICAL APPROACH FOR CURRENT ENDOVASCULAR AORTIC ANEURYSM REPAIR: TECHNICAL ASPECTS AND POTENTIAL COMPLICATIONS OF THE FEMORAL CUT-DOWN

Current aortic endografting devices require at least one femoral cut-down for deployment. The procedures most commonly occur in the sterile environment of the operating room, where any potential complication can be immediately treated such as AAA rupture, iliac artery perforation, femoral artery injury, distal embolization, or thrombosis. Also, when an iliofemoral conduit is required for access, the operating room environment is optimal. The patient is placed in the supine position and the abdomen and femoral regions are prepped and draped from the xiphoid to the midthigh. Although this extensive preparation is not required just for femoral exposure, it allows for the potential option of emergency open rescue interventions. Either vertical or transverse skin incisions are acceptable to expose the common femoral artery. The vertical incision is centered over the femoral pulse, with one-third of the incision above the inguinal crease and two-thirds below it. When the pulse is not palpable, the incision should extend vertically from a point midway between the anterior superior iliac spine and the pubic tubercle. The transverse incision is also centered over the femoral pulse, but it is located about 3 cm cephalad and parallel to the inguinal crease.

Upon carrying out the deeper dissection, the small superficial epigastric and superficial circumflex branches of the femoral vessels are usually encountered in the subcutaneous tissue and can be safely ligated and divided. Lymphatic vessels associated with the inguinal nodes should also be ligated prior to transaction so as to avoid a lymphocele. The fascia lata is opened over the medial margin of the sartorius muscle and the dissection is extended proximally to the level of the inguinal ligament. Lateral retraction of the sartorious muscle exposes the underlying funnel-shaped femoral sheath, which is incised longitudinally over the course of the femoral artery. The healing inflammatory changes observed after diagnostic arteriograms can sometimes render the femoral artery difficult to separate from the femoral vein. However, in general, only loose areolar tissue envelopes the artery under the opened femoral sheath. The common femoral artery is then easily separated from the femoral vein medially and the femoral nerve laterally, and then encircled proximally and distally with vessel loops. The common femoral artery divides into two major trunks: the deep and superficial femoral arteries that can be exposed by dissecting distally along the anterior, medial, and lateral surface of the parent trunk. Most commonly, the superficial femoral artery arises anteriorly and the profunda femoris artery arises posterolaterally, from the parent trunk. These vessels can be individually encircled with vessel loops, providing a longer segment of access to the common femoral artery. However, this more distal dissection is seldom necessary. The femoral cut-down procedure often needs to be repeated for contralateral femoral exposure. The remainder of the procedure is performed under full systemic heparin treatment, maintaining an ACT (activated clotting time) longer than 300 s.

Fairly standard catheter and wire techniques are then utilized to gain access to the suprarenal aorta and deliver the endograft. Because most devices are loaded on long, tapered delivery sheaths, the tip of the access wires are positioned high in the descending thoracic aorta. Modular devices are assembled within the aorta, one segment at a time. Most commonly, the main body of the device is delivered via one sheath containing the graft's main trunk with ipsilateral long limb (that anchors in the ipsilateral iliac artery) and a contralateral short limb. The short limb docks with a longer connecting iliac limb introduced separately from the contralateral femoral. In a unibody design, both ipsilateral and contralateral limbs are attached to the main trunk and main delivery system. In the unibody designs, after unsheathing within the aorta, the contraleral limb is guided and pulled into the proper side by means of a snared pull-through wire. Typically, heparin anticoagulation is reversed after removal of all catheters and wires and completed surgical repair of the femoral arteries (with interrupted nonabsorbable polypropylene sutures).

For bifurcated endograft designs, when a formal arteriotomy is required for introduction of the delivery sheath, it should be performed and repaired transversely to avoid narrowing

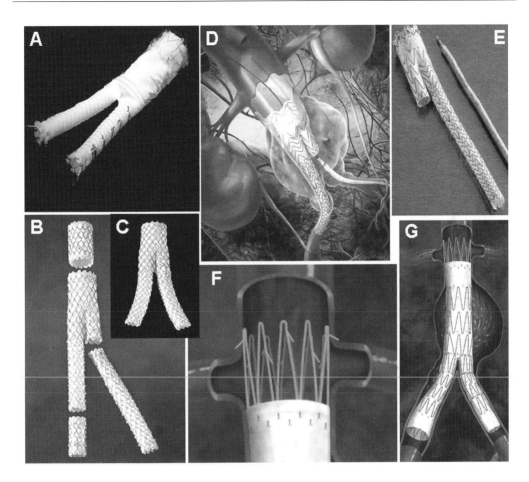

Fig. 2. The four FDA-approved devices: (**A**) Ancure, (**B, C**) AneuRx, (**D, E**) Excluder, and (**F, G**) Zenith.

of the femoral artery. In aorto-uni-iliac designs, where the need for a femoro-femoral bypass is anticipated, the arteriotomy is performed longitudinally to facilitate the femoral anastomoses.

Understanding the Differences in the Four FDA-Approved Devices

THE ANCURE DEVICE

The Ancure device (Fig. 2A) is a bifurcated unibody polyester graft that attaches proximally to the infrarenal aorta and iliac arteries distally by using sharp Elgiloy wire hooks that penetrate the arterial wall. A balloon is inflated at the attachment sites to ensure proper fixation. The entire device comes preloaded on a single delivery system. Bilateral femoral cut-downs are necessary: one side for the delivery system and the other side for a sheath utilized to retrieve and deploy the contralateral limb of the graft. The body of the graft is not reinforced by stents. This design closely mimics the grafts utilized in conventional open surgical repair of aortic aneurysms. The delivery system for the Ancure is 23.5F, thereby requiring one external iliac artery to be at least 7.9 mm in diameter. At the proximal fixation, the Ancure can attach to infrarenal aortic necks that are no wider than 26 mm and at least 15 mm in length. At the iliac arteries, distal fixation can be achieved in common iliac arteries that are no wider than 13 mm. Circumferential calcification in the infrarenal aortic neck might interfere with proper hook fixation. Calcified, tortuous, or stenotic external iliac arteries might interfere with the delivery of the device. These anatomic presentations are contraindications for using the Ancure device. Deployment of the Ancure, because it comes loaded on a single delivery system, is relatively complex and requires significant expertise. The learning curve tends to be slow.

THE ANEURX DEVICE

The AneuRx stent-graft is a modular bifurcated system (Figs. 2B and 2C). The graft is assembled within the aorta at the time of the aneurysm repair by using multiple catheter exchanges. The device consists of a polyester graft reinforced by an exoskeleton of diamond-shaped nitinol stent rings. The stent-graft is self-expanding and utilizes radial force as the mechanism for proximal and distal fixation. Proximal and distal modular extensions are available and can be ordered as needed, thus increasing flexibility for intraoperative design modifications such as extending the fixation zones or converting to aorto-uni-iliac design. The main bifurcated section of the device is prepackaged into a 21F delivery sheath. Therefore, at least one external iliac artery must be 7 mm or wider. At the infrarenal aorta, fixation can be obtained in diameters no wider than 26 mm and length of at least 10 mm. At the common iliac arteries, distal fixation can be accomplished in a more versatile range of diameters by the use of wide (aortic) extension cuffs that can flare out the distal fixation into a bell-bottom configuration. Although aortic cuffs are available as wide as 28 mm, it is not recommended to attempt fixation into aneurysmal iliac arteries that are wider than 20 mm. At 20 mm iliac artery diameter, a 22-mm aortic extension cuff can be utilized for adequate and safe distal fixation. However, this practice it is not endorsed by the company's IFU (instructions for use)

THE EXCLUDER DEVICE

The Excluder device is a modular device made of expanded polytetrafluoroethylene (ePTFE) graft materials bonded to the inside of a nitinol exoskeleton (Figs. 2D and 2E). There are no suture holes in the graft material because the exoskeleton is bonded with ePTFE/fluorinated ethylene propylene composite film. This feature decreases the risk of leakage through fabric tears. The main body is delivered through an 18F sheath and the contralateral portion is delivered through a 12F sheath; thus, the profile of the delivery system is smaller than the other FDA-approved devices. There is an external sealing cuff at the proximal fixation end. The deployment mechanism from the excluder device is very straightforward. Simply pulling on a deployment line (a PTFE fiber) that releases the constrained sleeve allows for self-expansion of the graft and deploys the device. There is no lengthening or shortening of the prosthesis with this fast deployment method. The proximal aortic neck must be smaller than 26 mm in diameter, longer than 15 mm, and less than 60° angulated. The distal iliac diameter can be no wider than 12 mm to achieve adequate fixation with this device. Aortic and iliac extension cuffs are also available with this device.

THE ZENITH DEVICE

The Zenith device consists of a bifurcated three-piece modular system (Figs. 2F and 2G). The endograft is made of woven polyester supported by self-expanding stainless-steel Z-stents. Bare proximal stents with barbs that expand radially upon deployment allow for suprarenal fixation. A trigger wire that holds it constrained to avoid premature deployment releases this proximal bare stent. The delivery system of the Zenith is characterized by a very long tapered tip with side holes that can be used for angiography through the sheath. Despite its suprarenal fixation mechanism, the Zenith device requires a nonaneurysmal infrarenal aortic neck of at least 15 mm length to ensure proper seal. The diameter of the neck cannot exceed 28 mm or be smaller than 18 mm. The angle of the aortic neck relative to the long axis of the aneurysm should not exceed 60° and relative to the axis of the suprarenal aorta should not exceed 45°. The iliac artery fixation zone should be at least 10 mm in length and 7.5–20 mm in diameter. Ancillary components are available for the Zenith device and include converters, iliac leg extensions, occluders, and main body extensions. Only the bifurcated endograft is FDA approved. However, with the aid of a converter, the flow-divider can be covered such as to create an aorto-uni-iliac configuration. The occluder can then be deployed at the contralateral common iliac artery level and a femoro-femoral bypass graft completes the procedure.

GENERAL CONSIDERATIONS AND OUTCOMES

Only one of the four FDA-approved devices (Ancure) has a unibody design, with sharp hook fixation against the infrarenal aorta and without metal stent support of the main trunk and limbs of the graft. The others (AneuRx, Excluder, Zenith) are fully supported, modular stent-grafts. Three of the four FDA-approved devices (Ancure, AneuRx, Excluder) are designed for infrarenal fixation. Only the Zenith has a suprarenal bare spring and barbs fixation component; however, the main proximal seal zone depends on the infrarenal neck in contact with the graft-covered part of the prosthesis. Figure 2 depicts the four FDA-approved devices.

All four devices that received FDA approval demonstrated technical success rates of aneurysm exclusion greater than 90%. Successful device deployment mandates the use of state-of-the-art intraoperative fluoroscopy equipment. X-ray exposure to patient and operating room team needs to be monitored and minimized. All these devices require surgical exposure of the femoral artery for insertion. They all eliminate the need for laparotomy. Although a definitive decrease in mortality has not been shown and the cases might be as long or longer in terms of operative time, the hospital length of stay and operative blood loss are decreased significantly when compared to open surgical controls. Patients recover faster, incur minor postoperative pain, and have decreased complications when compared to conventional open aneurysm repair (6). The very elderly and those with associated medical comorbidities prohibitive for open surgical aneurysm repair can be successfully treated by these minimally invasive techniques. This is believed to result from the fact that the major perioperative intravascular fluid shifts resulting in hemodynamic instability, seen in open aortic aneurysm repair, are not observed after endovascular repair. In addition, general anesthesia is not required for endovascular repair and the procedures can be performed under regional or even local anesthetic. Stay in the intensive care unit (ICU) is usually not needed after endovascular aneurysm exclusion. Because these procedures require the administration of contrast dye for adequate positioning of the endograft, contrast-dye-induced nephropathy can be a problem, particularly in those with pre-existing renal dysfunction.

Although the endovascular devices have added a significant dimension to the range of patients who could have repair of their aortic aneurysm in a minimally invasive manner, the technology is not applicable to all patients with aortic aneurysm. A limited number of sizes severely limits the types of aneurysm that can be successfully excluded, particularly in women (9). Anatomy-related exclusions include juxtarenal extension of the aneurysm, complicated proximal aortic necks (short, angulated, ulcerated, calcified, dilated), small tortuous or stenotic external iliac arteries, a calcified

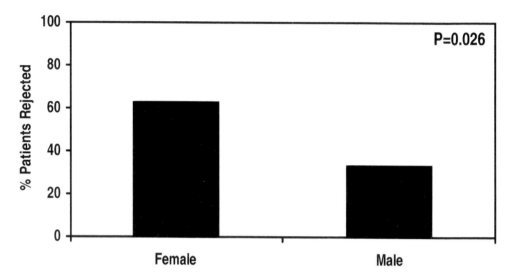

Fig. 3. Our center's initial experience ($n = 141$ patients) with Ancure and Talent devices showing the percent of patients rejected for endovascular AAA repair after initial evaluation because of unfavorable aorto-iliac and aneurysm anatomic features. (From ref. *7.*)

or narrowed aortic bifurcation, and coexistent extensive iliac artery aneurysms wherein endovascular exclusion could compromise pelvic circulation. In addition, the delivery systems for today's devices remain bulky and cumbersome. For example, when we looked at our initial experience with the Ancure and Talent (Medtronic AVE, Santa Rosa, CA), we noted that more female patients were excluded from endovascular repair because of small iliac arteries precluding access or because of an increased proportion of unfavorable proximal fixation features such as short, dilated, angulated infrarenal aortic necks (Fig. 3) *(7)*. Ongoing research, often industry sponsored, continues to improve materials and design in the hopes of developing lower-profile delivery systems with simpler deployment techniques. Alternatives to polyester fabric are being explored with the hopes of decreasing endograft profile and, ultimately, developing a completely percutaneous delivery system.

Preparations for Successful Device Implantation
to Achieve aneurysm Exclusion

The successful implantation of aortic endografts requires significant preoperative planning. Accurate radiographic imaging of the aneurysm, the fixation zones, and the access vessels is essential. Until recently, the gold standards for imaging in the preoperative evaluation for endovascular aortic aneurysm repair were spiral CT angiography with three-dimensional reconstruction and marker catheter arteriography. The latter, however, is not always necessary because of the advent of software-assisted centerline measurements from three-dimensional reconstruction of CT angiogram data *(8)*. Currently, these software assisted measurements are most commonly obtained with the aid of MMS (Medical Media Systems, West Lebanon, NH), obviating the need for a marker catheter arteriogram *(9)*. Unlike the standard open surgical repair, which can be planned even with limited non-contrast CT imaging, endovascular repair depends on detailed preoperative anatomic assessment. These assessments then lead to the choice of endograft make, the determination as to specific design configuration, and the needed device widths, lengths, and components to be ordered in order to accomplish successful aneurysm exclusion at the time of endovascular repair. This extensive preoperative planning is paramount for optimal short- and long-term outcome after endovascular aneurysm repair.

POST OPERATIVE FOLLOW-UP

The postoperative follow-up after endovascular aortic aneurysm repair focuses on surveillance of the fixation zones, the aneurysm volume, and the need to rule out evidence of blood flow outside the endograft and within the aneurysm sac (i.e., an endoleak). In addition, endograft limb patency is monitored. Follow-up surveillance usually includes a history and physical examination, plain abdomen/pelvis X-rays, and an abdomen/pelvis CT with and without contrast (including early- and late-phase imaging of the aneurysm sac). Lower extremity pulse volume recordings (PVRs) can be added to the standard vascular examination of peripheral pulses. These follow-ups are usually obtained at 1, 6, and 12 mo and yearly thereafter.

The topic of endoleaks will be covered in greater depth in the section Endoleaks. However, endoleaks are also relevant to the recommended follow-up. The search to rule out endoleak is routinely performed at 1, 6, and 12 mo and, thereafter, yearly, but can be performed more frequently for symptoms, aneurysm progression, or known fixation difficulties. An estimated 20% of patients will have an endoleak at 1 mo but most of those are type II endoleaks, related to flow through sac branches (inferior mesenteric artery, lumbar arteries, accessory renal arteries) and will spontaneously thrombose within the first year of follow-up. In the presence of symptoms or if the aneurysm sac is enlarging, embolization of these type II endoleaks might become necessary (10,11). In a standard open repair, all these branches would be surgically ligated. In endovascular repair, it is hoped that a low-flow situation resulting from complete proximal and distal endograft fixation (and thus aneurysm exclusion) will lead the sac branches to spontaneously thrombose. Unlike type II endoleaks, the type I endoleaks that result from inadequate proximal or distal fixation must be treated upon diagnosis, because they represent an unprotected aneurysm sac. Type I endoleaks can be treated by endovascular extensions, uncovered stents, or conversion to open repair.

Problems of endograft migration can be detected on follow-up imaging even before any evidence of endoleak and even as the aneurysm sac is actively remodeling and decreasing in volume (Fig. 4). Sudden exposure of a remodeling aneurysm sac to systemic pressure by migration of the endograft could lead to rupture even in aneurysms that have remodeled to small (less than 4 cm) diameters. Migration problems can be related to progression of aneurysmal dilatation at the fixation zones (12–16). Similar to type I endoleaks, migration can be treated by adding endovascular extensions or by conversion to open repair. Migration remains a concern during long-term follow-up, as we are now seeing patients in our own series developing radiologic evidence of migration in years 3–4 postimplant. Endoleaks also have an impact on aneurysm sac shrinkage (17). For Ancure and Zenith devices, the presence of an endoleak slows down the rate of AAA shrinkage. For the Excluder device, endoleaks are associated with an increase in size of the AAA sac (17).

Fatigue of the endograft components could become evident by fractures of the supporting metal components or by holes in the fabric (causing a type III endoleak). These could be detected by a combination of plain X-rays and CT angiogram. Another problem that might be detected on follow-up is disconnection of the modular components that also leads to a type III endoleak. Type III endoleaks, either from separation of graft junctions

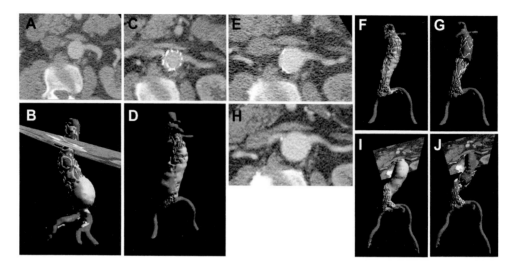

Fig. 4. Significant migration of a Talent endograft at 4 yr of follow-up, without evidence of endoleak and with full regression of the aneurysm sac. (**A, B**) Preoperative imaging on a 6-cm AAA showing the CT axial image at level of renal arteries (**A**) with minimal thrombus and MMS three-dimensional reconstruction (**B**) with a 22-mm length, 30-mm-diameter infrarenal aortic neck with mild angulation and thrombus. (**C, D**) Same patient 1 mo after successful endovascular repair with a Talent endograft, showing proximal fixation with suprarenal bare springs. (**E–J**) Progressive dilatation of infrarenal aortic neck resulting in significant distal migration at 1 yr (**E–G**) and 4 yr (**H–J**) of follow-up. At 4 yr of follow-up, the aneurysm has regressed to 3 cm, extensive circumferential thrombus extends up to the level of the renal arteries, and no endoleak can be observed on CT angiogram. However, the endograft has fallen into the sac and this AAA required conversion to open repair with explantation of the endograft. (Color illustration is printed in insert following page 236.)

or from material fatigue, could be treated by a graft-within-graft approach or conversion to open repair.

Another important aspect of follow-up relates to endograft limb patency. In our experience to date exceeding 500 endografts, we have observed delayed graft limb occlusions in both supported and unsupported endografts. However, unsupported limbs (Ancure) have a higher tendency to present with limb thromboses related to kinks *(18–20)*. Acute endolimb malperfusion can be treated by endovascular techniques *(18–20)* or could necessitate femoral–femoral bypass.

FDA-APPROVED ABDOMINAL AORTIC ENDOGRAFTS FOR ANEURYSM REPAIR: OUTCOMES OF THE CLINICAL TRIALS

Ancure

In prospective, nonrandomized, concurrent controlled phase II (18 US centers) and III studies (*n* = 305 patients in 21 US institutions) that compared the performance of the Ancure to open surgical AAA repair, the graft was found to be effective in preventing AAA rupture, with similar long-term survival to the open surgery group *(21,22)*. Of 573 patients, 531 (92.7%) underwent successful implantation of the endograft during the phase II and III trials. The combined major morbidity and mortality in the endovascular versus the open route were 28.8% versus 44.1%, respectfully. Significant benefits were noted in the endovascular group: shorter hospital stay (2 d vs 6 d), less surgical blood loss

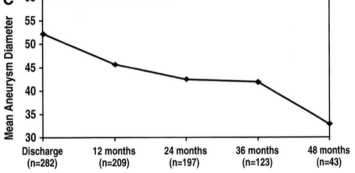

A

	12 Months	24 Months	36 Months	48 Months
# of Patients with Visit	272	242	157	64
Graft Migrations	1	0	0	0
Aneurysm Ruptures	0	0	0	0
Surgical Conversions (> 30 days)**	2	0	2	1

B

	Type I	Type II	Type Unknown
Discharge (n=300)	3.7%	30.3%	7.3%
48 months (n=53)	1.9%	11.3%	0.0%

C

Mean Aneurysm Diameter

(y-axis: 30, 35, 40, 45, 50, 55, 60)

Discharge (n=282) | 12 months (n=209) | 24 months (n=197) | 36 months (n=123) | 48 months (n=43)

Fig. 5. Summary of data for patients enrolled into the Ancure bifurcated US trial from December 1995 to November 1998. (**A**) Number of endograft migrations, AAA ruptures, and conversions to open. (**B**) Core lab data on endoleak rates at discharge and at 48 mo of follow-up. (**C**) Core lab data on mean AAA maximum diameters over time, up to 48 mo of follow-up. (Updated summary tables and figures provided by Ancure®, Guidant/EVT®, and courtesy of principal investigators.)

(400 mL vs 800 mL), and less intensive care unit use (33% vs 94%). Three hundred nineteen patients were followed for 5 yr. There were no aneurysm ruptures noted. Survival in the endovascular group was 68.1% compared to 77.2% in the surgical group (difference not significant). At 60 mo of follow-up, 74.4% of patients were free of endoleak and there were no type I or type III endoleaks and 97.6% of patients had aneurysm sacs that were decreasing in size or stable. One patient experienced an increase in the aneurysm sac and a conversion was required in nine patients (2.8%). Figure 5 summarizes the data on migrations, ruptures, conversions to open operations, endoleak rates, and aneurysm remodeling for the Ancure device.

AneuRx

There has been extensive clinical experience and relatively long follow-up (over 6 yr) with over 38, 000 patients treated from the United States, Europe, the Middle East, Australia, and the Far East on the outcomes achieved after endovascular AAA repair using the AneuRx endograft *(13,23–27)*. Whereas there have been a number of concerning reports of AAA ruptures *(24)*, ongoing infrarenal aortic neck dilatation, and significant migration rates *(13,15)*, the denominators are large as a result of thousands of patients treated world wide. As such, the overall outcome rates continue to appear favorable, as summarized in Fig. 6. However, it is of some concern that Conner et al. reported significant neck dilatation associated with migration in patients followed after treatment with

A

Clinical Trial	No. of Implants
US clinical trial	1193
Post-market US implants	>34, 000
EUROSTAR Registry*	924
Europe, Middle East, Australia, Far East	>2,500
Total	**>>38,000**

*October 2002 EUROSTAR Report

B

Kaplan Meier Estimates (%)	1 Yr	2 Yr	3 Yr	4 Yr	5 Yr
Freedom from aneurysm rupture	99.5	98.6	98.5	97.2	97.2
Freedom from conversion	98.5	97.0	95.2	92.6	91.1
Freedom from aneurysm related death	98.1	97.6	97.2	96.9	96.8
Probably of survival (all –cause mortality)	91.8	83.5	78.4	69.7	61.5

AneuRx Clinical Update Vol. II, January, 2004

C

Outcome	Operative (%)	≤30 Days (%)	>30 Days	Total
Aneurysm rupture	2/1193 (0.17)	3/1193 (0.25)	15/1193	20/1193
Conversion to surgical repair	11/1193 (0.92)	4/1193 (0.34)	45/1193	60/1193
Death (all-cause)	0	22/1193 (1.8)	228/1193	305/1193
Aneurysm-related death	0	22/1193 (1.8)	10/1193	32/1193

AneuRx Clinical Update, Vol. II, January2004

D

	Kaplan-Meier at 5 Yr (%)	Incidence (%)
Freedom from rupture	97.2	20/1193 (0.016%)
Freedom from surgical conversion	91.1	60/1193 (0.050%)
All-cause mortality	61.5	305/1193 (0.256%)
Freedom from aneurysm-related death	96.8	32/1193 (0.027%)

AneuRx Clinical Update, Vol. II, January2004

Fig. 6. Numbers of AneuRx devices implanted and key clinical results. (**A**) AneuRx devices implanted worldwide. (**B–D**) Key results from AneuRx US clinical trials. (Updated summary tables and Figures provided by AnuRx®, Medtronics ®, and courtesy of principal investigators.)

the AneuRx endograft with 7%, 20%, 42%, and 67% migration rates at 1, 2, 3, and 4yr of follow-up, respectively *(15)*. Oversizing of the proximal graft fixation by greater than 20% with its associated increase in radial force on the aortic wall was implicated as a significant factor in this problem. However, in an analysis of a much larger cohort of patients, Zarins et al. concluded that stent-graft migration appears to be largely related to short necks and low initial deployment of the AneuRx device and the global numbers were not as worrisome, although still significant (freedom from significant migration was only 81.2% at 3 yr) *(13,28)*.

Excluder

In the multicenter prospective trial comparing standard open repair of infrarenal AAA with Excluder bifurcated endoprosthesis treatment, the device was found to be safe and effective, with the most striking benefits in the reduction of operative blood loss and perioperative complications while allowing for faster recovery times *(29)*. The study included 19 US centers. Patients treated with the Excluder (*n* = 235) had a significantly lower chance of any major perioperative complication than the open surgical controls (*n* = 99) (Figs. 7A and 7B). After the immediate periprocedural difference in major adverse events, the complication curves become parallel (Fig. 7B), indicating similar rates of subsequent events. Compared with the operative group, early major adverse events were significantly reduced (Fig. 7C). Figure 7D shows the endoleak rates by type according to corelab-determined radiographic findings. Reintervention for further treatment of the AAA was required in 17 patients (7%) during the first year and in 14 patients (7%) in the second year of follow-up (Fig. 7E). All except four of these interventions were endovascular in nature. Three patients underwent conversion to open repair because of enlarging AAAs at 24, 28, and 29 mo of follow-up; none had a prior reintervention. Two of these three

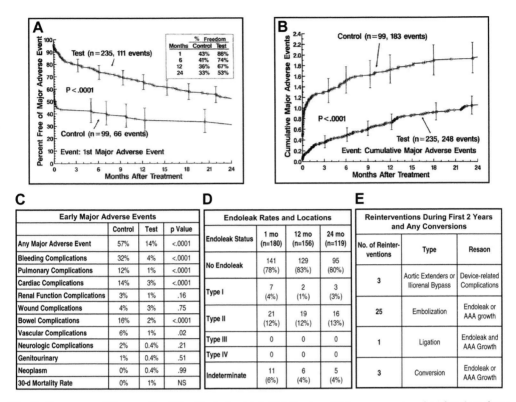

Fig. 7. Summary of the results of the Excluder trial. (**A**) Kaplan–Maier curves showing freedom from first major adverse event. (**B**) Kaplan–Maier curves showing cumulative major adverse events rates. (**C**) Detailed summary of early major adverse events. (**D**) Endoleak rates by types at 1, 12, and 24 mo follow-up (**E**) Details of reinterventions during the first 2 yr of follow-up. (From ref. *29*, with permission.)

patients had no radiographically identifiable endoleak and the third had an untreated type II endoleak.

Zenith

The Zenith US pivotal study evaluated the performance of the endograft in comparison to open surgical controls. Enrollment included 200 patients into a standard risk Zenith endograft arm, 80 patients into the surgical group, 100 patients into a high-risk Zenith endograft group, and 52 roll-in patients from January 2000 to July 2001. The overall results were very favorable for the Zenith-treated group, with significantly better clinical utility measures in the endovascular group than in the open repair group (Fig. 8). An update on the data that included 528 patients treated with the Zenith endograft with a mean follow-up of 18 mo *(30)* reported that 66% of those patients were considered to have associated medical comorbidity that would place them in a high-physiologic-risk group for open repair. Successful endograft implantation was accomplished in 524/228 (99.2%) of patients. Overall endoleak rate was low at 15%, of which 4% were type I and treated urgently. Only eight endograft migrations were detected after 2 yr of follow-up, mostly without clinical impact (<10 mm at 12 mo and subsequently stabilized, not requiring intervention). There were three (0.57%) late conversions to open repair and two (0.38%) AAA ruptures during the follow-up period *(30)*. Device migration

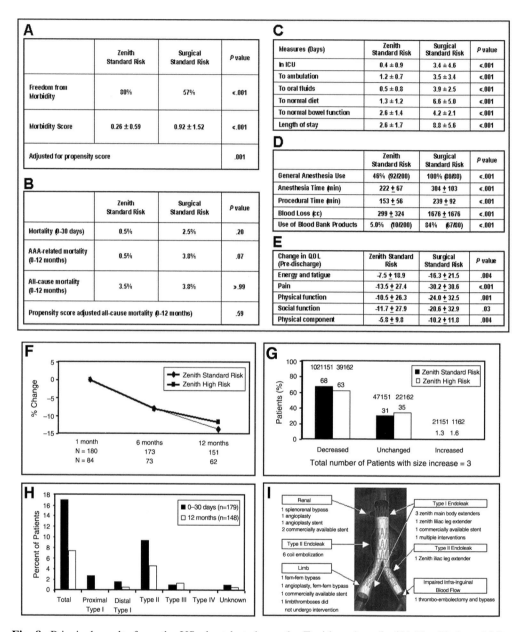

Fig. 8. Principal results from the US pivotal study on the Zenith endograft. (**A**) The 30-d morbidity rates. (**B**) Mortality rates at 30 d and 12 mo. Data on clinical utility in terms of recovery times (**C**), procedural measures (**D**), SF-36TM quality-of-life questionnaire (**E**), change in aneurysm size (remodeling) over time in terms of percent reduction in maximum AAA diameter (**F**), and in terms of the percentage of patients with larger than 5-mm reductions in maximum AAA diameter at 12 mo (**G**). (**H**) Rates of endoleaks by type. (**I**) Required secondary interventions by type. (Updated summary tables and figures provided by Zenith" AAA Endovascular Graft [COOK], and courtesy of principal investigators.)

and endoleaks are infrequent after treatment with the Zenith. However, endograft oversizing of greater than 30% is associated with a 14-fold increase in device migration (>5 mm) at 12 mo of follow-up and a 16-fold increased risk of AAA expansion at 1 yr of follow-up *(31)*.

COMMERCIALLY FABRICATED ABDOMINAL AORTIC ENDOGRAFTS UNDER CLINICAL TRIAL FOR ANEURYSM REPAIR: PROGRESS TO DATE

Trivascular

A completely novel device has been developed by Trivascular, Inc. (Santa Rosa, CA). Phase I trials are currently underway to evaluate the safety of this graft. It is a bifurcated unibody graft composed of ePTFE. In contrast to other endografts, there is no metal attached to the main-body fabric. Instead, the fabric is suited with hollow rings that are filled with a biopolymer that "cures" (hardens) after a certain time period. As a result, the graft is able to conform to the anatomy of the aorta or iliacs and subsequent "curing" of the rings establishes a seal. There are three nitinol stents attached to the ends of the graft (proximal suprarenal and both limbs), which aid in fixation. Delivery of the graft requires surgical access on the ipsilateral side. The contralateral side requires a 12F sheath, leaving the option of a percutaneous or open approach for that side. As this graft is only in the early stages of testing (phase I), efficacy data are not yet available.

Lifepath

The Lifepath AAA bifurcated graft system was developed by Edwards Lifesciences LLC (Irvine, CA). A phase II trial was completed across 23 centers. The Lifepath system consists of a bifurcated modular graft of woven polyester with an Elgiloy (Elgiloy Limited Partnership, Elgin, IL), endoskeleton. Unique to this graft is a balloon-expandable deployment technique. Similar to other endografts, the Lifepath requires bilateral groin cut-downs. The main body, contralateral limb, and ipsilateral limb are all delivered through sheaths. After unsheathing the graft, a balloon fixed at the attachment site is inflated. This allows for increased radial force as well as precise placement of the graft in the proximal or distal landing zone. Results from the trial demonstrated a technical success rate of 98.7% with five (2.2%) open conversions. At 1-mo follow-up, there were 25 (12.2%) endoleaks (7 type I; 18 type II), which decreased to 8 (5.9%) by 6 mo. Thirty-seven wireform fractures occurred in the first 79 grafts, with evidence of migration in 5 patients and an endoleak in 1. Afterward, the graft was modified by thickening the Elgiloy stents and, subsequently, only six patients demonstrated wireform fractures, with no evidence of migration or endoleak. The mean aneurysm diameter was decreased by 9 mm at 12 mo follow-up (9). There was no evidence of graft limb thromboses. Although the initial trial has been completed, follow-up data are still being collected and premarket approval (PMA) submission has not been filed to the FDA.

PowerLink

The Powerlink system was designed by Endologix, Inc. (Irvine, CA). Twelve centers participated in a phase II trial to evaluate this graft. The Powerlink system is a bifurcated unibody internally supported endograft made of ePTFE supported by a stainless-steel single-wire body endoskeleton. Because of the unibody design, surgical exposure of only the ipsilateral femoral artery needs to be obtained. A 9F sheath is used in the contralateral side, allowing recovery of the contralateral "limb cap." As opposed to modular aortic endografts, introduction of a contralateral limb is not necessary, as it is part of the main body (unibody design). Technical success in placement of this graft was 97.5% with four (3.3%) open conversions. At 30 d follow-up, only seven (5.9%) endoleaks were found (three type I; four type II). Three graft limb thromboses (two at 1 mo; one

Table 1
Key Procedural Outcome Indicators Comparing Treatment of Infrarenal AAA
with the Talent LPS AAA Stent-Graft Versus Open Repair.

Indicators	Surgical control group	Stent-graft group	p-Value
Procedure Duration (min)	221.2 ± 101.6	172.2 ± 77.1	<0.0001
Range	85–581	19–540	
Estimated blood loss (mL)	1541.6 ± 1218.5	345.5 ± 337.2	<0.0001
Transfusion required (%)	67	11	<0.0001
Length of stay			
Intensive Care Unit (h)			<0.0001
Mean	55.2	14.3	
Range	0–408	0–832	
Hospital (d)			<0.0001
Mean	8.7	4.6	
Range	3–47	1–69	

Source: ref. *33*, with permission.

at 15 mo) were all treated successfully. Only one patient demonstrated graft migration and there was no evidence of wireform fractures *(32)*. The mean aneurysm diameter was reduced by 6 mm at 12 mo follow-up. As of February 2004, the FDA has accepted the PMA submission by Endologix, Inc. Of note, this trial constituted their Powerlink system with infrarenal fixation. An ongoing trial now exists to evaluate the same technology with suprarenal fixation.

Talent

The Talent LPS stent-graft (Medtronic AVE, Santa Rosa, CA) is a self-expanding device made of nitinol and woven polyester. The bifurcated main trunk has a proximal end with a 15-mm-long uncovered (bare spring) designed for suprarenal fixation. This device can treat very wide infrarenal aortic necks ranging from 14 to 32 mm and iliac diameters ranging from 8 to 22 mm. Aortic and iliac extension modules are available as needed. The main trunk delivery system is 22F–24F and the iliac limb delivery system is 18F.

In a 17-center US pivotal clinical trial that enrolled 240 patients in the endovascular arm and 126 patients who underwent open surgical repair, the Talent LPS stent-graft had fewer complications and similar low operative mortality when compared to the open surgical controls *(33)*. The endovascular group fared significantly more favorably in the early perioperative period, as measured by several key procedural indicators (Table 1). The Talent is expected to be the next device to come into the FDA-approved market.

Anaconda

The Anaconda stent-graft system (Sulzer Vascutek, Austin, TX) is a modular device of nitinol and woven polyester (one-third thinner than conventional polyester graft material). The proximal fixation consists of a proximal ring stent made of multiple turns of nitinol wire shaped into a saddle configuration that exerts radial force against the aortic wall. This saddle configuration allows for the device to be deployed so that part of the graft material is flush with the renal ostia and part of it is also above the level of the renal arteries (while the renal ostia remain uncovered). Additionally, four pairs of sharp hooks provide extra fixation to the infrarenal aorta. The device makes use of a series of magnets to aid in the cannulation of the main body and the positioning of the contralateral limb. Using a control collar, the main bifurcation body device has a control mechanism that allows for retracting all hooks clear of the aortic wall and repositioning in a controlled fashion once deployed from the introducer sheath. After correct positioning, the main body of the device can be released by a series of release wires. Aortic and iliac cuffs can be utilized if needed. The main delivery system ranges from 18F to 20F. The delivery system for the iliac vessels is 16F. Proximal infrarenal aortic necks ranging from 18 to 30 mm in diameter and larger than 15 mm in length can be treated. At the distal fixation zone, iliac arteries less than 16 mm in diameter and greater than 30 mm in length can be treated. Access vessels have to be larger than 7.5 mm in diameter. The maximum aortic neck angulation that can be treated is 45° and the neck must have less than 50% contiguous calcification.

Teramed Ariba: Quantum LP

The Cordis Endovascular Quantum LP™ stent-graft system consists of a self-expandable nitinol and polyester modular design composed of an aortic trunk main body (that bifurcates into two 5-cm-long sockets) and flared ipsilateral and contralateral prostheses. Aortic and iliac extenders are also available. Similar to other modular devices, the main trunk and ipsilateral leg are deployed via one delivery system (20F–21F) and the contralateral leg is deployed through a separate, contralateral delivery system (19F). The endograft allows for transrenal fixation using bare nitinol stents. Sharp barbs enhance the proximal attachment to the aortic wall. Infrarenal aortic necks ranging from 22 to 30 mm in diameter and at least 15 mm in length can be treated. Iliacs ranging from 8 to 20 mm in diameter and a wide range of iliac lengths can be treated.

In pilot US and European clinical studies, 29 patients were treated from December 1999 to August 2003, with every patient followed for at least 6 mo. Twenty-seven patients completed 12 mo of follow-up and 2 patients died of AAA-unrelated causes. There were no type I endoleaks, AAA ruptures, stent-graft migrations, graft materials failure, or conversions to open surgery. There were three severe procedure-related adverse events (congestive heart failure, lower extremity ischemia, and renal failure).

RECENT REPORTS ON DEVICES-SPECIFIC OUTCOMES

Recently, device-specific outcomes have been reported after endovascular AAA repair in a study that followed 703 patients for over 6 yr *(34)* and 723 patients after a mean follow-up of 23.2 mo *(17)*. Although there were similar rates of freedom from rupture, conversion to open repair, migration, and need for secondary procedures, significant differences were noted for graft limb occlusions and rate of endoleak among patients treated with Ancure, AneuRx, Excluder, Talent, and Zenith *(34)*. Limb occlusions occurred most often with Ancure devices. Endoleaks of any type were most common with the Excluder and Ancure devices *(17,34)*. Modular separation was observed most frequently with the Zenith device *(34)*. Aneurysm shrinkage was most common with the Zenith and Talent devices and least common with the Excluder device *(17,34)*. Most interestingly, the behavior of the AAA sac appears to be not only dependent on the initial AAA size and the presence or absence of endoleak but also on the type of endoprosthesis utilized to exclude the aneurysm *(17)*. Specifically, reduction in sac size was greatest with the Zenith, followed by the Ancure, and then the Excluder endografts.

THORACIC AORTIC ENDOGRAFTS

Although thoracic aortic aneurysms are less common than AAA, conventional open thoracic aneurysm repair is associated with worse overall prognosis. The natural history of thoracic aortic aneurysms is also more worrisome, with less than 30% 2-yr survival rates, mostly related to aneurysm rupture (35). Surgical intervention improves 2-yr survival rates to as high as 70%, but carries high morbidity and mortality (36). Aortic endografting for thoracic aneurysms continues to be experimental but promises to become an important new modality for treatment for up to 50% or more of all thoracic aneurysms.

Initial studies with 'hand-made' or 'home-made' balloon-expandable devices (37–39) (series ranging from 13 to 108 patients) reported ranges of technical success rates of 78–100%, endoleak rates of 5.5–15%, procedure-related mortality rates of 0–14%, and procedure-related complications such as upper extremity ischemia (highest at 4.6%), stroke or transient ischemic attack (TIA) (as high as 7%), paraplegia (0–3.7%), migration (0–7%), and distal embolization (0–7%). More recently, clinical trials are ongoing with commercially manufactured thoracic aortic endografts (Vanguard, Boston Scientific Corp., Natick, MA; Excluder, W.L. Gore & Associates, Flagstaff, AZ; Talent, Medtronic, Santa Rosa, CA; Zenith, Cook, Bloomington, IN). These industry-fabricated devices are all self-expanding stents covered either externally or internally by dacron or PTFE material. In the thorax, cardiac motion is more pronounced and self-expandable deployment carries the advantage of being faster, safer, and likely less prone to distal migration. Proximal and distal fixation zones of normal caliber aorta 20 mm away from major branches are required for thoracic endografting. Because the devices are larger, the delivery sheaths are also larger, posing significant access vessel difficulties. In addition, the usual associated aortic tortuosity at the hiatus and the normal curve of the aortic arch present special challenges for successful delivery of endovascular devices for this region of the aorta. In time, prospective trials will tell if this technology will become as widely useful in the thoracic aorta as it has become for the abdominal aorta. Early reports comparing endovascular versus open controls for thoracic aneurysms treated with the Talent thoracic endograft are encouraging, including 30-d mortality (10% vs 31%), case duration (150 min vs 320 min), spinal cord injury (0% vs 12%), and ICU stay (4 d vs 13 d) for endovascular versus open surgery, respectfully (40–43).

SURGICAL OPTIONS FOR EXTENDING
THE PROXIMAL FIXATION ZONE

Reperfusing the Internal Iliac Arteries

The presence of common iliac artery aneurysms could significantly shorten the distal iliac fixation zones, contraindicating the endovascular approach to AAA repair. Increasingly however, reports indicate that it might be safe to intentionally occlude one or both internal iliac arteries without significant side effects (10,44–46). Occlusion of the internal iliac artery can then allow fixation at the level of the external iliac arteries, effectively lengthening the distal fixation zone to allow proper endovascular aneurysm exclusion. Although most vascular surgeons find no significant problem with the occlusion of only one internal iliac artery (if needed for endovascular AAA repair), most continue to have severe reservations about the intentional occlusion of both internal iliac arteries. In fact, potentially catastrophic symptoms of pelvic and colonic ischemia have been reported, with the simultaneous acute occlusion of both internal iliac arteries *(10)*. A surgical alternative has been successfully used and involves the reimplantation of one or both internal iliac arteries into the ipsilateral external iliac artery either by direct transposition or by a formal bypass conduit *(47,48)*. These procedures can be performed through a small pelvic incision via a retroperitoneal exposure and are reported to have minimal morbidity and mortality.

Splenorenal or Hepatorenal Bypass

In general, the most definitive contraindication to the endovascular approach for AAA repair has to do with a short (less than 15 mm) infrarenal aortic neck. However, there are patients that have prohibitive medical risk and would clearly not tolerate the extensive dissection and the severe hemodynamic changes associated with cross-clamping the aorta for a standard open surgical repair. Traditionally, such patients would be followed conservatively without a surgical option. When such a patient presents with an enlarging AAA (larger than 6 cm) or one that is symptomatic with abdominal or back pain, one could then opt for repair given otherwise certain impending rupture. If the only contraindication to endovascular exclusion is that of a short infrarenal neck, cross-clamping of the aorta could still be avoided by combining the extra-anatomic revascularization of one or both of the renal arteries with subsequent endovascular exclusion. Extra-anatomic revascularization of the renal arteries by splenorenal bypass (on the left) or hepatorenal bypass (on the right) is well documented to have low morbidity/mortality and faster recovery than would a standard open AAA repair. These procedures, although by necessity violate the peritoneal cavity, are associated with minimal blood loss and can be tolerated by most patients even with severe pre-existing cardiopulmonary comorbidity. There are no available data documenting the added risk of tandem operations, such as a splenorenal bypass followed shortly by an endovascular AAA repair; however, this potential option must be kept in mind. At our center, we have performed five such procedures for exceptional clinical situations, with excellent outcome in every case. There needs to be some distance between the SMA and renals. Furthermore, the procedure is more applicable when the renal arteries come off at different levels so that only one renal artery needs to be bypassed.

Transposition of the Subclavian Artery

An increasingly frequent clinical scenario is encountered when the proximal fixation zone above a descending thoracic artery aneurysm is shorter than 15 mm but otherwise the patient can be best served by an endovascular repair based on other favorable aneurysm anatomy features as well as pre-existing medical comorbidities that significantly increase the risk of standard open repair. In these cases, a well-known surgical option exists that carries minimal morbidity and close to no mortality and can be accomplished through a small transverse incision at the base of the neck (i.e., transposition of the subclavian artery to the common carotid artery). At our center, we have performed 15 subclavian artery transpositions for this indication without any procedure-related complications (unpublished data). Pursuing this option lengthens the proximal fixation zone by about 10–20 mm (Fig. 9).

ENDOLEAKS

Up to 20% of endovascular AAA patients will have contrast enhancement of the aneurysm (an endoleak) on the 1-mo postoperative CT scan. Endoleaks are classified by

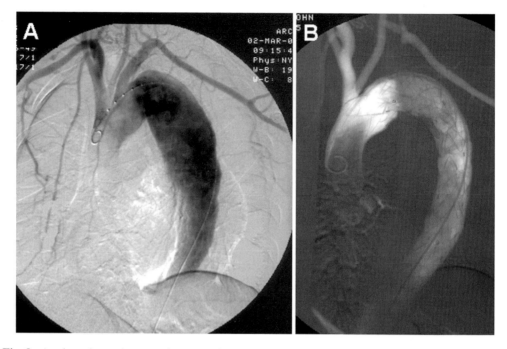

Fig. 9. Aortic arch arteriograms demonstrating a thoracic aortic aneurysm with a very short proximal landing zone (**A**) in a patient who underwent left subclavian artery to left common carotid artery transposition as seen in (**B**) and subsequent treatment of the aneurysm with a Talent thoracic endograft.

their site of origin *(49–50)*. Type I endoleaks originate from incomplete seal at the proximal or distal attachment sites. By definition, early-type I endoleak results from a failure in design, device, or deployment. Alternatively, late-type I endoleaks could be the result of aneurysmal disease progression or sac remodeling. Type II endoleaks originate from patent perfusing inferior mesenteric and/or lumbar arteries with a circuit of flow between these sac branches. These endoleaks are not caused by device or design failure. Successful endograft exclusion depends on spontaneous thrombosis of patent sac branches. During open aneurysm repair, these sac branches are usually vigorously backbleeding and require suture ligation. Type III endoleaks develop at graft junctions, and type IV endoleaks result from graft porosity.

Persistent endoleaks beyond 6 mo, late endoleaks, symptomatic aneurysms, or enlarging aneurysms (with or without endoleak) after endovascular AAA repair are cause for great concern and require diagnostic and therapeutic interventions. Type I endoleaks are of most concern because the aneurysm sac remains under systemic pressure. Type I endoleaks are treated by placing additional proximal or distal covered extensions or by increasing radial force with an uncovered stent; otherwise, the endograft must be explanted and the aneurysm repaired conventionally.

Type II endoleaks are thought to be of less concern unless the aneurysm sac expands over time. In that situation, elective transarterial or translumbar endovascular embolization of the endoleak within the sac and/or its feeding sac branches is indicated (Fig. 10) *(10,11,53)*. There is an approx 17–20% risk of needing further endovascular interventions related to type II endoleaks in the first 6 mo postrepair.

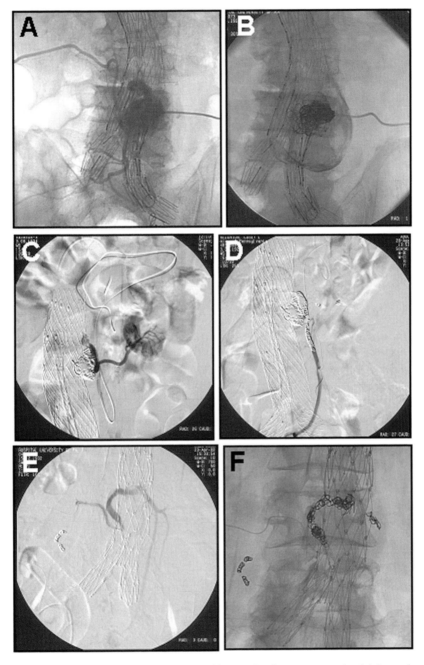

Fig. 10. Treatment options for type II endoleaks. **(A)** Translumbar access to the AAA sac demonstrating lumbar collaterals feeding a type II endoleak. **(B)** Coil embolization of the endoleak nidus (area of flow shown in A) within the AAA sac. **(C)** Recurrent type II endoleak after translumbar coil embolization of the AAA sac nidus. The endoleak is shown to be fed by IMA (inferior mesenteric artery) and left accessory renal artery flow. **(D)** Trans-SMA (superior mesenteric artery)/transarterial coil embolization of the IMA and left accessory renal collateral branches causing the recurrent endoleak seen in C. Transarterial embolization of iliolumbar branches **(E)** and IMA **(F)** via right internal iliac artery access for treatment of type II endoleak.

Of significant concern is the late development of an endoleak, defined as one that occurs 6 mo or longer after implantation. Late endoleaks must be studied with arteriography to determine the site of origin. The morphology of the aneurysm sac and proximal neck changes over time following endovascular repair. Sac shrinkage from aneurysm remodeling after endografting or neck angulation, lengthening, and dilatation (from progression of aneurysmal disease) could lead to late type I, type III, and, rarely, type II endoleaks. Late endoleaks usually result from migration of endograft components, dislodgment of fixation zones or modular junctions, or materials failure (fabric holes or metal fractures). Type I and III endoleaks can be treated by deployment of new endograft components to exclude the defect in the fabric or the junctional separation. Occasionally, explantation and open repair are required. Type IV endoleaks usually resolve spontaneously after reversal of heparin at the completion of the endovascular procedure.

ENDOVASCULAR APPROACH FOR RUPTURED AORTIC ANEURYSMS

Emergency open AAA repair for rupture is associated with high morbidity and mortality despite advances in diagnostic modalities and postoperative care (54). Currently, AAA rupture has an associated overall mortality in excess of 80% (55). At our center, we have explored the utility of the commercially available, FDA-approved endografts for emergency AAA presentations (56). Other centers have also examined this issue with their own experimental endografts (57–60). In most centers, however, the conditions of urgent aneurysm repair preclude the required detailed imaging and measurements for endograft design. In addition, commercial procurement of the designed endograft could take too long to meet the needs of an emergency AAA presentation. These devices are extremely costly and are not usually supplied by consignment, and, therefore, most centers do not carry "on-the-shelf" inventory in their operating rooms. As a result, in the setting of an emergency presentation, hemodynamic instability, and the prolonged time needed for endograft design and procurement, most vascular surgeons would not entertain the endovascular approach as a treatment option for ruptured AAA. Nevertheless, we have successfully treated five patients with contained ruptured AAA who were transferred and arrived hemodynamically stable to our medical center from neighboring centers (56). In these patients, pre-existing medical comorbidity placed them at very high morbidity/mortality risk with open AAA repair.

In these emergency settings, available imaging was usually less than optimal, including noncontrast CT scans or thick-cut CT scans. However, although commercially available endografts are certainly not "one-size-fits-all," these devices can prove to be sufficiently versatile to allow successful AAA exclusion in some emergency presentations, (Fig. 11). Others have adopted protocols for endovascular treatment of ruptured AAA, reporting improved morbidity and mortality over historical controls (57,61). The Montefiore group has reported very encouraging results with their home-made Montefiore Endovascular Grafting System (MEGS), which consists of a "one-size-fits-all" aorto-uni-iliac (AUI) design supplemented with a femoral–femoral bypass (57). Because of the in-house endograft availability, their protocol allows for the inclusion of patients with free rupture and hemodynamic instability. In their study, 31 patients presented with AAA rupture and 25 underwent endovascular graft repair. Six patients with unsuitable anatomy required open repair. Total operative mortality was 9.7% (three patients). The advantage of the Montefiore model is the immediate availability and "one-size-fits-all" design. Another group has reported their experience with the endovascular treatment of ruptured AAA (62,63). Although they report a 35% mortality, all patients receive detailed contrast-enhanced CT scans regardless of hemodynamic status. This group utilized both bifurcated

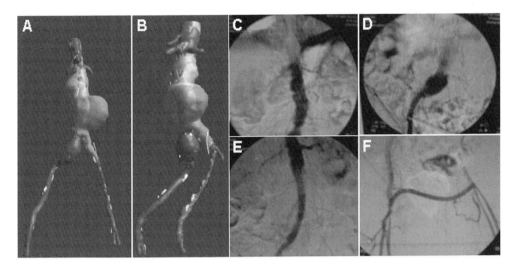

Fig. 11. A patient admitted with a contained ruptured AAA and hemodynamic stability is successfully treated with an AneuRx endograft converted to an aorto-uni-iliac design. **(A)** CT scan of contained ruptured AAA on presentation. **(B, C)** Retrospective three-dimensional reconstructions of CT data, showing left common iliac and right hypogastric artery occlusion. **(C)** Initial intraoperative arteriogram demonstrating left common iliac occlusion and a right common iliac aneurysm. **(D)** Initial deployment of the AneuRx graft body and retrograde injection of the right iliac system. **(E)** Conversion to an aorta-uni-iliac system with the use of an aortic extension cuff across the flow divider. **(F)** Completion arteriogram after femoral–femoral bypass with 8 mm reinforced PTFE. (Reprinted with permission from *J Vasc Surg*.)

grafts and AUI devices and seemed more tolerant of operative delay in favor of adequate imaging and a perfected preoperative stent-graft design. Although such an approach might initially seem unjustifiably risky, in fact patients with contained retroperitoneal rupture of AAA might be able to wait several hours for perioperative planning. A report by Walker et al. demonstrated the natural history of untreated ruptured AAA *(64)*. In this retrospective review of nonoperative cases, they found that patients had a mean life expectancy of 8 h from admission In this regard, it is important to view each case individually, balancing the risks of open repair in the setting of significant cardiopulmonary comorbidity versus the risk of any planned delays if an endovascular approach is considered safer for the patient. The role of endovascular repair for AAA with emergency presentations remains to be determined by further studies.

COMPLETELY PERCUTANEOUS ANEURYSM REPAIR

The initial Cordis endograft design clearly demonstrated feasibility for a completely percutaneous infrarenal AAA repair. Regrettably, efficacy was not to be reached, as difficulties with migration and fabric failure were soon encountered leading to the need to abort the phase I trial. However, endovascular technology is advancing rapidly and it is likely that we might soon see new devices developed that take on this ultimate challenge of completely percutaneous aortic aneurysm repair.

Percutaneous femoral closure devices such as that developed by Perclose Inc. (Redwood City, CA, USA) or SUB-Q Inc. (San Clemente, CA, USA) have yielded excellent success and minimal complication rates when utilized to close relatively small (6F–12F) femoral punctures *(65,66)*. Despite large introducer sizes (14F–27F) for the aortic endograft delivery sheaths, the endovascular femoral closure devices have the potential for making it possible to perform completely percutaneous endovascular aneurysm repair *(67,68)*. In a series of 14 patients with AAA repaired with AneuRx endografts, the Prostar (Perclose) device was successful in 75% of the attempted closures for the main-body femoral access (22F) and 71.4% of those attempted for the contralateral femoral access (the docking limb, 16F) *(67)*. However, conversion to open repair was required in six cases for hemorrhage, four cases for iliofemoral dissection, one case of device deployment failure, and one case of compromised distal flow. The authors sited patient selection as well as exact puncture technique and accurate device deployment as important factors in achieving success for these percutaneous femoral attempts in endovascular AAA repair. They noted higher success rates with larger iliac artery dimensions, decreased calcification, and minimal tortuosity *(67)*. This and other reports demonstrate that completely percutaneous endovascular AAA repair is feasible utilizing currently available femoral percutaneous closure devices. However, complication rates for the existing large delivery sheaths are high, and when they occur, they might be difficult to manage or disastrous (e.g., iliofemoral dissections and distal limb ischemia). Thus, the routine use of femoral percutaneous closure devices in endovascular AAA repair will likely await the development of smaller aortic endograft delivery sheaths and/or safer more accurate percutaneous femoral closure systems.

SUMMARY

With current technology and understanding of aortic endografting, this technique has replaced open surgical repair for many patients with AAA. New aortic stent-grafts will continue to be developed. These grafts can offer a smaller profile for delivery sheaths, more flexibility to treat angulation, increased ability to treat large aortic diameters, different methods of fixation and sealing, options for handling arterial branches, completely percutaneous delivery systems or other novel ideas. Certainly, new technology developed with the goal to meet deficiencies in current techniques will allow further progress and wider applicability of endovascular treatment for aortic aneurysms.

REFERENCES

1. Parodi, JC, Palmaz JC, Barone HD. Transfemoral intraluminal graft implantation for abdominal aortic aneurysms. Ann Vasc Surg 1991;5(6):491–499.
2. Edwards WH Jr, et al. Endovascular grafting of abdominal aortic aneurysms. A preliminary study. Ann Surg 1996;223(5):568–573; discussion 573–575.
3. Harris PL. The highs and lows of endovascular aneurysm repair: the first two years of the Eurostar Registry. Ann R Coll Surg Engl 1999;81(3):161–165.
4. Bertrand M, et al. Endovascular treatment of abdominal aortic aneurysms: is there a benefit regarding postoperative outcome? Eur J Anaesthesiol 2001;18(4):245–250.
5. Becquemin JP, et al. Mid-term results of a second generation bifurcated endovascular graft for abdominal aortic aneurysm repair: the French Vanguard trial. J Vasc Surg 1999;30(2):209–218.
6. Ceelen W, et al. Cost-benefit analysis of endovascular versus open abdominal aortic aneurysm treatment. Acta Chir Belg 1999;99(2):64–67.
7. Velazquez OC, et al. Gender-related differences in infrarenal aortic aneurysm morphologic features: issues relevant to Ancure and Talent endografts. J Vasc Surg 2001;33(2 Suppl):S77–S84.
8. Velazquez OC, Woo EY, Carpenter JP, et al. Decreased use of iliac extensions and reduced graft junctions with software-assisted centerline measurements in seclection of endograft components for endovascular aneurysm repair. J Vasc Surg in press. 2004;40:222–227.
9. Carpenter JP, et al. Multicenter pivotal trial results of the Lifepath System for endovascular aortic aneurysm repair. J Vasc Surg 2004;39(1):34–43.
10. Velazquez OC, et al. Relationship between preoperative patency of the inferior mesenteric artery and subsequent occurrence of type II endoleak in patients undergoing endovascular repair of abdominal aortic aneurysms. J Vasc Surg 2000;32(4):777–788.

11. Baum RA, et al. Diagnosis and treatment of inferior mesenteric arterial endoleaks after endovascular repair of abdominal aortic aneurysms. Radiology 2000;215(2):409–413.

12. Zarins CK, et al. Stent graft migration after endovascular aneurysm repair: importance of proximal fixation. J Vasc Surg 2003;38(6):1264–1272; discussion 1272.

13. Zarins CK, The US AneuRx Clinical Trial: 6-year clinical update 2002. J Vasc Surg 2003;37(4):904–908.

14. Cao P, et al. Device migration after endoluminal abdominal aortic aneurysm repair: analysis of 113 cases with a minimum follow-up period of 2 years. J Vasc Surg 2002;35(2):229–235.

15. Conner MS, 3rd, et al. Secondary procedures after endovascular aortic aneurysm repair. J Vasc Surg 2002;36(5):992–996.

16. Arko FR. Regarding "Endograft migration one to four years after endovascular abdominal aortic aneurysm repair with the AneuRx device: a cautionary note." J Vasc Surg 2003;37(4):916; author reply 916–918.

17. Greenberg RK, et al. Variable sac behavior after endovascular repair of abdominal aortic aneurysm: analysis of core laboratory data. J Vasc Surg 2004;39(1):95–101.

18. Fairman RM, et al. Limb interventions in patients undergoing treatment with an unsupported bifurcated aortic endograft system: a review of the Phase II EVT Trial. J Vasc Surg 2002;36(1):118–126.

19. Carpenter JP, et al. Failure of endovascular abdominal aortic aneurysm graft limbs. J Vasc Surg 2001; 33(2):296–302; discussion 302–303.

20. Baum RA, et al. Limb kinking in supported and unsupported abdominal aortic stent-grafts. J Vasc Intervent Radiol, 2000;11(9):1165–1171.

21. Moore WS, et al. Five-year interim comparison of the Guidant bifurcated endograft with open repair of abdominal aortic aneurysm. J Vasc Surg 2003;38(1):46–55.

22. Moore WS. The Guidant Ancure bifurcation endograft: five-year follow-up. Semin Vasc Surg 2003; 16(2):139–143.

23. Zarins CK, et al. AneuRx stent graft versus open surgical repair of abdominal aortic aneurysms: multi-center prospective clinical trial. J Vasc Surg 1999;29(2):292–305; discussion 306–308.

24. Zarins CK, White RA. Fogarty TJ. Aneurysm rupture after endovascular repair using the AneuRx stent graft. J Vasc Surg 2000;31(5):960–970.

25. Zarins CK, et al. The AneuRx stent graft: four-year results and worldwide experience 2000. J Vasc Surg 2001;33(2 Suppl.):S135–S145.

26. Ramaiah VG, et al. The AneuRx stent-graft since FDA approval: single-center experience of 230 cases. J Endovasc Ther 2002;9(4):464–469.

27. Ayerdi J, et al. Indications and outcomes of AneuRx Phase III trial versus use of commercial AneuRx stent graft. J Vasc Surg 2003;37(4):739–743.

28. Zarins CK, et al. Aneurysm enlargement following endovascular aneurysm repair: AneuRx clinical trial. J Vasc Surg 2004;39(1):109–117.

29. Matsumura JS, et al. A multicenter controlled clinical trial of open versus endovascular treatment of abdominal aortic aneurysm. J Vasc Surg 2003;37(2):262–271.

30. Greenberg RK, et al. An update of the Zenith endovascular graft for abdominal aortic aneurysms: initial implantation and mid-term follow-up data. J Vasc Surg 2001;33(2 Suppl.):S157–S164.

31. Sternbergh WC, 3rd, et al. Influence of endograft oversizing on device migration, endoleak, aneurysm shrinkage, and aortic neck dilation: results from the Zenith Multicenter Trial. J Vasc Surg 2004;39(1): 20–76.

32. Carpenter JP. Multicenter trial of the PowerLink bifurcated system for endovascular aortic aneurysm repair. J Vasc Surg 2002;36(6):1129–1137.

33. Criado FJ, Fairman RM, Becker GJ. Talent LPS AAA stent graft: results of a pivotal clinical trial. J Vasc Surg 2003;37(4):709–715.

34. Ouriel K, et al. Endovascular repair of abdominal aortic aneurysms: device-specific outcome. J Vasc Surg 2003;37(5):991–998.

35. Bickerstaff LK, et al. Thoracic aortic aneurysms: a population-based study. Surgery 1982;92(6):1103–1108.

36. Crawford ES, et al. Thoracoabdominal aortic aneurysms: preoperative and intraoperative factors determining immediate and long-term results of operations in 605 patients. J Vasc Surg 1986;3(3): 389–404.

37. Dake MD, et al. Transluminal placement of endovascular stent-grafts for the treatment of descending thoracic aortic aneurysms. N Engl J Med 1994;331(26):1729–1734.

38. Mitchell RS, Miller DC, Dake MD. Stent-graft repair of thoracic aortic aneurysms. Semin Vasc Surg 1997;10(4):257–271.

39. Temudom T, et al. Endovascular grafts in the treatment of thoracic aortic aneurysms and pseudoaneurysms. Ann Vasc Surg 2000;14(3):230–238.

40. Ehrlich M, et al. Endovascular stent graft repair for aneurysms on the descending thoracic aorta. Ann Thorac Surg 1998;66(1):19–24; discussion 24–25.

41. Criado FJ, et al. Technical strategies to expand stent-graft applicability in the aortic arch and proximal descending thoracic aorta. J Endovasc Ther 2002;9(Suppl. 2):II32–II38.

42. Criado FJ, Clark NS, Barnatan MF. Stent graft repair in the aortic arch and descending thoracic aorta: a 4-year experience. J Vasc Surg 2002;36(6):1121–1128.

43. Fairman RM, Stent grafting in the thoracic aorta. Endovasc Today 2003:3–5.

44. Razavi MK, et al. Internal iliac artery embolization in the stent-graft treatment of aortoiliac aneurysms: analysis of outcomes and complications. J Vasc Interv Radiol 2000;11(5):561–566.

45. Criado FJ, et al. Safety of coil embolization of the internal iliac artery in endovascular grafting of abdominal aortic aneurysms. J Vasc Surg 2000;32(4):684–688.

46. Velmahos GC, et al. Angiographic embolization of bilateral internal iliac arteries to control life-threatening hemorrhage after blunt trauma to the pelvis. Am Surg 2000;66(9):858–862.

47. Yano OJ, et al. Ancillary techniques to facilitate endovascular repair of aortic aneurysms. J Vasc Surg 2001;34(1):69–75.

48. Chuter TA, Reilly LM. Surgical reconstruction of the iliac arteries prior to endovascular aortic aneurysm repair. J Endovasc Surg 1997;4(3):307–311.

49. White GH, et al. Type III and type IV endoleak: toward a complete definition of blood flow in the sac after endoluminal AAA repair. J Endovasc Surg 1998;5(4):305–309.

50. White GH, Yu, W, May J. Endoleak—a proposed new terminology to describe incomplete aneurysm exclusion by an endoluminal graft. J Endovasc Surg 1996;3(1):124–125.

51. White GH, et al. Endoleak as a complication of endoluminal grafting of abdominal aortic aneurysms: classification, incidence, diagnosis, and management. J Endovasc Surg 1997;4(2):152–168.

52. White GH, et al. Endotension: an explanation for continued AAA growth after successful endoluminal repair. J Endovasc Surg 1999;6(4):308–315.

53. Kasirajan K, et al. Technique and results of transfemoral superselective coil embolization of type II lumbar endoleak. J Vasc Surg 2003;38(1):61–66.

54. Heller JA, et al. Two decades of abdominal aortic aneurysm repair: have we made any progress? J Vasc Surg 2000;32(6):1091–1100.

55. Taylor LM, Jr., and Porter JM. Basic data related to clinical decision-making in abdominal aortic aneurysms. Ann Vasc Surg 1987;1(4):502–504.

56. Lombardi JV, Fairman RM, Carpenter JC, et al. The utility of commercially available endografts in the treatment of contained-ruptureed AAA with hemodynamic stability. J Vasc Surg 2004;40:154–160.

57. Ohki T, Veith FJ. Endovascular therapy for ruptured abdominal aortic aneurysms. Adv Surg 2001;35: 131–151.

58. Veith FJ, Gargiulo NJ 3rd, Ohki T. Endovascular treatment of ruptured infrarenal aortic and iliac aneurysms. Acta Chir Belg 2003;103(6):555–562.

59. Veith FJ, et al. Endovascular grafts and other catheter-directed techniques in the management of ruptured abdominal aortic aneurysms. Semin Vasc Surg 2003;16(4):326–331.

60. Veith FJ, et al. Treatment of ruptured abdominal aneurysms with stent grafts: a new gold standard? Semin Vasc Surg 2003;16(2):171–175.

61. Greenberg RK, et al. An endoluminal method of hemorrhage control and repair of ruptured abdominal aortic aneurysms. J Endovasc Ther 2000;7(1):1–7.

62. Hinchliffe RJ, et al. Endovascular repair of ruptured abdominal aortic aneurysm—a challenge to open repair? Results of a single centre experience in 20 patients. Eur J Vasc Endovasc Surg 2001;22(6): 528–534.

63 Hinchliffe RJ, Hopkinson BR. Ruptured abdominal aortic aneurysm. Time for a new approach. J Cardiovasc Surg (Torino) 2002;43(3):345–347.

64. Walker EM, Hopkinson BR, Makin GS. Unoperated abdominal aortic aneurysm: presentation and natural history. Ann R Coll Surg Engl 1983;65(5):311–313.

65. Tron C, et al. A randomized comparison of a percutaneous suture device versus manual compression for femoral artery hemostasis after PTCA. J Intervent Cardiol 2003;16(3):217–221.

66. Yadav JS, et al. Comparison of the QuickSeal Femoral Arterial Closure System with manual compression following diagnostic and interventional catheterization procedures. Am J Cardiol 2003; 91(12):1463–1466.

67. Traul DK, et al. Percutaneous endovascular repair of infrarenal abdominal aortic aneurysms: a feasibility study. J Vasc Surg 2000;32(4):770–776.

68. Torsello GB, et al. Endovascular suture versus cutdown for endovascular aneurysm repair: a prospective randomized pilot study. J Vasc Surg 2003;38(1):78–82.

V ASSOCIATED IMAGING MODALITIES

20

Interventional Echocardiography

Frank E. Silvestry, MD

CONTENTS

INTRODUCTION

As percutaneous noncoronary interventional cardiology procedures move toward an increasing complex, anatomically based paradigm, procedural guidance with real-time echocardiography has become an important aspect of their successful performance. Traditionally, fluoroscopy as well as angiography has been used for noncoronary procedural guidance in the catheterization laboratory, but significant limitations exist. Fluoroscopy alone is unable to identify important anatomic structures such as the cardiac valves as well as structures such as the coronary sinus ostium, vena cava, and pulmonary veins. Angiography offers some improvement over fluoroscopic-only guidance, but often cannot delineate complex anatomical structures and the relationship between two structures that do not share the same cardiac chamber requires the use of radiographic contrast agents and cannot be performed continuously in real time during the procedure. Furthermore, important targets of therapy such as the mitral valve and fossa ovalis are complex three-dimensional structures, and therapeutic devices must be deployed in a precise fashion relative to their anatomy for proper function. During percutaneous noncoronary interventions, echocardiographic guidance assists the interventional cardiologist in the performance of

From: *Contemporary Cardiology: Interventional Cardiology:*
Percutaneous Noncoronary Intervention
Edited by: H. C. Herrmann © Humana Press Inc., Totowa, NJ

transseptal catheterization, in monitoring guide wire, delivery sheath, and balloon or device position relative to anatomic structures, as well as in the evaluation for thrombus, pericardial effusion, and other procedural complications. This chapter will review the echocardiographic modalities (transthoracic echocardiography, transesophageal echocardiography, and intracardiac echocardiography) used to guide these procedures in the catheterization laboratory. Real-time computed tomography (CT) and magnetic resonance imaging (MRI) guidance of percutaneous noncoronary interventions will be covered in a separate chapter.

ACC/AHA/ASE GUIDELINES FOR THE CLINICAL APPLICATION OF ECHOCARDIOGRAPHY

In 1997, a report of the American College of Cardiology, American Heart Association, and American Society of Echocardiography Task Force on Practice Guidelines was developed to provide a framework for the use of echocardiography in a wide variety of clinical settings, and these guidelines were updated in 2003 *(1)*. These guidelines cover the use of transthoracic echocardiography (TTE) and transesophageal echocardiography (TEE); however, to date, no such guidelines have been developed for intracardiac echocardiography (ICE). Recommendations for use of TTE and TEE in specific clinical settings are based on the strength of the supporting evidence in the medical literature and are divided into four categories: class I indicates conditions for which there is evidence or general agreement that a given procedure or treatment is useful and effective; class II indicates that a divergence of opinion or conflicting evidence exists regarding the efficacy or usefulness of a procedure or treatment and is divided into class IIa and IIb (class IIa indicates that despite the divergent opinion, the weight of the evidence or opinion favors usefulness/efficacy, whereas class IIb indicates that the usefulness/efficacy is less well established); class III denotes that there is evidence that the procedure or treatment is not useful and in come cases might be harmful. Wherever applicable, this chapter will note the task force recommendations in the sections that follow.

ECHOCARDIOGRAPHIC MONITORING OF INTERVENTIONAL PROCEDURES

Real-time or on-line echocardiographic guidance of a variety of interventional procedures has been previously described (see Table 1). As TTE is widely available and can be easily and readily performed in the catheterization laboratory, it has been used to guide a wide variety of interventional procedures. Common uses of TTE in interventional cardiology include guidance of subxiphoid pericardiocentesis, percutaneous balloon mitral valvuloplasty, and selecting appropriate myocardium upon which to perform alcohol septal ablation in hypertrophic obstructive cardiomyopathy. It might also be useful as an adjunct imaging modality in specific situations, such as supplementing ICE during percutaneous atrial–septal defect (ASD) closure in patients with deficient atrial–septal rims *(2)* or supplementing TEE during percutaneous mitral valve repair with the edge-to-edge clip repair system *(3)*. TEE and ICE can be used to facilitate the deployment of percutaneous ASD and patent foramen ovale (PFO) closure devices, perform percutaneous valvuloplasty, as well as guide more complex, noncoronary interventions such as transseptal catheterization, percutaneous mitral repair, placement of LAA occlusion devices, and placement of stented valves.

Table 1
Procedures Guided by Echocardiography

Pericardiocentesis
Transseptal catheterization
Percutaneous balloon valvuloplasty
Percutaneous transcatheter closure of septal defects
Alcohol septal ablation in hypertrophic obstructive cardiomyopathy
Placement of percutaneous left ventricular support devices
Percutaneous repair of mitral regurgitation with the edge-to-edge repair system
Percutaneous repair of mitral regurgitation with the coronary sinus devices
Placement of LAA occlusion devices
Placement of stented valve replacement
Echocardiographically guided RV and LV biopsies
Laser lead extraction of pacemaker and defibrillator leads
Congenital heart disease applications such as completion of Fontan, coarctation repair
Electrophysiologic procedures such as pulmonary vein isolation for atrial fibrillation, sinoatrial node
  modification for inappropriate sinus tachycardia, and ablation of LV tachycardia

Note: LV = left ventricular; RV = right ventricular.

TTE-GUIDED PERICARDIOCENTESIS

In the early 1980s, TTE-guided percutaneous therapeutic pericardiocentesis was first described by Seward et al. at the Mayo Clinic, and in 2002, they described the outcomes of this procedure performed in 1127 patients during a 21-yr period since their initial report *(4,5)*. Echo-guided pericardiocentesis is listed as a class IIa indication in the ACC/AHA/ASE task force guidelines, indicating despite conflicting evidence or divergence of opinion; the body of evidence in the medical literature favors its usefulness.

Transthoracic endocardiography offers an excellent preprocedural assessment of the size and location of the pericardial effusion and can determine whether the effusion is free-flowing or organized; Doppler interrogation of the atrioventricular and ventriculoarterial valves provide physiologic evidence for increased intrapericardial pressure *(6–10)*. With increased intrapericardial pressure, respirophasic variation in mitral and tricuspid inflow (as well as in pulmonic and aortic outflow) velocities develops. Increased intrapericardial pressure is said to be present when mitral and aortic velocities vary by more than 30% with respiration and tricuspid and pulmonic velocities vary by more than 50%. With frank tamponade, diastolic collapse of the right ventricle is seen, and this finding has a greater than 80% specificity for tamponade physiology *(7)*. Clearance for subxiphoid pericardiocentesis is assessed by determining whether there is greater than 1 cm of clearance between the epicardial and parietal pericardial surfaces at the apex of the heart.

To guide pericardiocentesis, images are typically obtained from the apical views to image the apical entry of the pericardiocentesis needle while preserving the subxiphoid sterile field. Some centers use echocardiography to guide the optimal entry point for the needle (chest wall vs subcostal), whereas others use traditional anatomical landmarks and perform pericardiocentesis via a subcostal approach, using echocardiography to confirm that the pericardium has been appropriately cannulated *(11)*. Although the pericardiocentesis needle tip (or sheath) might not be easily visualized on TTE, once a small amount of fluid (i.e., 8–10 cm^3) is removed, confirmation that the needle or sheath is in the pericardial space is achieved by the injection of an equal amount of agitated saline mixed with air to form contrast bubbles that are easily imaged by TTE *(12–15)*. If a non-pericardial space has been cannulated, the needle or smaller sheath is removed prior to placing any additional catheters, thus avoiding the risk of perforation. Once confirmation by contrast injection that the pericardial space has been appropriately cannulated, a larger drainage catheter is placed to evacuate the pericardial fluid. Postprocedure, confirmation of the adequacy of drainage as well as changes in the hemodynamic effect of the effusion can be obtained to guide further therapy.

Practical advantages of echo-guided pericardiocentesis include its ability to be performed portably and rapidly. It can be performed at the bedside in unstable patients. The necessary equipment is widely available, and the technique is applicable to a wide variety of clinical situations. As such, it offers distinct advantages over fluoroscopic guidance when performed by experienced operators. In patients with poor acoustic windows, TEE or ICE can be substituted, although the apex is not typically well visualized by either of these modalities.

TRANSSEPTAL CATHETERIZATION

Although imaging is not invariably required for the successful performance of transseptal catheterization, it offers some potential advantages over traditional fluoroscopic guidance *(16–20)*. Anatomic variability in the position and orientation of the fossa ovalis and its surrounding structures might present specific challenges to even those interventional cardiologists with significant transseptal experience, and imaging offers the potential for increased safety, with lower risk of cannulating other spaces adjacent to the fossa. Similarly, imaging can decrease the time required for the transseptal to be performed as well as minimizing the fluoroscopy required for the procedure. In patients who are pregnant, for example, radiation exposure can be reduced with echocardiographic transseptal guidance *(21–24)*. Imaging might also assist those operators without significant transseptal experience who are learning the procedure *(17,25)*.

Transthoracic endocardiography does not offer sufficient imaging resolution in most cases to guide transseptal catheterization and, as such, is rarely used solely for this purpose. Typically, TEE (see Fig. 1.1) and, more recently, ICE are used when imaging is required. As ICE imaging can be performed without additional sedation or general anesthesia, as well as with minimal additional patient risk and discomfort, ICE is becoming the "gold standard" if imaging is required for this procedure *(21–24)*.

PERCUTANEOUS BALLOON VALVULOPLASTY

Echocardiography can be used to assist in the guidance of percutaneous balloon valvuloplasty (PBV) of stenotic mitral, aortic, tricuspid, and pulmonic valves, to assess the adequacy of the result, and to monitor for complications *(26,27)*. The greatest experience has been in using echocardiography to guide percutaneous balloon mitral valvuloplasty, which serves as a model for how echocardiography can be used to guide interventional procedures. In the updated ACC/AHA/ASE guidelines, echocardiography (and particularly TEE) has been given a class I indication for use in guiding percutaneous mitral balloon valvuloplasty. Although both TTE and TEE are typically used in concert prior to the procedure to evaluate the suitability for PBV and exclude LAA thrombus, TTE often provides acceptable image quality for assessment of the mitral valvuloplasty score

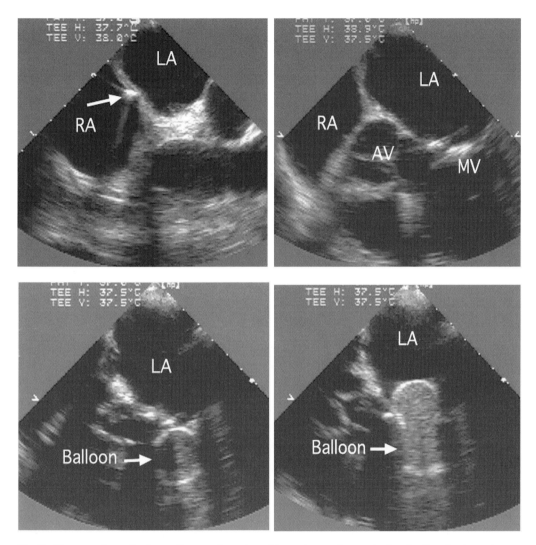

Fig. 1. Transesophageal echocardiogram from the mid-esophagus demonstrating the Brockenbrough needle position in the right atrium (RA) at the fossa ovalis, prior to entry into the left atrium (LA). Transesophageal echocardiogram from the mid esophagus demonstrating a calcified and rheumatically deformed mitral valve (MV) prior to balloon valvuloplasty. Left atrium = LA; right atrium = RA; aortic valve = AV. Transesophageal echocardiogram from the mid-esophagus demonstrating the valvuloplasty balloon beginning to inflate, initially distally in the left ventricle. Left atrium = LA. Transesophageal echocardiogram from the mid-esophagus demonstrating the valvuloplasty balloon inflation, both distally in the left ventricle and proximally in the left atrium (LA). Transesophageal echocardiogram from the mid esophagus demonstrating full inflation of the valvuloplasty balloon. Intracardiac echocardiographic view from the high right atrium (RA), with slight anterior flexion, demonstrating rheumatically deformed posterior and anterior MV leaflets (PL, AL), prior to percutaneous balloon valvuloplasty. Coronary sinus = CS; left ventricle = LV. Intracardiac echocardiographic view from the RV imaging through the interventricular septum (IVS), demonstrating the left ventricle (LV) as well as rheumatically deformed anterior mitral valve leaflet (arrow) with the classic "hockey-stick deformity" typical of rheumatic mitral stenosis. Intracardiac echocardiographic view from the high right atrium (RA), with slight anterior flexion, demonstrating full inflation of the valvuloplasty balloon across the mitral valve. Coronary sinus = CS; left atrium = LA. Intracardiac echocardiographic view from the high right atrium (RA), with slight anterior flexion, demonstrating improved posterior and anterior MV leaflet mobility (PL, AL), immediately following percutaneous balloon valvuloplasty. Coronary sinus = CS; left ventricle = LV.

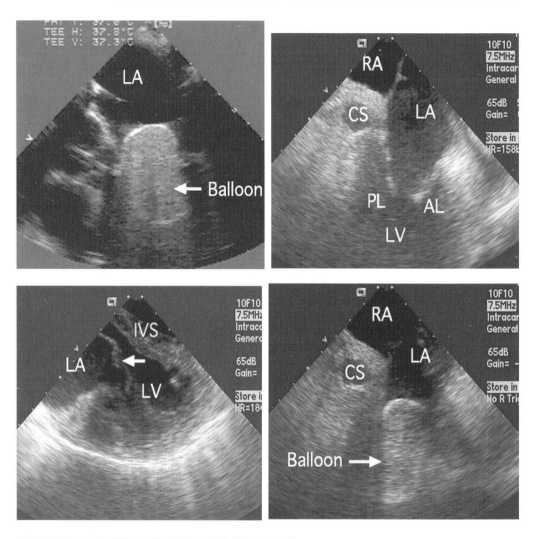

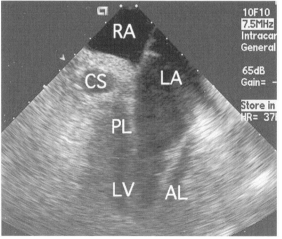

Fig. 1. *(Continued)*

Table 2
Mitral Valve Scoring by Echocardiography Prior to PBV

The extent and severity of valvular and subvalvular deformity can be assessed by assigning a
  score of 1 to 4 for each of the following:
  • Degree of leaflet rigidity
  • Amount of leaflet calcification
  • Severity of leaflet thickening
  • Extent of subvalvular thickening and calcification

Note: The maximum score is 16; higher scores indicate more severe anatomic disease and reduced likelihood of success.

(see Table 2) and could provide suitable information for real-time procedural guidance
in the interventional laboratory. Prevalvuloplasty, TEE can also be used to calculate the
mitral valvuloplasty score (see Table 2) if TTE images are not diagnostic, assess for significant preprocedural mitral regurgitation, and, most importantly, is required to exclude
LA or LAA thrombus that may preclude PBV *(28–30)*. LAA thrombus is a contraindication to the procedure, because of the risk of stroke resulting from catheter dislodgement. The mitral valvuloplasty echo score can be used to identify appropriate anatomical candidates for the procedure, identify those at risk for development of severe mitral
regurgitation after valvuloplasty, and predict the long-term outcome of the procedure
(see Chapter 1 and ref. *31*).

Interventionalists performing PBV who are experienced in transseptal catheterization
might not require any additional imaging to perform this part of the procedure. Early on,
real-time TTE was attempted to assist the transseptal puncture, although the resolution of
TTE limits its utility in many cases. More often, TEE and ICE are used when imaging is
required for transseptal catheterization during mitral PBV *(16,20,25,32,33)* (see Fig. 1.1).

Once left atrial access is achieved, both TTE and TEE can be used in real time to assess
balloon position, estimate mitral valve diastolic gradients, and estimate mitral valve area
after balloon inflation, as well to monitor for an increase in mitral regurgitation that might
preclude subsequent inflations *(27,34–42)* (see Figs. 1B–1E). Typically, apical long-axis
or esophageal four-chamber views are used to measure pulsed or continuous-wave Doppler
gradients and to assess for mitral regurgitation with color Doppler. The pressure half-time
method for mitral valve area estimation might not correlate with the hemodynamically
derived mitral valve area estimate using the Gorlin formula immediately following balloon
valvuloplasty if a transseptal approach is used *(43–45)*, and, therefore, the peak and mean
gradients estimated by pulsed or continuous-wave Doppler might be more useful in assessing the adequacy of the result in this setting. It has been suggested that that these discrepancies between Doppler and hemodynamically estimated mitral valve area calculations
might be attributable to the overestimation of the cardiac output with hemodynamic measurements, caused by the presence of the iatrogenic ASD associated with transseptal
catheterization. If a retrograde nontransseptal approach is used, the Doppler-derived pressure half-time method appears to be accurate. Planimetry of the mitral valve in the
parasternal short-axis on TTE or transgastric short-axis view on TEE can also be used to
estimate mitral valve area and supplement the estimation of pressure gradients, thereby
assessing the adequacy of the procedure. Short-axis views of the mitral valve at the commissural level might also provide information as to the mechanism of improvement in
degree of stenosis immediately after valvuloplasty, as well as determining whether addi-

tional commissural separation is required for an adequate result. TTE and TEE can also be used to monitor for complications such as left atrial thrombus, pericardial effusion, tamponade, left ventricular or left atrial perforation, and severe mitral regurgitation. Similarly, TEE can assess the hemodynamic impact of the residual ASD resulting from the transseptal puncture. TEE could be of particular benefit when attempting to minimize the fluoroscopic exposure during the entire procedure (i.e., in pregnancy) or when initial attempts at fluoroscopically guided transseptal puncture are unsuccessful. As of this writing, there are no studies to suggest that TEE or ICE can reduce complications associated with PBV.

Intracardiac endocardiography has recently been used to guide mitral valve PBV (46–48). ICE offers advantages over TEE in that it does not require additional sedation or general anesthesia and it improves patient comfort. With ICE, the transseptal catheterization can be monitored in real time, thereby potentially reducing the risk of complications. With ICE, assessment of balloon position, mitral gradients, and severity of mitral regurgitation (MR) is feasible, and some operators have begun using this imaging modality during PBV (see Figs. 1F–1I). Direct comparison to TTE or TEE is lacking and requires further study to determine whether it provides sufficient advantage to justify its additional cost (see Videos 1–9 on accompanying CD-ROM of ICE guidance of PBV).

ALCOHOL SEPTAL ABLATION IN HYPERTROPHIC OBSTRUCTIVE CARDIOMYOPATHY

In the management of hypertrophic obstructive cardiomyopathy (HOCM), surgical myectomy and dual-chamber pacemaker implantation are considered to be established extensions to medical treatment. Percutaneous transluminal septal myocardial ablation by alcohol-induced septal branch occlusion has been introduced as an alternative nonsurgical procedure for reducing the left ventricular outflow tract gradient (49–53). TTE can be used in alcohol septal ablation for patients with HOCM to localize an optimal site for ablation as well as assess the adequacy of the hemodynamic result (see Fig. 2). Echocardiographic views typically used include the parasternal long-axis view, which is used to determine the maximum region of septal hypertrophy as well as the contact point between the interventricular septum and the systolic anterior motion of the anterior leaflet of the mitral valve (SAM contact point). Similarly, the apical three- and five-chamber views offer similar anatomic delineation of the left ventricular outflow tract as well as offering the ability to measure left ventricular outflow tract gradients by continuous-wave Doppler interrogation. Caution must be used to avoid measuring the signal from any associated mitral regurgitation, as this could result in an overestimation of the LVOT gradients. As with pericardiocentesis, the injection of a small amount of agitated saline mixed with air microbubbles (or other echocardiographic contrast agent) into the septal perforator vessel with balloon occlusion allows confirmation that the ablation site will incorporate the region of maximum septal hypertrophy and involve the SAM contact point. In rare cases, opacification of the medial papillary muscle or the left ventricular posterolateral free wall might be seen, suggesting that an alternate ablation target vessel should be sought (50), thus avoiding potentially fatal complications resulting from induction of a necrosis of myocardium distant from the septal target area. Postablation, gradients can be remeasured, although postablation edema could result in an elevated gradient for several weeks following ablation. Because harmonic imaging can be used for detection of ultrasound contrast agents in myocardial perfusion studies, superharmonic imaging has

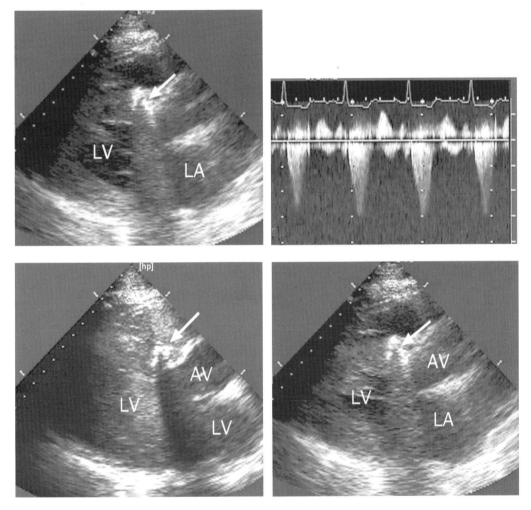

Fig. 2. Transthoracic echocardiographic view from the parasternal long axis demonstrating inflation of an occluder balloon in the first septal perforator to confirm position prior to alcohol septal ablation for HOCM. Left ventricle = LV; left atrium = LA. Continuous-wave Doppler velocity profile prior to alcohol septal ablation for hypertrophic cardiomyopathy confirming left ventricular outflow tract obstruction, with a resting 36 mm Hg predicted gradient. (Each of the vertical markers represents 1-m/s velocity.) Transthoracic echocardiographic view from the parasternal long axis demonstrating inflation of an occluder balloon in the first septal perforator as well as injection of left ventricular contrast (Optison) to confirm position prior to alcohol septal ablation for HOCM. Left ventricle = LV; left atrium = LA; aortic valve = AV. With injection of contrast, the region to be ablated becomes increasingly echogenic, with prominent shadowing noted over the mitral valve. Postablation gradients are now normal, with each of the small vertical markers representing 20-cm/s velocity.

been recently used to differentiate treated and nontreated myocardium in HOCM ethanol ablation *(54)*. This technique detects the third, fourth, and fifth harmonics, which are not created in tissue, resulting, hence, in a high contrast-to-tissue ratio. Whether this technique offers advantages in the real-time guidance of these procedures is not known.

As with mitral valve (MV) PBV, procedural complications, including pericardial effusion and tamponade, can be quickly identified. In patients with poor transthoracic

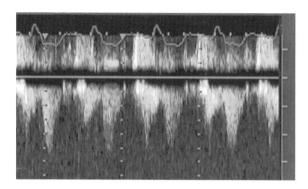

Fig. 2. *(Continued)*

echocardiographic windows, TEE can occasionally be substituted, although measurement of the LVOT gradients is more challenging because of differences in alignment in the transducer with the direction of flow in the LVOT *(55)*. Limited studies exist examining the role of TEE in guiding alcohol septal ablation in HOCM. Although ICE guidance of septal ablation is theoretically possible, this has not been systematically evaluated.

TRANSESOPHAGEAL ECHOCARDIOGRAPHY IN ASD AND PFO CLOSURE

Preprocedural transesophageal echocardiographic (TEE) measurement of the size and location of ASD and PFO has been helpful in the selection of the appropriate patients for percutaneous transcatheter closure (PTC) as well as selecting the appropriate device to use. In addition, TEE can be used to guide the procedure in real time, an approach that could eliminate the need for fluoroscopy *(46,47)*. The insertion of more than one device to close multiple ASDs is safe and effective; both two- and three-dimensional TEE has been shown to be particularly helpful when multiple devices are used *(4)*. TEE provides an accurate assessment of atrial–septal anatomy and assists in guide-wire placement, transseptal puncture (if necessary), closure device sizing, and deployment. Furthermore, it gives immediate information regarding the adequacy of closure *(4,46–49)*. Drawbacks of TEE are potential patient discomfort and the risk of aspiration in the supine patient with prolonged esophageal intubation. As a result, TEE-guided PTC is often performed under general anesthesia with endotracheal intubation, which requires the expertise of an anesthesiologist and adds to the time and cost of the procedure *(50)*. TEE can be supplemented by TTE in patients with attenuated or deficient anterior septal rims and unusual septal morphology, as was shown in a small number of patients undergoing PTC *(51)*.

TEE IN COMPLEX MV PROCEDURES

A newer MV repair system has been developed as an alternative to surgical repair, using the concepts of the edge-to-edge technique developed by Alfieri but performed with a percutaneous endovascular repair system. The endovascular Mitral Repair System (Evalve™; Redwood City, CA) uses a steerable guide catheter to position a two-armed V-shaped clip to approximate the leaflet tissue near the midline of the valve, thus reducing or eliminating mitral regurgitation. The delivery of the Evalve clip has five major steps that require echocardiographic guidance: transseptal catheterization, alignment of the clip delivery system perpendicular to the plane of the MV and centered with reference to the line of coaptation, alignment of the approximation implant device with the open arms perpendicular to the coaptation line of the mitral valve, closing of the arms and approximation of the tips of the mitral valve, and release of the implant device. A combination of transesophageal echo (TEE) and transthoracic echo (TTE) has been used to guide the entire procedure. TEE has been instrumental during transseptal crossing, clip alignment perpendicular to the mitral valve, closing of the clip, and release of the device; TTE was helpful in perpendicular clip alignment and essential in short-axis clip alignment. At the end of the procedure, it was possible to image the "figure-of-8" diastolic profile of the double MV orifice. TEE monitoring also allows an assessment of the degree of MR and transmitral gradients before the procedure, prior to clip removal, and immediately after the device was deployed *(3)*.

Newer coronary sinus devices are also being developed to perform a percutaneous mitral annuloplasty repair, thereby reducing MR by enhancing mitral coaptation *(56)*. TEE and/or ICE can be used to cannulate the coronary sinus ostium, place the device, monitor for procedural complications, as well as to assess the degree of MR and transmitral gradients before and after the procedure.

INTRACARDIAC ECHOCARDIOGRAPHY

Intracardiac echocardiography is a newer modality that can also provide excellent imaging of the atrial septum and associated structures *(50)*. It utilizes a single-use ICE catheter and requires additional 10F–11F venous access. Benefits in using ICE for radiofrequency ablation of atrial fibrillation and, more recently, for transcatheter septal closure procedures have been demonstrated *(53,54)*. An advantage over TEE is that ICE obviates the need for general anesthesia, as well as additional echocardiography support, because the operator performing the percutaneous closure can also manipulate the ICE catheter. In some centers, however, additional echocardiography expertise is employed to assist in the ICE examination of the interatrial septum (IAS) during closure.

There are three currently available ICE systems for the guidance of percutaneous procedures. Each has unique features. The Boston Scientific UltraICE utilizes radial ICE imaging, is not steerable, and is presently limited to two-dimensional imaging. Both Siemens AcuNav and the newer EP Medsystems ImageMate are steerable and deflectable and have two-dimensional, color, and spectral Doppler capabilities.

Other advantages of ICE in the guidance of intracardiac procedures when compared to TEE include shorter procedure and fluoroscopy times and, as such, it is emerging as the standard imaging modality for guiding septal closure procedures *(55–58)*. ICE can be used as the primary imaging modality, without supplemental TTE or TEE. Recently, ICE has been shown to offer comparable cost to TEE in guiding septal closure procedures, when general anesthesia is used *(57)*.

In guiding closure of ASD and PFO, images are typically obtained from the mid-right atrium (see Figs. 3 and 4). In the case of the steerable and deflectable catheters, posterior and rightward tilting of the transducer away from the interatrial septum provides excellent imaging of the septum and surrounding structures. The devices currently in use are typically double-disk devices with or without a self-centering mechanism. The method of implantation is variable and unique to each device. The mechanism of closure of all devices ultimately involves stenting the defect, with subsequent thrombus formation and neo-endothelialization.

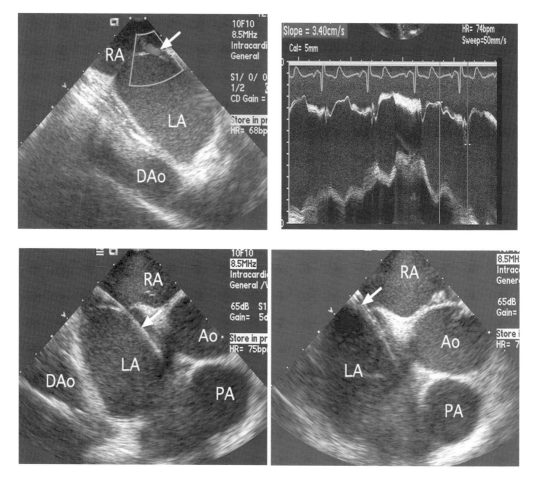

Fig. 3. Intracardiac echo image from the mid-right atrium (RA) with posterior and rightward tilting demonstrating left-to-right color Doppler flow (arrow) through a stretched patent foramen ovale. Left atrium = LA; descending thoracic aorta = DAo. M-mode recording through the interatrial septum demonstrating increased mobility (greater than 1.5 cm) consistent with atrial septal aneurysm. Intracardiac echo image from the mid right atrium (RA) with posterior and rightward tilting demonstrating guide wire (arrow) crossing through a patent foramen ovale into the left atrium (LA). Aorta = Ao; pulmonary artery = PA; descending thoracic aorta = DAo. Intracardiac echo image from the mid right atrium (RA) with posterior and rightward tilting demonstrating the delivery sheath (arrow) crossing through a patent foramen ovale into the left atrium = LA; Aorta = Ao; pulmonary artery = PA; descending thoracic aorta = DAo. Intracardiac echo image from the mid right atrium (RA) with posterior and rightward tilting demonstrating a CardioSeal closure device with its upper arms malpositioned such that the are folding within the PFO tunnel (arrow). Left atrium = LA; Aorta = Ao; descending thoracic aorta = DAo. Intracardiac echo image from the mid-right atrium (RA) with posterior and rightward tilting demonstrating a CardioSeal closure device with its upper arms now appropriately positioned such that the are compressing against the PFO tunnel (arrow) in the left atrium (LA). Intracardiac echo image from the mid-right atrium (RA) with posterior and rightward tilting demonstrating a CardioSeal closure (arrow) with both sides of the disk fully deployed. The device is still attached to the guiding cable. Left atrium = LA; aorta = Ao; descending thoracic aorta = DAo. Intracardiac echo image from the mid-right atrium (RA) with posterior and rightward tilting demonstrating a CardioSeal closure after release from the guiding cable. Left atrium = LA; descending thoracic aorta = DAo.

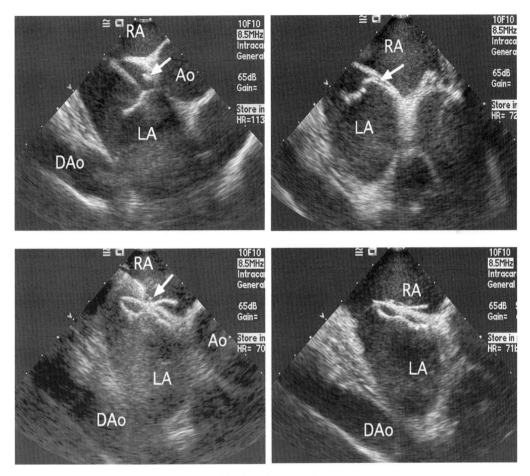

Fig. 3. *(Continued)*

The preprocedural assessment of the interatrial septum by ICE includes evaluation of the entire interatrial septum. PFO is defined as a right-to-left communication through the fossa ovalis, and a stretched PFO is defined as the same anatomical defect with resting or intermittent left-to-right flow by color Doppler imaging. Right-to-left shunting is typically demonstrated by the injection of agitated saline at rest and with provocative maneuvers such as Valsalva. An atrial–septal aneurysm is defined as 15 mm of total movement of a 15-mm base of atrial–septal tissue. (See Videos 1–8 of ICE-guided PFO closure on the accompanying CD-ROM.)

The ASD type (ostium secundum, ostium primum, sinus venosus, coronary sinus), maximum ASD diameter, and defect number if multiple defects are present are easily assessed with ICE evaluation. Presently, only ostium secundum ASDs are amenable to percutaneous closure. Defects up to 38 mm in diameter have been closed successfully with percutaneous devices, as well as multiple ASDs and those associated with atrial–septal aneurysm. Associated abnormalities of the pulmonary veins, IVC, SVC, coronary sinus, and AV valves should be excluded. Consideration of the size of the atrial–septal rim of tissue surrounding the defect is important in evaluating patients for successful closure, and a rim of 5 mm is generally considered adequate. The inferior and superior rims can be particularly important for this technique, although small series have

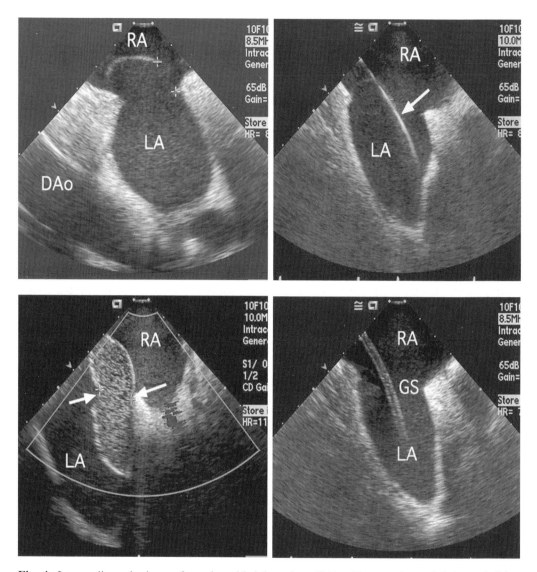

Fig. 4. Intracardiac echo image from the mid right atrium (RA) with posterior and rightward tilting demonstrating a moderate size ostium secundum atrial septal defect. Left atrium = LA; descending thoracic aorta = DAo. Intracardiac echo image from the mid right atrium (RA) with posterior and rightward tilting demonstrating the guide wire crossing the atrial septal defect into the left atrium (LA). Intracardiac echo image from the mid right atrium (RA) with posterior and rightward tilting demonstrating a sizing balloon (arrows at balloon waist) across the ASD. Color Doppler is used to ensure stoppage of flow, thus confirming that the balloon fully occludes the defect. Intracardiac echo image from the mid right atrium (RA) with posterior and rightward tilting demonstrating the guiding sheath (GS) crossing the defect into the left atrium (LA). Intracardiac echo image from the mid right atrium (RA) with posterior and rightward tilting demonstrating the left atrial disk of an Amplatzer septal occluder (ASO) opening. The Amplatzer septal occluder is pulled back to the interatrial septum (IAS) in the left atrium (LA), prior to opening the right atrial (RA) disk. After both disks are deployed, a push–pull maneuver is performed to confirm a stable position without risk of dislodgement prior to release. The device is being pulled on in this image. Prior to release, the device is shown appropriately positioned. Following release of the guiding cable, the device typically migrates as it is no longer under tension from the guiding cable. Right atrium = RA; left atrium = LA; interatrial septum = IAS.

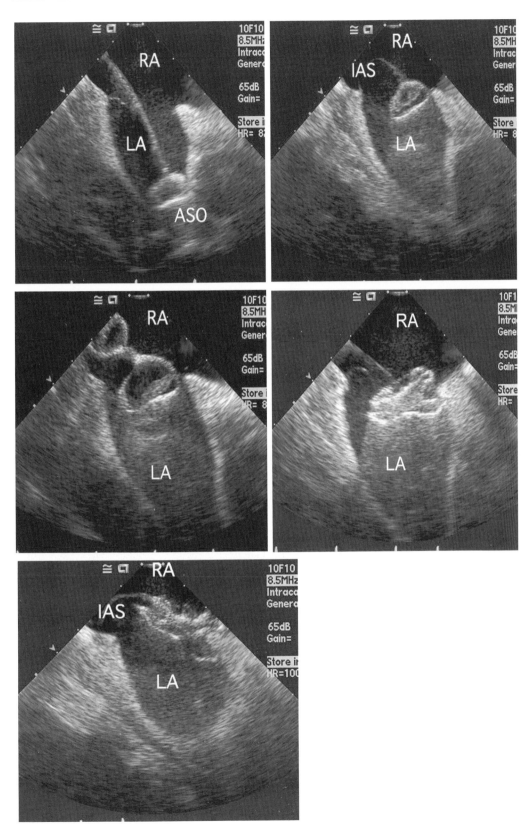

Fig. 4. *(Continued)*

reported success in patients with deficient rims. Balloon sizing of the ASD can be achieved with a balloon by one of two methods.

A "pulling technique" is one in which a sizing balloon is inflated in the left atrium to a size larger than the ASD and pulled toward the defect until flow is occluded (documented by color Doppler on either TEE or ICE). The balloon is then deflated until it moves from the left atrium to the right atrium. The amount of fluid inside the balloon at the time the balloon crosses the defect is measured and, once removed, it is compared with a sizing plate that corresponds to the diameter of the defect.

Alternatively, the simpler "stationary balloon dilation" involves the use of a low-pressure balloon that is placed across the ASD and inflated. Imaging with TEE or ICE as well as fluoroscopy monitors the inflation, and when the defect is completely occluded, there will be no color Doppler flow shunting seen, and a waist appears in the balloon contour. The balloon waist diameter is measured by echocardiography or fluoroscopy, and this size corresponds to the stretched diameter of the ASD.

The balloon is then removed, leaving the guide wire in place, and the proper-sized device delivery sheath is passed over the wire into the left upper pulmonary vein (for stability) under echocardiographic guidance. The closure device is then delivered through the sheath into the left atrium. The individual insertion technique vary at this point, but typically employs opening the left atrial disk or arms and pulling them back to the interatrial septum. Once the LA aspect of the device is in position, the RA aspect is opened, thereby "sandwiching" the septum. The arms of the device rest on the rims of atrial tissue surrounding the defect. For this reason, in ASDs associated with deficiencies in these rims, a stable position can be more difficult to achieve. A stable device position for certain devices (i.e., Amplatzer Septal Occluder) is confirmed by moving the connecting cable (and, thus, the device attached to it) forward and backward.

When the device is confirmed to be in a satisfactory position, surrounding structures are evaluated. Large devices might threaten the patency of the right upper pulmonary vein, superior vena cava, inferior vena cava, coronary sinus, and, occasionally, the function of the tricuspid and mitral valves. The device is then released and reimaged with echocardiography to assess for immediate ASD closure, as its position often changes once the traction of the connecting cable is no longer present. (See Videos 1–7 of ICE-guided ASD closure on accompanying CD-ROM.)

FUTURE DIRECTIONS

Newer imaging modalities currently being developed include on-line real-time three-dimensional TEE and ICE, which offers the potential for additional advantages in the guidance of percutaneous noncoronary interventions. These modalities could offer the advantage of being able to delineate the complex relationships among intracardiac anatomy, physiology, and device function, although they have not been systematically evaluated in these settings (58–72).

As echocardiographically guided interventions become more complex, collaboration between the interventional cardiologist and interventional echocardiographer becomes increasingly vital to the success of these procedures. Communication must be facilitated in such a way to ensure that both operators are speaking "the same language" and referring to the same anatomic landmarks or targets. Both the echocardiographer and the interventionalist must become familiar with the other's subspecialty in order to facilitate successful cooperation and collaboration. The time required for performing complex procedures such as percutaneous mitral valve repair are significant and require commitment on the part of the echocardiographer to be present for the duration of the proceure. Finally, future goals for advanced echocardiography training include an interventional echocardiographic subspeciality, with training in all modalities used to guide these procedures, including intracardiac echocardiography.

REFERENCES

1. Cheitlin MD, et al. ACC/AHA/ASE 2003 guideline update for the clinical application of echocardiography: summary article: a report of the American College of Cardiology/American Heart Association Task Force on Practice Guidelines (ACC/AHA/ASE Committee to Update the 1997 Guidelines for the Clinical Application of Echocardiography). Circulation 2003;108(9):1146–1162.
2. Du ZD, et al. Comparison of transcatheter closure of secundum atrial septal defect using the Amplatzer septal occluder associated with deficient versus sufficient rims. Am J Cardiol 2002;90(8):865–869.
3. Rodriguez L, et al. Echocardiographic guidance of Percutaneous repair for mitral regurgitation with Evalve system. Initial clinical experience. J Am Coll Cardiol 2004, in press.
4. Callahan JA, et al. Pericardiocentesis assisted by two-dimensional echocardiography. J Thorac Cardiovasc Surg 1983;85(6):877–879.
5. Callahan JA, Seward JB, Tajik AJ. Two-dimensional echocardiography during pericardiocentesis. Am J Cardiol 1984;54(1):246.
6. Shah PM, Nanda NC. Echocardiography in the diagnosis of pericardial effusion. Cardiovasc Clin 1976; 7(3):125–130.
7. Singh S, et al. Right ventricular and right atrial collapse in patients with cardiac tamponade—a combined echocardiographic and hemodynamic study. Circulation 1984;70(6):966–971.
8. Appleton CP, Hatle LK, Popp RK. Cardiac tamponade and pericardial effusion: respiratory variation in transvalvular flow velocities studied by Doppler echocardiography. J Am Coll Cardiol 1988;11(5): 1020–1030.
9. Leeman DE, Levine MJ, Come PC. Doppler echocardiography in cardiac tamponade: exaggerated respiratory variation in transvalvular blood flow velocity integrals. J Am Coll Cardiol 1988;11(3): 572–578.
10. Chandraratna PA. Echocardiography and Doppler ultrasound in the evaluation of pericardial disease. Circulation 1991;84(3 Suppl.):I303–I310.
11. Tsang TS, et al. Consecutive 1127 therapeutic echocardiographically guided pericardiocenteses: clinical profile, practice patterns, and outcomes spanning 21 years. Mayo Clin Proc 2002;77(5):429–436.
12. Chabdraratna PA, et al. Echocardiographic contrast studies during pericardiocentesis. Ann Inter Med 1977;87(2):199–200.
13. O'Sullivan J, Heads A, Hunter S. Microbubble image enhancement and pericardiocentesis. Int J Cardiol 1993;42(1):95–96.
14. Weisse AB, et al. Contrast echocardiography as an adjunct in hemorrhagic or complicated pericardiocentesis. Am Heart J 1996;131(4):822–825.
15. Betts TR, Radvan JR. Contrast echocardiography during pericardiocentesis. [see comment]. Heart (Br Cardiac Soc) 1999;81(3):329.
16. Kronzon I, et al. Use of two-dimensional echocardiography during transseptal cardiac catheterization. J Am Coll Cardiol 1984;4(2):425–428.
17. Doorey AJ, Goldenberg EM. Transseptal catheterization in adults: enhanced efficacy and safety by low-volume operators using a "non-standard" technique. Cathet Cardiovasc Diagn 1991;22(4):239–243.
18. Goldstein SA, et al. Feasibility of on-line transesophageal echocardiography during balloon mitral valvulotomy: experience with 93 patients. J Heart Valve Dis 1994;3(2):136–148.
19. Harrison JK, et al. Complications related to percutaneous transvenous mitral commissurotomy. Cathet Cardiovasc Diagn 1994;Suppl(2): 52–60.
20. Hahn K, et al. Transesophageal echocardiographically guided atrial transseptal catheterization in patients with normal-sized atria: incidence of complications. Clin Cardiol 1995;18(4):217–220.
21. Ben Farhat M, et al. Percutaneous balloon mitral valvuloplasty in eight pregnant women with severe mitral stenosis. Euro Heart J 1992;13(12):1658–1664.
22. Mangione JA, et al. Percutaneous double balloon mitral valvuloplasty in pregnant women. Am J Cardiol 1989;64(1):99–102.

23. Uygur D, Beksac MS. Mitral balloon valvuloplasty during pregnancy in developing countries. Eur J Obstet Gynecol Reprod Biol 2001;96(2):226–228.
24. Nercolini DC, et al. Percutaneous mitral balloon valvuloplasty in pregnant women with mitral stenosis. [see comment]. Cathet Cardiovasc Intervent 2002;57(3):318–322.
25. Hurrell DG, et al. Echocardiography in the invasive laboratory: utility of two-dimensional echocardiography in performing transseptal catheterization. Mayo Clini Proc 1998;73(2):126–131.
26. Kultursay H, et al. Mitral balloon valvuloplasty with transesophageal echocardiography without using fluoroscopy. Cathet Cardiovasc Diagn 1992;27(4):317–321.
27. Kronzon I, et al. Transesophageal echocardiography during percutaneous mitral valvuloplasty. J Am Soc Echocardiogr 1989;2(6):380–385.
28. Olson JD, et al. Exclusion of atrial thrombus by transesophageal echocardiography. J Am Soc Echocardiogr 1992;5(1):52–56.
29. Kamalesh M, Burger AJ, Shubrooks SJ. Jr. The use of transesophageal echocardiography to avoid left atrial thrombus during percutaneous mitral valvuloplasty. [see comment]. Cathet Cardiovasc Diagn 1993;28(4):320–322.
30. Krishnamoorthy KM, et al. Usefulness of transthoracic echocardiography for identification of left atrial thrombus before balloon mitral valvuloplasty. Am J Cardiol 2003;92(9):1132–1134.
31. Padial LR, et al. Echocardiography can predict the development of severe mitral regurgitation after percutaneous mitral valvuloplasty by the Inoue technique. Am J Cardiol 1999;83(8):1210–1213.
32. Hung JS, et al. Usefulness of intracardiac echocardiography in complex transseptal catheterization during percutaneous transvenous mitral commissurotomy. Mayo Clin Proc 1996;71(2):134–140.
33. Daoud EG, Kalbfleisch SJ, Hummel JD. Intracardiac echocardiography to guide transseptal left heart catheterization for radiofrequency catheter ablation. J Cardiovasc Electrophysiol 1999;10(3):358–363.
34. Casale PN, et al. Transesophageal echocardiography in percutaneous balloon valvuloplasty for mitral stenosis. Cleve Clin J Med 1989;56(6):597–600.
35. Chen CG, et al. Value of two-dimensional echocardiography in selecting patients and balloon sizes for percutaneous balloon mitral valvuloplasty. J Am Coll Cardiol 1989;14(7):1651–1658.
36. Chan K, et al. Role of transesophageal echocardiography in percutaneous balloon mitral valvuloplasty. Echocardiography 1990;7(2):115–123.
37. Jaarsma W, et al. Transesophageal echocardiography during percutaneous balloon mitral valvuloplasty. J Am Soc Echocardiogr 1990;3(5):384–391.
38. Parro A Jr, et al. Value and limitations of color Doppler echocardiography in the evaluation of percutaneous balloon mitral valvuloplasty for isolated mitral stenosis. Am J Cardiol 1991;67(15):1261–1267.
39. Arora R, et al. Role of transesophageal echocardiography during balloon mitral valvuloplasty. Indian Heart J 1992;44(6):391–394.
40. Pavlides GS, et al. The value of transesophageal echocardiography in predicting immediate and long-term outcome of balloon mitral valvuloplasty: comparison with transthoracic echocardiography. J Intervent Cardiol 1994;7(5):401–408.
41. Robinson NM, et al. The value of transthoracic echocardiography during percutaneous balloon mitral valvuloplasty. J Am Soc Echocardiogr 1995;8(1):79–86.
42. Park SH, Kim MA, Hyon MS. The advantages of on-line transesophageal echocardiography guide during percutaneous balloon mitral valvuloplasty. J Am Soc Echocardiogr 2000;13(1):26–34.
43. Shiran A, et al. Accuracy of two-dimensional echocardiographic planimetry of the mitral valve area before and after balloon valvuloplasty. Cardiology 1998;90(3):227–230.
44. Pitsavos CE, et al. Assessment of accuracy of the Doppler pressure half-time method in the estimation of the mitral valve area immediately after balloon mitral valvuloplasty. Eur Heart J 1997;18(3):455–463.
45. Fredman CS, et al. Comparison of hemodynamic pressure half-time method and Gorlin formula with Doppler and echocardiographic determinations of mitral valve area in patients with combined mitral stenosis and regurgitation. Am Heart J 1990;119(1):121–129.
46. Schwartz SL, et al. Intracardiac echocardiography during simulated aortic and mitral balloon valvuloplasty: in vivo experimental studies. Am Heart J 1992;123(3):665–674.
47. Salem MI, et al. Intracardiac echocardiography using the AcuNav ultrasound catheter during percutaneous balloon mitral valvuloplasty. J Am Soc Echocardiogr 2002;15(12):1533–1537.
48. Bruce CJ, Friedman PA. Intracardiac echocardiography. Eur J Echocardiogr 2001;2(4):234-244.
49. Faber L, et al. [Percutaneous transluminal septal myocardial ablation in hypertrophic obstructive cardiomyopathy: acute results in 66 patients with reference to myocardial contrast echocardiography]. Zeitschr f Kardiol 1998;87(3):191–201.

50. Faber L, et al. Intraprocedural myocardial contrast echocardiography as a routine procedure in percuta- neous transluminal septal myocardial ablation: detection of threatening myocardial necrosis distant from the septal target area. Cathet Cardiovasc Intervent 1999;47(4):462–466.

51. Mutlak D, et al. Non-surgical myocardial reduction in hypertrophic obstructive cardiomyopathy. [see comment]. Israel Med Assoc J Imaj 2002;4(2):86–90.

52. Nielsen CD, Spencer WH. 3rd. Role of controlled septal infarct in hypertrophic obstructive cardiomy- opathy. Cardiol Rev 2002;10(2):108–118.

53. Sakakibara M, et al. [Percutaneous transluminal septal ablation with ethanol in hypertrophic obstructive cardiomyopathy: a case report]. J Cardiol 1999;34(1):35–40.

54. Ten Cate FJ, et al. Visualization of myocardial perfusion after percutaneous myocardial septal ablation for hypertrophic cardiomyopathy using superharmonic imaging. J Am Soc Echocardiogr 2003;16(4): 370–372.

55. Widimsky P, et al. Potential applications for transesophageal echocardiography in hypertrophic car- diomyopathies. J Am Soc Echocardiogr 1992;5(2):163–167.

56. Condado JA, Velez-Gimon M. Catheter-based approach to mitral regurgitation. J Intervent Cardiol 2003;16(6):523–534.

57. Koenig P, et al. Role of intracardiac echocardiographic guidance in transcatheter closure of atrial septal defects and patent foramen ovale using the Amplatzer device. J Intervent Cardiol 2003;16(1):51–62.

58. De Castro S, et al. Qualitative and quantitative evaluation of mitral valve morphology by intraoperative volume-rendered three-dimensional echocardiography. J Heart Valve Dis 2002;11(2):173–180.

59. Gunasegaran K, et al. Three-dimensional transesophageal echocardiography (TEE) and other future directions. Cardiol Clin 2000;18(4):893–910.

60. Hozumi T, Yoshikawa J. Three-dimensional echocardiography using a multiplane transesophageal probe: the clinical applications. Echocardiography 2000;17(8):757–764.

61. Yu TH, Fu M, Chua S. Three-dimensional echocardiographic image of atrial septal aneurysm: report of two cases. Changgeng Yi Xue Za Zhi 2000;23(11):701–705.

62. Chauvel C, et al. Usefulness of three-dimensional echocardiography for the evaluation of mitral valve prolapse: an intraoperative study. J Heart Valve Dis 2000;9(3):341–349.

63. Applebaum RM, et al. Utility of three-dimensional echocardiography during balloon mitral valvuloplasty. J Am Coll Cardiol 1998;32(5):1405–1409.

64. Magni G, et al. Two- and three-dimensional transesophageal echocardiography in patient selection and assessment of atrial septal defect closure by the new DAS-Angel Wings device: initial clinical experi- ence. Circulation 1997;96(6):1722–1728.

65. Binder T, et al. Value of three-dimensional echocardiography as an adjunct to conventional trans- esophageal echocardiography. Cardiology 1996;87(4):335–342.

66. Salustri A, et al. Three-dimensional echocardiography of normal and pathologic mitral valve: a com- parison with two-dimensional transesophageal echocardiography. J Am Coll Cardiol 1996;27(6):1502–1510.

67. Szili-Torok T, et al. Interatrial septum pacing guided by three-dimensional intracardiac echocardiogra- phy. J Am Coll Cardiol 2002;40(12):2139–2143.

68. Light ED, et al. Feasibility study for real time three-dimensional Doppler intracardiac echocardiography. Ultrason Imaging 2002;24(1):36–46.

69. Smith SW, et al. Feasibility study of real-time three-dimensional intracardiac echocardiography for guidance of interventional electrophysiology. Pacing Clin Electrophysiol 2002;25(3):351–357.

70. Szili-Torok T, Roelandt JR, Jordaens LJ. Bachmann's bundle pacing: a role for three-dimensional intracardiac echocardiography? [comment]. J Cardiovasc Electrophysiol 2002;13(1):97–98.

71. Light ED, et al. Real-time three-dimensional intracardiac echocardiography. Ultrasound Med Biol 2001;27(9):1177–1183.

72. Foster GP, Picard MH. Intracardiac echocardiography: current uses and future directions. Echocardiography 2001;18(1):43–48.

21

3D Angiography

Nathan E. Green, MD, S.-Y. James Chen, PhD,
John C. Messenger, MD,
and John D. Carroll, MD

CONTENTS

INTRODUCTION

The clinical application of three-dimensional (3D) imaging technology represents a powerful advancement in the diagnosis and treatment of patients with vascular disease. From its initial use with noninvasive imaging modalities like computed tomography (CT), 3D imaging technology is now used during invasive angiographic procedures for the diagnosis of vascular disease and guidance during therapeutic interventions. Three-dimensional angiography resolves and streamlines many of the challenges of traditional two-dimensional (2D) angiography. Whereas traditional angiography relies heavily upon the experience of the operator to minimize the imaging limitations introduced by its 2D format, 3D angiography provides an objective, operator-independent method of acquiring more angiographic information to guide clinical decisions and patient care. As an interventional imaging tool, 3D angiography has the potential to simplify complex procedures, reduce radiation exposure, and improve patient outcomes. In this chapter, we explore the techniques and development of 3D angiography and the potential clinical and research applications of this powerful technology.

From: *Contemporary Cardiology: Interventional Cardiology:*
Percutaneous Noncoronary Intervention
Edited by: H. C. Herrmann © Humana Press Inc., Totowa, NJ

3D IMAGING: HISTORY AND RECONSTRUCTION TECHNIQUES

Imaging in three dimensions is critical to understanding the dynamic spatial relationships of complex geometric structures. In medicine, the application of powerful 3D imaging tools that are capable of accurate anatomic delineation is paramount to continued improvements in patient care. Additionally, 3D imaging is a more effective and intuitive method to interpret diagnostic imaging studies and could decrease the volume of 2D images needed for traditional imaging interpretation. Because of the clinical need for precisely characterizing small tortuous vessels and vascular pathology, angiography is well suited for the application of 3D imaging technology.

Historically, imaging studies have relied upon transverse cuts or X-ray projections through a selected area of interest to generate 2D images. After acquiring the cuts or projections with X-ray, ultrasound, or other techniques, these images are then displayed in sequence and reviewed by the interpreting physician. Traditional 2D imaging studies acquire large volumes of data that can be used for diagnostic and therapeutic decisions. Unfortunately, the interpretation of the study is dependent on the physician's ability to dynamically reconstruct an accurate, mental 3D image of the structure from the 2D image dataset. Although this technique works well with smaller image sets, a diagnostic CT angiogram of the lower extremities can generate over 900 transverse reconstructions and require a significant amount of time for accurate image interpretation (1).

Interest in improving the topographical display of structures by visualizing in the third dimension culminated in the late 1970s with the development of 3D software. Using images of the spine obtained with CT, Herman and Coin created 3D dynamic images to assist with planning of spinal disk surgeries (2). As computer processing and imaging technology improved over the following decades, 3D imaging of nearly any organ became possible with a variety of imaging techniques including CT, electron beam CT (EBCT), magnetic resonance imaging (MRI), or ultrasound (3–7).

The development and widespread application of noninvasive imaging techniques has reduced the need for invasive angiography except coronary arteriography. Invasive angiography still remains the gold standard for the diagnosis and treatment of most vascular disease. The combination of small vessel size, tortuosity, vessel motion, and superior imaging with arterial contrast injections have contributed to the persistence of angiography as the primary imaging tool for assessing vascular structures. Similar to noninvasive imaging techniques, interest in using 3D techniques during angiography also began in the 1970s with stereoscopic views obtained of the cerebral vessels through rotation of X-ray tubes (8–9). As computer processing power increased and imaging techniques improved, digital subtraction angiography (DSA) was combined with rotational acquisitions to generate 3D angiographic images (10–13). Similar interest in the coronary and peripheral circulations has resulted in the clinical application of 3D reconstruction techniques that have been used to identify vascular obstructions, simulate vascular procedures, and guide complex interventions (14–20).

3D Reconstruction Techniques

Several postprocessing techniques or computer algorithms capable of generating images from CT, MRI, and angiographic data have been described. In general, these methods can be divided into either 2D projectional techniques or 3D rendering techniques. The multiplanar reformation (MPR) and maximum intensity projection (MIP) techniques are simplistic methods for producing 2D images from 3D datasets (1). Although images with

MPR or MIP are fast and easy to generate, visualization is limited to external structural modeling and not intraluminal imaging. To visualize the lumen of a tubular structure, the shaded surface display (SSD) technique uses an operator-defined threshold of pixel intensity values to reconstruct surface reflections *(21)*. Using an imaginary light source and different thresholds, images are displayed with or without adjacent structures in a 3D format. In the coronary circulation, a technique similar to SSD has been used for accurate 3D modeling of the coronary arterial tree *(14)*. The SSD technique has also been successfully used to reconstruct cerebral and peripheral arteries, airways, and bowel *(22–28)*. Volume rendering (VR) is the most complex of the developed 3D reconstruction techniques *(1,26)*. In contrast to SSD, VR uses the entire acquired dataset to generate a 3D structure with preservation of all spatial relationships. Although the VR technique has been used with CT, MRI, and angiographic data, the significant computer processing time for reconstructions has limited its widespread application *(20,27,28)*. However, as the technical and reconstruction limitations are resolved, the VR technique will likely occupy an important role in imaging of vascular structures in the very near future.

TRADITIONAL ANGIOGRAPHY: TECHNIQUES AND LIMITATIONS

Despite the growth and development of powerful noninvasive imaging techniques, invasive angiography remains an essential tool in the diagnosis and treatment of vascular disease. In the circulatory system, noninvasive tests have been limited by suboptimal resolution *(29)*, limited sensitivity *(30)*, imaging artifacts from vessel tortuosity *(31)*, lack of functional information such as vessel flow, and limited utility in patients with metallic clips, stents, or sternal wires *(32,33)*. Furthermore, only angiography is currently capable of imaging guidance during percutaneous revascularization procedures of the cerebral, coronary, and peripheral vasculature. In contrast to the marked advances in noninvasive imaging over the last decade, there have been relatively few advances in image acquisition or postprocessing techniques with traditional angiography.

The imaging characteristics of traditional angiography introduce significant artifacts into the accurate representation of vascular structures. Angiography, through the injection of radiopaque contrast, produces a 2D silhouette that could misrepresent the true anatomic characteristics of the 3D vessel lumen. Vessel overlap and vessel foreshortening are two of the inherent recognized limitations of angiography. Vessel overlap occurs with superimposition of two images and is usually recognized by experienced angiographers. In contrast, foreshortening of a vessel segment could be unrecognized *(18)* and result in missed lesions, underestimation of stenosis severity, and inaccurate lesion length measurements. Because of the multiple imaging artifacts introduced by this technique and its simplistic depiction of the lumen, traditional angiography has been termed "luminology" *(34)*. In addition to inherent imaging artifacts, traditional angiographic studies and the interpretation of vessel pathology are also challenged by tortuosity of vessels, suboptimal imaging projections, and eccentricity of lesions *(35–39)*.

Clinically, traditional angiography has important limitations that are partially dependent on the imaged vascular system. During coronary angiography, selection of the optimal view is dependent on each patient's anatomy and the ability of the angiographer to efficiently identify the optimal imaging projection in which to view a specific segment of the coronary artery. Typically, this entails 6–10 fixed views and several additional views that could subjectively minimize artifacts. In the cerebral circulation, a similar technique is utilized to adequately image the area of interest and minimize the amount of vessel foreshortening, vessel overlap, or other artifacts. This traditional technique has several disadvantages. First, each supplementary image that is required to identify the optimal view exposes the patient to additional contrast and radiation and increases the risk of procedural complications. Second, the placement and measurement of intracoronary devices is estimated with traditional angiography and could result in incomplete coverage or misplacement. Finally, because traditional angiography is a subjective imaging examination, the selection of inadequate views or their inaccurate interpretation could result in inappropriate therapy *(40,41)*.

The imaging limitations of traditional angiography have generated interest in the development of improved imaging techniques and modalities. Biplane imaging systems were initially adopted to minimize artifacts through the acquisition of two orthogonal views of the vessel segment of interest *(34,42)*. As experience with angiography increased, "optimal" gantry projections in which to image specific vessel segments were defined *(43,44)*. However, despite these initial advancements, traditional angiography has remained a subjective, operator-dependent imaging modality. The advancement of imaging techniques and computer processing power over the last decade have resulted in the development of safer, more powerful, and more precise imaging techniques of vascular structures and pathology.

ROTATIONAL ANGIOGRAPHY

The principle of acquiring multiple projections to improve the diagnostic accuracy of angiography has been described *(8,45)*. From these and other initial investigations, the technique of acquiring multiple images through an arc, or rotational angiography, was developed. Angiographic techniques using manual rotations, automated rotations, and automated rotations with 3D reconstruction have been described *(19,27,46–48)*. Although the same images as traditional angiography are acquired, rotational angiography can be automated and standardized and provides significantly more angiographic information than traditional angiography. Furthermore, because of the acquisition technique rotational angiography uses, image data can be utilized for 3D volumetric reconstruction.

Several automated rotational angiography techniques have been previously described *(19,20,48)*. In general, images are acquired over a large arc using high-speed isocentric rotation at 30°–45° per second of a ceiling-suspended or floor-mounted C-arm. For a typical diagnostic angiogram of the coronary arteries, two cineangiograms of the left and one cineangiogram of the right coronary artery are performed. Each cineangiogram is acquired over 4 s, requires approximately 10 cm^3 of intravenous contrast per injection, and results in 360 different images of the coronary arterial tree. In the cerebral and peripheral circulations, rotational angiography is performed with an initial rotational mask acquisition and a second acquisition during manual or automatic injection *(13)*. In addition to its unique role during angiography, rotational imaging systems can also be used to acquire images of intracardiac or intraluminal devices such as stents, aneurysm clips, or interatrial septal occluder devices (Fig. 1).

Rotational angiography has several important imaging advantages over traditional angiography. First and perhaps most importantly for the next generation of imaging techniques, the data acquired with rotational angiography are three dimensional and can be reconstructed into true 3D images. Second, rotational angiography provides a less operator-dependent method of acquiring angiographic images that, as experience with the technique increases, can result in better standardization of angiographic imaging. Third,

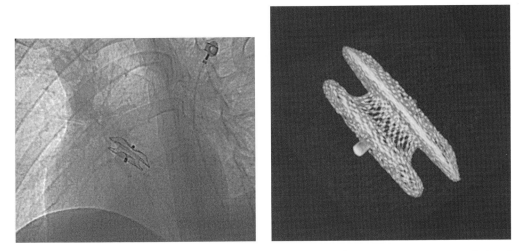

Fig. 1. Still image from a rotational angiogram of an Amplatzer® Septal Occluder device **(left)**. On the right, rotational angiography has been used to generate a volumetric 3D reconstruction of an Amplatzer device.

rotational angiography acquires markedly more information than traditional angiography (up to 20 times as many images for coronary angiography) that can be used for patient care decisions. Although the images are displayed in 2D, the rotating confluence of structures results in a pseudo-3D image that might be easier to interpret than static images. Furthermore, the rotating image can be stopped at any single image to permit easy and rapid identification of important projections.

From a safety standpoint, rotational angiography has several advantages over traditional angiography. In the coronary circulation, rotational angiography has been demonstrated to require less radiation and contrast than traditional angiography (19,47,48). In a prospective study of patients undergoing diagnostic coronary angiography, rotational angiography decreased total contrast dye usage by 33% and total radiation exposure by 31% (19). From an interventional standpoint, rotational angiography also could be useful in identifying the optimal view with the least amount of radiation exposure to the patient and angiographer (49).

Clinically, rotational angiography could improve the diagnostic accuracy of invasive imaging examinations by providing additional views with which to identify and treat vascular disease. In the cerebral circulation, rotational angiography has been used successfully with digital subtraction angiography (DSA) to generate 3D images and improve the accuracy of traditional biplane DSA (11,50–52). As Hochmuth et al. demonstrated, rotational angiography combined with DSA demonstrated additional cerebral aneurysms that were not visible with standard imaging and assisted with delineating the anatomy of the aneurysms (50). In the coronary circulation, rotational angiography has several important applications during diagnostic and therapeutic procedures. As a diagnostic tool, rotational angiography provides significantly more images than traditional angiography and is able to accurately display and identify the best angle at which to visualize complex, eccentric stenoses, including bifurcation lesions. In patients with saphenous vein bypass grafts, a single injection is usually adequate to display the graft, anastomosis, and native vessel. During percutaneous coronary interventions, rotational angiography can be used to identify the view with the least amount of foreshortening and overlap for accurate stent placement. Similar to the experience in the cerebral circulation, rotational angiography is also capable of identifying coronary stenoses that can be underrepresented or unidentified using traditional angiography (47). In the peripheral circulation, rotational angiography of the thoracic aorta, cerebral, iliac, and renal arteries has also been described (20).

Rotational angiography represents an important step in the development of more powerful angiographic imaging techniques. Despite the additional images acquired with rotational angiography, the inherent limitations of 2D imaging are still present and could impact clinical decisions. Even if rotational angiography has a modest impact on patient outcomes, it provides a 3D volumetric dataset that can be used in combination with computer algorithms to generate true 3D images.

3D ANGIOGRAPHY

Since the initial description of radiographic imaging, there has been significant interest in the development of technologies that were capable of displaying objects in three dimensions. Historically, there has been limited success in accurately displaying vessels in 3D with angiography because of inadequate angiographic acquisition techniques and insufficient computer processing power. Over the last decade, the combination of well-defined rotational techniques and powerful computer technology has resulted in clinically useful 3D rotational angiography (3D-RA) systems. The development of 3D-RA has created new interest in the clinical applicability and potential implications of this powerful technology for training, patient care, and research.

Because of the volumetric data obtained with rotational angiography, several 3D algorithms have been described with 3D-RA. In the cerebral and peripheral circulations, rotational acquisitions have been combined with the MIP technique and the SSD technique to generate 3D images. In contrast, the coronary circulation has been more challenging to image because of its dynamic, perpetual motion during the acquisition phase. To produce 3D images of the coronaries, several "modeling" rather than reconstruction techniques that are dependent on a separate calibration object have been described (7,13,53–64). These techniques are limited by the need for a phantom calibration of the imaging system, acquisition with predefined gantry orientations, and biplane imaging systems. A 3D modeling algorithm that does not require a calibration object has also been described (14–17,20,53). Using a computer-based, four-step algorithm, the technique integrates 2D projections into a 3D image, which can be then be used for interpretation, procedural planning, and simulation (Fig. 2 and video of Fig. 2 right panel on CD). This latter technique has been prospectively validated (18), can be applied to peripheral and cerebral image sets, and can be used to accurately measure 3D vessel lengths, vessel foreshortening, curvature, and bifurcation angles.

Although the modeling and other described techniques provide 3D images that can be used for clinical decision-making, limited progress has been made in creating true 3D images with volumetric reconstruction techniques. Because of the relatively stationary nature of the cerebral and peripheral vessels, 3D volumetric reconstructions derived from angiographic datasets have been described in these vascular systems (28,65). In contrast, the constant motion and small size of the coronary vessels have impeded the extension of similar techniques to the cardiac circulation. Recently, volumetric reconstruction using ECG-gated rotational angiography of porcine coronary arteries and a hybrid 3D modeling–3D volumetric reconstruction technique in human coronary arteries has been described (27,66). As the technical limitations are resolved,

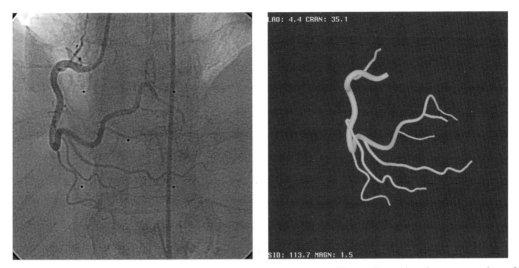

Fig. 2. Two-dimensional angiogram of the right coronary artery. Three-dimensional reconstruction of the artery demonstrates the tortuosity and bifurcation points in 3D detail **(right)**.

volumetric reconstruction will likely assume an important role in the accurate reconstruction of 3D vessels in the near future.

3D ANGIOGRAPHY: CLINICAL APPLICATIONS

The potential clinical applications of a powerful, more accurate, and safer imaging technique than traditional angiography are significant. Whereas noninvasive imaging will likely occupy an essential role in the initial diagnosis of peripheral, cerebral, and coronary vascular disease, there will be an even more important role for angiographic imaging during interventional procedures. Not only will 3D angiography improve on the accuracy of traditional techniques, but procedural efficiency will increase, contrast and radiation exposure will decrease, and interventions will be performed with precision guidance using this new imaging technique (Table 1).

In general, 3D angiographic techniques will eliminate or minimize many of the clinical limitations of traditional angiography. Using 3D angiography, the angiographer will be able to identify inaccurate 2D vessel lengths, quantify the tortuosity of a vessel, and identify the best angle in which to view a complex lesion at a vessel bifurcation *(18,67)*. The ability to accurately and efficiently identify the exact gantry angle at which to view a specific vessel segment will also be possible with 3D angiography. Using an Optimal View Map™ *(16)*, the angiographer will be able to select a specific vessel segment and, through a computer algorithm, the optimal view with the least amount of foreshortening and overlap will be generated. Not only will interventional procedures be more efficient with this tool, but patients would be exposed to less radiation and contrast while their procedure was performed with computer-generated precision.

Currently, experience with 3D imaging techniques is the most advanced in the cerebral circulation. Using rotational angiography and CT- or MRI-based techniques, 3D imaging was pioneered for clinical use in the cerebrovascular system. In the 1970s, the use of DSA was introduced to improve the accuracy of identifying complex cerebrovascular pathology. Traditionally, multiple oblique views were required to adequately identify the complex architecture of an aneurysm. If percutaneous interventional coiling or treatment was planned,

Table 1
Advantages and Clinical Uses of 3D Rotational Angiography

Imaging advantage	Clinical benefit
Improved 3D measurements	Accurately sized intracardiac devices
Minimization of imaging artifacts	Prediction of optimal views
Less contrast and radiation	Reduced risk of nephrotoxicity
Operator-independent acquisition	Standardization of imaging studies
3D images	Facilitated interpretation

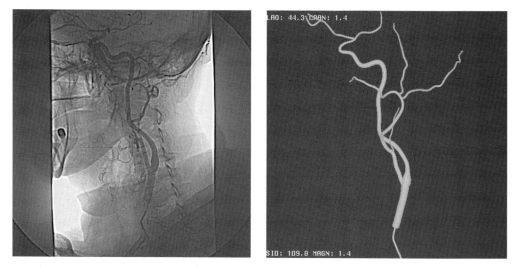

Fig. 3. Carotid angiogram and 3D reconstruction image. (Original angiographic image courtesy of Dan McCormick, Hahnemann University Hospital.)

additional views were frequently essential to identify the location of the neck, accessory vessels, or other procedurally important anatomy. Rotational angiography has been combined with 3D reconstruction techniques to improve the display of cerebral anatomy (Figs. 3 and 4 and see videos of these figures on the accompanying CD [original angiogram courtesy of Daniel McCormick DO, Hahnemann University Hospital]). As Hochmuth et al. demonstrated, rotational angiography provided important clinical information and was superior to the traditional imaging technique of DSA in the angiographically characterizing cerebral aneurysms (50). Three-dimensional angiography also might have an important impact on patient outcomes. As Albuquerque et al. demonstrated in a group of patients undergoing cerebral aneurysm coiling, 3D rotational angiography facilitated the performance of the procedure and provided critical information that modified the treatment technique or eliminated unnecessary therapy (68). Given the visual, technical, and clinical advantages of 3D angiography over traditional angiography, 3D-RA is becoming a standard imaging modality in many interventional neuroradiology laboratories.

Because of the many challenges of imaging the coronary arterial tree, 3D coronary angiography is less advanced than 3D imaging of cerebrovascular circulation. As the technical limitations are resolved and powerful 3D angiography programs are included in the next product cycle of angiographic imaging systems, visualizing and treating cardiovascular

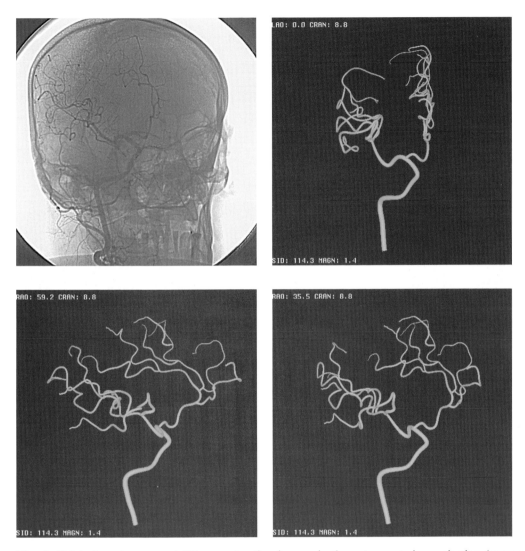

Fig. 4. Original angiogram and 3D reconstruction images in the anteroposterior projection **(upper right panel)** and right anterior oblique projections **(lower panels)**. (Original angiogram courtesy of Dan McCormick, Hahnemann University Hospital.)

pathology will advance. Three-dimensional angiography can be used during routine diagnostic procedures to improve the diagnostic accuracy or clarify an indeterminate stenosis identified during noninvasive imaging. During interventional procedures, 3D angiography can be used to identify the optimal view in which to image an eccentric lesion and accurately identify and assist with the placement of an exactly sized coronary stent. Concurrently, the patient will require less intravenous contrast for the completion of the procedure and spend less time in the cardiac catheterization laboratory and the operator, staff, and patient will be exposed to less radiation. Given the growing number of patients with cardiovascular disease *(69)*, 3D angiography has the potential to profoundly impact practice patterns and patient care during invasive and interventional procedures.

Imaging of the peripheral vasculature has traditionally been performed with angiography. Recently, as experience with CT- and MRI-based techniques has expanded, noninvasive

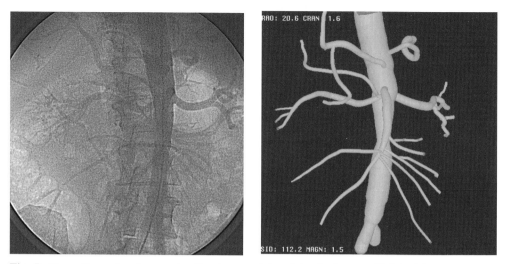

Fig. 5. Three-dimensional reconstruction image of the abdominal aorta. (Original image courtesy of Medical Simulation Corporation and Krishna Rocha-Singh, Prairie Cardiovascular Consultants, Springfield, IL.)

imaging techniques have assumed an important role in the diagnosis of aortic aneurysms, renal artery stenoses, and peripheral arterial disease. Interventional procedures have been performed with angiography as the primary imaging modality. Initial clinical experiences with 3D angiography in the diagnosis and treatment of peripheral vascular disease are now being published *(65,70,71)*. Given the relative ease of imaging the stationary peripheral vessels, 3D angiography will likely assume an important role in the future endovascular treatment of aortic aneurysms, renal artery stenoses, and iliac or femoral artery occlusions (Fig. 5 and video on accompanying CD [original image courtesy of Medical Simulation Corp. and Krishna Rocha-Singh, Prairie Cardiovascular Consultants, Springfield, IL]).

CONCLUSIONS

Three-dimensional imaging of the cardiovascular, cerebrovascular, and peripheral vascular systems is a rapidly changing and developing field. Although traditional angiography has been used for decades, 3D angiography resolves many of the historical limitations introduced by 2D imaging of 3D structures. The use of 3D angiography in the cerebral circulation has provided more clinically important information than traditional digital subtraction angiography. Although experience with 3D angiography of the coronary and peripheral arteries is limited, initial investigations have demonstrated improvements in diagnostic imaging compared with traditional angiography. This new imaging technique has the potential to improve patient outcomes by reducing radiation and contrast exposure during diagnostic procedures. From a therapeutic standpoint, 3D angiography provides an accurate and efficient method of objectively guiding complex interventional procedures that could translate into additional patient outcome improvements. Three-dimensional angiography is a significant imaging technology advancement and has the potential to positively impact the diagnosis and treatment of patients with all forms of vascular disease.

ACKNOWLEDGMENTS

We acknowledge the graphic design contributions of Adam Hansgen, M.S. and Kathy Kioussopoulos, R.N. for her programmatic support. This work was supported in part by grants from the Blount Scholar Endowed Fellowship and the National Institutes of Health (grant HL60220).

REFERENCES

1. Rubin GD. 3-D imaging with MDCT. Euro J Radiol 2003;45:S37–S41.
2. Herman GT, Coin CG. The use of three-dimensional computer display in the study of disk disease. J Comput Assist Tomogr 1980;4:564–567.
3. Knapp RH, Vannier MW, Marsh JL. Generation of three dimensional images from CT scans: technological perspective. Radiol Technol 1985;56:391–398.
4. Ravenel JG, McAdams HP. Multiplanar and three-dimensional imaging of the thorax. Radiol Clin North Am 2003;41:475–489.
5. Klingensmith JD, Schoenhagen P, Tajaddini A, et al. Automated three-dimensional assessment of coronary artery anatomy with intravascular ultrasound scanning. Am Heart J 2003;145:795–805.
6. Horton KM, Fishman EK. The current status of multidetector CT and three-dimensional imaging of the small bowel. Radiol Clin North Am 2003;41:199–212.
7. Frangi AF, Niessen WJ, Viergever MA. Three-dimensional modeling for functional analysis of cardiac images: a review. IEEE Trans Med Imaging 2001;20:2–25.
8. Cornelis G, Bellet A, van Eygen B, et al. Rotational multiple sequence roentgenography of intracranial aneurysms. Acta Radiol Diagn (Stockh) 1972;13:74–76.
9. Voigt K, Stoeter P, Petersen D. Rotational cerebral roentgenography. Evaluation of the technical procedure and diagnostic application with model structures. Neuroradiology 1975;10:95–100.
10. Thron A, Voigt K. Rotational cerebral angiography: procedure and value. Am J Neuroradiol 1983;4:289–291.
11. Schumacher M, Kutluk K, Ott D. Digital rotational radiography in neuroradiology. Am J Neuroradiol 1989;10:644–649.
12. Hoff DJ, Wallace MC, terBrugge KG, Gentili F. Rotational angiography assessment of cerebral aneurysms. Am J Neuroradiol 1994;15:1945–1948.
13. Fahrig R, Fox AJ, Lownie S, Holdsworth DW. Use of a C-arm system to generate true three-dimensional computed rotational angiograms: preliminary in vitro and in vivo results. Am J Neuroradiol 1997;18:1507–1514.
14. Chen SYJ, Hoffman KR, Carroll JD. Three-dimensional reconstruction of coronary arterial tree based on biplane angiograms. Proc SPIE Med Imaging: Image Process 1996;2710:103–114.
15. Chen SYJ, Metz CE. Improved determination of biplane imaging geometry from two projection images and its application to three-dimensional reconstruction of coronary arterial trees. Med Phys 1997;24:633–654.
16. Chen SYJ, Carroll JD. 3-D reconstruction of coronary arterial tree to optimize angiographic visualization. IEEE Trans Med Imaging 2000;19:318–336.
17. Chen SYJ, Carroll JD, Messenger JC. Quantitative analysis of reconstructed 3-D coronary arterial tree and intracoronary devices. IEEE Trans Med Imaging 2002;21:724–740.
18. Messenger JC, Chen SYJ, Carroll JD, et al. 3-D coronary reconstruction from routine single-plane coronary angiograms: clinical validation and quantitative analysis of the right coronary artery in 100 patients. Int J Cardiac Imaging 2000;16:413–427.
19. Maddux JT, Wink O, Messenger JC, et al. randomized study of the safety and clinical utility of rotational angiography versus standard angiography in the diagnosis of coronary artery disease. Cathet Cardiovasc Interv 2004;62:167–174.
20. Green NE, Chen SYJ, Messenger JC, et al. Three-dimensional vascular angiography. Curr Probl Cardiol 2004;29:104–142.
21. Magnusson M, Lenz R. Evaluation of methods for shaded surface display of CT volumes. Comput Med Imaging Graph 1991;15:247–256.
22. Fenlon HM, Nunes DP, Schroy PC, et al. A comparison of virtual and conventional colonoscopy for the detection of colorectal polyps. N Engl J Med 1999;341:1496–1503.

23. Kimura F, Shen Y, Date S, et al. Thoracic aortic aneurysm and aortic dissection: new endoscopic mode for three-dimensional CT display of the aorta. Radiology 1996;198:573–578.

24. Vining DJ, Liu K, Choplin RH, et al. Virtual bronchoscopy. Relationships of virtual reality endobronchial simulations to actual bronchoscopic findings. Chest 1996;109:549–553.

25. Anxionnat R, Bracard S, Ducrocq X, et al. Intracranial aneurysms: clinical value of 3D digital subtraction angiography in the therapeutic decision and endovascular treatment. Radiology 2001;218:799–808.

26. Rubin GD, Beaulieu EF, Argiro V, et al. Perspective volume rendering of CT and MR images: applications for endoscopic imaging. Radiology 1996;199:321–330.

27. Wink O, Kemkers R, Chen SYJ, Carroll JD. Intra-procedural coronary intervention planning using hybrid 3; dimensional reconstruction techniques. Acad Radiol 2003;10:1433–1441.

28. Piotin M, Gailloud P, Bidaut L, et al. CT angiography, MR angiography, and rotational digital subtraction angiography for volumetric assessment of intracranial aneurysms. An experimental study. Neuroradiology 2003;45:404–409.

29. Lu B, Zhuang N, Mao S, Bakhsheshi H, et al. Image quality of three-dimensional electron beam coronary angiography. J Comput Assist Tomogr 2002;26:202–209.

30. Kim WY, Danias PG, Stuber M, et al. Coronary magnetic resonance angiography for the detection of coronary stenoses. N Engl J Med 2001;345:1863–1869.

31. Gerber TC, Kuzo RS, Karstaedt N, et al. Current results and new developments of coronary angiography with use of contrast-enhanced computed tomography of the heart. Mayo Clin Proc 2002;77:55–71.

32. Katzen BT. The future of catheter-based angiography: implications for the vascular interventionalist. Radiol Clin North Am 2002;40:689–692.

33. Nieman K, van Geuns R-JM, Wielopolski P, et al. Noninvasive coronary imaging in the new millenium: a comparison of computed tomography and magnetic resonance techniques. Rev Cardiovasc Med 2002;3:77–84.

34. Topol EJ, Nissen SE. Our preoccupation with coronary luminology: the dissociation between clinical and angiographic findings in ischemic heart disease. Circulation 1995;92:2333–2342.

35. Galbraith JE, Murphy ML, de Soyza N. Coronary angiogram interpretation. Interobserver variability. JAMA 1978;240:2053–2056.

36. Arnett EN, Isner JM, Redwood CR, et al. Coronary artery narrowing in coronary heart disease: comparison of cineangiographic and necropsy findings. Ann Intern Med 1979;91:350–356.

37. De Scheerder I, De Man F, Herregods MC, et al. Intravascular ultrasound versus angiography for measurement of luminal diameters in normal and diseased coronary arteries. Am Heart J 1994;127:243–251.

38. Mizuno K, Miyamoto A, Satomura K, et al. Angioscopic coronary macromorphology in patients with acute coronary disorders. Lancet 1991;337:809–812.

39. Schwarts JN, Kong Y, Hackel DB, Bartel AG. Comparison of angiographic and postmortem findings in patients with coronary artery disease. Am J Cardiol 1975;36:174–178.

40. Banerjee S, Crook AM, Dawson JR, Timmis AD, Hemingway H. Magnitude and consequences of error in coronary angiography interpretation (The ACRE Study). Am J Cardiol 2000;85:309–341.

41. Leape LL, Park RE, Bashore TM, Harrison JK, Davidson CJ, Brook RH. Effect of variability in the interpretation of coronary angiograms on the appropriateness of use of coronary revascularization procedures. Am Heart J 2000;139:106–113.

42. Dumay ACM, Reiber JHC, Gerbrands JJ. Determination of optimal angiographic viewing angles: basic principles and evaluation study. IEEE Trans Med Imaging 1994;13:13–24.

43. Pepine CJ, Lambert CR, Hill JA. Coronary angiography. In: Pepine CJ, Lambert CR, Hill JA, eds. Diagnostic and therapeutic cardiac catheterization. Baltimore, MD: Williams & Wilkins 1994:238–274.

44. Bashore TM, Bates ER, Berger PB, et al. American College of Cardiology/Society for Cardiac Angiography and Interventions Clinical Expert Consensus Document on Cardiac Catheterization Laboratory Standards: A report of the American College of Cardiology Task Force on Clinical Expert Consensus Documents endorsed by the American Heart Association and the Diagnostic and Interventional Catheterization Committee of the Council on Clinical Cardiology of the AHA. J Am Coll Cardiol 2001;37:2170–2214.

45. Spears JR, Sandor T, Baim DS, Paulin S. The minimum error in estimating coronary luminal cross-sectional area from cineangiographic diameter measurements. Cathet Cardiovasc Diagn 1983;9:119–128.

46. Kuon E, Niederst PN, Dahm JB. Usefulness of rotational spin for coronary angiography in patients with advanced renal insufficiency. Am J Cardiol 2002;90:369–373.

47. Tommasini G, Camerni A, Gatti A, et al. Panoramic coronary angiography. J Am Coll Cardiol 1998;31: 871–877.

48. Raman SV, Magorien RD, Vaillant R, et al. Rotational cardiovascular x-ray imaging for left coronary artery angiography using a digital flat-panel cardiac imaging system. Am J Cardiol 2002;90 (Suppl 6A):129H (abstract).

49. Pitney MR, Allan RM, Giles RW, et al. Modifying fluoroscopic views reduces operator radiation exposure during coronary angioplasty. J Am Coll Cardiol 1994;24:1660–1663.

50. Hochmuth A, Spetzger U, Schumacher M. Comparison of three-dimensional rotational angiography with digital subtraction angiography in the assessment of ruptured cerebral aneurysms. Am J Neuroradiol 2002;23:1199–1205.

51. Heautot JF, Chabert E, Gandon Y, et al. Analysis of cerebrovascular diseases by a new 3-dimensional computerised X-ray angiography system. Neuroradiology 1998;40:203–209.

52. Tanoue S, Kiyosue H, Kenai H, et al. Three-dimensional reconstructed images after rotational angiography in the evaluation of intracranial aneurysms: surgical correlation. Neurosurgery 2000;47:866–871.

53. Hoffman KR, Metz CE, Chen SYJ. Determination of 3D imaging geometry and object configurations from two biplane views: an enhancement of the Metz–Fencil technique. Med Phys 1995;22:1219–1227.

54. Parker DL, Pope DL, Van Bree R, Marshall HW. Three-dimensional reconstruction of moving arterial beds from digital subtraction angiography. Comput Biomed Res 1987;20:166–185.

55. Pellot C, Herment A, Sigelle M, et al. A 3D reconstruction of vascular structures from two x-ray angiograms using an adapted simulated annealing algorithm. IEEE Trans Med Imaging 1994;13:48–60.

56. Wahle A, Wellnhofer E, Mugaragu I, et al. Assessment of diffuse coronary artery disease by quantitative analysis of coronary morphology based upon 3D reconstruction from biplane angiograms. IEEE Trans Med Imaging 1995;14:230–241.

57. Nguyen TV, Sklansky J. Reconstructing the 3D medial axes of coronary arteries in single-view cineangiograms. IEEE Trans Med Imaging 1994;13:61–73.

58. Delaere D, Smets C, Suetens P, et al. Knowledge-based system for the three-dimensional reconstruction of blood vessels from two angiographic projections. Med Biol Eng Comput 1991;29:NS27–NS36.

59. Liu I, Sun Y. Fully automated reconstruction of three-dimensional vascular tree structures from two orthogonal views using computational algorithms and production rules. Opt Eng 1992;31:2197–2207.

60. Rougee A, Picard C, Saint-Felix D, et al. Three-dimensional coronary arteriography. Int J Cardiac Imaging 1994;10:67–70.

61. Metz CE, Fencil LE. Determination of three-dimensional structures in biplane radiography without prior knowledge of the relationship between two views: theory. Med Phys 1989;16:45–51.

62. Weng J, Ahuja N, Huang TS. Optimal motion and structure estimation. IEEE Trans PAMI 1993;15: 864–884.

63. Blondel C, Vaillant R, Devernay F, et al. Automatic trinocular 3D reconstruction of coronary artery centerlines from rotational x-ray angiography. In: Computer Assisted Radiology and Surgery 2002 Proceedings, New York: Springer-Verlag, 2002.

64. Finet G, Masquet C, Eifferman A, et al. Can we optimize our angiographic views every time? Qualitative and quantitative evaluation of a new functionality. Invest Radiol 1996;31:523–531.

65. Boccalandro F, Giesler G, Amhad M, Smalling RW. Rotational aortogram with three-dimensional reconstruction in a case of celiac artery stenosis. Circulation 2003;108:2153.

66. Rasche V, Buecker A, Grass M, et al. ECG-gated 3D-rotational coronary angiography (3DRCA). In: Computer Assisted Radiology and Surgery 2002 Proceedings. New York: Springer-Verlag, 2002.

67. Wellnhofer E, Wahle A, Mugaragu I, et al. Validation of an accurate method for three-dimensional reconstruction and quantitative assessment of volumes, lengths and diameters of coronary vascular branches and segments from biplane angiographic projections. Int J Cardiac Imaging 1999;15:339–353.

68. Albuquerque FC, Spetzler RF, Zabramski JM, McDougall CG. Effects of three-dimensional angiography on the coiling of cerebral aneurysms. Neurosurgery 2002;51:597–606.

69. American Heart Association. Heart disease and stroke statistics—2003 Update. Dallas; TX: American Heart Association, 2002.

70. Aziz I, Lee J, Lee JT, et al. Accuracy of three-dimensional simulation in the sizing of aortic endoluminal devices. Ann Vasc Surg 2003;17:129–136.

71. van den Berg JC, Overtoom TTC, de Valois JC, Moll FL. Using three-dimensional rotational angiography for sizing of covered stents. Am J Radiol 2002;178:149–152.

22

Interventional Cardiovascular MRI

Current Status and Future Directions

Milind Y. Desai, MD, Albert C. Lardo, PhD, and Joao A. C. Lima, MD, MBA

CONTENTS

INTRODUCTION

Cardiovascular disease continues to be the leading cause of death in the Western world and the incidence is projected to increase in the future *(1)*. Traditionally, X-ray techniques have been the mainstay in terms of imaging modality for diagnostic and therapeutic cardiovascular procedures. However, there are inherent limitations to this technology including inability to perform three-dimensional imaging, poor soft tissue contrast, and exposure to ionizing radiation and nephrotoxic contrast, agents, which has prompted the exploration

From: *Contemporary Cardiology: Interventional Cardiology:*
Percutaneous Noncoronary Intervention
Edited by: H. C. Herrmann © Humana Press Inc., Totowa, NJ

for new image-guided modalities. These techniques include ultrasound (transesophageal, intracardiac, and intravascular), laser spectroscopy, computed tomography (CT), optical coherence tomography (OCT), angioscopy, and magnetic resonance (MR) imaging. Of these, in recent years, ultrasound-based techniques have played an important role in diagnostic imaging as well as guiding both cardiac and vascular interventions (2). However, ultrasound is limited by low spatial resolution, inability to easily prescribe multiple imaging planes, and inability to provide detailed functional information related to the physiologic response of catheter or pharmacologic intervention.

Magnetic resonance imaging (MRI) has several distinct advantages over other imaging modalities, including no ionizing radiation, no nephrotoxic contrast, high spatial resolution, excellent soft tissue characterization, and ability to define any tomographic plane. Despite these advantage, MR-guided invasive cardiovascular medicine has been slow to develop because of the following challenges: magnet and hardware compatibility, cardiac and respiratory gating, patient access, need to localize catheters and devices accurately, and need for rapid imaging reconstruction and display. However, with the improvements in scanner hardware, superfast interactive MRI, development of miniature MR-compatible internal catheters, guide wires, and ablation catheters, the field of therapeutic MRI is expanding at a very rapid rate.

This chapter will attempt to cover the current state of the art in different diagnostic capabilities of semi-invasive/invasive MRI, real-time MRI, techniques of catheter tracking, and different appilcations of interventional and therapeutic MRI and, finally, discuss the safety aspects of invasive cardiovascular MRI.

REAL-TIME MRI

Magnetic resonance imaging thus far has been a static modality requiring relatively long acquisition times to provide high-resolution images (3). However, in recent years, with an increasing ability to rapidly acquire multiple images at different times in successive cardiac cycles, cine MRI has become a reality and has formed the basis for many MR-based techniques such as assessment of myocardial perfusion, angiography, and myocardial function. The need for higher temporal resolution for these applications and the growing interest in interventional MRI has been the impetus for the development of real-time MRI. The largest stumbling block for real-time MR techniques was the inability of the imaging hardware to perform these tasks, as they were not designed for this purpose. Further advancement in the MR gradient hardware has made it possible to rapidly encode spatial information of the imaging data required to produce a 256×256 image of a 24-cm field-of-view (about 1 mm spatial resolution) in about 120 ms. If the spatial resolution is reduced to 128×128, this time is further reduced to 50 ms (20 frames/s). Thus, the era of real-time MRI was ushered in with the development of many new pulse sequences with the ability to perform rapid spatial information encoding. These include keyhole imaging (4), spiral imaging (5), multiecho imaging (6), local look reduced field-of-view imaging (7), wavelet-encoded data acquisition (8), and steady-state free precession (e.g. FIESTA).

The next important development in this field was the ability to perform real-time interactive manipulations of the imaging data utilizing a user interface in conjunction with a short-bore cardiovascular scanner and fast spiral imaging. This leads to (1) rapid data acquisition, data transfer, image reconstruction, and real-time display, (2) interactive real-time control of the image slice, and (3) high-quality images without cardiac or respiratory gating. Thus, slices can be prescribed in any plane at 12 frames/s without scan interruption (Fig. 1).

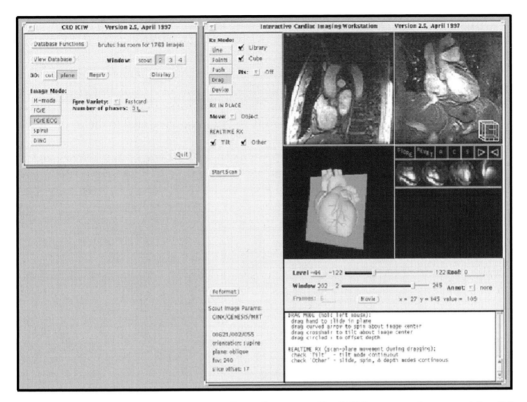

Fig. 1. Real-time interactive software interface. The two cardiac MR images on the upper right of the panel represent two orthogonal slice prescriptions that serve as scout images for later prescriptions. The drawing of the heart shown in the lower left panel serves as an anatomic landmark that shows the position and orientation of the slice. Using mouse or trackball control, the slice can be altered in real time and imaging parameters such as slice thickness and field-of-view can be defined.

The real-time hardware platform consists of a workstation and a bus adapter and can be adapted onto the conventional scanner at a reasonable cost.

DEVICE NAVIGATION FOR REAL-TIME MRI

Accurate visualization and positioning of the interventional devices in relation to the surrounding anatomy is critical for a successful and safe image-guided interventional procedure. Also important is the ability to easily identify the interventional devices and achieve real-time imaging for good maneuverability. There are primarily two methods that have evolved over the years to aid endovascular navigation of interventional devices: *passive MR tracking* and *active MR tracking (9,10)*.

Passive MR Tracking

Passive MR tracking techniques are based on visualization of the signal void and susceptibility artifacts caused by the interventional instruments themselves because of displacement of the protons. This form of tracking constitutes the normal imaging process and does not require any extra postprocessing or hardware. The magnetic susceptibility artifact is generated by magnetic field inhomogeneities, and the severity of the artifact is directly proportional to the magnetic susceptibility (μ) of the material. The ideal passive

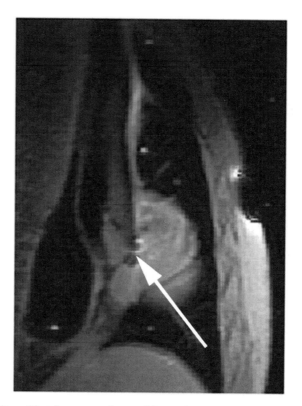

Fig. 2. A susceptibility artifact from a passive tracking catheter placed retrogradely from the aorta into the heart.

tracking device produces an artifact that is visible enough to track but small enough not to obscure underlying anatomy. The artifact generated by a particular material is dependent on a multitude of factors, like the magnetic field strength, spatial orientation of the device with respect to the magnetic field, physical cross-section of the device, pulse sequence, and imaging parameters. Thus, careful attention needs to be paid to obtain an optimum tracking artifact. To date, different types of passive MR tracking catheter and guide wire have been developed.

A susceptibility-based device (Fig. 2) is designed by constructing paramagnetic materials, such as dysprosium oxide rings, into the wall or onto the surface of a conventional catheter or guide wire. These dysprosium oxide rings produce susceptibility artifacts, which then can be passively tracked under MRI *(9,11)*.

Coating the surface or filling the guide-wire lumen of interventional devices with gadolinium is another technique to monitor catheter positioning *(12,13)*. This technique combines high temporal resolution, independence of orientation within the magnetic field, and visibility of the entire length of conventional angiographic catheters. A recent study tested the ability to passively track various commercially available interventional devices with four different pulse sequences *(14)*. They found that cobalt/nickel/steel alloy wires present the best and most consistent results.

Passive tracking offers some advantages, such as allowing visualization of the entire device as well as no safety or maneuverability problems with the catheters *(9)*. However, because of the dependence of the passive tracking technique on field strength,

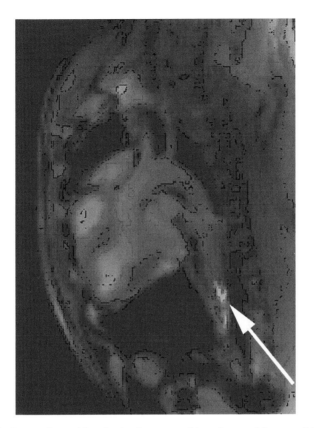

Fig. 3. A vascular guide wire in the aorta with active tracking capabilities.

device orientation, and the particular pulse sequence parameters, susceptibility artifacts are often inconsistent and the temporal resolution is usually inadequate *(10,11)*.

A field inhomogeneity catheter consists of a copper wire mounted on the entire length of a device to induce local field artifacts for visualizing devices *(15,16)*. The copper wire (50–80 μm in diameter) is attached to the catheter and is connected to a battery through which direct current is passed, leading to local field causing intravoxel spin dephasing and a signal loss around the catheter, which allows the entire catheter to be visualized. The degree of the artifact is proportional to strength of the current (usually between 50 and 150 mA). The movement of the catheter in the main magnetic field as a result of the forces on the wires is a drawback, which can be minimized by an antiparallel configuration of the wires *(15)*. However, the inhomogeneity catheter presents visualization problems in small and tortuous vessels *(16)*.

Active Tracking

In contrast to the passive imaging techniques, active tracking requires the creation of a signal that is actively detected or emitted by the device to identify its location (Fig. 3). This can be achieved by visualizing a signal from a miniature radio-frequncy (RF) coil that is incorporated into the commercially available interventional devices such as embolization catheters and balloon catheters *(10,17–19)*. The miniature coils are connected, through a fully insulated coaxial cable embedded in the catheter wall, onto the surface coil reception port for signal reception.

A coil-tipped catheter is made by winding the miniature coil, which is a copper wire spiral, for 16–20 turns around the tips of interventional devices to actively identify their position *(10,18)*. The miniature coil detects MR signals from only those spins near the coil, so that a single sharp peak is observed in the power spectrum and is indicative of the location of the coil in real space *(20)*. A primary drawback with this catheter is the fact that only the tip of the device can be seen on the MR image *(10,21)*. Visualization of only a single point might not be sufficient for steering devices in complex vascular territory *(22)*.

Generally, a guide wire is usually placed first to either guide interventional devices or to directly recanalize severely stenotic or occluded vessels in routine interventional procedures. Making the guide wire visible under MR fluoroscopy has been attempted *(22,23)*. Electrically coupled antennas with loop or stub shapes, which offered the potential to incorporate these antennas into conventional sterile guide wires, have been tested *(23)*. Efforts have also been made to incorporate miniature coils with different geometries onto the tips of commercially available guide wires *(21,24)*. The miniature coils are attached to a coaxial cable running through the center of the guide wire, and the entire assembly is enclosed in a sheath of fluoroethylenepropylene (FEP) to protect the coil and make the guide wire smooth *(22)*. The miniature RF coil delivers a high-contrast signal over its full length, enabling visualization of the position and curvature of the tip of the guide wire *(24)*. Because a guide wire has limited space to place a tuning and coupling component at the distal (neck) portion (between the coil and the long coaxial cable), the coil-tipped guide wire is tuned and matched at its proximal end (at the interface between the coaxial cable and the surface coil input of the scanner) *(22)*. As with coil-tipped catheters, the problems with the coil-tipped guide wires are that the signal is limited to the coil at the guide-wire tip and that there is a possible local heating risk from the coils attached to the tip *(24)*.

In the active tracking technique, the position of the device is derived from the signal received by a miniature RF coil that is attached to the instrument itself *(10,22,25)*. As the body coil excites the slice, the miniature coil detects the signal and gradient recall echoes are generated in three orthogonal axes to frequency encode the location of the coil. Thus, the 3D coordinates of the coil can be tracked in real time at 20 frames/s, with a spatial resolution of 1 mm. The position of the coil is used to control the motion of a cursor over a scout (road map) image. Active MR tracking provides high-contrast signal and robust determination of device position and higher tracking speeds, but requires hardware modification of the MR scanner and seems to be limited to road-map techniques *(22)*. The miniature coils and electric wires can reduce the maneuverability of an interventional device *(11)*, and active tracking of coil-tipped guide wires and microcatheters remains challenging because the signal-to-noise (SNR) decreases as the size of the miniature RF coil is decreased *(21)*.

In order to permit effective manipulation, particularly through tortuous vessels, a guide wire needs to be visualized along its entire length. Another technique in active tracking utilizes the loopless antenna *(26)*, which is made from a coaxial cable, consisting of a conducting wire that is an extended inner conductor from the coaxial cable. The tip is a dipole leading to a very thin-diameter antenna. This device has the following characteristics: (1) high sensitivity to the MR signal along the entire length of the antenna; (2) sensitivity inversely proportional to the distance from the antenna; (3) production of very high signal around the antenna when it is used as a transmitter/receiver probe; (4) creation of a projection image because the antenna localizes the MR signal around itself and does not require slice selection *(27)*.

With this technique, the entire body of the loopless antenna can be observed under MRI. Because the electronic circuits are placed outside the vessels at the proximal end of the coaxial cable, the physical dimensions of the loopless antenna can be constructed without limitations. Currently, the thinnest loopless antenna that can be manufactured easily is 0.014 in. in diameter. This antenna can be either directly inserted into small or tortuous vessels or placed into the central channel of interventional devices. Because the loopless antenna is expected to function not only as an intravascular MR receiver probe for intravascular MR imaging and for creation of intravascular MR fluoroscopy but also as a conventional guide wire for interventional MR imaging, it is called an MRI guide wire (MRIG) (28). Indeed, for reasons of safety and for technical purposes, such as torque control and subselective placement as well as negotiation of hard atherosclerotic lesions, this antenna/guide wire must also function as an imaging receiver probe when performing intravascular MR-guided interventional procedures. The MRIG has been tested in vivo and found to be useful for both intravascular MRI and cardiovascular interventional MRI (29,30). A recent study also demonstrated the possibility of 3D visualization of the MRIG by depth reconstruction from projection MR images (31).

MR-GUIDED DIAGNOSTIC AND THERAPEUTIC PROCEDURES

Over the last decade, MR guided cardiovascular diagnosis and therapy has slowly evolved from a research tool into a clinically applied tool with significant promise as an alternative to traditional invasive surgical procedures and x-ray based radiologic techniques. To date, different MR imaging-guided diagnostic and therapeutic cardiovascular procedures, including atherosclerotic plaque imaging, interventional and diagnostic electrophysiology, balloon angioplasty, endovasuclar stenting, arterial embolization, transjugular intrahepatic portocaval shunt procedures (TIPS), vena cava filter placement, and vascular gene delivery/tranfection, have been tested and evaluated in both animals and humans, with promising results.

IMAGING OF THE ATHEROSCLEROTIC PLAQUE

Atherosclerosis continues to be the leading cause of morbidity and mortality in the Western world and the incidence is projected to increase in the future (1). Clinicians have traditionally focused on flow-limiting stenoses originating from the atherosclerotic process. However, it has been shown that the onset of atherosclerosis begins in the vessel wall as an extraluminal phenomenon, also known as positive arterial remodeling or the Glagov phenomenon, and significant obstruction to the coronary blood flow does not occur until the later stages of disease (32). Therefore, the notion of flow-limiting stenoses has been challenged and studies now focus away from the vessel lumen and toward the diagnosis of subclinical atherosclerosis (SA) in the vessel wall (33). MRI, because of its unparalleled resolution, 3D capabilities, and the capacity for soft tissue characterization, is emerging as a powerful modality to assess the atherosclerotic plaque burden in the cardiovascular system. Traditionally, cardiovascular MRI is performed using external receivers that are placed on the chest and back of the patient. This has shortcomings inherent to their design, which places an upper limit on spatial resolution, making it difficult to visualize deeper-seated vessels. Hence, in recent years, intravascular receiver coils have been developed that can be placed directly into the vessel of interest and a high SNR is generated in the voxels adjacent to the coil. Zimmerman et al. have shown in a rabbit model that intravascular MRI enables significantly improved detection of early atherosclerosis and plaque characterization as compared to surface MRI *(34)*. They used a loop of wire enclosed by a polymeric water-filled balloon, which, when expanded, increases the coil diameter, hence improving the imaging capabilities of the coil. Martin et al. were able to study the aorta by placing the RF receiver coil in the inferior vena cava rather than in the aorta *(35)*. However, because these techniques involve invasion of the vascular space, attempts have been made to obtain high-resolution vascular and intracardiac images using transesophageal (TE) MRI *(36)*. These probes consist of either the loopless antenna design inserted into a standard nasogastric tube or balloon expandable loop design (Fig. 4). The spatial resolution is better than that obtained by surface MRI but less than obtained with intravascular coils. In our institution, we have applied this technique to monitor the effect of statin therapy on plaque regression in the aorta. We were able to show that the plaque volume was reduced by 9% at 6 mo and 14% at 12 mo ($p = 0.007$ and 0.01, respectively) *(37)*. Thus, this technique could have potential in terms of serial assessment of atherosclerotic plaque burden in the aorta.

MR-GUIDED BALLOON ANGIOPLASTY

With the development of newer active and passive tracking techniques, ultrafast imaging, gadolinium-filled balloons, and small-diameter coils, performance and monitoring of balloon angioplasty using MRI has become technically feasible. Different techniques to create experimental stenoses have evolved including cable tie *(28,29)*, use of ameroid constrictors or titanium clips *(38),* and balloon overdilatation and de-endothelialization *(39)*. Using the cable-created stenotic model, monitoring of inflation/deflation of an angioplasty balloon catheter when opening an experimentally created stenosis of a rabbit aorta has been tested. In this study, a 1.5F loopless antenna was used as a guide wire with a standard 4-cm, 4F balloon angioplasty catheter. The intravascular antenna was also used as a high-resolution imaging probe to monitor vessel dilatation using an MR fluoroscopy sequence. The margin of the balloon was tracked using two tantalum alloy rings. A subsequent study with the same stenotic model demonstrated the feasibility of performing intravascular MR-guided balloon angioplasty in vivo. This technical development provides an on-line methodology to (1) adequately monitor the entire process of selective catheterization and the dilation of stenotic vessels and (2) immediate confirmation of the success of the primary balloon angioplasty treatment by assessing distal organ function using MR perfusion imaging *(28)*. Recently, the feasibility of using MRI to guide balloon angioplasty of renal artery stenosis generated by a constrictor has been demonstrated using a passive tracking approach with MR angiography *(40)*.

The success of MRI-guided percutaneous transluminal coronary angioplasty (PTCA) in living animals has also been reported. Using active tracking methods, investigators performed the entire process, including (1) catheterization of the targeted coronary artery, (2) generation of selective coronary MR angiography, (3) creation of high-resolution MR images of the target coronary arterial wall, and (4) positioning and inflation/deflation of an angioplasty balloon, all under MRI guidance *(41)*.

MR-GUIDED STENT IMAGING AND PLACEMENT

Endovascular stents have become front-line therapy for the treatment of obstructive peripheral and coronary disease *(42–44)*. The emerging ability to perform MR angiography, including coronary MR angiography, and the advent of fast imaging techniques that permit

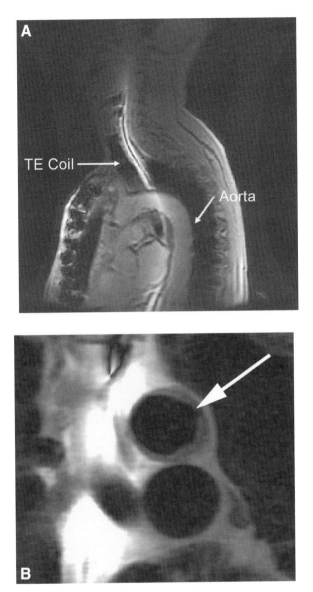

Fig. 4. (A) the transesophageal antenna is advanced through the nose and placed in the vicinity of the aortic arch and descending aorta. Note also the thoracic surface coil and the back coil signal. **(B)** Cross-sectional image of the transverse aorta delineating the atherosclerotic plaque (arrows). Note the bright signal from the transesophageal coil.

real-time imaging *(45,46)* and catheter tracking have opened new prospects for MRI to guide stent placement (Figs. 5 and 6).

With the exponential growth in the number of implanted stents and an ever-increasing role of cardiovascular MRI in the clinical arena, it is becoming commonplace to perform MR scans on patients with endoluminal stents. In general, the concerns regarding stent heating and safety have been adequately addressed, but traditional stainless-steel stents generate significant susceptibility artifacts that preclude reliable MR imaging of the vessel wall *(47)*. These artifacts appear much larger than actual size of the device and often

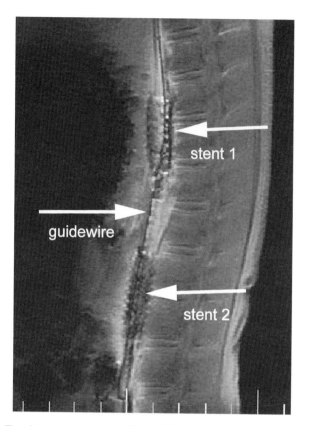

Fig. 5. Two intra-aortic stents with an MR imaging guide wire in between.

obliterate the vessel wall and nearby structures. Radio-frequency-based artifacts, including the generation of eddy currents and radio-frequency shielding (Faraday effect), serve to further decrease the signal inside the stent lumen, independent of susceptibility effects. This has led many stent manufacturers to develop stents with new MRI-compatible materials (such as nitinol and tantalum) that eliminate torque and aim to permit assessment of the vessel wall. Also, materials with lower conductivity have a better imaging profile during MRI, as strut susceptibility artifacts are small and largely reflect the true physical cross-section of the stent *(48)*. Further, the signal inside the stent improves greatly in materials with lower conductivity compared with stents with more conductive materials. Thus, with the avoidance of these artifacts, the ability to assess in-stent restenosis using noninvasive MRI can greatly reduce the need for coronary catheterization in these patients.

The feasibility of stent deployment in coronary and peripheral vasculature using MRI has also been tested in both animals and humans. Buecker et al. have demonstrated the feasibility of MRI-guided iliac nitinol stent placement in pigs using radial scanning together with a sliding window reconstruction technique *(49)*. Stainless-steel balloon expandable coronary stents have recently been placed in animals under real-time MRI guidance using a newly developed real-time steady-state free-procession sequence with radial *k*-space sampling *(50)*. In a porcine model, 10 of 11 stents were successfully placed in the left main coronary artery without complication.

Manke et al. described the first human MRI-guided nitinol stent placement study in 13 patients with iliac artery stenosis *(51)*. For enhanced visualization during imaging,

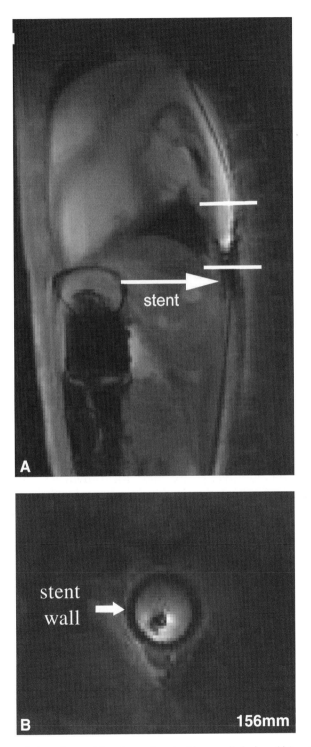

Fig. 6. An intra-aortic imaging guide wire and a stent in saggital view (**A**) and axial view (**B**).

the angioplasty balloon was inflated with a water/gadolinium solution. Images were evaluated both with digital subtraction angiography and contrast-enhanced MR angiography. Ten of 13 patients were treated successfully by MRI-guided intervention alone and 11 of 12 stents were placed correctly. There was a steep learning curve and the investigators attributed the relatively high complication rate and long procedure time to the lack of real-time monitoring during the procedure. Lardo recently performed MRI-guided stent placement in the iliac arteries of pigs with the assistance of an intravascular MRI guide wire *(52)*. Following real-time monitoring of a self-expandable biliary stent using a steady-state fast precession sequence, an intravascular MRI coil was placed inside the stent lumen and high-resolution in-stent imaging performed. The increased signal generated by the local intravascular coil greatly improved visualization of the stent wall and vessel compared with external coil imaging of the same vascular segment.

MRI-GUIDED INTERVENTIONAL ELECTROPHYSIOLOGY

Recently, the clinical indications for RF catheter ablation have expanded to include atrial flutter and curative procedures for atrial fibrillation based on the surgical MAZE procedure as well as ablation of atrial fibrillation foci in the pulmonary veins *(53,54)*. The procedure is extremely time-consuming, requires prolonged fluoroscopy exposure, and has been associated with a high incidence of recurrence and complications. Most of these problems stem from the difficulty associated with creating and confirming the presence of continuous linear lesions within the atrium. The ablation sites required for catheter ablation of atrial flutter and atrial fibrillation are identified almost entirely on an anatomic basis. The presence of gaps between these lesions can allow the activation impulse to pass through the gap and complete a re-entrant circuit, thereby sustaining atrial fibrillation or flutter. MRI (Fig. 7) can offer a number of advantages as compared to X-ray fluoroscopic techniques: (1) real-time catheter placement with detailed endocardial anatomic information; (2) rapid high-resolution 3D visualization of cardiac chambers; (3) high-resolution functional atrial imaging to evaluate atrial function and flow dynamics during therapy; (4) the potential for real-time spatial and temporal lesion monitoring during therapy; (5) elimination of patient and physician radiation exposure.

Our institution has described the use of a MRI-compatible interventional electrophysiology hardware system in conjunction with a real-time interactive cardiac MRI system to perform a comprehensive cardiac radiofrequency ablation study *(55)*. Using a standard external surface coil, it was shown that (1) MR images and intracardiac electrograms could be acquired *during* radio-frequency ablation therapy using special filtering techniques, (2) nonmagnetic MR-compatible catheters could be successfully visualized and placed at right atrial and right ventricular targets using real-time MRI sequences with interactive scan plane modification, and (3) regional changes in ablated cardiac tissue can be detected. The following sections outline our experience performing MR-guided cardiac ablation.

MR-Guided Catheter Placement

Current techniques to map and identify arrhythmogenic foci are based on low-resolution voltage maps generated by catheter movements under X-ray fluoroscopy, which generate only limited anatomic information and catheter placement is arduous and poorly repro-

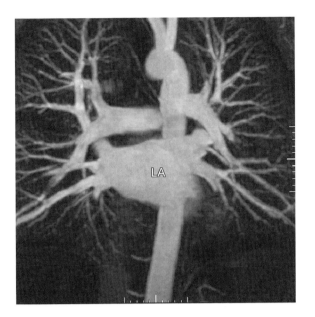

Fig. 7. Post gadolinium maximum intensity projection of all four pulmonary veins. LA = left atrium.

ducible. Anatomic MRI-guided electrophysiologic mapping can significantly improve the localization accuracy of critical arrhythmogenic substrate because of high-resolution imaging of endocardial anatomy and the ability to interactively modify the scan plane, using a graphical interface (55,56). MR-guided catheter placement leads to direct visualization of the electrodeendocardial tissue interface, thus increasing lesion size by improving the efficiency of RF tissue delivery (57). MR-guided catheter placement is limited by the fact that catheter can move out of the imaging plane and, therefore, make the full trajectory of the catheter difficult to visualize. Additionally, it is necessary to define optimal standard imaging planes and protocols for specific procedures and to develop software for rapid three-dimensional reconstruction of atrial chambers with direct interactive manipulation of the rendered volume.

In Vivo Lesion Visualization

Magnetic resonance imaging guided ablation therapy has the ability to visualize and monitor lesion formation with high temporal and spatial resolution. Lesions appear as elliptical hyperintense regions (most likely the result of interstitial edema) directly adjacent to the catheter tip on T2-weighted FSE images. MRI can detect changes because of heat-induced biophysical changes in cardiac tissue, such as interstitial edema, hyperemia, conformational changes, cellular shrinkage, and tissue coagulation. Additionally, lesion detection 1–2 min following ablation with subsequent formation over 10–15 min is consistent with the temporal physiologic response of local acute interstitial edema.

FUNCTIONAL IMAGING

Another important and practical advantage of MRI-guided ablation therapy is the potential to perform functional imaging. Preservation of atrial transport function is a concern in patients undergoing atrial radio-frequency catheter ablation. In patients with dilated left atria secondary to mitral regurgitation undergoing right- and/or left-sided atrial fibrillation ablation, high-resolution cine atrial imaging can be easily performed to assess atrial mechanical function and flow.

IN VIVO MR IMAGING OF VASCULAR GENE THERAPY

Gene therapy is rapidly emerging as a viable modality and has shown a tremendous potential in the treatment of atherosclerotic diseases. Preclinical studies have demonstrated that many genes could prove useful for stimulating angiogenesis to improve cardiac and limb vascular insufficiency, for preventing postangioplasty or in-stent restenosis, for preventing acute thrombosis to avoid organ infarction, for stabilizing plaques to reduce plaque progression and the risk of plaque rupture, and for correcting the levels of low-density lipoproteins and high-density lipoproteins to treat hypercholesterolemia (58–63). Precise delivery of genes into targeted atherosclerotic plaques, efficient transfer of genes into the endothelial and smooth muscle cells of the target, and prompt assessment of gene expression over time are three challenging tasks for successful vascular gene therapy. Catheter-based endovascular delivery of genes offers a promising therapeutic approach to delivering highly concentrated genetic materials and minimizing undesirable systemic toxicity. MR technology offers great potential in this field.

Imaging of gene therapy of the cardiovascular system can be very challenging because of the following: (1) thin vessel walls, which require high-resolution imaging modalities; (2) cardiac beating/vessel pulses, which require specific methods to reduce motion artifacts; (3) blood flow, which requires strategies to enhance the interaction between genes/vectors and the targeted vessel lesions; and (4) relatively complicated endovascular interventional procedures. Recently, MRI has been tested for monitoring and guiding vascular gene delivery, tracking vascular gene expression, and enhancing vascular gene transfection/transduction (64).

MR IMAGING OF CARDIOVASCULAR GENE TRANSFER

Monitoring vascular gene delivery and tracking vascular gene expression are critical. One study has demonstrated that catheter-based vascular gene delivery can be monitored by MRI in vivo In this study, Magnevist (a gadolinium-based MRI contrast agent) was mixed with either a blue dye or a third-generation lentiviral vector carrying a green fluorescent protein (GFP) gene (64). Gadolinium was used as an imaging marker for MRI to visualize vessel wall enhancement, the blue dye/GFP was used as a tissue stain marker to confirm the success of the transfer, and the entire primary delivery procedure was monitored under high-resolution MRI. Thus, MRI can visualize the site of gadolinium/gene delivery, how the target portion is marked, and whether the gene transfer procedure causes complications, such as perforation.

MR IMAGING ENHANCED CARDIOVASCULAR
GENE TRANSFECTION/TRANSDUCTION

Gene transfer into a target-specific cell is a major challenge in this field, with a very low success rate (1%) (65). Several studies have shown that gene transfection or expression can be significantly enhanced onefold to fourfold with heating, as tested in different cells, such as prostate tumor cells, chondrocytes, and kidney cells (66–68). Local heat generation at the target site using an easily placed internal heating source could be a logical way of achieving that. An MRI-guide wire, called an MRI-heating guide wire (MRIHG) *(26,69)* can be used to deliver external thermal energy into the target vessels and has the following functions: (1) as a receiver antenna to generate intravascular high-resolution MRI of atherosclerotic plaques of the vessel wall *(70,71)*; (2) as a conventional guide wire to guide endovascular interventions under MRI *(28)*; and (3) as an intravascular heating source to deliver external thermal energy into the target vessel wall during MRI of vascular gene delivery, and, thereby, enhance vascular gene transfection *(69)*. With this technique, transduction of GFP–lentiviral is increased threefold to fivefold in heated arteries as compared with unheated arteries *(72,73)*.

MR TRACKING OF VASCULAR GENE EXPRESSION

Tracking gene expression involves imaging methods to assess gene function by detecting functional transgene-encoding proteins (referred to as "imaging downstream") at the targets over time. To date, different exogenous imaging marker genes, also termed imaging reporter genes, have been developed: (1) marker genes encoding for intracellular proteins (such as enzymes) to modify imaging prodrugs, so that tissue accumulation of such drugs reflects gene expression, and (2) marker genes encoding for cell surface, ligand-binding proteins or peptides (such as receptors) that can then be targeted using corresponding imaging tracers *(74)*. MRI can be used to monitor overexpression of the transferrin gene, which produces a cell surface transferrin receptor. The transferrin receptor is then probed specifically by a superparamagnetic transferrin that can be subsequently detected under MRI *(75)*.

MR IMAGING OF PHENOTYPIC CONSEQUENCES OF VASCULAR GENE THERAPY

Magnetic resonance imaging, along with other methods, enables convenient assessment of reperfusion of the vasculature in the tissues/organs distal to the gene-targeted vessels. For example, gene transfer of plasmid DNA-encoding vascular endothelial growth factor (VEGF) brings about clinical benefits associated with angiographic evidence of new collateral vessels as well as improved leg blood flow as monitored by MR angiography *(76)*. Functional MRI, such as perfusion MRI, can also provide sensitive imaging methods to evaluate the circulatory improvement in tissues/organs *(76,77)*.

SAFETY

With the development of any new diagnostic and therapeutic modality, its safety has to be ascertained. The obvious concerns include electromagnetic exposure and internal heating on top of intervention-related issues. Studies have found that conventional MRI is safe in this regard *(78)*. However, interventional procedures present new challenges, including the placement of monitoring equipment and surgical instruments in close proximity to a high magnetic field, in vivo placement of long conductive wires and electrical components in rapidly changing magnetic fields, all of which can lead to local heating *(79)*. Such heating effects can be minimized by incorporating decoupling circuitry into the device, thus limiting the transfer of energy through the probe/wire by the transmit coil. Also, the careful use of imaging sequences that limit RF power disposition and duration also help reduce the possibility of excessive heating. Existing studies do point toward the safety of this technology, but further comprehensive studies are required for confirmation.

CONCLUSION

Intravascular MR technology, including intravascular MRI and intravascular MR-guided interventions, represents a new and promising imaging modality with unique properties for characterizing atherosclerotic plaque structures and guiding vascular interventional therapy. The use of intravascular MR techniques, combined with other advanced MRI techniques, such as MR angiography and functional MRI, will open up new avenues for the future comprehensive management of cardiovascular atherosclerotic disease. The further improvements in MR fluoroscopy with true real-time display (analogous to X-ray fluoroscopy), open high-field-strength MR units, and faster pulse sequences will establish the role of intravascular MR technology in modern medicine.

REFERENCES

1. American Heart Association. 2001 heart and stroke statistical update. Dallas, TX.: American Heart Association.
2. Isner JM, Rosenfield K, Losordo DW, et al. Percutaneous intravascular US as adjunct to catheter-based interventions: preliminary experience in patients with peripheral vascular disease. Radiology 1990;175:61–70.
3. Lardo AC. Real-time magnetic resonance imaging: diagnostic and interventional pplications. Pediatr Cardiol 2000;21(1):80–98.
4. van Vaals JJ, Brummer ME, Dixon WT, et al. "Keyhole" method for accelerating imaging of contrast agent uptake. J Magn Reson Imaging 1993;3:671–675.
5. Meyer CH, Hu BS, Nishimura DG, Macovski A. Fast spiral coronary artery imaging. Magn Reson Med 1992;28:202–213.
6. Reeder SB, Atalar E, Faranesh AZ, McVeigh ER. Multi- echo segmented k-space imaging: an optimized hybrid sequence for ultrafast cardiac imaging. Magn Reson Med 1994;41:375–385.
7. Hu X, Parrish T. Reduction of field of view for dynamic imaging. Magn Reson Med 1994;31:691–694.
8. Weaver JB, Xu Y, Healy DM, Driscoll JR. Waveletencoded MR imaging. Magn Reson Med 1992; 24:275–287.
9. Bakker CJ, Hoogeveen RM, Hurtak WF, et al. MR-guided endovascular interventions: susceptibility-based catheter and near-real-time imaging technique. Radiology 1997;202:273–276.
10. Leung DA, Debatin JF, Wildermuth S, et al. Intravascular MR tracking catheter: preliminary experimental evaluation. Am J Radiol 1995;164:1265–1270.
11. Bakker CJ, Smits HF, Bos C, et al. MR-guided balloon angioplasty: in vitro demonstration of the potential of MRI for guiding, monitoring, and evaluating endovascular interventions. J Magn Reson Imaging 1998;8:245–250.
12. Frayne R, Strother CM, Unal O, et al. Signal-emitting coatings for interventional MR. In:1998 Scientific Program, Annual meeting of RSNA, 1998;281.
13. Omary R, Unal O, Koscielski D, et al. Real-time MR imaging-guided passive catheter tracking with use of gadolinium-filled catheters. J Vasc Interv Radiol 2000;11:1079–1085.
14. Kochli VD, McKinnon GC, Hofmann E, von Schulthess GK. Vascular interventions guided by ultrafast MR imaging: evaluation of different materials. Magn Reson Med 1994;31:309–314.
15. Glowinski A, Adam G, Bucher A, et al. Catheter visualization using locally induced, actively controlled field inhomogeneities. Magn Reson Med 1997;38:253–258.
16. Adam G, Glowinski A, Neuerburg J, et al. Visualization of MR compatible catheters by electrically induced local field inhomogeneities: evaluation in vivo. J Magn Reson Imaging 1998;8:209–213.
17. Kandarpa K, Jakab P, Patz S, et al. Prototype miniature endoluminal MR imaging catheter. J Vase Interv Radiol 1993;4:419–427.
18. Aoki S, Nanbu A, Araki T, et al. Active MR tracking on a 0.2 Tesla MR imager. Radiat Med 1999; 17:251–257.
19. Wildermuth S, Dumoulin C, Pfammatter T, et al. MR guided percutaneous angioplasty: assessment of tracking safety, catheter handling and functionality. Cardiovasc Intervent Radiol 1998;21:404–410.
20. Dumoulin CL, Souza SP, Darrow RD. Real-time position monitoring of invasive devices using magnetic resonance. Mago Reson Med 1993;29:411–415.

21. Ladd ME, Zimmermann GG, McKinnon GC, et al. Visualization of vascular guidewires using MR tracking. J Magn Reson Imaging 1998;8:251–253.
22. Ladd ME, Erhart P, Debatin JF, et al. Guidewire antennas for MR fluoroscopy. Magn Reson Med 1997;37:891–897.
23. McKinnon GC, Debatin JF, Leung DA, et al. Towards active guidewire visualization in interventional magnetic resonance imaging. Magma 1996;4:13–18.
24. Ladd ME, Zimmermann GG, Quick HH, et al. Active MR visualization of a vascular guidewire in vivo. J Magn Reson Imaging 1998;8:220–225.
25. Wendt M, Busch M, Wetzler R, et al. Shifted rotated keyhole imaging and active tip tracking for interventional procedure guidance. J Magn Reson Imaging 1998;8:258–261.
26. Ocali O, Atalar E. Intravascular magnetic resonance imaging using a loopless catheter antenna. Magn Reson Med 1997;37:112–118.
27. Atalar E, Kraitchman DL, Carkhuff B, et al. Catheter-tracking FOV MR fluoroscopy. Magn Reson Med 1998;40:865–872.
28. Yang X, Atalar E. Intravascular MR-guided balloon angioplasty using an MR imaging-guidewire: an in vivo feasibility study. Radiology 2000;217:501–506.
29. Yang X, Bolster B, Kraitchman D, Atalar E. Intravascular MR-monitored balloon angioplasty: an in vivo feasibility study. J Vasc Intervent Radiol 1998;9:953–959.
30. Yang X, Atalar E. On-line management of ischemic disease using intravascular MR guided intervention combined with MR perfusion imaging and MR angiography. Circulation 1999;100:I–799.
31. Solaiyappan M, Lee J, Atalar E. Depth reconstruction from projection images for 3D visualization of intravascular MRI probes. In: 7th scientific meeting and exhibition, ISMRM, 1999.
32. Glagov S, Weisenberg E, Zarins CK, et al. Compensatory enlargement of human atherosclerotic coronary arteries. N Engl J Med. 1987;316(22):1371–1375.
33. George BS. Combined coronary and peripheral intervention: The oculo-stenotic-dilatory reflex or good medicine? Cathet Cardiovasc Intervent 2001;52(1):105.
34. Zimmermann-Paul GG, Quick HH, Vogt P, et al. High-resolution intravascular magnetic resonance imaging monitoring of plaque formation in heritable hyperlipidemic rabbits. Circulation 1999; 99:1054–1061.
35. Martin AJ, McLoughlin RF, Chu KC, et al. An expandable intravenous RF coil for arterial wall imaging. J Magn Reson Imaging 1998;8:226–234.
36. Shunk KA, Lima JA, Heldman AW, Atalar E. Transesophageal magnetic resonance imaging. Magn Reson Med 1999;41:722–726.
37. Steen H, Warren WP, Gautam S, et al. Combined transesophageal–surface MRI monitors progressive reverse remodelling in patients with aortic atherosclerosis after 6 and 12 months of statin therapy. Abstract presented at AHA, 2003.
38. Godart F, Beregi J, Nicol L, et al. MR-guided balloon angioplasty of stenosed aorta: in vivo evaluation using near-standard instruments and a passive tracking technique. J Magn Reson Imaging 2000; 12:639–644.
39. Le-Blanche A, Rossert J, Wassef M, et al. MR-guided PTA in experimental bilateral rabbit renal artery stenosis and MR angiography follow-up versus histomorphometry. Cardiovasc Intervent Radiol 2000;23:368–374.
40. Omary R, Frayne R, Unal O, et al. MR-guided angioplasty of renal artery stenosis in a pig model: a feasibility study. J Vasc Intervent Radiol 2000;11:373–381.
41. Serfaty JM, Yang X, Foo TK, et al. MRI-guided coronary catheterization and PTCA: A feasibility study on a dog model. Magn Reson Med 2003;49:258–263.
42. Serruys PW SB, Beatt KJ, et al. Angiographic follow upafter placement of self expanding coronary artery stents. N Engl J Med 1991;324:13–17.
43. Mehta RH, Bates ER. Coronary stent implantation in acute myocardial infaction. Am Heart J 1999;137:603–611.
44. De Feyter PJ FD. Coronary stent implantation: a panacea for the interventional cardiologist? Eur Heart J 2000;21:1719–1726.
45. Sodickson DK, McKenzie CA, Li W, et al. Contrast enhanced 3D MR angiography with simultaneous acquisition of spatial harmonics: a pilot study. Radiology 2000;217:284–289.
46. Sodickson DK, McKenzie CA. A generalized approach to parallel magnetic resonance imaging. Med Phys 2001;28:1629–1643.
47. Hug J, Nagel E, Bornstedt A, et al. Coronary arterial stents: safety and artifacts during MR imaging. Radiology 2000;216:781–787.

48. Buecker A, Spuentrup E, Ruebben A, Gunther R. Artifact-free in-stent lumen visualization by standard magnetic resonance angiography using a new metallic magnetic resonance imaging stent. Circulation 2002;105:1772–1775.

49. Buecker A, Neuerburg J, Adam G, et al. Real-time MR fluoroscopy for MR-guided iliac artery stent placement. J Magn Reson Imaging 2000;12:616–622.

50. Spuentrup E, Ruebben A, Schaeffter T, et al. Magnetic resonance- guided coronary artery stent placement in a swine model. Circulation 2002;105:874–879.

51. Manke C, Nitz W, Djavidani B, et al. MR imaging-guided stent placement in iliac arterial stenoses: a feasibility study. Radiology 2001;219:527–534.

52. Lardo A. High resolution intravascular imaging following magnetic resonance guided aortic stent placement. Circulation 2001.

53. Swartz JF, Pellersels G, Silvers J, et al. A catheter-based curative approach to atrial fibrillation in humans. Circulation 1994;90(Suppl. I):I-335 (abstract).

54. Haissaguerre M, Gencel L, Fischer B, et al. Successful catheter ablation of atrial fibrillation. J Cardiovasc Electrophysiol 1994;5:1045–1052.

55. Lardo AC, McVeigh ER, Atalar E, et al. Magnetic resonance guided radiofrequency ablation: visualization and temporal characterization of thermal lesions. Circulation 1998;98:3385.

56. Halperin HR, Lardo AC, McVeigh ER, et al. Catheter placement and high fidelity electrophysiologic signal acquisition during magnetic resonance imaging. PACE;1999.

57. Kalman JM, Fitzpatrick AP, Olgin JE, et al. Biophysical characteristics of radiofrequency lesion formation in vivo: dynamics of catheter tip-tissue contact evaluated by intracardiac echocardiography. Am Heart J 1997;133:8–18.

58. Nabel E. Gene therapy for cardiovascular disease. Circulation 1995;91:541–548.

59. Isner J. Manipulating angiogenesis against vascular disease. Hosp Pract 1999;34:69–74.

60. Crystal R. Transfer of genes to humans: early lessons and obstacles to success. Science 1995; 270:404–410.

61. Leiden J. Beating the odds: a cardiomyocyte cell line at last. J Clin Invest 1999;103:591–592.

62. Dzau V. The concept and potentials of cardiovascular gene therapy. Indian Heart J 1998;50:23–33.

63. Sinnaeve P, Varenne O, Collen D, Janssens S. Gene therapy in the cardiovascular system: an update. Cardiovasc Res 1999;44:498–506.

64. Yang X, Atalar E, Li D, et al. Magnetic resonance imaging permits in vivo monitoring of catheter based vascular gene delivery. Circulation 2001;104:1588–1590.

65. Nabel E, Leiden J. Gene transfer approaches for cardiovascular disease. In: Chien K, ed. Molecular basis of cardiovascular disease. Philadelphia: WB Saunders; 1999;86–112.

66. Takai T, Ohmori H. Enhancement of DNA transfection efficiency by heat treatment of cultured mammalian cells. Biochem Biophys Acta 1992;1129:161–165.

67. Greenleaf W, Bolander M, Sarkar G, et al. Artificial cavitation nuclei significantly enhance acoustically induced cell transfection. Ultrasound Med Biol 1998;24:587–595.

68. Blackburn R, Galoforo S, Corry P, Lee Y. Adenoviral-mediated transfer of a heat inducible double suicide gene into prostate carcinoma cells. Cancer Res 1998;58:1358–1362.

69. Qiu B, Yeung C, Du X, Atalar E, Yang X. Using an MR imging-guidewire as an intravascular heating source: toward thermal enhancement of vascular gene transfection under MR guidance. In 10th Scientific Meeting and Exhibition Program, International Society for Magnetic Resonance in Medicine, 2002 (abstract).

70. Yang X, Atalar E, Zerhouni EA. Intravascular MR imaging and intravascular MR guided interventions. Int J Cardiovasc Intervent 1999;2:85–96.

71. Yang X, Serfaty J, Quick H, et al. Intracoronary high-resolution MR imaging using an loopless receiver antenna: An initial in vivo study. In 2000 Scientific Program, annual meeting of RSNA, 2000:286.

72. Du X, Qiu B, Wang D, Yang X. MR imaging-guidewire as a heating source for enhancement of gene transduction in human vascular smooth muscle cells. In: 10th Scientific Meeting and Exhibition Program, International Society for Magnetic Resonance in Medicine, 2002 (abstract).

73. Du X, Qiu B, Yang X. Intravascular MR imaging/RF heating-enhanced vascular gene transduction: an in vivo feasibility study. In: 11th Scientific Meeting and Exhibition Program, International Society for Magnetic Resonance in Medicine, 2003.

74. Bogdanov A, Weissleder R. The development of in vivo imaging systems to study gene expression. Trends Biotechnol 1998;16:5–10.

75. Weissleder R, Moore A, Mahmood U, et al. In vivo magnetic resonance imaging of transgene expression. Nature Med 2000;6:351–354.

76. Lewin M, Bredow S, Sergeyev N, et al. In vivo assessment of vascular endothelial growth factor-induced angiogenesis. Int J Cancer 1999;83:798–802.

77. Pearlman J, Laham R, Simons M. Coronary angiogenesis: detection in vivo with MR imaging sensitive to collateral neocirculation—preliminary study in pigs. Radiology 2000;214:801–807.

78. Budinger TF. Nuclear magnetic resonance (NR) in vitro studies: known thresholds for health effects. J Comput Assist Tomogr 1981;5:800–811.

79. Wildermuth S, Dumoulin CL, Pfammatter T, et al. MR-guided percutaneous angioplasty: assessment of tracking safety, catheter handling and functionality. Cardiovasc Intervent Radiol 1998;21:404–410.

INDEX